ANNALS OF
THE NEW YORK ACADEMY
OF SCIENCES

Volume 835

EDITORIAL STAFF

Executive Editor
BILL BOLAND

Managing Editor
JUSTINE CULLINAN

Associate Editor
MARION L. GARRY

The New York Academy of Sciences
2 East 63rd Street
New York, New York 10021

FRONTIERS OF NEUROLOGY
A SYMPOSIUM IN HONOR OF FRED PLUM

ANNALS OF THE NEW YORK ACADEMY OF SCIENCES
Volume 835

FRONTIERS OF NEUROLOGY
A SYMPOSIUM IN HONOR OF FRED PLUM

Edited by Donald J. Reis and Jerome B. Posner

The New York Academy of Sciences
New York, New York
1997

Library of Congress Cataloging-in-Publication Data

Frontiers of neurology: a symposium in honor of Fred Plum / edited by
  Donald J. Reis and Jerome B. Posner.
      p.   cm. — (Annals of the New York Academy of Sciences, ISSN
  0077-8923: v. 835)
    Includes bibliographical references and index.
    ISBN 1-57331-096-4 (cloth: alk. paper). — ISBN 1-57331-097-2
  (paper)
    1. Neurology—Congresses.   2. Nervous system—Diseases—
  Congresses.   3. Cognitive neuroscience—Congresses.
  4. Cerebrovascular disease—Congresses.   5. Plum, Fred, 1924–   .
  I. Plum, Fred, 1924–   . II. Reis, Donald J.   III. Posner, Jerome
  B., 1932–   . IV. Series.
    [DNLM: 1. Nervous System Diseases—congresses.   W1 AN626YL v. 835
  1997 / WL 140 F935 1997]
  Q11.N5 vol. 835
  [RC346]
  500 s—dc21
  [612.8]
  DNLM/DLC
  for Library of Congress   97-32679
                                                                        CIP

BiC/PCP
Printed in the United States of America
ISBN 1-57331-096-4 (cloth)
ISBN 1-57331-097-2 (paper)
ISSN 0077-8923

ANNALS OF THE NEW YORK ACADEMY OF SCIENCES
Volume 835
December 19, 1997

FRONTIERS OF NEUROLOGY: A SYMPOSIUM IN HONOR OF FRED PLUM[a]

Editors
DONALD J. REIS AND JEROME B. POSNER

CONTENTS

[a] This volume comprises papers presented at a meeting entitled Frontiers of Neurology: A Symposium in Honor of Fred Plum, held on October 5, 1996 at Cornell University Medical College in New York City.

Part IV. Cognitive, Integrative, and Clinical Neuroscience

Financial assistance was received from:

THE CHARLES A. DANA FOUNDATION

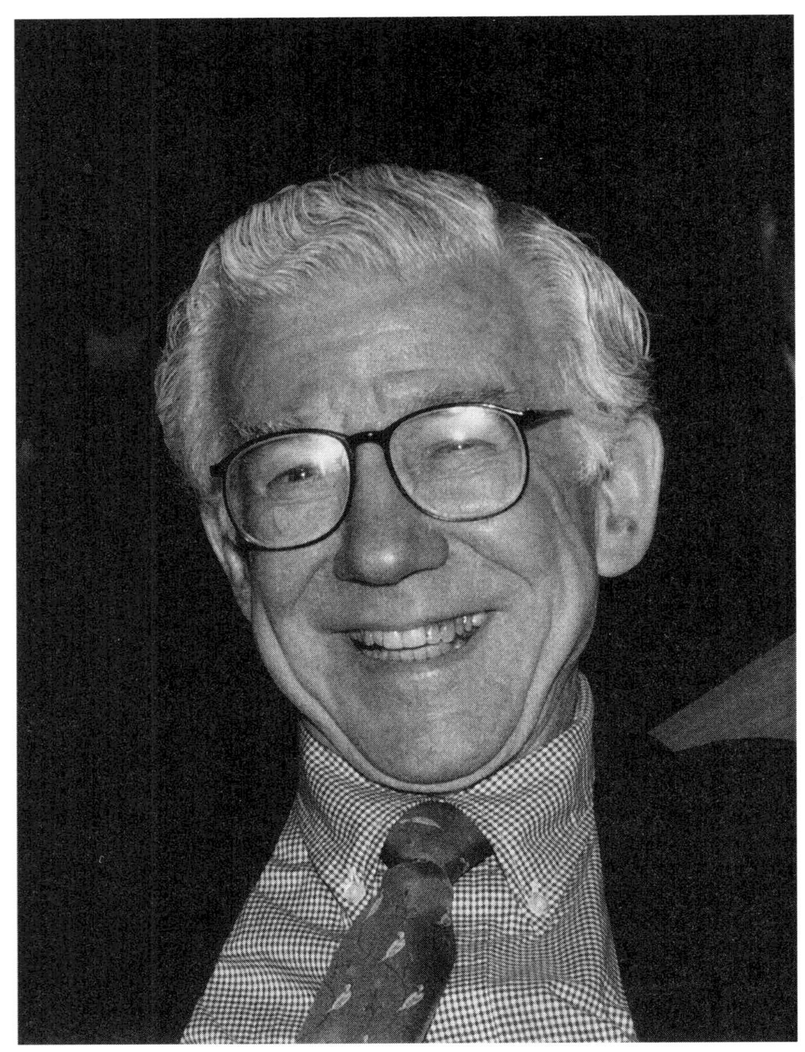

FRED PLUM, M.D.

Preface

DONALD J. REIS[a] AND JEROME B. POSNER[b]

[a]Department of Neurology and Neuroscience
Cornell University Medical College
411 East 69th Street
New York, New York 10021

[b]Department of Neurology
Memorial Sloan-Kettering Cancer Center
1275 York Avenue
New York, New York 10021

Fred Plum has been a major force in neurology ever since he joined the faculty of the Department of Medicine of the University of Washington in 1953. His appointment as the Neurology Division Chief at age 29 and just out of training was one of the many inspired appointments made by Robert Williams, then chair of the Department of Medicine. Dr. Plum's impact in the field grew even greater when he became chairman of the Department of Neurology at Cornell University Medical College in 1963. His accomplishments as a consummate clinician, a productive clinical investigator, and an electrifying teacher are known not only to all neurologists and neuroscientists, but also to many physicians and investigators not otherwise knowledgeable in neurologic realms. Perhaps his most important accomplishment has been the training of a generation of clinician/investigators, many of whom have achieved substantial eminence in their own right. Among Dr. Plum's former trainees—some of whom came to him as residents, others as postdoctoral fellows—are senior professors in departments of neurology and of basic sciences throughout the United States and Europe, as well as 20 chairs of departments in neurology in the United States.

However much time these individuals spent training with Fred Plum, the experience left an indelible mark on the work they have subsequently accomplished. Dr. Plum's trainees themselves have now trained a new generation of clinician/investigators, whose work continues to show marks of Dr. Plum's indirect influence.

This symposium *Frontiers of Neurology* addressed Fred Plum's contributions to neurology and neuroscience, with his former trainees presenting their latest work. Because the number of Dr. Plum's trainees is so large and their contributions diverse, the symposium encompassed many of the modern developments in neurology and neuroscience. The four sections of the symposium were chaired by offspring of Dr. Plum, all of whom have gone on to chair their own departments of neurology.

The first section on developmental and cellular neuroscience includes presentations ranging from studies of neuronal precursors to gene therapy for neurologic disease. The section on neuroimmunology and degenerative disease includes topics ranging from Alzheimer's disease to paraneoplastic syndromes, and addresses both basic and clinical treatment of issues. The third section focuses on cerebral metabolism and cerebrovascular disease and includes topics such as stroke, ischemic brain injury, and the general area of molecular neural protection. The final section on cognitive, integrative, and clinical neuroscience covers work ranging from studies on the molecular level to those of the human brain by imaging.

Each paper presented in this volume represents an attempt by the author to recognize the large debt owed to Fred Plum for the role he has played in each of our careers, not only in our training (whether at the graduate, postgraduate, or junior faculty level), which taught us that anything less than excellence was unacceptable, but also because throughout our careers he has guided and nurtured us, some close at hand, others from afar. Those who read these papers and who know Dr. Plum will see his influence in every one of them.

We wish to thank The Charles A. Dana Foundation for their financial support of the symposium; the other members of the symposium Organizing Committee—Drs. John Caronna, Kathleen Foley, and Frank Petito; the symposium section chairs— Drs. James N. Davis, Robert W. Hamill, Richard W. Price, William R. Shapiro, Robert C. Collins, J. Donald Easton, Alexander G. Reeves, Thomas R. Swift, and G. Frederick Wooten; and Kathleen Koenig for administration of the symposium. Finally, we wish to acknowledge the Editorial Department of the New York Academy of Sciences for seeing this volume through the press.

Gene Therapy for Nervous System Disease[a]

MARK H. TUSZYNSKI[b]

Department of Neurosciences
University of California-San Diego
La Jolla, California 92093-0608

and

Veterans Affairs Medical Center
San Diego, California 92161

INTRODUCTION

Recent advances in molecular biology have led to the development of *gene therapy*, a potential means of treating a variety of medical disorders. By genetically modifying cells to express either natural or novel genes at augmented levels, it may be possible to correct metabolic deficiencies, regulate the immune system, alter malignant cell properties, or deliver therapeutic molecules such as growth factors or neurotransmitters to the diseased nervous system. Gene manipulation could also be used to prevent the expression of deleterious genes, including gene mutations, oncogenic genes, or abnormally processed natural gene products such as the β-amyloid precursor protein. Several neurological disorders could benefit from these treatment approaches.

Two approaches to gene therapy have been used to date in animal models and in human clinical trials. *In vivo* gene therapy refers to the genetic alteration of host cells *in vivo*, whereas *ex vivo* gene therapy refers to the genetic alteration of cells in the culture dish, followed by the *in vivo* transplantation of these genetically altered cells to a specific parenchymal site (see refs. 1–3). Each approach has unique benefits and drawbacks.

In vivo gene therapy techniques are generally simple, requiring only the *in vivo* injection of a transgenic "vector" such as deactivated adenovirus, adeno-associated virus, herpes virus, retrovirus, or lentivirus.[4–9] Vector particles can be injected in relatively high titers, resulting in efficient but transient infection of host cells with the new genes (transgenes). Current drawbacks of *ex vivo* gene therapy methods include the following: (1) Transgene expression by genetically modified host cells occurs for relatively brief periods, on the order of only weeks. (2) There is a lack of specificity of target cell infection; that is, in the nervous system both neuronal and nonneuronal cells are infected by the transgene, resulting in uncertain and potentially diverse biological effects. (3) Some viral vectors for *in vivo* gene therapy are toxic to the host cell or elicit immune responses, particularly herpes virus and

[a] This work was supported by the National Institute for Aging, Veterans Affairs Research, Hollfelder Foundation, American Paralysis Association, and International Spinal Research Trust.
[b] Address correspondence to Mark H. Tuszynski, M.D., Ph.D., Department of Neurosciences-0608, University of California-San Diego, La Jolla, CA 92093-0608. E-mail: mtuszyns@ucsd.edu

1

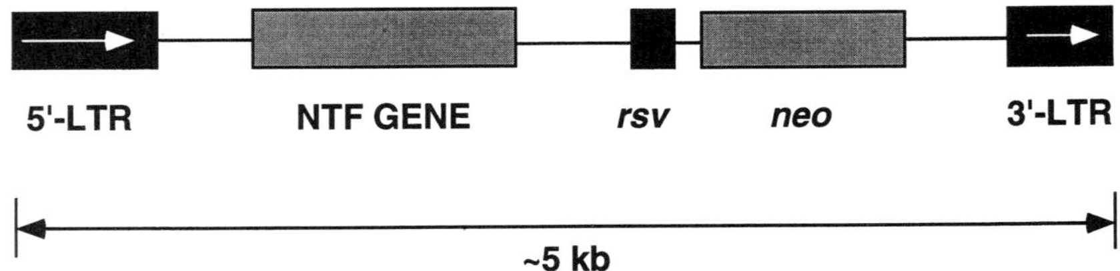

FIGURE 1. Prototypical vector design for gene therapy. The viral wild-type promoter (5'-long terminal repeat, or 5'-LTR) constitutively expresses the first transgene, in this case a neurotrophic factor (NTF) gene. This is followed by a second "internal" promoter from Rous sarcoma virus (*rsv*) that constitutively expresses a second transgene for neomycin resistance (*neo*). Cells that contain the neomycin resistance gene will survive the addition of this antibiotic to the cell culture media; thus, cells that have successfully incorporated the vector can be selected *in vitro*. The transgene is completed by the wild-type 3'-long terminal repeat (3'-LTR) sequence. The entire construct is approximately 5 kb in size.

adenovirus vectors. Advances in *in vivo* vector design are likely to overcome these drawbacks in the near future.

At the present time the chief advantage of *ex vivo* gene therapy relative to *in vivo* gene therapy lies in a greater base of experimental animal model experience in the nervous system using *ex vivo* methods, and solid evidence for long-term gene expression in cells genetically modified *ex vivo*. The most commonly used vector for *ex vivo* gene therapy experiments is derived from the Moloney murine leukemia virus (MLV).[1] Wild-type genes from MLV that are necessary for viral replication and viral envelope formation are deleted from the viral genome and replaced with new genes of interest (FIG. 1). The transgene vectors are then "packaged" into viral envelopes, and these particles are subsequently added to cultures of host cells that are targeted for genetic modification. Host cells that successfully incorporate the transgenes and express their gene products are then selected *in vitro*; these cells are amplified in number (cloned), and are then transplanted back into the host animal. In this manner, a new gene product is delivered to a specific site in the nervous system to support a biological function.

There are several advantages to *ex vivo* gene therapy techniques.

1. Host cells that express the desired transgene at high levels can be selected *in vitro*, prior to transplantation. Thus, the odds of sustaining efficient transgene expression *in vivo* are improved; this selection procedure cannot be utilized with *in vivo* gene therapy methods.
2. Expression of the transgene product has been shown to persist for at least 18 months after transplantation into the host using *ex vivo* methods,[10] a duration that greatly exceeds that observed to date with *in vivo* gene therapy methods. Clinical trials for human disease are more readily justifiable when transgene expression of this duration is attained.
3. Correction of abnormal phenotypes has been documented in several animal models of diseases of the nervous system using *ex vivo* methods, including correlational models of Parkinson's disease (PD),[11–14] Alzheimer's disease (AD),[15–19] and spinal cord injury.[10,20,21]
4. An extremely low risk exists of genetically modifying *nontargeted* cells in the nervous system, because no replication-competent viral vectors are placed *in vivo*.

5. Although cells are transplanted into the brain when *ex vivo* methods of gene therapy are used, there is no risk of grafted cell rejection because the individual's own cells are modified and transplanted (autografts).

There are also several potential disadvantages of *ex vivo* gene therapy methods.

1. Vectors that have achieved the greatest duration of transgene expression using *ex vivo* methods, MLV vectors, can only genetically modify dividing cells. Thus, the most inherently attractive target cell types for gene therapy in the nervous system, including the neuron and oligodendrocyte, cannot be infected with this type of vector, and other cell types must be targeted for gene therapy. Most *ex vivo* gene therapy experiments in the nervous system have targeted fibroblasts, immortalized cell lines, neural progenitor cell lines, and Schwann cells for gene therapy and transplantation to the nervous system.[17,22,23]
2. Cell transplantation is a more invasive procedure for introducing novel genes into the nervous system than *in vivo* gene therapy. Whereas *in vivo* gene therapy injects a relatively small volume of fluid containing transgene viral particles, *ex vivo* gene therapy transplants relatively larger fluid volumes that contain cells rather than viral particles. The grafting procedure itself, the volume of cells introduced, and the risk of malignant transformation of the transplanted cells present a risk that probably exceeds the risk of secondary damage encountered with *in vivo* gene therapy methods.

GENE THERAPY FOR ALZHEIMER'S DISEASE

A correlational model of AD was one of the first animal models to assess the potential use of gene therapy to treat neurological disease.[15] In AD, multiple neuronal populations undergo degeneration, including basal forebrain cholinergic, noradrenergic, serotonergic, and peptidergic neurons.[24] The degeneration of several of these neuronal phenotypes is preventable in animal models by the delivery of neuronal growth factors, or neurotrophic factors (NTFs), to degenerating neurons.[25-29] The best characterized NTF, nerve growth factor (NGF), specifically prevents the degeneration of basal forebrain cholinergic neurons after injury or as a result of spontaneous, age-related atrophy.[25-27] Degeneration of basal forebrain cholinergic systems is a regular and severe component of neuronal loss in AD and is likely to contribute to cognitive dysfunction in the disease. Thus, one therapeutic approach to AD is to prevent neuronal degeneration by the delivery of NTFs to the brain.[30,31]

Early investigations into NTF delivery to the brain to prevent cholinergic neuronal degeneration utilized intracerebroventricular (i.c.v.) infusions of NGF.[25,26] Although this method of NTF delivery was capable of preventing the degeneration of 100% of injured cholinergic neurons, other types of cells in the nervous system also responded to the NGF delivery, producing several toxic effects. These toxic effects included the migration of Schwann cells into the subpial space of the brain stem and spinal cord, and their subsequent proliferation in this region.[32] Further, sensory axons and sympathetic axons, both NGF-responsive systems, abnormally sprouted into the subpial space and cerebral vasculature, respectively.[32,33] Recipients of NGF infusions also suffered weight loss.[34] Thus, whereas delivery of NTFs to the nervous system is a powerful means of preventing neuronal degeneration in animal models, their nontargeted delivery produces unacceptable adverse effects from nontargeted neurotrophin-responsive systems. Clearly, a specifically targeted, regionally restricted form of neurotrophin delivery to the central nervous system (CNS) is needed.

Gene therapy may be an effective method of achieving regionally restricted and sustained delivery of therapeutic substances to the CNS. To explore this possibility, primary rat fibroblasts were genetically modified to produce and secrete human NGF (hNGF) using the MLV vectors described above. *In vitro*, genetically modified rat fibroblasts produced approximately 10 ng hNGF/10^5 cells/day, an amount that greatly exceeded physiological levels of NGF production in the adult brain, whereas nonmodified fibroblasts produced no detectable NGF.[15] The rats' genetically modified cells were then harvested from *in vitro* cultures and transplanted to the septal nucleus after inducing lesions of basal forebrain cholinergic neurons. Whereas this type of lesion ordinarily causes the degeneration of approximately 75% of cholinergic neurons, rats that received grafts of hNGF-producing cells showed a loss of only 5% of neurons. Thus, the transplantation of genetically modified cells to the brain was an effective means of preventing neuronal degeneration. In later experiments, aged rats that showed spontaneous atrophy of basal forebrain cholinergic neurons and associated deficits in learning and memory also received grafts of hNGF-producing fibroblasts to the brain.[35] Animals that received NGF-producing cells, but not control, nonmodified fibroblasts, showed reversal of mnemonic deficits and improvement of cholinergic neuronal morphology.[35] Subsequently, other investigations have verified these findings using grafts of other genetically modified cell types.[17]

To determine whether this approach was a practical means of protecting neurons in the larger primate brain, the degeneration of basal forebrain cholinergic neurons in adult monkeys was induced by unilaterally transecting the fornix. Monkeys then received transplants of autologous fibroblasts genetically modified to produce human NGF, or, in control subjects, nongenetically modified fibroblast grafts (FIG. 2). Transplants were placed intraparenchymally, directly into the region of degenerating cell bodies. The placement of cells intraparenchymally maximized neurotrophin delivery to degenerating neurons and shielded other potentially NGF-responsive neurons from the neurotrophin exposure encountered by delivery techniques such as i.c.v. infusions. One month after the lesion, control-lesioned monkeys showed degeneration of 75% of basal forebrain cholinergic neurons, whereas monkeys that received NGF-secreting autologous genetically modified cell grafts showed an average loss of immunolabeling in only 28% of cholinergic neurons.[18] The grafted monkey with the largest and most accurately targeted NGF-producing transplant showed a loss of only 8% of immunolabeled cholinergic neurons. Subsequent experiments have shown that monkeys with hNGF-producing intraparenchymal grafts do not experience weight loss, Schwann cell migration into the CNS, or abnormal sprouting of sympathetic and sensory systems for periods of at least eight months after genetically modified cell placement. Transgene expression is also maintained for at least eight months *in vivo*.

To date, approximately 60 NGF-secreting grafts have been placed into 12 monkeys. In no case have grafted cells formed tumors, caused hydrocephalus, or resulted in other obvious adverse effects. No monkey has become ill as a result of the presence of an NGF-producing or control fibroblast graft. Thus, NGF delivery by transgenic approaches is a potentially practical means of delivering molecules to specific intraparenchymal sites in the brain. The feasibility of gene therapy for the treatment of human diseases such as AD requires verification of the preceding efficacy and safety data in additional primates. Further, questions remain to be resolved regarding the placement and number of NGF-secreting grafts that will be

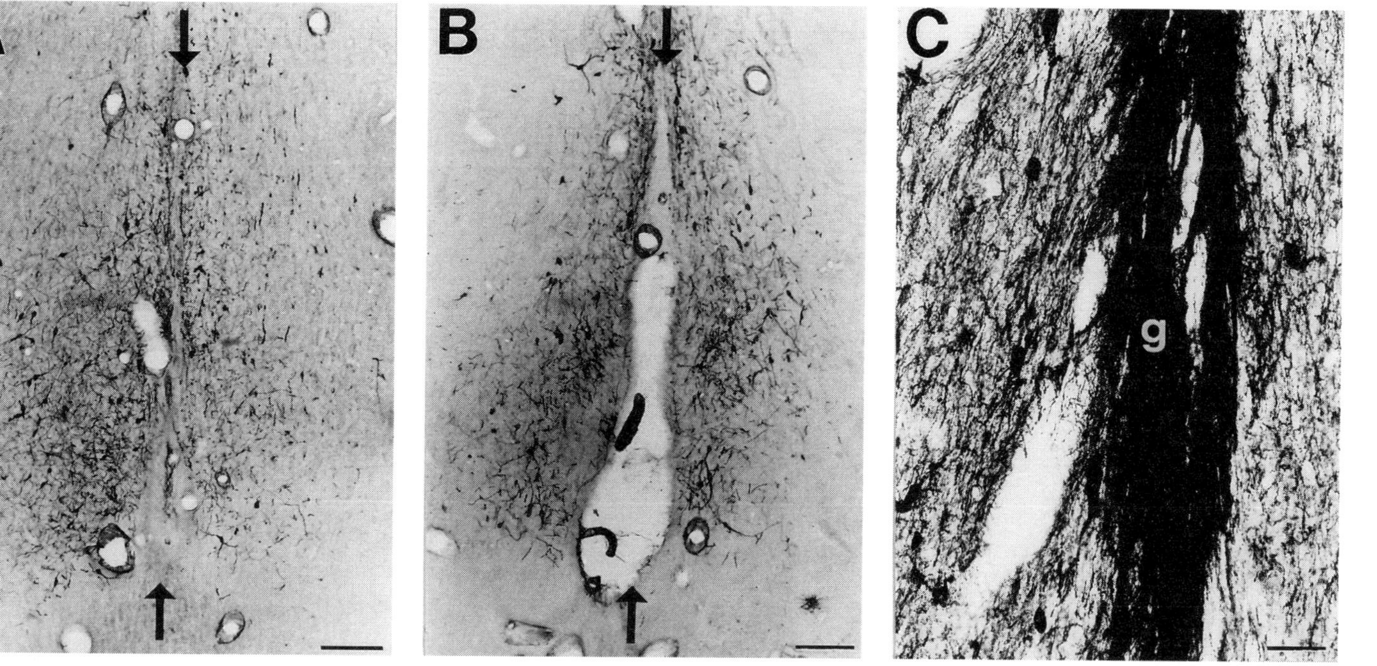

FIGURE 2. Photomicrograph illustrating effects of grafts of cells genetically modified to produce human nerve growth factor (hNGF) to the adult primate brain. (**A**) Following right-sided transections of the fornix, the number of cholinergic neurons immunolabeled for the p75 low-affinity neurotrophin receptor is reduced in the right medial septal region. The left side, unaffected by the lesion, shows a normal number of p75-immunolabeled neurons. This monkey received an intraseptal graft of autologous control fibroblasts that were *not* genetically modified to produce NGF. Arrow indicates midline; scale bar in **A** and **B** = 250 μm. (**B**) In a monkey that has undergone a right-sided fornix transection and has received a graft of NGF-producing autologous fibroblasts, cholinergic neuronal degeneration is prevented on the right side of the medial septal nucleus. (**C**) The NGF-secreting graft in the septal region is penetrated by cholinergic axons (acetylcholinesterase stain), indicating tropic (growth) responses of adult primate cholinergic axons to an NGF source. g, graft. Scale bar = 50 μm.

required in the Alzheimer's brain, the duration of gene expression beyond eight months, the duration of neuronal protection after transgene expression ceases, and the feasibility of repeating the grafting procedure should down-regulation of gene expression occur.

Other means of delivering NGF or agumenting NGF function in the brain may accomplish neurotrophin delivery in a manner that is less invasive than gene therapy. For example, delivery of NGF peptide analogues, NGF release-stimulators or NGF attached to shuttle molecules are under investigation;[36] a limitation of these methods remains their nonselective delivery of NGF or NGF analogues to both basal forebrain and nonbasal forebrain NGF-responsive neurons, potentially causing the unacceptable adverse effects observed after NGF i.c.v. infusion studies.[34,37] Additional preclinical toxicity testing and clinical trials in patients will be required to clarify these possibilities. Should a method of NGF delivery to the brain other than gene therapy be found to result in significant efficacy, the techniques developed in gene therapy experiments conducted to date may prove to be beneficial for the treatment of other neurological diseases.

GENE THERAPY FOR OTHER NEURODEGENERATIVE DISORDERS

Parkinson's disease (PD) offers one example of an alternative treatment model for gene therapy. In PD as in AD, neuronal degeneration occurs in relatively focal brain regions. Gene therapy may be a means of intraparenchymally delivering neuroprotective substances such as NTFs,[38,39] or compensatory substances such as neurotransmitters,[11,14] to these specific regions. Pioneering rat experiments demonstrated that primary fibroblasts, genetically modified to produce and secrete the dopamine biosynthetic enzyme tyrosine hydroxylase (TH), could augment *in vivo* extracellular brain levels of TH and dopamine after grafting to the striatum.[11] Functional deficits were ameliorated. Subsequent grafting experiments using another dopamine biosynthetic enzyme, dopamine β-hydroxylase, confirmed these findings.[14] Primate studies also showed that primary fibroblasts genetically modified to produce and secrete TH could elevate brain dopamine levels.[40] Gene therapy approaches similar to those outlined for NGF delivery in models of AD could also be used in PD or Huntington's disease to deliver NTFs that prevent degeneration of the cells in the substantia nigra (e.g., brain-derived neurotrophic factor, glial cell-line derived neurotrophic factor[38,39]) and striatum (e.g., NGF, leukemia inhibitory factor, and others[41,42]). Genetically modified primary or immortalized neural stem cells and biopolymer-encapsulated cells, like genetically modified fibroblasts, have also been shown to protect the neuronal phenotype in animal models of PD and Huntington's disease.[17,41,42]

GENE THERAPY FOR AXONAL REGENERATION

In addition to neuroprotective functions, gene therapy may be an effective means of promoting reconstruction of injured CNS projections. In rat models of spinal cord injury (SCI), cells genetically modified to produce and secrete NGF, neurotrophin-3 (NT-3), and basic fibroblast growth factor (bFGF) have been shown to promote axonal growth from several classes of neurons.[10,20,21] Fibroblasts genetically modified to produce NGF elicit extremely robust growth from dorsolateral fasciculus sensory axons originating from dorsal root projections in the injured rat spinal cord,[20] and also elicit significant growth responses from putative local motor axons and supraspinal noradrenergic axons.[10] Cells genetically modified to produce NT-3 elicit significant growth of primary sensory afferent axons from the dorsal root after grafting to the unlesioned spinal cord;[43] however, after grafting to the injured spinal cord, NT-3-producing cell grafts elicit robust sprouting of supraspinal corticospinal axons,[44] resulting in partial functional recovery on a motor task assessing conditioned locomotion in rats. Cells transduced to produce bFGF elicit axon growth from dorsolateral fasciculus axons;[45] responses from other axonal systems are under investigation. Many of these growth effects were predictable, based upon previously published reports using direct neurotrophin delivery to the injured spinal cord or based upon developmental patterns of neurotrophin dependence.[46,47] An appealing aspect of gene therapy for treating SCI lies in its ability to deliver growth factors to injured targets specifically, leading to directed rather than random axonal growth responses. The combination of gene therapy and the placement of synthetic axon guidance channels in the injured spinal cord could lead to superior orientation of quantitatively large numbers of injured axons. Studies in progress support this possibility.

GENE THERAPY AND MALIGNANCY

Tumors in the brain are unique in that they constitute a population of dividing cells. Thus, vectors such as MLV that can infect only dividing cells are ideally suited for genetically modifying tumor cells without affecting normal CNS cells. In animal models, transgenes have been constructed that introduce "suicide" genes such as the herpes simplex gene thymidine kinase (TK) into brain tumor cells.[8,48-51] When the dividing cells incorporate the TK gene, they become vulnerable to death when exposed to the antiviral drug gancyclovir.[50] In animal studies, MLV vectors containing the TK gene have been injected into the brains of rats with glioma cells, resulting in incorporation of the TK gene only into the dividing tumor cells. When the animals are subsequently fed oral gancyclovir, tumor cell death occurs, resulting in reduction of tumor size.[49] In addition, the death of some cells in the region of the tumor that have not been infected with the transgene also occurs, a so-called bystander effect.[8] By using strategies of this sort, techniques are being developed for targeting the treatment of human brain tumors. Current preclinical studies are focusing upon efficiently infecting a large percentage of tumor cells with the transgenic suicide genes, and exploring the use of vectors other than MLV.[48]

FUTURE DIRECTIONS

Ideally, it would be possible to control the amount of a transgene product that is produced *in vivo* in much the same way that one can manipulate oral or invasively administered drug dosages. Retroviral vectors used in the studies described above contain promoter elements that constitutively, or continuously, express transgenes at relatively high levels, and the amounts of gene products expressed by these vectors cannot currently be varied. Thus, significant effort in the field of gene therapy is devoted to achieving regulation of transgene expression.

Several methods for achieving regulatable transgene expression are being tested experimentally.

1. The introduction of steroid response elements into transgene constructs can alter transgene expression.[2] In these vectors, the exposure of a genetically modified cell to steroids will alter the activity of the transgene *promoter*, or the portion of the gene that controls the expression of the gene of interest such as a neurotrophin gene. Thus, a cell exposed to steroids will increase the efficiency with which it expresses the transgene.
2. Other transgene constructs contain an element that responds to tetracycline. This so-called tetracycline response element can be engineered in such a way as to either enhance or repress transgene expression in the presence of tetracycline.[52] Thus, an animal can be fed oral tetracycline as a means of controlling transgene expression.
3. The production of some transgene products depends on the availability of sufficient amounts of precursor molecules. Thus, one means of controlling the synthesis of some compounds is to limit the amount of precursor availability. For example, cells can be genetically modified to produce enhanced amounts of the cholinergic neurotransmitter acetylcholine (ACh) by introducing into them the gene for ACh synthesis, choline acetyltransferase (ChAT). In these transduced cells, it has been reported that ChAT production and ACh synthesis can be regulated by feeding animals varying amounts of the ACh precursor choline.[53]

An extension of the concept of regulatable gene expression is possessing the capability to completely shut off transgene expression. Discontinuation of transgene expression might be necessary if the biological function served by the transgene is no longer necessary, or if transgene expression actually becomes deleterious. Suicide genes such as thymidine kinase or the pro-apoptotic (programmed cell death-inducing) genes *p53* or *bax* could be inserted into transgene vectors to induce death in genetically modified cells.[48,49] Studies of these approaches are ongoing.

CONCLUSIONS

Gene therapy is a potential means of achieving intraparenchymal, specifically targeted and regionally restricted delivery of neuroactive substances to the nervous system. Neuronal growth-promoting substances, neurotransmitters, and biosynthetic enzymes could be delivered to prevent development of abnormal phenotypes, to deliver cytotoxic substances for tumor therapy, to intervene in the course of neurodegenerative disorders, and to promote nervous system reconstruction after injury. Improvements in vector design, duration of gene expression, and regulation of gene expression will lead to further refinements in the practicality and safety of gene therapy.

REFERENCES

1. MILLER, D. A. 1990. Retrovirus packaging cells. Hum. Gene Ther. **1:** 5–14.
2. SUHR, S. & F. H. GAGE. 1993. Gene therapy for neurologic disease. Arch. Neurol. **50:** 1252–1268.
3. BLAU, H. M. & M. L. SPRINGER. 1995. Gene therapy—A novel form of drug delivery. N. Engl. J. Med. **333:** 1204–1207.
4. KREMER, E. J. & M. PERRICAUDET. 1995. Adenovirus and adeno-associated virus mediated gene transfer. Br. Med. Bull. **51:** 31–44.

5. NALDINI, L., U. BLOMER & P. GALLAY, *et al.* 1996. In vivo gene delivery and stable transduction of nondividing cells by a lentiviral vector. Science **272:** 263–267.
6. WILSON, J. M. 1996. Adenoviruses as gene-delivery vehicles. N. Engl. J. Med. **334:** 1185–1187.
7. GLORIOSO, J. C., N. A. DeLUCA & D. J. FINK. 1995. Development and application of herpes simplex virus vectors for human gene therapy. Annu. Rev. Microbiol. **49:** 675–710.
8. HAMEL, W., L. MAGNELLI, V. P. CHIARUGI & M. A. ISRAEL. 1996. Herpes simplex virus thymidine kinase/gancyclovir-mediated apoptotic death of bystander cells. Cancer Res. **56:** 2697–2702.
9. TENENBAUM, L., J. L. DARLING & E. HOOGHE-PETERS. 1994. Adeno-associated virus (AAV) as a vector for gene transfer into glial cells of the human central nervous system. Gene Ther. **1(Suppl. 1):** S80.
10. TUSZYNSKI, M. H., K. GABRIEL, F. H. GAGE, S. SUHR, S. MEYER & A. ROSETTI. 1996. Nerve growth factor delivery by gene transfer induces differential outgrowth of sensory, motor and noradrenergic neurites after adult spinal cord injury. Exp. Neurol. **137:** 157–173.
11. WOLFF, J. A., L. J. FISHER, L. XU, *et al.* 1989. Grafting fibroblasts genetically modified to produce L-dopa in a rat model of Parkinson disease. Proc. Natl. Acad. Sci. USA **86:** 9011–9014.
12. HORELLOU, P., C. LUNDBERG, B. LeBOURDELLES, *et al.* 1991. Behavioural effects of genetically engineered cells releasing dopa and dopamine after intracerebral grafts in a rat model of Parkinson's disease. J. Physiol. (Paris) **85:** 158–170.
13. HORELLOU, P., P. BRUNDIN, P. KALEN, J. MALLET & A. BJORKLUND. 1990. In vivo release of dopa and dopamine from genetically engineered cells grafted to the denervated striatum. Neuron **5:** 393–402.
14. KANG, U. J., L. J. FISHER, T. H. JOH, K. L. O'MALLEY & F. H. GAGE. 1993. Regulation of dopamine production by genetically modified primary fibroblasts. J. Neurosci. **13:** 5203–5211.
15. ROSENBERG, M. B., T. FRIEDMANN, R. C. ROBERTSON, *et al.* 1988. Grafting genetically modified cells to the damaged brain: Restorative effects of NGF expression. Science **242:** 1575–1578.
16. CHEN, K. S. & F. H. GAGE. 1995. Somatic gene transfer of NGF to the aged brain: Behavioral and morphological amelioration. J. Neurosci. **15:** 2819–2825.
17. MARTINEZ-SERRANO, A., W. FISCHER & A. BJORKLUND. 1995. Reversal of age-dependent cognitive impairments and cholinergic neuron atrophy by NGF-secreting neural progenitors grafted to the basal forebrain. Neuron **15:** 473–484.
18. TUSZYNSKI, M. H., J. ROBERTS, M. C. SENUT, H.-S. U & F. H. GAGE. 1996. Gene therapy in the adult primate brain: Intraparenchymal grafts of cells genetically modified to produce nerve growth factor prevent cholinergic neuronal degeneration. Gene Ther. **3:** 305–314.
19. STRÖMBERG, I., C. J. WETMORE, T. EBENDAL, P. ERNFORS, H. PERSSON & L. OLSON. 1990. Rescue of basal forebrain cholinergic neurons after implantation of genetically modified cells producing recombinant NGF. J. Neurosci. Res. **25:** 405–411.
20. NAKAHARA, Y., M.-C. SENUT, F. H. GAGE & M. H. TUSZYNSKI. 1996. Grafts of fibroblasts genetically modified to secrete NGF, BDNF, NT-3 or basic FGF elicit differential responses in the adult spinal cord. Cell Transplant. **5:** 191–204.
21. TUSZYNSKI, M. H., K. MURAI, A. BLESCH, R. GRILL & I. MILLER. 1997. Functional characterization of NGF-secreting cell grafts to the acutely injured spinal cord. Cell Transplant. **6:** 361–368.
22. FRIEDMANN, T. & R. ROBLIN. 1972. Gene therapy for human genetic disease? Science **175:** 949–955.
23. SPENCER, D. D., R. J. ROBBINS, F. NAFTOLIN, *et al.* 1992. Unilateral transplantation of human fetal mesencephalic tissue into the caudate nucleus of patients with Parkinson's disease. N. Engl. J. Med. **327:** 1541–1548.
24. TERRY, R. D., R. KATZMAN & K. L. BICK. 1994. Alzheimer Disease. Raven Press. New York.

25. HEFTI, F. 1986. Nerve growth factor (NGF) promotes survival of septal cholinergic neurons after fimbrial transection. J. Neurosci. **6:** 2155–2162.

26. FISCHER, W., K. WICTORIN, A. BJORKLUND, L. R. WILLIAMS, S. VARON & F. H. GAGE. 1987. Amelioration of cholinergic neuron atrophy and spatial memory impairment in aged rats by nerve growth factor. Nature **329:** 65–68.

27. TUSZYNSKI, M. H., H.-S. U & F. H. GAGE. 1991. Recombinant human nerve growth factor infusions prevent cholinergic neuronal degeneration in the adult primate brain. Ann. Neurol. **30:** 625–636.

28. MORSE, J. K., S. J. WIEGAND, K. ANDERSON, *et al.* 1993. Brain-derived neurotrophic factor (BDNF) prevents the degeneration of medial septal cholinergic neurons following fimbria transection. J. Neurosci. **13:** 4146–4156.

29. WIDMER, H. R., B. KNUSEL & F. HEFTI. 1993. BDNF protection of basal forebrain cholinergic neurons after axotomy: Complete protection of p75 NGFR-positive cells. Neuroreport **4:** 363–366.

30. HEFTI, F. & W. J. WEINER. 1986. Nerve growth factor and Alzheimer's disease. Ann. Neurol. **20:** 275–281.

31. TUSZYNSKI, M. H. & F. H. GAGE. 1994. Neuotrophic factors and neuronal loss: Potential relevance to Alzheimer's disease. *In* Alzheimer's Disease. R. Terry, R. Katzman & K. L. Bick, Eds.: 405–418. Raven Press. New York.

32. WINKLER, J., G. A. RAMIREZ, H. G. KUHN, *et al.* 1996. Reversible induction of Schwann cell hyperplasia and sprouting of sensory and sympathetic neurites in vivo after continuous intracerebroventricular administration of nerve growth factor. Ann. Neurol. **40:** 128–139.

33. MENESINI, M. G., J. S. CHEN & R. LEVI-MONTALCINI. 1978. Sympathetic nerve fiber ingrowth in the central nervous system of neonatal rodent upon intracerebral nerve growth factor injections. Arch. Ital. Biol. **116:** 53–84.

34. WILLIAMS, L. R. 1991. Hypophagia is induced by intracerebroventricular administration of nerve growth factor. Exp. Neurol. **113:** 31–37.

35. FISCHER, W., A. BJORKLUND, K. CHEN & F. H. GAGE. 1991. NGF improves spatial memory in aged rodents as a function of age. J. Neurosci. **11:** 1889–1906.

36. FRIDEN, P. M., L. R. WALUS, P. WATSON, *et al.* 1993. Blood-brain barrier penetration and in vivo activity of an NGF conjugate. Science **259:** 373–377.

37. GAFFAN, D. & S. HARRISON. 1989. A comparison of the effects of fornix transection and sulcus principalis ablation upon spatial learning by monkeys. Behav. Brain. Res. **31:** 207–220.

38. SPINA, M. B., C. HYMAN, S. SQUINTO & R. M. LINDSAY. 1992. Brain-derived neurotrophic factor protects dopaminergic cells from 6-hydroxydopamine toxicity. Ann. N. Y. Acad. Sci. **648:** 348–350.

39. LIN, L. F., D. H. DOHERTY, J. D. LILE, S. BEKTESH & F. COLLINS. 1993. GDNF: A glial cell-line derived neurotrophic factor for midbrain dopaminergic neurons. Science **260:** 1130–1132.

40. LEFF, S. E., F. WU, C. UNRUH, *et al.* 1995. Coexpression of human GTP cyclohydrolase I (GTPCH1) and human tyrosine hydroxylase cDNAs to potentiate L-DOPA production by fibroblasts: Applications to Parkinson's disease gene therapy. Soc. Neurosci. Abstr. **21:** 1272.

41. EMERICH, D. F., J. P. HAMMANG, E. E. BAETGE & S. R. WINN. 1994. Implantation of polymer-encapsulated human nerve growth factor-screening fibroblasts attenuates the behavioral and neuropathological consequences of quinolinic acid injections into rodent striatum. Exp. Neurol. **130:** 141–150.

42. KORDOWER, J. H., E. Y. CHEN, E. J. MUFSON, S. R. WINN & D. F. EMERICH. 1996. Intrastriatal implants of polymer encapsulated cells genetically modified to secrete human nerve growth factor: trophic effects upon cholinergic and noncholinergic striatal neurons. Neuroscience **72:** 63–77.

43. SENUT, M.-C., M. H. TUSZYNSKI, H. K. RAYMON, *et al.* 1995. Regional differences in responsiveness of adult CNS axons to grafts of cells expressing human neurotrophin-3. Exp. Neurol. **135:** 36–55.

44. GRILL, R., K. MURAI, A. BLESCH, F. H. GAGE & M. H. TUSZYNSKI. 1997. Cellular

delivery of neurotrophin-3 promotes corticospinal axonal growth and partial functional recovery after spinal cord injury. J. Neurosci. **17:** 5560–5572.

45. TUSZYNSKI, M. H., D. A. PETERSON, J. RAY, A. BAIRD, Y. NAKAHARA & F. H. GAGE. 1994. Fibroblasts genetically modified to produce nerve growth factor induce robust neuritic ingrowth after grafting to the spinal cord. Exp. Neurol. **126:** 1–14.

46. SCHNELL, L., R. SCHNEIDER, R. KOLBECK, Y. A. BARDE & M. E. SCHWAB. 1994. Neurotrophin-3 enhances sprouting of corticospinal tract during development and after adult spinal cord lesion. Nature **367:** 170–173.

47. LEVI-MONTALCINI, R. 1987. The nerve growth factor 35 years later. Science **237:** 1154–1162.

48. EZZEDDINE, Z. D., R. L. MARTUZA, D. PLATIKA, *et al.* 1991. Selective killing of glioma cells in culture and in vivo by retrovirus transfer of the herpes simplex virus thymidine kinase. New Biol. **3:** 608–614.

49. BARBA, D., J. HARDIN, J. RAY & F. H. GAGE. 1993. Thymidine kinase-mediated killing of rat brain tumors. J. Neurosurg. **79:** 729–735.

50. VINCENT, A. J., R. VOGELS, G. V. SOMEREN, *et al.* 1996. Herpes simplex virus thymidine kinase gene therapy for rat malignant brain tumors. Hum. Gene Ther. **7:** 197–205.

51. GE, L., N. M. RESNICK, L. K. ERNST, L. A. SALVUCCI, D. C. ASMAN & D. L. COOPER. 1995. Gene therapeutic approaches to primary and metastatic brain tumors: II. Ribozyme-mediated suppression of CD44 expression. J. Neurooncol. **26:** 251–257.

52. GOSSEN, M., A. L. BONIN, S. FREUNDLIEB & H. BUJARD. 1994. Inducible gene expression systems for higher eukaryotic cells. Curr. Opin. Biotechnol. **5:** 516–520.

53. WINKLER, J., S. T. SUHR, F. H. GAGE, L. J. THAL & L. FISCHER. 1995. Essential role of neocortical acetylcholine in spatial memory. Nature **375:** 484–487.

Trophic Factors, Synaptic Plasticity, and Memory

ERIC S. LEVINE[a] AND IRA B. BLACK

Department of Neuroscience and Cell Biology
Robert Wood Johnson Medical School
University of Medicine and Dentistry of New Jersey
675 Hoes Lane
Piscataway, New Jersey 08854

One of the central issues in neuroscience concerns the cellular foundations of memory. How are brief environmental experiences translated into stable, long-lasting changes in brain function? Conversely, how are learning and memory processes disrupted by degenerative disease or injury? At a mechanistic level, this is a question of how brain activity itself modifies the functional connections between neurons, the synapses. Activity-dependent modulation of synaptic transmission has assumed primacy in most formulations of memory. The synaptic apparatus simultaneously subserves millisecond-to-millisecond interneuronal communication and stores long-term information, thereby participating in the mnemonic process. Although there is an ever-expanding list of transmitters, peptides, and hormones that function as synaptic messengers, little is known about the intercellular signals that regulate the strength and efficacy of synaptic transmission.

One potentially rewarding approach is to focus on the signals that regulate nervous system development, when maximal synaptic and neural plasticity occurs. During development, the functional circuitry of the brain is established through processes of axonal and dendritic outgrowth, synapse formation and stabilization, and the loss of neurons that fail to make appropriate connections. Growth and trophic factors are important classes of signals involved in these events. In particular, nerve growth factor (NGF) and related neurotrophins are essential for the selective survival and differentiation of specific neurons within the peripheral and central nervous systems.[1,2]

In this brief overview, we focus on our recent studies suggesting a novel role for these trophic factors in the dynamic modulation of synaptic efficacy, both during development and in maturity. Most importantly, trophins acutely modulate both pre- and postsynaptic mechanisms regulating synaptic transmission. Additionally, trophin gene expression itself is regulated by neuronal impulse activity, indicating that external stimuli modulate trophin availability. Thus, signaling mechanisms that participate in the formation of neuronal circuits during development appear to operate throughout life to modulate interneuronal communication.

The neurotrophin gene family includes NGF, brain-derived neurotrophic factor (BDNF), neurotrophin-3 (NT-3), and neurotrophin-4/5 (NT-4/5). Three *trk* family members, *trk*A, *trk*B, and *trk*C, encode essential components of receptors for these neurotrophins.[3] NGF acts upon trkA, BDNF and NT-4/5 on trkB, and NT-3 acts primarily on trkC, but also interacts with trkA and trkB.[3-5] All neurotrophins also bind to p75, a widely distributed receptor of uncertain function.[6] Neurotrophin

[a] E-mail: levine@mbcl.rutgers.edu; black@mbcl.rutgers.edu

"

receptors exist in several isoforms. The full-length, active forms of the trk family are necessary for the normal development and maintenance of specific neuronal populations. It remains to be determined whether the truncated trkB and trkC receptors, which lack tyrosine kinase catalytic domains, play roles in neurotrophin-mediated function.

Neurotrophins and their receptors are expressed throughout the central nervous system. Our studies focus on the hippocampus, in which synaptic plasticity and memory appear to be closely associated. Several forms of activity-dependent synaptic plasticity have been demonstrated in this brain structure, including long-term potentiation, considered to be a cellular model of memory mechanisms. The hippocampus is also the site of highest expression in the brain for neurotrophins and their receptors during development and maturity. Thus, trophin modulation of synaptic transmission in the hippocampus may have consequences for plasticity underlying mnemonic processes.

ACTIVITY-DEPENDENT REGULATION OF NEUROTROPHIN GENE EXPRESSION

One important requirement for involvement in activity-dependent plasticity is increased availability of a molecule in response to heightened neuronal activity. Several different lines of investigation have shown that neurotrophin gene expression is modulated by neuronal impulse activity. Trophin expression *in vivo* in both the hippocampus and neocortex is increased by limbic seizures. Dramatic increases in NGF and BDNF mRNA levels are produced by distinct methods of seizure induction, including dentate gyrus lesions, kainic acid injections, and electrical stimulation.[7–10] Specific mechanisms underlying activity-dependent regulation of trophin gene expression have been characterized in dissociated neuronal cultures. We and others have shown that direct depolarization or activation of glutamate receptors markedly increases hippocampal neuron NGF and BDNF mRNAs.[11–14]

Electrical stimulation of intrinsic pathways also regulates neurotrophin gene expression, providing a critical physiologic context. Stimuli that elicit long-term potentiation (LTP), for example, increase BDNF and NT-3 messages in the hippocampus.[15,16] LTP has been invoked as a requisite for learning and memory. Additionally, the recent description of a deficit in LTP in null mutations of the BDNF gene in (knockout) mice supports the contention that neurotrophins play critical roles in synaptic plasticity and, perhaps, memory.[17,18]

SPECIFIC NEUROTROPHINS INCREASE SYNAPTIC EFFICACY

Recent studies from our laboratory and others have shown that neurotrophins directly enhance efficacy of synaptic transmission. The exact mechanisms by which trophins modulate synaptic activity remain to be established. In several neuronal populations, specific neurotrophins enhance both spontaneous and evoked synaptic currents.[19–23] These effects involve modulation of pre- and postsynaptic mechanisms, suggesting actions at multiple loci. Presynaptic effects have been best characterized at the *Xenopus* neuromuscular junction, where BDNF and NT-3 potentiate evoked synaptic currents within minutes of exposure by enhancing presynaptic acetylcholine release.[20]

A

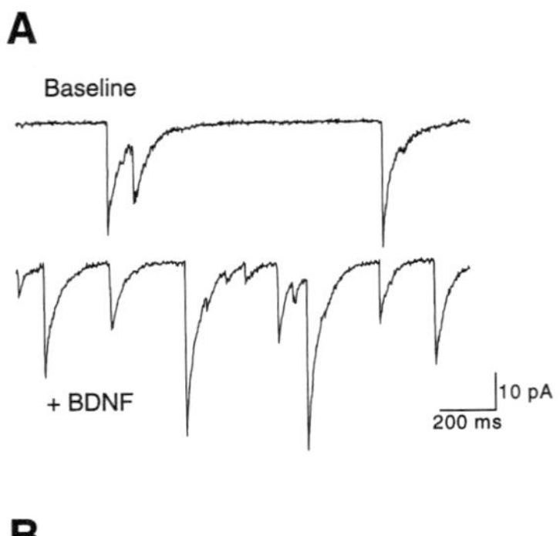

B

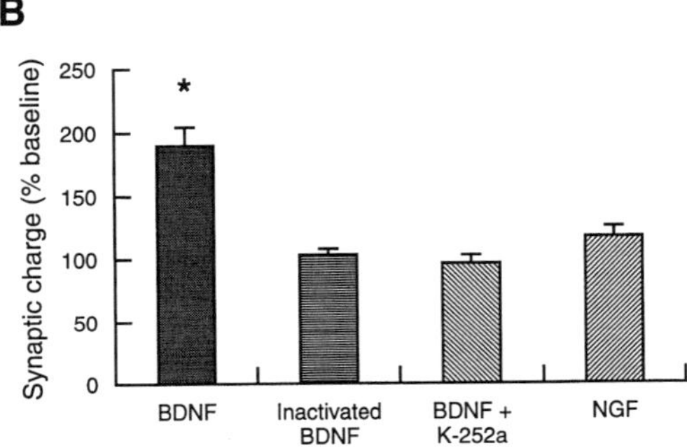

FIGURE 1. Potentiation of synaptic transmission by brain-derived neurotrophic factor (BDNF). (**A**) Whole-cell voltage-clamp recordings from a hippocampal neuron before and three minutes after exposure to BDNF (V_{hold} = −60 mV). (**B**) Effects on synaptic charge after bath application of BDNF (50 ng/mL; n = 10 cells), heat-inactivated BDNF (50 ng/mL; n = 9 cells), or NGF (50 ng/mL; n = 13 cells). In some experiments, cultures were pretreated for one hour with K-252a in the bath solution (200 nM; n = 7 cells). *p < 0.001 compared to baseline levels for that condition. Recordings were obtained from multiple platings.

We examined trophic modulation of synaptic transmission in the hippocampus. Patch-clamp recordings were made from neuronal cultures obtained from embryonic rat hippocampus, grown in serum-free, fully defined medium. Under these conditions, neurons form extensive connections, display spontaneous synaptic activity, and fire action potentials in response to synaptic inputs. In the first set of studies, impulse activity was recorded using the whole-cell current clamp configuration. Application of BDNF caused an immediate, twofold increase in the firing rate of hippocampal neurons.[21] This increase was sustained in the presence of BDNF, and firing rate returned to baseline levels 10–15 min following removal of the factor.

To investigate underlying synaptic mechanisms, the effect of BDNF was characterized in a series of whole-cell voltage clamp experiments. Recordings of excitatory postsynaptic currents (EPSCs) revealed a marked enhancement within 2–3 min of BDNF exposure (FIG. 1A). These synaptic currents were not spontaneous miniature potentials and were action potential dependent, because their occurrence was eliminated by the sodium channel blocker tetrodotoxin. Currents were quantified by measuring the integrated current, or synaptic charge. BDNF application elicited a twofold increase in synaptic charge with a time course similar to the increase in action potential activity (FIG. 1B). In contrast, treatment with heat-inactivated BDNF had no effect on synaptic charge. Additionally, bath application of the relatively specific *trk* tyrosine kinase inhibitor K-252a, which prevents biological responses to neurotrophins,[24–26] completely blocked the effect of BDNF on synaptic charge.[21]

RECEPTOR SPECIFICITY

Related members of the neurotrophin gene family often have overlapping effects on responsive populations. To examine the specificity of the effect of BDNF on synaptic currents, we examined responses to other trophic factors. TrkB receptor activation appears critical for the synaptic enhancement, because NT-4, another trkB ligand, elicits effects similar to BDNF. In contrast, the related neurotrophins, NGF and NT-3, which primarily interact with other trk receptors, did not share this effect. Additionally, we found that the unrelated growth factors, epidermal growth factor and basic fibroblast growth factor, were also without effect.[27]

MECHANISMS OF ACTION: POSTSYNAPTIC LOCI

We investigated the role of postsynaptic events in trophin-induced synaptic plasticity. In these experiments we took advantage of the possibility of injecting drugs selectively into the postsynaptic cell by inclusion of the drug in the internal solution of the patch pipette. FIGURE 2 shows individual examples of the time course of the BDNF effect on synaptic charge under various conditions. Intracellular injection of K-252a significantly decreased the magnitude of the effect compared

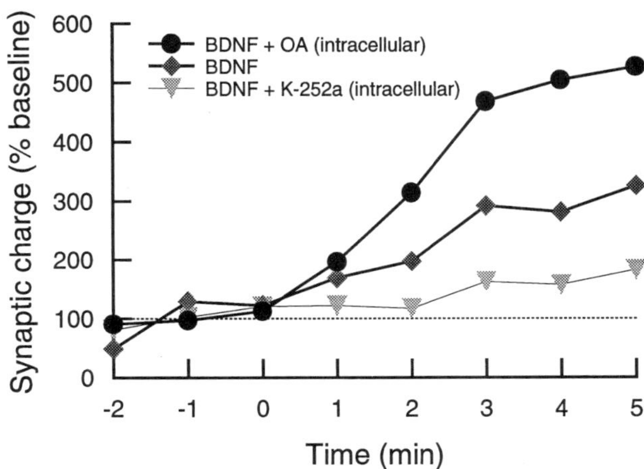

FIGURE 2. Time courses of recordings from individual neurons for the effect of either bath-applied BDNF alone (50 ng/mL; *diamonds*), or in combination with intracellular injection of K-252a (200 nM; *triangles*) or okadaic acid (OA; 0.5 μM; *circles*). Recordings were obtained from sister cultures. Each point represents the average synaptic charge for a 1-min period.

to BDNF alone. Conversely, intracellular injection of the phosphatase inhibitor okadaic acid, which prolongs phosphorylation events, enhanced the magnitude of the effect.[21] Baseline synaptic charge was not affected by inclusion of either K-252a or okadaic acid in the internal solution. These results indicate that phosphorylation-dependent changes in postsynaptic responsiveness are required for the trophin effect on synaptic currents.

Exposure to BDNF, in fact, produced increases in both the frequency and amplitude of synaptic currents (see FIG. 1A). We analyzed these components individually. Because the EPSCs were action potential dependent, the frequency of synaptic currents was increased as a direct consequence of increased impulse activity of the presynaptic inputs to the recorded cell. Intracellular injection of K-252a or okadaic acid directly into the postsynaptic cell, therefore, had no effect on BDNF-induced increase in frequency. Conversely, the increase in synaptic current amplitude was enhanced by intracellular injection of the phosphatase inhibitor okadaic acid, and completely abolished by injection of the tyrosine kinase inhibitor K-252a. These results indicate that the effect of BDNF on EPSC amplitude, in particular, is a direct result of postsynaptic modulation.

The synaptic effects of the trkB ligands are mediated postsynaptically, but little is known of the distribution of neurotrophin receptors. To define the subcellular locus of synaptic modulation and delineate underlying mechanisms, we examined the localization of trkB receptors in the hippocampus. Western blot analyses revealed that full-length, functional trkB receptors are an intrinsic component of the postsynaptic density (PSD), a specialization of the postsynaptic membrane, in both the developing and adult hippocampus.[28] The truncated, nonsignaling form of the trkB receptor, although present in the synaptic membrane fraction, was undetectable in the PSD.

The PSD is a proteinaceous, disc-shaped subcellular organelle apposed to the inner surface of the postsynaptic membrane of chemical synapses. Several characteristics suggest that the PSD plays a pivotal role in synaptic function and synaptic plasticity.[29,30] Neurotransmitter receptors, protein kinases, phosphoprotein phosphatases, and ion channel proteins are anchored to the PSD.[31] These findings suggest that the PSD participates in signal transduction and, potentially, receptor regulation. Indeed, recent studies revealed that neurotransmitter receptors, including NMDA (*N*-methyl-D-aspartate) and AMPA (D,L-a-amino-3-hydroxy-5-methyl-4-isoaxazole propionic acid) receptors can be phosphorylated by intrinsic PSD kinases, resulting in enhanced synaptic transmission.[32–34] Many of the same protein kinases are known to be involved in trkB signal transduction pathways.[35,36] Thus, neurotrophins may modulate synaptic transmission by phosphorylation of these and other receptors in the PSD. Our findings represent a first step in understanding the roles of neurotrophin signaling in brain synaptic communication.

A ROLE FOR BDNF IN MEMORY *IN VIVO*?

Recent studies from our laboratory raise the possibility that hippocampal BDNF is associated with spatial memory function. Unilateral hippocampal lesions result in spatial memory deficits in the neonatal rat, while having far fewer effects in adults.[37] These results indicate that the contralateral, unlesioned hippocampus is dysfunctional after neonatal lesions. This model provides the opportunity to examine trophin gene expression in the remaining, apparently dysfunctional hippocampus of rats with deranged memory function. In fact, BDNF mRNA was decreased significantly, whereas NGF message was unchanged. Moreover, measures of cholinergic and GABAergic function were normal.[37] These initial studies raise the possibility that BDNF, which regulates synaptic plasticity *in vitro*, also plays a role in memory mechanisms *in vivo*. We are presently extending these studies.

In summary, the neurotrophins, BDNF and NT-4, ligands of the trkB receptor, rapidly increase both the frequency and amplitude of excitatory synaptic currents in hippocampal neurons. The potentiation of synaptic current amplitude, in particular, results from a phosphorylation-dependent change in postsynaptic responsiveness. Neurotrophins also enhance synaptic transmission by increasing presynaptic transmitter release. These results suggest that trophic factors play a central role in the dynamic modulation of synaptic efficacy. Acute modulation by neurotrophins may constitute an intermediary stage, preceding more stable changes (e.g., in synaptic morphology or ion channel expression) that depend on alterations in gene expression and/or protein synthesis. The precise role(s) of neurotrophins in memory mechanisms is presently under active investigation.

REFERENCES

1. LEVI-MONTALCINI, R. & P. U. ANGELETTI. 1968. Nerve growth factor. Physiol. Rev. **48:** 534–569.
2. THOENEN, H., C. BANDTLOW & R. HEUMANN. 1987. The physiological function of nerve growth factor in the central nervous system: Comparison with the periphery. Rev. Physiol. Biochem. Pharmacol. **109:** 145–178.
3. MEAKIN, S. O. & E. M. SHOOTER. 1992. The nerve growth factor family of receptors. Trends Neurosci. **15:** 323–331.
4. KLEIN, R., S. Q. JING, V. NANDURI, E. O'ROURKE & M. BARBACID. 1991. The trk proto-oncogene encodes a receptor for nerve growth factor. Cell **65:** 189–197.
5. LAMBALLE, F., R. KLEIN & M. BARBACID. 1991. trkC, A new member of the trk family of tyrosine protein kinases, is a receptor for neurotrophin-3. Cell **66:** 967–979.
6. CHAO, M. V. 1994. The p75 neurotrophin receptor. J. Neurobiol. **25:** 1373–1385.
7. GALL, C. M. & P. J. ISACKSON. 1989. Limbic seizures increase neuronal production of messenger RNA for nerve growth factor. Science **245:** 758–761.
8. GALL, C., K. MURRAY & P. J. ISACKSON. 1991. Kainic acid-induced seizures stimulate increased expression of nerve growth factor mRNA in rat hippocampus. Mol. Brain Res. **9:** 113–123.
9. ISACKSON, P. J., M. M. HUNTSMAN, K. D. MURRAY & C. M. GALL. 1991. BDNF mRNA expression is increased in adult rat forebrain after limbic seizures: Temporal patterns of induction distinct from NGF. Neuron **69:** 937–948.
10. LINDHOLM, D., E. CASTREN, M. BERZAGHI, A. BLOCHL & H. THOENEN. 1994. Activity-dependent and hormonal regulation of neurotrophin mRNA levels in the brain—Implications for neuronal plasticity. J. Neurobiol. **2:** 1362–1372.
11. LU, B., M. YOKOYAMA, C. F. DREYFUS & I. B. BLACK. 1991. Depolarizing stimuli regulate nerve growth factor gene expression in cultured hippocampal neurons. Proc. Natl. Acad. Sci. USA **88:** 6289–6292.
12. ZAFRA, F., B. HENGERER, J. LEIBROCK, H. THOENEN & D. LINDHOLM. 1990. Activity dependent regulation of BDNF and NGF mRNAs in the rat hippocampus is mediated by non-NMDA glutamate receptors. Embo J. **9:** 3545–3550.
13. ZAFRA, F., D. LINDHOLM, E. CASTREN, J. HARTIKKA & H. THOENEN. 1992. Regulation of brain-derived neurotrophic factor and nerve growth factor mRNA in primary cultures of hippocampal neurons and astrocytes. J. Neurosci. **12:** 4793–4799.
14. ELLIOTT, R. C., C. E. INTURRISI, I. B. BLACK & C. F. DREYFUS. 1994. An improved method detects differential NGF and BDNF gene expression in response to depolarization in cultured hippocampal neurons. Mol. Brain Res. **26:** 81–88.
15. CASTREN, E., M. PITKANEN, J. SIRVIO, A. PARSADANIAN, D. LINDHOLM, H. THOENEN &

P. J. RIEKKINEN. 1993. The induction of LTP increases BDNF and NGF mRNA but decreases NT-3 mRNA in the dentate gyrus. Neuroreport **4:** 895–898.

16. PATTERSON, S. L., L. M. GROVER, P. A. SCHWARTZKROIN & M. BOTHWELL. 1992. Neurotrophin expression in rat hippocampal slices: A stimulus paradigm inducing LTP in CA1 evokes increases in BDNF and NT-3 mRNAs. Neuron **9:** 1081–1088.

17. KORTE, M., P. CARROLL, E. WOLF, G. BREM, H. THOENEN & T. BONHOEFFER. 1995. Hippocampal long-term potentiation is impaired in mice lacking brain-derived neurotrophic factor. Proc. Natl. Acad. Sci. USA **92:** 8856–8860.

18. PATTERSON, S. L., T. ABEL, T. A. DEUEL, K. C. MARTIN, J. C. ROSE & E. R. KANDEL. 1996. Recombinant BDNF rescues deficits in basal synaptic transmission and hippocampal LTP in BDNF knockout mice. Neuron **16:** 1137–1145.

19. KIM, H. G., T. WANG, P. OLAFSSON & B. LU. 1994. Neurotrophin 3 potentiates neuronal activity and inhibits gamma-aminobutyratergic synaptic transmission in cortical neurons. Proc. Natl. Acad. Sci. USA **91:** 12341–12345.

20. LOHOF, A. M., N. Y. IP & M. M. POO. 1993. Potentiation of developing neuromuscular synapses by the neurotrophins NT-3 and BDNF. Nature **363:** 350–353.

21. LEVINE, E. S., C. F. DREYFUS, I. B. BLACK & M. R. PLUMMER. 1995. Brain-derived neurotrophic factor rapidly enhances synaptic transmission in hippocampal neurons via postsynaptic tyrosine kinase receptors. Proc. Natl. Acad. Sci. USA **92:** 8074–8077.

22. KANG, H. J. & E. M. SCHUMANN. 1995. Neurotrophin-induced modulation of synaptic transmission in the adult hippocampus. J. Physiol. (Paris) **89:** 11–22.

23. FIGUROV, A., L. D. POZZO-MILLER, P. OLAFSSON, T. WANG & B. LU. 1996. Regulation of synaptic responses to high-frequency stimulation and LTP by neurotrophins in the hippocampus. Nature **381:** 706–709.

24. OHMICHI, M., S. J. DECKER, L. PANG & A. R. SALTIEL. 1992. Inhibition of the cellular actions of nerve growth factor by staurosporine and K252A results from the attenuation of the activity of the trk tyrosine kinase. Biochemistry **31:** 4034–4039.

25. TAPLEY, P., F. LAMBALLE & M. BARBACID. 1992. K252a is a selective inhibitor of the tyrosine protein kinase activity of the trk family of oncogenes and neurotrophin receptors. Oncogene **7:** 371–381.

26. BERG, M. M., D. W. STERNBERG, L. F. PARADA & M. V. CHAO. 1992. K-252a inhibits nerve growth factor-induced trk proto-oncogene tyrosine phosphorylation and kinase activity. J. Biol. Chem. **267:** 13–16.

27. LEVINE, E. S., C. F. DREYFUS, I. B. BLACK & M. R. PLUMMER. 1996. Selective role for trkB neurotrophin receptors in rapid modulation of hippocampal synaptic transmission. Mol. Brain Res. **38:** 300–303.

28. WU, K., J. L. XU, P. C. SUEN, E. S. LEVINE, Y. Y. HUANG, H. T. J. MOUNT, S. Y. LIN & I. B. BLACK. 1996. Functional trkB neurotrophin receptors are intrinsic components of the adult brain postsynaptic density. Mol. Brain Res. **43:** 286–290.

29. SIEKEVITZ, P. 1985. The postsynaptic density: A possible role in long-lasting effects in the central nervous system. Proc. Natl. Acad. Sci. USA **82:** 3494–3498.

30. WU, K. & I. B. BLACK. 1988. Transsynaptic impulse activity regulates postsynaptic density molecules in developing and adult rat superior cervical ganglion. Proc. Natl. Acad. Sci. USA **85:** 6207–6210.

31. WU, K. & P. SIEKEVITZ. 1988. Neurochemical characteristics of a postsynaptic density fraction isolated from adult canine hippocampus. Brain Res. **457:** 98–112.

32. GREENGARD, P., J. JEN, A. C. NAIRN & C. F. STEVENS. 1991. Enhancement of the glutamate response by cAMP-dependent protein kinase in hippocampal neurons. Science **253:** 1135–1138.

33. RAYMOND, L. A., W. G. TINGLEY, C. D. BLACKSTONE, K. W. ROCHE & R. L. HUGANIR. 1994. Glutamate receptor modulation by protein phosphorylation. J. Physiol. (Paris) **88:** 181–192.

34. TAN, S. E., R. J. WENTHOLD & T. R. SODERLING. 1994. Phosphorylation of AMPA-type glutamate receptors by calcium/calmodulin-dependent protein kinase II and protein kinase C in cultured hippocampal neurons. J. Neurosci. **14:** 1123–1129.

35. ZIRRGIEBEL, U., Y. OHGA, B. CARTER, B. BERNINGER, N. INAGAKI, H. THOENEN & D. LINDHOLM. 1995. Characterization of TrkB receptor-mediated signaling pathways

in rat cerebellar granule neurons: Involvement of protein kinase C in neuronal survival. J. Neurochem. **65:** 2241–2250.

36. MARSH, H. N., W. K. SCHOLZ, F. LAMBALLE, R. KLEIN, V. NANDURI, M. BARBACID & H. C. PALFREY. 1993. Signal transduction events mediated by the BDNF receptor gp 145trkB in primary hippocampal pyramidal cell culture. J. Neurosci. **13:** 4281–4292.

37. VAN PRAAG, H., P. M. QU, R. C. ELLIOTT, H. WU, C. F. DREYFUS & I. B. BLACK. Unilateral hippocampal lesions in newborn and adult rats: Effects on spatial memory and BDNF gene expression. Behav. Brain Res. In press.

Findings about the Cholinergic Basal Forebrain Using Immunotoxin to the Nerve Growth Factor Receptor

RONALD G. WILEY[a]

Departments of Neurology and Pharmacology
Vanderbilt University, and Neurology Service
VAMC
Nashville, Tennessee

INTRODUCTION

The cholinergic hypothesis of dementia in aging and Alzheimer's disease (AD)[1] has stimulated interest in the cholinergic neurons of the basal forebrain (CBF) and pointed attention to the need for better understanding of the normal function of the CBF. The search for animal models of AD has included attempts to produce cholinergic hypofunction using various lesioning techniques on the CBF. Before 1991, several authors noted that attempts to use conventional lesioning techniques on the CBF did not reproduce the neuropathology of AD.[2–11] Studies using excitotoxin lesions of the CBF in rats raised questions about the significance of CBF degeneration in AD because a correlation did not exist between extent of behavioral impairment and loss of cortical cholinergic innervation.[12–16] The obvious concern was that excitotoxin lesions of the CBF produce behavioral deficits because of damage to noncholinergic neurons in the basal forebrain. A method for producing selective destruction of the CBF was clearly needed.

CBF neurons are unique in the forebrain of healthy, adults rats in abundantly expressing the low-affinity neurotrophin receptor ($p75^{NTr}$).[17–19] Based upon observations by Schweitzer[20,21] that a monoclonal antibody (192 IgG) to $p75^{NTr}$ was selectively taken up and concentrated in rat CBF neurons after intracerebroventricular (i.c.v.) injection, we made an immunotoxin (192-saporin) with this antibody.[22] 192-saporin consists of the 192 IgG[23] disulfide conjugated to the ribosome-inactivating protein, saporin.[24] We chose saporin because a 192-IgG immunotoxin made with ricin A chain[25] was inactive *in vivo*; because at least one immunotoxin made with saporin was more potent and effective than a similar conjugate made with ricin A chain;[26] and because we had previous success lesioning neurons *in vivo* with OX7-saporin.[27] Thus, 192-saporin was developed in order to make selective lesions of the CBF in rats for the purpose of analyzing the function of the CBF and any relationship between loss of CBF neurons and cognitive dysfunction. Reviews of some of this material have appeared previously.[28–30]

[a] Address correspondence to Ronald G. Wiley, M.D., Ph.D., Neurology Service (127), VAMC, 1310 24th Avenue, South, Nashville, TN 37212-2637. E-mail: ronald.g.wiley@vanderbilt.edu

ANATOMICAL STUDIES

Numerous reports have documented the loss of choline acetyltransferase (ChAT)+ and p75[NTr]+ neurons from the CBF after i.c.v. or local intraparenchymal injection of 192-saporin. The findings of several anatomical studies of rats injected with 192-saporin also include:

1. The lesion that results from i.c.v. injection of 192-saporin includes the CBF and Purkinje neurons of the cerebellum[22,29,31–33] (this correlates with the distribution of p75[NTr] expression in adult rat brain[17–19]).
2. Neurons that express tyrosine hydroxylase,[22] glutamic acid dehydrogenase,[34] parvalbumin,[35–38] galanin,[39] neuropeptide Y,[39,40] and neurotensin[39] appear unaffected by 192-saporin injections (i.c.v. or intraparenchymal).
3. The cholinergic innervation of the amygdala is preserved, even after destruction of all neurons expressing p75[NTr], supporting the conclusion that the cholinergic afferents to the amygdala do not express p75[NTr].[32,41,42]
4. Two bands of acetylcholinesterase+ (AChE+) fibers remain in the cingulate cortex in animals with all p75[NTr]+ neurons destroyed leading to a similar conclusion.[32,41]
5. The noncholinergic neurons in the region of the nucleus basalis magnocellularis (Nbm) that stain for calbindin D-28k or NADPH-diaphorase were unaffected by 192-saporin.[32]
6. Prelabeling cortically projecting Nbm neurons with fluoro-gold showed that only those that also labeled for ChAT were destroyed by 192-saporin.[43]
7. *In situ* hybridization studies showed that loss of staining for p75[NTr] after 192-saporin is accompanied by loss of mRNA for p75[NTr][44] in the CBF.
8. Destruction of CBF neurons by 192-saporin produces very little tissue reaction except a brisk, transient microglial infiltrate in the CBF.[37,45]
9. Cortical AChE+ fibers are depleted by local cortical infusions of 192-saporin.[46]
10. Glutamic acid dehydrogenase immunocytochemical staining is decreased in the septae between whisker barrels in somatosensory cortex after 192-saporin lesions of CBF.[47]

In conclusion, the anatomical studies support the specificity and efficacy of 192-saporin when used to destroy the CBF. The only significant reservation is that i.c.v. injections also damage some cerebellar Purkinje cells. One group has reported a very delayed decrease in striatal ChAT+ interneurons after local Nbm injection,[32,33] which has not been confirmed by subsequent studies. Cholinergic neurons (ChAT+) in other brain regions are uniformly unaffected by 192-saporin injections.[22,29,32,41]

NEUROCHEMICAL STUDIES

In general, the neurochemical studies have consistently supported the anatomical data showing substantial loss of ChAT activity from the CBF and terminal fields of CBF projections to the hippocampus,[48–50] olfactory bulb,[48,49] and neocortex.[48,49] In parallel, AChE activity in these same structures is also reduced.[51] Assays of ChAT activity in regions containing or innervated by cholinergic neurons that do not express p75[NTr], such as thalamus, striatum and brain stem, have shown no effect of the immunotoxin.[38,49] Binding of radiolabeled hemicholinium-3 (HC-3), a marker for cholinergic terminals, is selectively and profoundly decreased in the terminal fields of the CBF after injection of 92-saporin.[52,53] Other neurotransmitters that have been studied are not consistently affected by injections of 192-saporin; these include norepinephrine, dopamine, and serotonin.[36,38,49,50,53,54] Although some studies have reported increased norepinephrine in the hippocampus[36,50] and neocortex,[36,54] one study reported decreased norepinephrine in the hippocampus.[53] In addition, one study reported increased dopamine in the neocortex[36] and another in the olfactory bulb.[49] Given the numbers of assays of monoamine neurotransmitters and metabolites, the significance of the occasional report of increased levels or turnover in a specific terminal field is uncertain. Certainly the neurochemical studies have not shown any evidence that 192-saporin injections consistently ablate any neurotransmitter other than acetylcholine. Grafting of nerve growth factor (NGF)-secreting fibroblasts into rats with partial CBF lesions from 192-saporin can restore levels of ChAT, AChE, and HC-3 binding.[55] Studies of muscarinic receptors using immunocytochemistry have reported that 192-saporin injections (i.c.v.) decrease the number of m2 reactive fibers in the fimbria/fornix; however, no other significant changes in m1–m4 distribution or abundance were noted in either the septum or hippocampus,[56,57] indicating that the great majority of these receptors are not on the processes of CBF neurons. *In situ* hybridization and radioligand receptor binding assays were used to analyze the effects of i.c.v. 192-saporin; the only change found in muscarinic receptors was a 40% loss of m2 mRNA in the CBF.[52]

Changes in neural chemistry other than neurotransmitter metabolism have been reported after 192-saporin injection. Rossner and colleagues[58] have observed increased c-fos mRNA levels by *in situ* hybridization in the medial and lateral septum after i.c.v. injection of 192-saporin. They also reported increased c-jun nRNA in the medial septum and layer IV of parietal and occipital neocortex. Treatment with 192-saporin blocks the induction of NGF mRNA produced by generalized seizures produced (from hippocampal kindling).[59] These authors also reported that 192-saporin injection abolished the seizure-induced increase in trkC and decrease in neurotrophin-3 mRNAs while partially blocking the seizure-induced increase in BDNF mRNA (exons I and III, but not II). They found no change in expression of trkB mRNA. In summary, the neurochemical studies support the specificity of 192-saporin for CBF neurons and are just beginning to reveal the consequences of this lesion on other neural systems. An unexpected finding is the lack of effect of CBF lesions on muscarinic receptor distribution.

ELECTROPHYSIOLOGICAL STUDIES

192-Saporin lesions of the CBF produce an overall decrease in the amplitude of cortical electroencephalogram (EEG) at all frequencies.[60] Injection of 192-saporin into the septum produces a decrease in the amplitude of hippocampal theta activity that begins after three days and reaches maximum by seven days.[61] This effect persists for at least eight weeks. Injections (i.c.v.) also decrease theta power and amplitude,[62] but neither type of injection affected theta frequency suggesting that the pacemaker is noncholinergic. Recently, CBF lesions made with 192-saporin injections have been shown to have no effect on long-term potentiation (LTP) in hippocampal region CA1,[63] but these lesions do eliminate the presumed cholinergic slow excitatory postsynaptic potential in CA1 pyramidal neurons while enhancing the afterhyperpolarization seen following a train of spikes.[64]

Sleep studies in rats injected with 192-saporin i.c.v. have shown transient changes but very few long-term effects.[60,62] The only effect that persisted after seven days was shortening of REM sleep epochs without an overall change in total amount of REM sleep. However, 192-saporin lesions have been reported to decrease slow event-related cortical potentials seen in a classical conditioning paradigm,[65] and the initial stages of hippocampal kindling are enhanced by 192-saporin lesions of the CBF.[59]

Initial studies indicate a decrease in whisker barrel field plasticity in response to whisker pairing[66,67] after 192-saporin lesions of the CBF. These studies successfully utilized local cortical infusions of 192-saporin to produce a restricted, unilateral denervation of the somatosensory cortex. Others have reported that mean response rates from the barrel of a whisker being stimulated increased after CBF lesion (i.c.v. 192-saporin), but only in old rats.[68] Lastly, forcing rats to use the remaining two whiskers after 192-saporin injection produced some pairing bias in adjacent barrels of the intact whiskers similar to rats without CBF lesions,[69] suggesting that experience can overcome the effects of CBF lesions on barrel field plasticity.

The most notable aspect of the electrophysiological data with 192-saporin is probably the lack of effects on sleep, fully developed kindled seizures, LTP, and the absence of neocortical EEG slow waves that are characteristic of muscarinic antagonist effects.

BEHAVIORAL STUDIES

By using i.c.v. injections that affect all portions of the CBF, deficits have been reported in passive avoidance[38,41] and water maze[33,36,38,70] performance. These deficits have consisted primarily of impaired acquisition without major abnormalities in motor performance such as spontaneous locomotor activity[31,38] or swim speed.[31,70] However, some motor deficits have been described at the doses necessary to completely ablate the CBF,[31,53] and cued navigation was reported to be impaired in one study[33] suggesting a nonmnemonic performance deficit. The motor abnormalities tend to diminish or even disappear with time and probably reflect the cerebellar damage that results from i.c.v. injections of 192-saporin. Dose-response studies indicate that behavioral deficits most consistently correlate with very extensive cell loss in the CBF. One study reported that passive avoidance deficits after i.c.v. 192-saporin were only evident in animals with >85% ChAT+ cell loss in the CBF, particularly the Nbm.[71] Others have reported water-maze deficits only at doses that produce maximal loss of cortical and/or hippocampal ChAT activity.[31,38,53] Dose-related radial maze deficits also have been reported.[54] Combining water maze and radial maze data, one can conclude that working memory tasks are impaired by 192-saporin lesions of the CBF. With use of various delays, the radial maze studies show a deficit in all internal delays that gets more severe at longer delays in rats injected with 192-saporin than in controls, suggesting deficits in both mnemonic and nonmnemonic processes.

Other behavioral findings with i.c.v. 192-saporin injections include:

- Less habituation of the startle reaction to acoustic stimuli than in controls.[31]
- Delayed nonmatch to position or sample tasks are impaired by high-grade CBF lesions made by i.c.v. injections of 192-saporin[54,72] with both delay-dependent and delay-independent deficits.
- Decreased acquisition, but relatively less impaired retention on an object-memory task.[73]

Restricted lesions of the Nbm bilaterally have been reported to produce either no effect[34,39,74] or

- Impaired acquisition of passive avoidance behavior,[34] which also was inferred to be related to the extent of Nbm lesion in animals injected i.c.v. with 192-saporin[71]
- Decreased water-maze acquisition and performance[33] in one study and no effect in another[34]
- Decreased behavioral vigilance as determined by decreased ability to detect the correct visual cues without a deficit in rejection of noncues[75]
- Decreased attention to an inconsistent conditioned stimulus (CS) in a classical conditioning paradigm, but also decreased development of latent inhibition by repeated presentation of the CS without the unconditioned stimulus (UCS)[76]
- Decreased nocturnal activity[34]
- No change in delayed alternation in a T-maze with partial Nbm lesions[39]

By comparison, restricted septal lesions have been reported to produce:

- No effect in the water maze[34] or mild impairment of initial acquisition without effect on asymptotic performance level[33]
- Impaired delayed nonmatch to position performance[34]
- Dose-related deficits in radial maze performance[54] with both delay-dependent and delay-independent components
- Decreased nocturnal activity[34]

Although still in the early stages, analysis of the behavioral effects of selective CBF lesions using 192-saporin has revealed several insights:

1. Incomplete lesions (<85% ablation) of the CBF are not reliably associated with behavioral deficits in the various tasks that have been examined (passive avoidance, water maze, radial maze, delayed nonmatch to position).
2. Deficits in several paradigms appear to have delay-dependent and delay-independent components suggesting both mnemonic and nonmnemonic dysfunction as a result of the lesions.
3. The most robust abnormalities are consistently seen with complete ablations of the CBF which until recently have required i.c.v. injections, but may be achievable with bilateral injections into the midportion of the diagonal band of Broca (unpublished data). Local injections that completely ablate the CBF would avoid possible confounding of the results by damage to cerebellar Purkinje neurons.

CONCLUSIONS

It is premature to conclude with assurance that CBF function is an obligatory component of memory formation. The hypothesis that the CBF mediates selective attention,[77-79] which may be a required precondition for formation of associations that later are stored in memory, remains a viable possibility on the basis of current behavioral data with 192-saporin. Indeed, the CBF may contribute to memory formation in more than one way, perhaps by providing necessary input to structures where association links are forged and memory traces stored while also modulating cortical responsiveness to sensory inputs. Thus, any behavioral deficits after CBF lesions might reflect the sum of effects on several different processes. Lesions of the CBF using local injections have not produced uniformly significant behavioral deficits; this may reflect that the CBF functions as a unitary entity with considerable redundancy or reserve capacity. Perhaps there is no strict localization of specific behavioral functions within the CBF. The sparing of cholinergic innervation to the amygdala with 192-saporin lesions leaves open questions about the role of this component of the CBF. Similarly, sparing of the midbrain cholinergic cell groups that project to the forebrain may explain some of the differences between the effects of 192-saporin lesions compared to systemic muscarinic antagonists. It is hoped that innovative behavioral studies with 192-saporin and development of additional immunolesioning tools, such as anti-DβH-saporin, which selectively destroys noradrenergic and adrenergic neurons,[80] will continue to advance the process of unraveling the functional neuroanatomy of behavior.

REFERENCES

1. COYLE, J. T., D. L. PRICE & M. R. DeLONG. 1983. Alzheimer's disease: A disorder of cortical cholinergic innervation. Science **219:** 1184–1190.
2. SHIOSAKA, S. 1992. Attempts to make models for Alzheimer's disease. Neurosci. Res. **13:** 237–255.
3. BALL, M. J. 1982. Alzheimer's disease: A challenging engima. Arch. Pathol. Lab. Med. **106:** 157–162.
4. JARRARD, L. E., A. LEVY, J. L. MEYERHOFF & G. J. KANT. 1985. Intracerebral injections of AF64A: An animal model of Alzheimer's disease? Ann. N. Y. Acad. Sci. **444:** 520–522.
5. SMITH, G. 1988. Animal models of Alzheimer's disease: Experimental cholinergic denervation. Brain Res. **472:** 103–118.
6. THAL, L. J., R. J. MANDEL, R. D. TERRY, G. BUZSAKI & F. H. GAGE. 1990. Nucleus basalis lesions fail to induce senile plaques in the rat. Exp. Neurol. **108:** 88–90.
7. WENK, G. L. 1990. Animal models of Alzheimer's disease: Are they valid and useful? Acta Neurobiol. Exp. (Warsz.) **50:** 219–223.
8. FISHER, A. & I. HANIN. 1986. Potential animal models for senile dementia of Alzheimer's type, with emphasis on AF64A-induced cholinotoxicity. Annu. Rev. Pharmacol. Toxicol. **26:** 161–181.
9. SARTER, M. 1987. Animal models of brain ageing and dementia. Compr. Gerontol. A **1:** 4–15.
10. PEPEU, G., I. M. PEPEU & F. CASAMENTI. 1990. The validity of animal models in the search for drugs for the aging brain. Drug Des. Deliv. **7:** 1–10.
11. WALSH, T. J. & J. J. CHROBAK. 1991. Animal models of Alzheimer's disease: Role of hippocampal cholinergic systems in working memory. *In* Brain, Emotion and Cognition. L. Dalhowski & C. F. Flaherty, Eds.: 347–378. Lawrence Erlbaum Associates. Hillsdale, NJ.
12. DUNNETT, S. B., I. G. WHISHAW, G. H. JONES & S. T. BUNCH. 1987. Behavioural, biochemical and histochemical effects of different neurotoxic amino acids injected into nucleus basalis magnocellularis of rats. Neuroscience **20:** 653–669.
13. FIBIGER, H. C. 1991. Cholinergic mechanisms in learning, memory and dementia: A review of recent evidence. Trends Neurosci. **14:** 220–223.
14. DUNNETT, S. B., B. J. EVERITT & T. W. ROBBINS. 1991. The basal forebrain-cortical cholinergic system: Interpreting the functional consequences of excitotoxic lesions. Trends Neurosci. **14:** 494–501.
15. DUNNETT, S. B. & H. C. FIBIGER. 1993. Role of forebrain cholinergic systems in learning and memory: Relevance to the cognitive deficits of aging and Alzheimer's dementia. Prog. Brain Res. **98:** 413–420.
16. FIBIGER, H. C. 1991. Cholinergic mechanisms in learning, memory and dementia: A review of recent evidence [see comments]. Trends Neurosci **14:** 220–223.
17. KOH, S. & G. A. HIGGINS. 1991. Differential regulation of the low-affinity nerve growth

factor receptor during postnatal development of the rat brain. J. Comp. Neurol. **313:** 494–508.

18. PIORO, E. P., A. RIBEIRO-DA-SILVA & A. C. CUELLO. 1991. Similarities in the ultrastructural distribution of nerve growth factor receptor-like immunoreactivity in cerebellar Purkinje cells of the neonatal and colchicine-treated adult rat. J. Comp. Neurol. **305:** 189–200.

19. CUELLO, A. C., E. P. PIORO & A. RIBEIRO-DA-SILVA. 1990. Cellular and subcellular localization of nerve growth factor receptor-like immunoreactivity in the rat CNS. Neurochem. Int. **17:** 205–213.

20. SCHWEITZER, J. B. 1987. Nerve growth factor receptor-mediated transport from cerebrospinal fluid to basal forebrain neurons. Brain Res. **423:** 309–317.

21. SCHWEITZER, J. B. 1989. Nerve growth factor receptor-mediated transport from CSF labels cholinergic neurons: Direct demonstration by a double-labeling study. Brain Res. **490:** 390–396.

22. WILEY, R. G., T. N. OELTMANN & D. A. LAPPI. 1991. Immunolesioning: Selective destruction of neurons using immunotoxin to rat NGF receptor. Brain Res. **562:** 149–153.

23. CHANDLER, C. E., L. M. PARSONS, M. HOSANG & E. M. SHOOTER. 1984. A monoclonal antibody modulates the interaction of nerve growth factor with PC12 cells. J. Biol. Chem. **259:** 6882–6889.

24. STIRPE, F., A. CASPERI-CAMPANI, L. BARBIERI, A. FALASCA, A. ABBONDANZA & W. A. STEVENS. 1983. Ribosome-inactivating proteins from the seeds of *Saponaria officinalis* L. (soapwort) of *Agrostemma githago* L. (corn cockle) and of *Asparagus officinalis* (asparagus) and from the latex of *Hura crepitans* L. (sandbox tree). Biochem. J. **216:** 617–625.

25. DISTEFANO, P. S., J. B. SCHWEITZER, M. TANIUCHI & E. M. JOHNSON, JR. 1985. Selective destruction of nerve growth factor receptor-bearing cells in vitro using a hybrid toxin composed of ricin A chain and a monoclonal antibody against the nerve growth factor receptor. J. Cell Biol. **101:** 1107–1114.

26. THORPE, P. E., A. N. F. BROWN, J. A. G. BREMMER, B. M. J. FOXWELL & F. STIRPE. 1985. An immunotoxin composed of monoclonal anti-Thy 1.1 antibody and a ribosome-inactivating protein from Saponaria officinalis: Potent antitumor effects in vitro and in vivo. J. Natl. Cancer Inst. **75:** 151–159.

27. WILEY, R. G., F. STIRPE, P. THORPE & T. N. OELTMANN. 1989. Neuronotoxic effects of monoclonal anti-Thy 1 antibody (OX7) coupled to the ribosome inactivating protein, saporin, as studied by suicide transport experiments in the rat. Brain Res. **505:** 44–54.

28. WILEY, R. G. 1992. Neural lesioning with ribosome-inactivating proteins: Suicide transport and immunolesioning. Trends Neurosci. **15:** 285–290.

29. WILEY, R. G. & D. A. LAPPI. 1994. Suicide Transport and Immunolesioning. R. G. Landes Medical Publishers, Austin, TX.

30. GALLAGHER, M. & P. J. COLOMBO. 1995. Ageing: The cholinergic hypothesis of cognitive decline. Curr. Opin. Neurobiol. **5:** 161–168.

31. WAITE, J. J., A. D. CHEN, M. L. WARDLOW, R. G. WILEY, D. A. LAPPI & L. J. THAL. 1995. 192 immunoglobulin G-saporin produces graded behavioral and biochemical changes accompanying the loss of cholinergic neurons of the basal forebrain and cerebellar Purkinje cells. Neuroscience **65:** 463–476.

32. HECKERS, S., T. OHTAKE, R. G. WILEY, D. A. LAPPI, C. GEULA & M. M. MESULAM. 1994. Complete and selective cholinergic denervation of rat neocortex and hippocampus but not amygdala by an immunotoxin against the p75 NGF receptor. J. Neurosci. **14:** 1271–1289.

33. BERGER-SWEENEY, J., S. HECKERS, M. M. MESULAM, R. G. WILEY, D. A. LAPPI & M. SHARMA. 1994. Differential effects on spatial navigation of immunotoxin-induced cholinergic lesions of the medial septal area and nucleus basalis magnocellularis. J. Neurosci. **14:** 4507–4519.

34. TORRES, E. M., T. A. PERRY, A. BLOKLAND, L. S. WILKINSON, R. G. WILEY, D. A. LAPPI & S. B. DUNNETT. 1994. Behavioural, histochemical and biochemical consequences of

selective immunolesions in discrete regions of the basal forebrain cholinergic system. Neuroscience **63:** 95–122.

35. ROSSNER, S., W. HÄRTIG, R. SCHLIEBS, G. BRÜCKNER, K. BRAUER, J. R. PEREZ-POLO, R. G. WILEY & M. BIGL. 1995. 192 IgG-saporin immunotoxin-induced loss of cholinergic cells differentially activates microglia in rat basal forebrain nuclei. J. Neurosci. Res. **41:** 335–346.

36. LEANZA, G., O. G. NILSSON, G. NIKKHAH, R. G. WILEY & A. BJORKLUND. 1996. Effects of neonatal lesions of the basal forebrain cholinergic system by 192 IgG-saporin: Biochemical, behavioural and morphological characterization. Neuroscience **74:** 119–141.

37. ROSNER, S., W. HARTIG, R. SCHLIEBS, G. BRUCKNER, K. BRAUER, J. R. PEREZ-POLO, R. G. WILEY & V. BIGL. 1995. 192 IgG-saporin immunotoxin-induced loss of cholinergic cells differentially activates microglia in rat basal forebrain nuclei. J. Neurosci. Res. **41:** 335–346.

38. LEANZA, G., O. G. NILSSON, R. G. WILEY & A. BJÖRKLUND. 1995. Selective lesioning of the basal forebrain cholinergic system by intraventricular 192 IgG-saporin: Behavioural, biochemical and stereological studies in the rat. Eur. J. Neurosci. **7:** 329–343.

39. WENK, G. L., J. D. STOEHR, G. QUINTANA, S. MOBLEY & R. G. WILEY. 1994. Behavioral, biochemical, histological, and electrophysiological effects of 192 IgG-saporin injections into the basal forebrain of rats. J. Neurosci. **14:** 5986–5995.

40. STOEHR, J. D., S. L. MOBLEY, D. ROICE, R. BROOKS, L. M. BAKER, R. G. WILEY & G. L. WENK. 1997. The effects of selective cholinergic basal forebrain lesions and aging upon expectancy in the rat. Neurobiol. Learn. Mem. **67:** 214–227.

41. WILEY, R. G., T. G. BERBOS, T. DECKWERTH, E. M. JOHNSON, JR. & D. A. LAPPI. 1995. Destruction of the cholinergic basal forebrain using immunotoxin to rat NGF receptor: Modeling the cholinergic degeneration of Alzheimer's disease. J. Neurol. Sci. **128:** 157–166.

42. HECKERS, S. & M.-M. MESULAM. 1994. Two types of cholinergic projections to the rat amygdala. Neuroscience **60:** 383–397.

43. BOOK, A. A., R. G. WILEY & J. B. SCHWEITZER. 1994. 192 IgG-saporin. I. Specific lethality for cholinergic neurons in the basal forebrain of the rat. J. Neuropathol. Exp. Neurol. **53:** 95–102.

44. SINGH, V. & J. B. SCHWEITZER. 1995. Loss of p75 nerve growth factor receptor mRNA containing neurons in rat forebrain after intraventricular IgG 192-saporin administration. Neurosci. Lett. **194:** 117–120.

45. BOOK, A. A., R. G. WILEY & J. B. SCHWEITZER. 1995. 192 IgG-saporin. 2. Neuropathology in the rat brain. Acta Neuropathol. (Berl.) **89:** 519–526.

46. HOLLEY, L. A., R. G. WILEY, D. A. LAPPI & M. SARTER. 1994. Cortical cholinergic deafferentiation following the intracortical infusion of 192 IgG-saporin: A quantitative histochemical study. Brain Res. **663:** 277–286.

47. HERRON, P., L. ZHANG, Z. C. LI & J. B. SCHWEITZER. 1996. Effects of cholinergic depletion on GAD immunoreactivity in rat PMBSF cortex. Soc. Neurosci. Abstr. **22:** 1358 (Abstr.).

48. YU, J., R. G. WILEY & R. J. PEREZ-POLO. 1996. Altered NGF protein levels in different brain areas after immunolesion. J. Neurosci. Res. **43:** 213–223.

49. WAITE, J. J., M. L. WARDLOW, A. C. CHEN, D. A. LAPPI, R. G. WILEY & L. J. THAL. 1994. Time course of cholinergic and monoaminergic changes in rat brain after immunolesioning with 192 IgG-saporin. Neurosci. Lett. **169:** 154–158.

50. PAPPAS, B. A., C. M. DAVIDSON, T. FORTIN, S. NALLATHAMBY, G. A. S. PARK & R. G. WILEY. 1996. 192 IgG-saporin lesion of the forebrain cholinergic neurons in neonatal rats. Dev. Brain Res. **96:** 52–61.

51. HÄGE, B., M. FROTSCHER & T. NAUMANN. 1996. Activity of choline acetyltransferase in the rat medial septal nucleus following fimbria-fornix transection or selective immunolesioning with 192 IgG-saporin. Neurosci. Lett. **205:** 119–122.

52. ROSSNER, S., R. SCHLIEBS, J. R. PEREZ-POLO, R. G. WILEY & V. BIGL. 1995. Differential changes in cholinergic markers from selected brain regions after specific immunolesion of the rat cholinergic basal forebrain system. J. Neurosci. Res. **40:** 31–43.

53. WALSH, T. J., R. M. KELLY, K. D. DOUGHERTY, R. W. STACKMAN, R. G. WILEY & C. L. KUTSCHER. 1995. Behavioral and neurobiological alterations induced by the immunotoxin 192-IgG-saporin: Cholinergic and non-cholinergic effects following icv injection. Brain Res. **702:** 233–245.
54. WALSH, T. J., C. D. HERZOG, C. GANDHI, R. W. STACKMAN & R. G. WILEY. 1996. Injection of IgG 192-saporin into the medial septum produces cholinergic hypofunction and dose-dependent working memory deficits. Brain Res. **726:** 69–79.
55. ROSSNER, S., J. YU, D. PIZZO, K. WERRBACH-PEREZ, R. SCHLIEBS, V. BIGL & J. R. PEREZ-POLO. 1996. Effects of intraventricular transplantation of NGF-secreting cells on cholinergic basal forebrain neurons after partial immunolesion. J. Neurosci. Res. **45:** 40–56.
56. LEVEY, A. I., S. M. EDMUNDS, S. M. HERSCH, R. G. WILEY & C. J. HEILMAN. 1995. Light and electron microscopic study of m2 muscarinic acetylcholine receptor in the basal forebrain of the rat. J. Comp. Neurol. **351:** 339–356.
57. LEVEY, A. I., S. M. EDMUNDS, V. KOLIATSOS, R. G. WILEY & C. J. HEILMAN. 1995. Expression of m1–m4 muscarinic acetylcholine receptor proteins in rat hippocampus and regulation by cholinergic innervation. J. Neurosci. **15:** 4077–4092.
58. ROSNER, S., J. R. PEREZ-POLO, R. G. WILEY, R. SCHLIEBS & V. BIGL. 1995. Differential expression of immediate early genes in distinct layers of rat cerebral cortex after selective immunolesion of the forebrain cholinergic system. J. Neurosci. Res. **40:** 31–43.
59. KOKAIA, M., I. FERENCZ, G. LEANZA, E. ELMÉR, M. METSIS, Z. KOKAIA, R. G. WILEY & O. LINDVALL. 1996. Immunolesioning of basal forebrain cholinergic neurons facilitates hippocampal kindling and perturbs neurotrophin messenger RNA regulation. Neuroscience **70:** 313–327.
60. KAPÁS, L., F. OBÁL, JR., A. A. BOOK, J. B. SCHWEITZER, R. G. WILEY & J. M. KRUEGER. 1996. The effects of immunolesions of nerve growth factor-receptive neurons by 192 IgG-saporin on sleep. Brain Res. **712:** 53–59.
61. LEE, M. G., J. J. CHROBAK, A. SIK, R. G. WILEY & G. BUZSÁKI. 1994. Hippocampal theta activity following selective lesion of the septal cholinergic system. Neuroscience **62:** 1033–1047.
62. BASSANT, M. H., E. APARTIS, F. R. JAZAT-POINDESSOUS, R. G. WILEY & Y. A. LAMOUR. 1995. Selective immunolesion of the basal forebrain cholinergic neurons: Effects on hippocampal activity during sleep and wakefulness in the rat. Neurodegeneration **4:** 61–70.
63. JOUVENCEAU, A., J. M. BILLARD, Y. LAMOUR & P. DUTAR. 1996. Persistence of CA1 hippocampal LTP after selective cholinergic denervation. Neuroreport **7:** 948–952.
64. JOUVENCEAU, A., J.-M. BILLARD, R. G. WILEY, Y. LAMOUR & P. DUTAR. 1994. Cholinergic denervation of the rat hippocampus by 192-IgG-saporin: Electrophysiological evidence. Neuroreport **5:** 1781–1784.
65. STOEHR, J. D., S. I. HECK, R. G. WILEY & G. L. WENK. 1997. The role of basal forebrain cholinergic cells in cortical event-related slow potentials: Effects of selective lesions and aging. Brain Res. In press.
66. SACHDEV, R., S.-M. LU, R. G. WILEY & F. F. EBNER. 1995. Effects of acetylcholine depletion in the rat barrel cortex. Soc. Neurosci. Abstr. **21:** 123 (Abstr.).
67. BASKERVILLE, K. A., N. R. HEASTON, J. B. SCHWEITZER & P. HERRON. 1995. Role of acetylcholine in experience-dependent plasticity in the somatosensory cortex of the rat. Soc. Neurosci. Abstr. **21:** 123 (Abstr.).
68. LI, Z. C., J. B. SCHWEITZER, L. ZHANG & P. HERRON. 1996. Effects of cholinergic depletion on the cortical functions in Fisher hybrid rats. Soc. Neurosci. Abstr. **22:** 158 (Abstr.).
69. SACHDEV, R. N. S., M. STONECYPHER, M. EGLI, R. G. WILEY, S.-M. LU & F. F. EBNER. 1996. Gap crossing training enhances whisker pairing bias in acetylcholine depleted rats. Soc. Neurosci. Abstr. **22:** 1357 (Abstr.).
70. NILSSON, O. G., G. LEANZA, C. ROSENBLAD, D. A. LAPPI, R. G. WILEY & A. BJORKLUND. 1992. Spatial learning impairments in rats with selective immunolesion of the forebrain cholinergic system. Neuroreport **3:** 1005–1008.

71. Zhang, Z. J., T. G. Berbos, C. C. Wrenn & R. G. Wiley. 1996. Loss of nucleus basalis manocellularis, but not septal, cholinergic neurons correlates with passive avoidance impairment in rats treated with 192-saporin. Neurosci. Lett. **203:** 214–218.
72. Steckler, T., A. B. Keith, R. G. Wiley & A. Sahgal. 1995. Cholinergic lesions by 192 IgG-saporin and short-term recognition memory: Role of the septohippocampal projection. Neuroscience **66:** 101–114.
73. Vnek, N., L. F. Kromer, R. G. Wiley & L. A. Rothblat. 1997. The basal forebrain cholinergic system and object memory in the rat. Behav. Brain Res. In press.
74. Baxter, M. G., D. J. Bucci, L. K. Gorman, R. G. Wiley & M. Gallagher. 1995. Selective immunotoxic lesions of basal forebrain cholinergic cells: Effects on learning and memory in rats. Behav. Neurosci. **109:** 714–722.
75. McGaughy, J., T. Kaiser & M. Sarter. 1996. Behavioral vigilance following infusions of 192 IgG-saporin into the basal forebrain: Selectivity of the behavioral impairment and relation to cortical AChE-positive fiber density. Behav. Neurosci. **110:** 247–265.
76. Chiba, A. A., D. J. Bucci, P. C. Holland & M. Gallagher. 1995. Basal forebrain cholinergic lesions disrupt increments but not decrements in conditioned stimulus processing. J. Neurosci. **15:** 7315–7322.
77. Stone, E. A. & Y. Zhang. 1995. Adrenoreceptor antagonists block c-fos response to stress in the mouse brain. Brain Res. **694:** 279–286.
78. Inglis, F. M., J. C. Day & H. C. Fibiger. 1994. Enhanced acetylcholine release in hippocampus and cortex during the anticipation and consumption of a palatable meal. Neuroscience **62:** 1049–1056.
79. Acquas, E., C. Wilson & H. C. Fibiger. 1996. Conditioned and unconditioned stimuli increase frontal cortical and hippocampal acetylcholine release: Effects of novelty, habituation, and fear. J. Neurosci. **16:** 3089–3096.
80. Wrenn, C. C., M. J. Picklo, D. A. Lappi, D. Robertson & R. G. Wiley. 1996. Central noradrenergic lesioning using anti-DBH-saporin: Anatomical findings. Brain Res. **740:** 175–186.

Neural Precursors and Neuronal Production in the Adult Mammalian Forebrain[a]

STEVEN A. GOLDMAN,[b,i] MAIKEN NEDERGAARD,[c]
RONALD G. CRYSTAL,[d] RICHARD A. R. FRASER,[e]
ROBERT GOODMAN,[f]
CATHERINE HARRISON-RESTELLI,[b] JINWEN JIANG,[b]
H. MICHAEL KEYOUNG,[b,g] CAROLINE LEVENTHAL,[b,g]
DAVID W. PINCUS,[b,f] ABRAHAM SHAHAR,[b,h]
AND SU WANG[b]

*[b]Departments of Neurology and Neuroscience, and
Medicine[d] and Surgery (Neurosurgery)[e]
Cornell University Medical College
New York, New York 10021*

*[c]Departments of Cell Biology and Neurosurgery
New York Medical College
Valhalla, New York 10590*

*[f]Department of Neurosurgery
Columbia-Presbyterian Medical Center
New York, New York 10029*

*[g]Aitken Neuroscience Center
New York, New York 10021*

*[h]Department of Virology
Israel Biological Institute
Nes-Ziona, Israel*

The damaged brain is largely incapable of structural self-repair, in part because of the failure of the mature brain to generate new neurons. Yet the absence of neuronal production in the adult forebrain appears to reflect not a lack of appropriate neuronal precursor cells, but rather their tonic inhibition and/or lack of postmitotic trophic and migratory support: Recent studies have indicated that neuronal precursor cells are distributed widely throughout the ventricular subependymal zone (SZ), which includes the ependymal and subependymal layer of the adult vertebrate forebrain. These cells continue to produce neurons in some species, but even then only in selected regions, and appear more generally to become vestigial. Thus, adult precursors appear to be more ubiquitous than the limited occurrence of adult

[a] Work in the Goldman laboratory was supported by grants from the National Institute of Neurological Disorders and Stroke (R01NS33106 and R01NS29813), and by the Mathers Charitable Foundation, Lookout Foundation, Hirschl/Weill-Caulier Trust, Aitken Charitable Trust, American Paralysis Association, and the National Multiple Sclerosis Society.
[i] Address correspondence to Steven Goldman, M.D., Ph.D., Dept. of Neurology and Neuroscience, Cornell University Medical College, New York, NY 10021.

neurogenesis might indicate. This suggested that neurogenesis might be restricted by the loss of permissive signals for daughter cell survival in the adult brain. In this report, we review the evidence for persistent neuronal progenitors in the postnatal mammalian brain, in particular that of the adult human. We will focus on strategies for inducing neuronal production from these cells *in vivo*, as well as on methods for isolating and enriching defined populations of progenitor cells for both transplantation and experimental study.

ADULT NEUROGENESIS IN NON-MAMMALIAN VERTEBRATES

For almost two decades, it has been clear that both bony and cartilaginous fish, as well as amphibia and lizards, possess the capacity during adulthood to form new nerve cells in response to both growth and injury (reviewed previously in ref. 1). With Fernando Nottebohm, we reported a similar process of adult neurogenesis in adult passerine songbirds,[2] a group of birds previously reported to exhibit seasonal, gonadal steroid-dependent central neuroplasticity in parallel with the development of song.[3] While examining the basis for this androgen-associated regional hypertrophy of the principal vocal control center (HVC), we found that new neurons, as well as glia and endothelial cells, could be recruited to the HVC of adult canaries.[2] This process of ongoing neuronal addition to an adult neostriatal nucleus was as robust as it was then novel, and prompted a decade of intensive study thereafter. We and others found that songbirds generated new nerve cells from precursor cells within the ventricular zone abutting the neostriatal wall, and did so in both a seasonally regulated and hormone-dependent manner. The new neurons migrated not only into HVC, but also more widely into the neostriatal parenchyma, along radial guide fibers (reviewed in refs. 1, 4–6).

The production of neurons from these precursors could be supported in cultured explants of the adult songbird SZ,[7] a preparation which allowed the early events in adult neurogenesis to be examined in greater detail.[8-10] Retroviral introduction of the *lacZ* gene first demonstrated that single precursor cells co-generated neurons and radial guide cells together.[11] Combined [^{3}H]thymidine autoradiography and immunolocalization of the early neuronal RNA-binding protein Hu then revealed that the newly generated neuronal daughter cells departed the SZ to enter the brain parenchyma only after a week or so of postmitotic development,[12] at which point they down-regulated expression of the surface adhesion molecule N-cadherin.[13] The new neurons then up-regulated expression of another cell adhesion molecule, NgCAM, the blockade of which abrogated migration. NgCAM was then found to transduce an NgCAM-dependent calcium response in the migrating neuron, the elicitation of which was necessary for both neuronal migration and survival during migration.[14] The postmitotic survival of these new neurons was enhanced by gonadal steroids, which acted upon a layer of subventricular, estrogen-receptive neurons traversed by the new neurons immediately after their initial departure from the SZ.[15] Among other actions, estrogen was found to be required for development of NgCAM-dependent calcium signaling by the new neuronal migrants, and was associated with a decrease in the incidence and rate of apoptosis within the newly generated neuronal population.[16] Besides the gonadal steroids, several neurotrophic agents were found to be critical for the differentiation and outgrowth of new neurons from the adult SZ: In particular, insulin-like growth factor (IGF-1) was found to support the outgrowth of new neurons from explants of the adult SZ; in addition, IGF-1 was associated with the very radial guide cells upon which the new neurons migrated.[17]

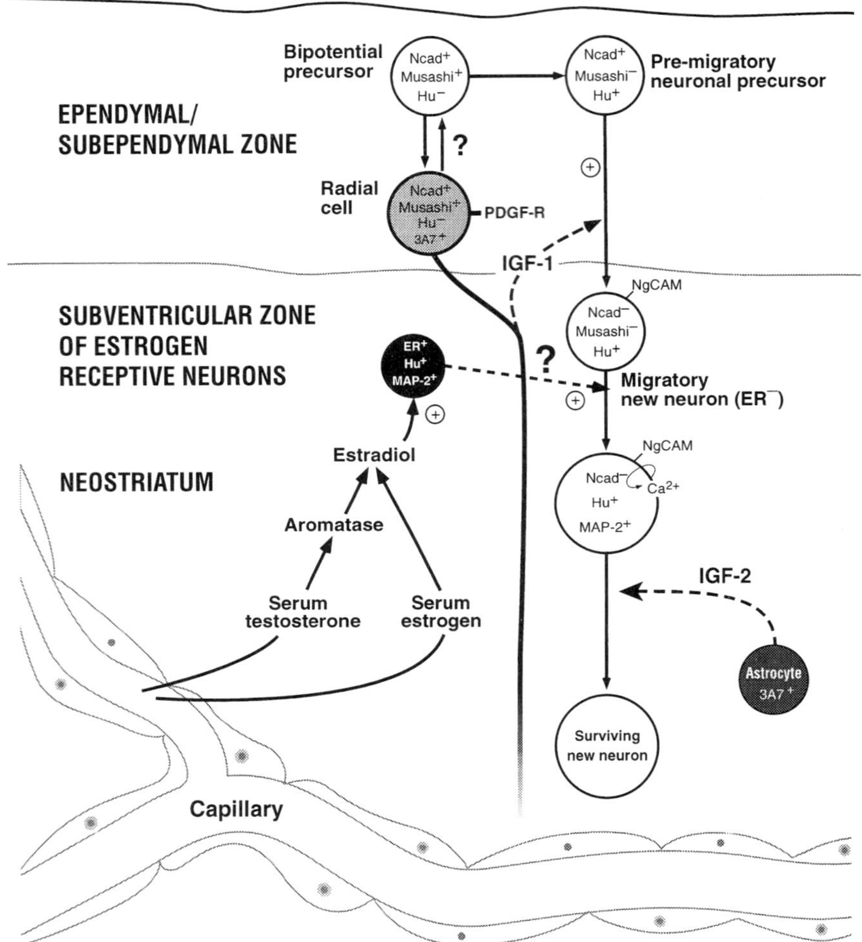

FIGURE 1. Neuronal migration into the adult songbird neostriatum. This schematic summarizes much of what is known about neuronal recruitment into the avian forebrain (*see text*). *Abbreviations*: 3A7, a vimentin-associated filament recognized by mAb 3A7;[10,63] ER, estrogen receptor; musashi, an RNA-binding protein expressed by neural progenitors;[64] IGF-1 and IGF-2, insulin-like growth factors 1 and 2; MAP-2, microtubule-associated protein-2; Ncad, N-cadherin; NgCAM, neuro-glial cell adhesion molecule.

These events have been reviewed elsewhere[1,4,18] and will not be further discussed here. Their salient message is that a number of humoral agents and contact-mediated events, presented in a closely timed and interdependent sequence, are associated with the recruitment of new neurons into the adult avian neostriatum (see FIG. 1). The complex interaction of these events in the songbird brain provided us a model of what might be needed to reconstitute functional neurogenesis in the adult mammalian brain, and in doing so provided a conceptual basis for subsequent studies of neuronal precursor cells and neurogenesis in the adult mammalian brain.

NEUROGENESIS IN THE ADULT MAMMALIAN BRAIN

In contrast to the widespread nature of neurogenesis in the adult avian brain, the adult mammalian forebrain generates new neurons in only a few regions, including the hippocampal dentate gyrus and olfactory bulb.[19-21] These sites differ substantially from one another, in that although dentate granule neurons appear to divide *in situ*, rodent olfactory bulb neurons are long-distance migrants from the forebrain SZ.[22] Neurogenesis in the olfactory bulb is in some respects similar to that of the avian brain—both comprise the SZ-based production of new neurons, followed by their parenchymal migration and target recruitment. *In vivo*, the principal neurogenic segment of the adult rodent SZ is the rostral 1 mm giving rise to neurons destined for the olfactory bulb;[22-24] however, mitosis within the SZ persists throughout the adult rodent's lateral ventricular lining.[25] In the adult mouse forebrain, some of the progeny of these dividing SZ cells may die shortly after their genesis, never initiating migration or differentiation.[26] Yet once removed in culture, the adult murine SZ, like its avian counterpart, generates a MAP-2$^+$ neuronal outgrowth.[27,28] Together, these results suggested that the dying daughter cells of the adult SZ might be committed to neuronal phenotype, but die before leaving the SZ. If so, one might predict that neuronal daughter cells could be rescued with the provision of appropriate postmitotic support, whether in the form of a permissive migratory path or cognate humoral neurotrophins.

Neuronal Precursor Cells Persist in the Adult Mammalian Forebrain

Neural precursor cells may be found in the adult mammalian brain, just as in birds. Reynolds and Weiss[29] reported the existence of precursor cells in the adult rodent striatum, which proliferated under the influence of epidermal growth factor (EGF), and which generated neurons upon differentiation. These precursors were exquisitely sensitive to both ambient serum and the presence of any adhesion-competent substrate, and as a result were propagated in suspension. Although all major cell types could be generated from these precursor cells, it remains unclear whether new neurons, astrocytes, and oligodendrocytes arise from a common stem cell in this preparation, or from distinct, lineage-restricted progenitor lines. Richards *et al.* similarly demonstrated the production of neurons from dissociated adult rat forebrain, with precursor division in basic fibroblast growth factor (FGF2) and astrocyte-conditioned media.[30] Other workers have reported that adult neural progenitors, like their embryonic counterparts,[31,32] divide in response to FGF2.[33,34]

Neuronal Precursor Cells of the Adult Forebrain Reside in the SZ

The SZ restriction of neuronal precursors in the songbird brain[7-9] suggested that the neural precursors of the adult rodent brain might be similarly restricted to the SZ. Lois and Alvarez-Buylla[27] examined this issue in mice, and found that although explants of adult neostriatal SZ generated neuronal outgrowth *in vitro*, neocortical explants did not. These SZ-derived neurons could be prelabeled with

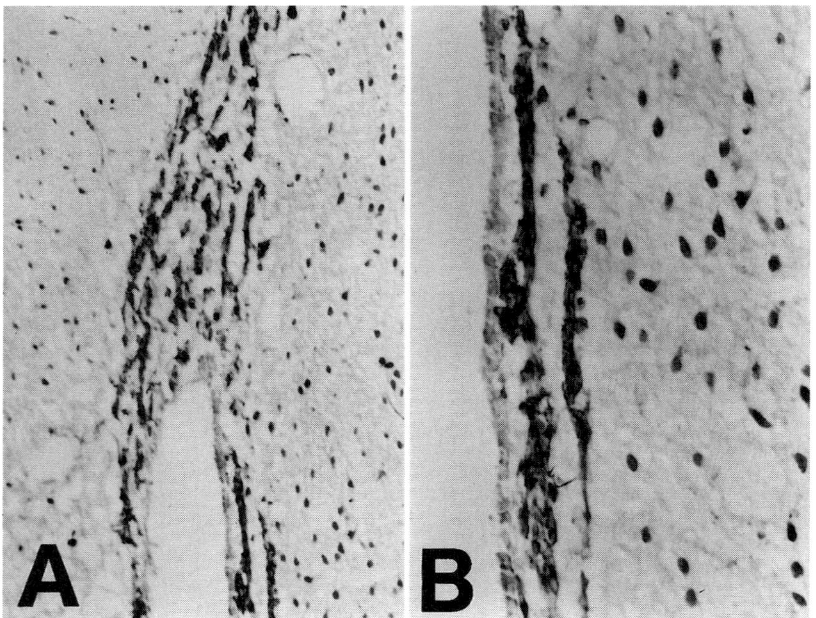

FIGURE 2. Hu expression identifies newly specified neurons in the adult rat SZ. These photomicrographs show coronal views of the anterolateral horn of the lateral ventricle of an adult rat, stained for Hu protein with monoclonal antibody 16A11.[12,56,65–67] **(A)** Abundant Hu+, presumably neuronally specified cells, are apparent in the SZ. **(B)** Chains of Hu+ SZ cells arrayed in their typical linear configuration; [3H]thymidine radiography with serial sacrifice confirmed that these cells were migratory to the olfactory bulb.

[3H]thymidine in the days before sacrifice, indicating that they arose from progenitors that were actively cycling *in vivo*. Morshead *et al.*[35] similarly reported that EGF-expandable neural precursors were limited to the striatal SZ. We also found that the adult rat SZ generated neuronal outgrowth *in vitro*, whereas subcortical and cortical explants failed to do so.[28] Importantly, explants derived from a wide expanse of the rat ventricular epithelium, spanning roughly its anterior two-thirds, generated neuronal outgrowth in culture. This region included, but was not limited to, the area of the SZ that gives rise to olfactory bulb neurons in adulthood.

In vivo, neuronally specified cells were mapped using antibodies against the early neuronal determinants βIII tubulin and Hu, and were found distributed widely throughout the lateral ventricular wall of postnatal mice,[36,37] rats,[4] and humans[38] (FIG. 2). In addition, less-committed neural precursors have been identified in cultures of the SZ taken throughout the neuraxis.[39] Thus, neuronal progenitor cells appear to be distributed over the adult ventricular system to a far greater extent than the limited occurrence of actual neurogenesis would suggest.

BDNF Supports the Survival of Neurons Arising from the Adult Rat SZ

These studies suggested the persistence into adulthood of a relatively widespread SZ progenitor cell population which, although neurogenic in selected regions, more generally became vestigial. On that basis, we reasoned that in those areas which do not exhibit neurogenesis, its absence might in part reflect a lack of postmitotic trophic support. We therefore sought to identify humoral agents capable of promoting the survival of neurons generated from adult precursors. To this end, we examined members of the neurotrophin family, including NGF, BDNF, NT-3, and NT-4/5. These agents promote the survival of postmitotic neurons in a variety of systems (reviewed in refs. 40 and 41). Among them, however, only BDNF is expressed to a significant extent in adult cortex;[42] we therefore asked whether BDNF might affect the differentiation or survival of new neurons in the adult rat brain. We did so by comparing neuronal outgrowth in BDNF-treated to untreated SZ explants, as well as to plates treated with NGF or NT-3. BDNF, alone among the neurotrophins, enhanced both the number of neurons arising from adult SZ explants and the survival of these neurons—almost twice as many neurons arose from explants treated with 40 ng/mL BDNF as from unsupplemented controls. BDNF then promoted the survival of these new neurons, rescuing over one-third from otherwise predictable death by 3 weeks *in vitro*.[28] Notably, BDNF exerted its survival effect on neurons arising throughout the entire expanse of the adult SZ (FIG. 3).

BDNF Acts to Support Neuronal Differentiation, Maturation, and Survival, but Does Not Influence Neuronal Phenotype Specification

To better understand the role of BDNF in supporting adult neurogenesis, we asked the following: (1) Does BDNF act to influence the commitment to neuronal phenotype of SZ daughter cells, or are BDNF's actions limited to the support of neuronal maturation and survival; (2) is the neuronal requirement for BDNF transient during maturation or continuous thereafter; and (3) is another *trkB* ligand, NT-4, also capable of supporting the production of neurons by the adult rat SZ? By comparing neuronal outgrowth and survival from explants of the adult rat SZ exposed to either BDNF, NT4, or BDNF and NT4 together, to that of untreated controls, we found that BDNF and NT4 both prolonged the outgrowth and enhanced the survival of new neurons. Neither, however, promoted neuronal specification or phenotypic commitment: BDNF withdrawal precipitated rapid neuronal death relative to controls, as did the addition of its antagonist trkB-Fc. Furthermore, the initial rate of neuronal outgrowth was identical in BDNF-treated cultures and untreated controls, and for the first week *in vitro*, neither differed from cultures treated from the outset with trkB-Fc. Delayed addition of BDNF was as effective in maintaining neuronal survival as was early exposure, through the eighth day *in vitro*[4,43] (also, Goldman, Kirschenbaum, and Restelli, manuscript submitted). Thus, BDNF acted as a survival factor for adult SZ-derived neurons, but did not influence neuronal specification. As such, BDNF enhanced neuronal numbers selectively rather than instructively.

Neuronal Progenitors Persist in the Senescent SZ

We asked next whether either the (1) spatial distribution, (2) abundance, or (3) BDNF responsiveness of the neuronal precursor population was affected by age. SZ explants were taken from both 4- and 20-month old rats, from segments sampled across the rostrocaudal extent of the ventricular surface. Explants from each region were taken from young and old rats and were cultured in media with or without added BDNF (20 ng/mL). The extent of neuronal production by these

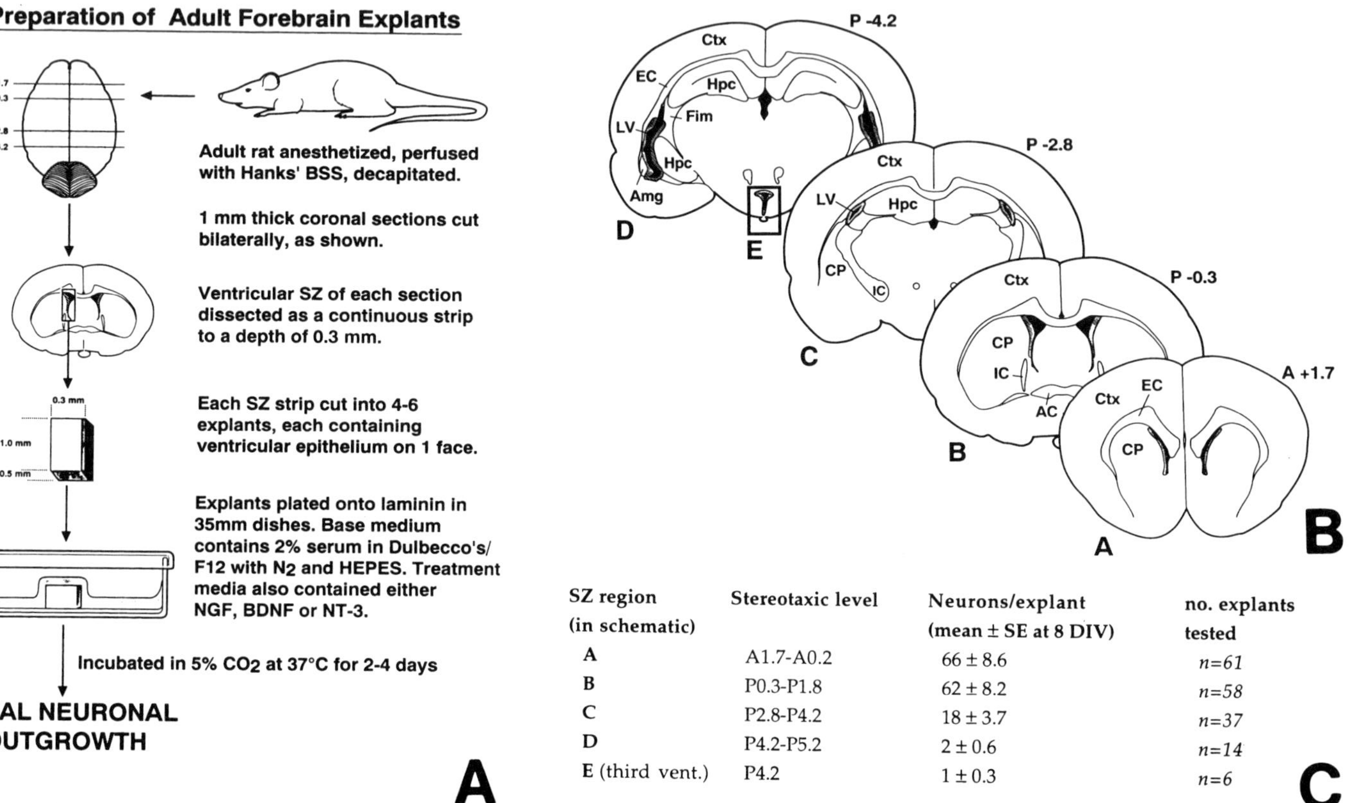

SZ region (in schematic)	Stereotaxic level	Neurons/explant (mean ± SE at 8 DIV)	no. explants tested
A	A1.7-A0.2	66 ± 8.6	n=61
B	P0.3-P1.8	62 ± 8.2	n=58
C	P2.8-P4.2	18 ± 3.7	n=37
D	P4.2-P5.2	2 ± 0.6	n=14
E (third vent.)	P4.2	1 ± 0.3	n=6

C

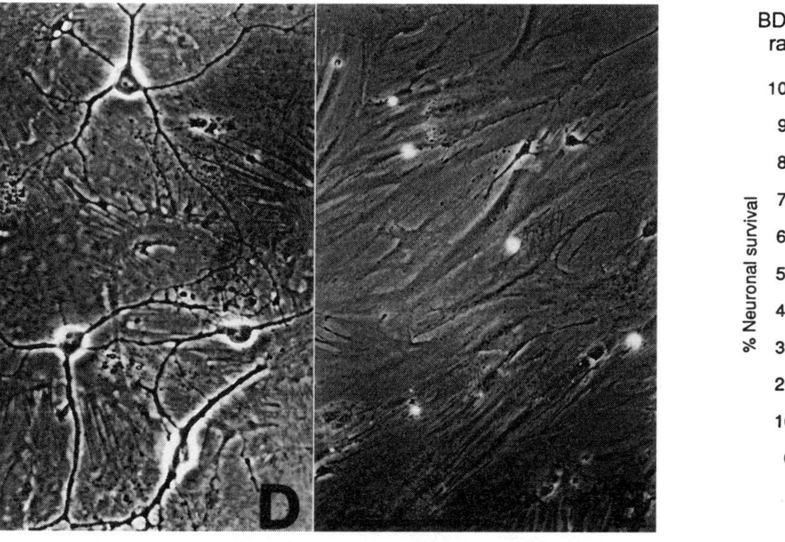

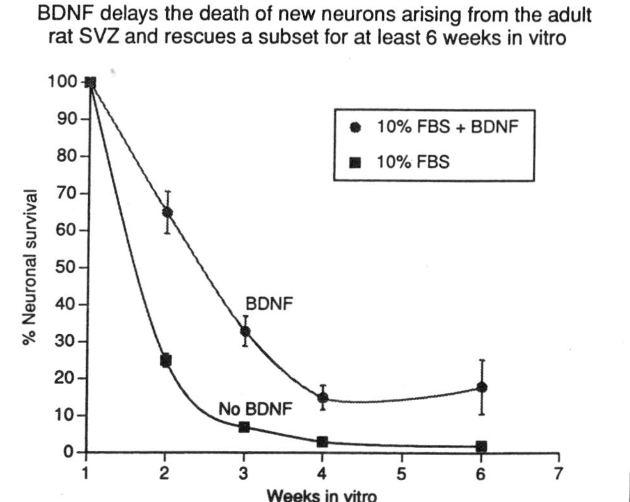

FIGURE 3. In the adult rat forebrain, a wide area of the subependymal zone (SZ) harbors neuronal precursor cells, which produce BDNF-responsive neurons *in vitro*. (**A**) The basic methodology for preparing these adult SZ explant cultures is outlined. (**B**) When explants were sampled from five regions of the adult rat SZ, significant neuronal outgrowth was observed from roughly the rostral two-thirds of the lateral ventricular system. (**C**) The extent of neuronal outgrowth as a function of the level of derivation of each sample is tabulated. In (**D**) and (**E**), BDNF supported the survival of new neurons. From 11 DIV onwards, BDNF-supplemented cultures enjoyed greater neuronal survival than their controls. Shown in **D** are typical healthy, interconnected neurons in a BDNF-supplemented SZ explant outgrowth at 36 DIV; displayed in **E** is a sister culture raised without added BDNF, in which no neurons survived to 21 DIV. In (**F**) neuronal survival is compared in cultures exposed to BDNF (20 ng/mL), relative to their unsupplemented controls. The graph plots the percentage of neuronal survival (relative to the maximal neuronal outgrowth for each group), as a function of the number of weeks *in vitro*. BDNF-treated neurons experienced a significant prolongation of their survival, and a fraction (roughly one-quarter of the population) remained viable for at least six weeks *in vitro*, having been rescued from otherwise likely death by the end of the second week in culture. Scale = 25 μm.

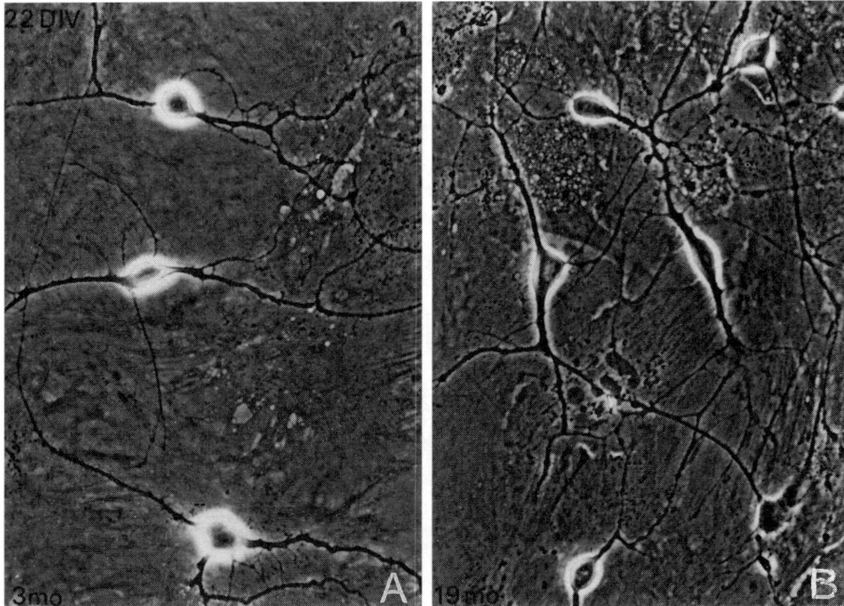

FIGURE 4. Neuronal progenitors persist in the senescent forebrain. SZ explants derived from both young and old rats generated substantial neuronal outgrowth. These phase micrographs show neurons arising from the SZ of young and elderly rats. Neurons are recognizable by their ovoid somata, phase birefringence, and typical bi- and tripolar morphologies with a few non-tapering primary neurites arborizing into extensive fiber networks. (**A**) Neuronal outgrowth from an SZ explant taken from a 3-month-old rat, 22 DIV. (**B**) The corresponding outgrowth from a 19-month-old rat forebrain SZ, after 19 DIV. Scale = 25 μm.

explants varied with their level of derivation; although the most anterior samples exhibited the most neuronal outgrowth, some was observed at every level. The extent of neuronal outgrowth was moderately attenuated with age, with the senescent SZ exhibiting >60% of the neuronal outgrowth of its younger counterpart (FIG. 4). The duration of neuronal survival did not differ between the young and old rats, nor did the extent of their BDNF responses. In fact, the BDNF response was so robust in the aged rat SZ that BDNF supplementation effectively restored neuronal outgrowth from the aged SZ explants to that of their juvenile counterparts. Thus, the neuronal precursors of the rat brain persist into senescence, and remain responsive to BDNF; the size of the precursor pool attenuates minimally with age, and its spatial extent remains constant.[44]

NEURAL PRECURSORS IN THE ADULT HUMAN BRAIN

Neuronal Precursor Cells Reside in the Adult Human Forebrain SZ

In adult infrahuman primates, including both marmosets and rhesus monkeys, the lateral ventricular SZ continues to harbor dividing cells, in a distribution analo-

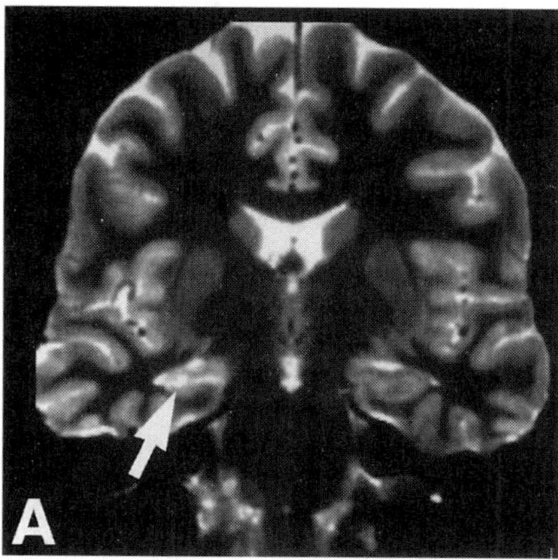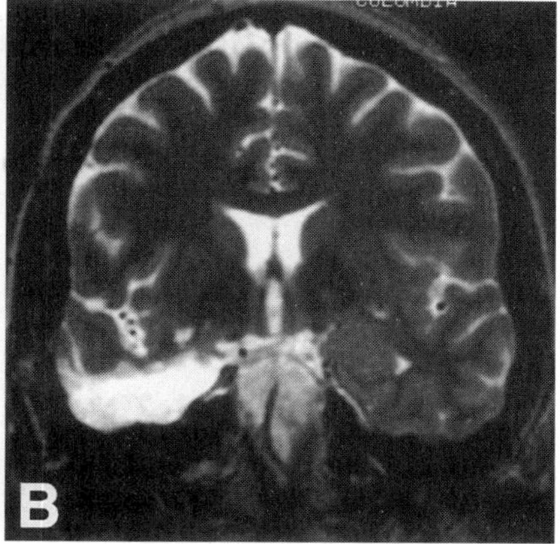

FIGURE 5. The adult human temporal lobe provides a ready source of subependymal progenitor cells. Samples were obtained from patients with refractory epilepsy during temporal lobectomy. (**A**) A magnetic resonance image of typical mesial temporal sclerosis (1.5 tesla, T2 image) is shown, with an atrophic right hippocampus and dentate gyrus (*arrow*), in a 37-year-old female; (**B**) after anterior lobectomy.

gous to that of the adult rodent SZ. No evidence of *in situ* neuronal production by these cells has yet been found despite several studies intended to test that possibility. Nonetheless, our results in the avian and rat brain suggested the persistence in adults of an SZ neuronal precursor cell population, which remains actively neurogenic in selected groups such as the songbirds, but which more generally becomes vestigial, yielding short-lived or rare progeny. We therefore postulated that the adult human forebrain might retain a reservoir of such cells, which cease generating neurons *in vivo* yet retain the capacity for neurogenesis *in vitro*. To test this possibility, we sought evidence of neurogenesis in cultures of adult human temporal lobe. Both explants and dissociates were prepared from fresh brain, obtained in the course of anterior temporal resection (FIG. 5); these samples were dissected into cortical, subcortical, and periventricular zone, and cultured under conditions conducive for adult neuronal differentiation in the canary and rat. Whether raised by explantation or enzymatic dissociation into monolayer culture, the SZ samples gave rise to neurons, as identified both antigenically (as MAP-2$^+$, MAP-5$^+$, NF$^+$, and/or N-CAM$^+$) and physiologically. However, *only* those explants derived from the SZ generated new neurons, whereas those taken from adjacent cortex failed to do so. We concluded on that basis that adult humans, like their avian and rodent counterparts, continue to harbor periventricular neural progenitors (FIGS. 6 and 7).[45]

Adult Human Precursor Cells Are Capable of Mitotic Neurogenesis and Maturation **in Vitro**

The majority of antigenically identified human neurons were postmitotic *in vitro*. Although it is difficult to distinguish whether the unlabeled neurons in these cultures derived from surviving parenchymal cells or from the neuronal maturation of precursors induced to differentiate by the culture conditions, the overall restriction of

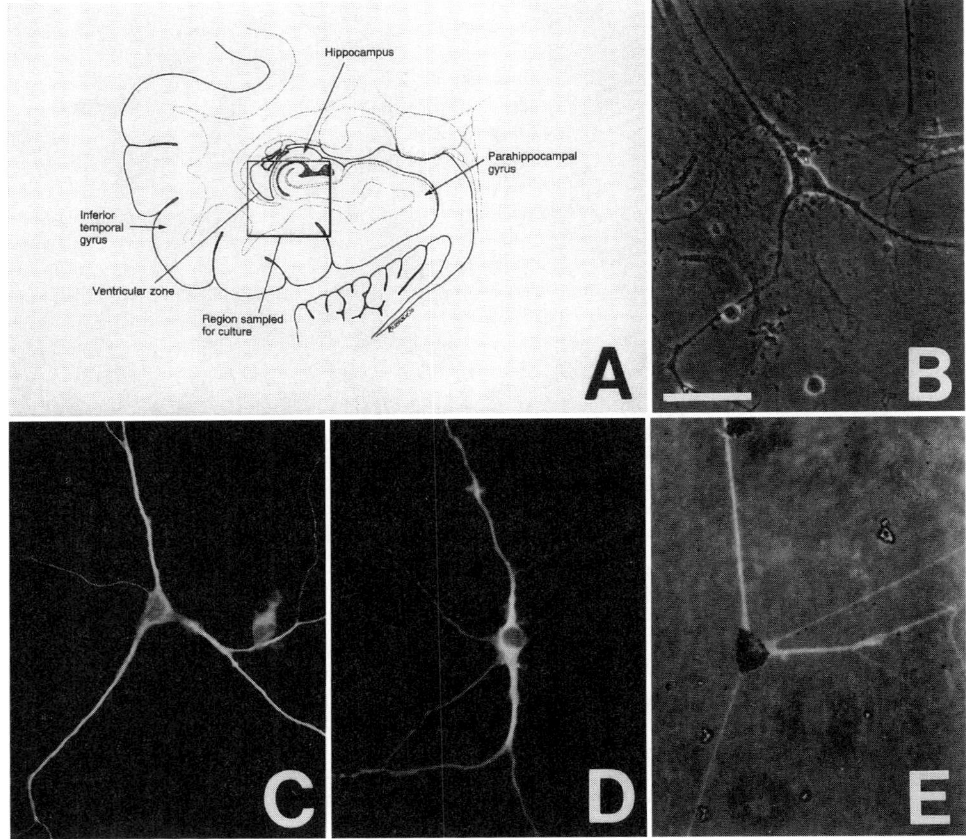

FIGURE 6. Neuronal precursor cells persist in the adult human SZ. (**A**) The borders of a typical inferior temporal lobe resection are outlined, and correspond roughly to the resection imaged in FIGURE 5. Each sample included cortical, subcortical and periventricular portions, the latter including the ependyma and adjacent subventricular tissue. (**B**) The outgrowth from an adult SZ explant is displayed, in which a presumptive neuron is seen upon a layer of flat substrate cells at 19 DIV. (**C**) A MAP-2[+] neuron, found in a subcortical culture at 18 DIV, is shown; (**D**) an N-CAM[+] neuron in an SZ dissociate at 12 DIV. (**E**) A MAP-5[+] cell that incorporated [3H]thymidine *in vitro* is displayed, suggesting its origin from precursor cell mitosis. Scale = 50 μm.

neuronal outgrowth to SZ explants suggested the latter. Accordingly, when dissociates of adult temporal SZ were exposed to [3H]thymidine, antigenically verified neurons that incorporated thymidine were found, suggesting the origin of these cells from precursor mitosis *in vitro*. These adult SZ-derived neurons were functionally as well as antigenically neuronal: When SZ outgrowths with neuron-like cells were loaded with the calcium dye fluo-3, then depolarized during confocal imaging, they exhibited depolarization-induced increments in cytosolic calcium (Ca^{2+}_i). Whereas astrocytic and oligodendrocytic responses to 60 mM KCl were minimal, neurons displayed rapid and reversible, >fourfold elevation in their cal-

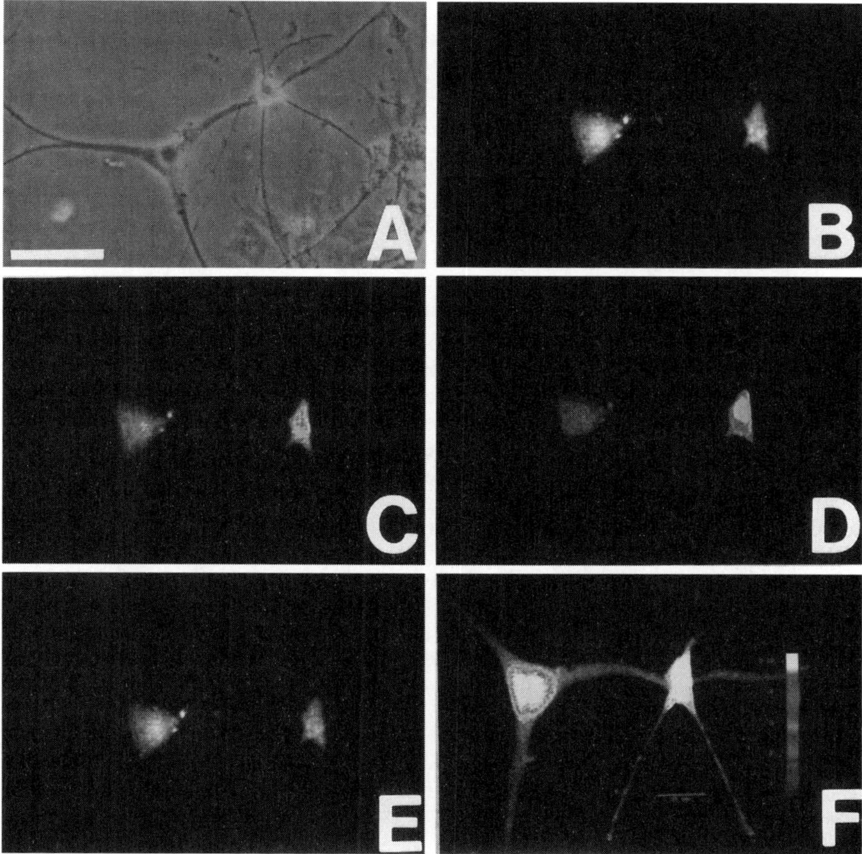

FIGURE 7. Adult human SZ-generated neurons are physiologically functional. Voltage-gated calcium channels were demonstrated by challenging these cells with K$^+$-induced depolarization. In this plate, an adult temporal SZ culture was tested at 28 DIV, after loading with the Ca^{2+}-sensitive dye fluo-3. A neuron's response to K$^+$-depolarization is contrasted with that of a neighboring astrocyte. (**A**) A phase micrograph of two adjacent cells, one neuron-like and the other astrocytic. (**B**) Shown are their baseline levels of Ca^{2+}$_i$, as viewed by confocal microscopy upon argon laser scanning at 488 nm. (**C**) The same two cells within seconds after exposure to 60 mM K$^+$. The neuron-like cell increased its Ca^{2+}$_i$ rapidly and reversibly, in contrast to the co-cultured astrocyte. (**D**) Upon addition of tetrodotoxin (TTX; 1 mM), K$^+$-stimulation yielded a >sixfold increase in neuronal Ca^{2+}$_i$, whereas astrocytic Ca^{2+}$_i$ increased <twofold. The depolarization-induced Ca^{2+}$_i$-increment of this cell suggested its neuronal phenotype, as did the TTX-accentuation of its Ca^{2+}$_i$ response. (**E**) Upon withdrawal of K$^+$, each cell returned to its resting Ca^{2+}$_i$ level. (**F**) Image taken after addition of the calcium ionophore lasalocid (50 mM), which revealed the presence of functional calcium channels in both cell types. Scale = 25 μm. (From Goldman[4] and Kirschenbaum *et al.*[45] Reprinted with permission from *Cerebral Cortex*.)

cium signals in response to K^+, consistent with the activity of neuronal voltage-gated calcium channels. The presence of new neurons in these cultures suggested that precursors persist in the human brain, just as in rats and birds.[45]

Adult Human Precursor Cells Respond to FGF2 and BDNF with Neuronal Differentiation and Long-term Survival

Previous studies have found that the proliferation of adult rodent SZ precursors derived is promoted by FGF2, whereas the survival of their neuronal daughters is supported by BDNF. We next applied these observations on the control of neurogenesis by adult rat SZ precursor cells to their human counterparts by sequentially treating adult human brain tissue with FGF2 followed by BDNF. When we compared neuronal number and survival in human temporal SZ explants raised in FGF2 (20 ng/mL; 1 week, in the presence of [³H]thymidine as a marker of cell division) followed by BDNF (40 ng/mL; 1–8 weeks) to either unsupplemented plates or those given *either* FGF2 *or* BDNF, we found a substantial increment in neuronal survival in the FGF2/BDNF-treated cultures. After as long as 9 weeks *in vitro*, many explants raised in FGF2/BDNF exhibited elaborate networks, including scores of neurons. These cells were MAP-2$^+$ and displayed sharp calcium increments to K^+-depolarization, suggesting their functional maturation. Many incorporated [³H]thymidine, indicating their genesis during the week in bFGF, 8 weeks earlier. In contrast, no surviving neurons were noted beyond 2 weeks *in vitro* in plates not treated with bFGF and BDNF. Although we have not yet defined the respective contributions of FGF2-driven precursor expansion and BDNF-supported survival to this result, it is clear that FGF2/BDNF together allowed the production and survival of relatively complex networks of new neurons in cultures of the adult human brain (FIG. 8).[38,46,47]

The Adult Mammalian SZ Harbors Oligodendrocyte Precursors

In explants of both the adult rat and human SZ, we noted immature migrants (N-CAM$^+$/G$_{D3}$$^+$/O4$^\pm$/O1) that developed into mature oligodendrocytes over the course of several weeks *in vitro* (FIG. 9). The SZ specificity of these cells, and their absence from cortical explant outgrowths, argued that they arose from precursors rather than from mature oligos that dedifferentiated *in vitro*. In both rat and human SZ cultures, a minor but significant fraction of O4$^+$ cells incorporated [³H]thymidine *in vitro*, suggesting their origin from precursor division. In adult human subcortical white matter, oligo precursors have been described, and conditions appropriate for their *in vitro* division have been characterized.[48,49] Whether these subcortical precursors are co-derived with the SZ-based progenitors that we found is unknown. It is also unclear whether these precursors are pluripotent for neurons and oligos, as in development, or whether they constitute more narrowly restricted oligodendrocyte precursors.[45]

POTENTIAL ENDOGENOUS ACTIVATORS OF NEUROGENESIS

Adult Human Astrocytes Express the Neurotrophins

These studies suggested that the permissiveness of adult brain to neurogenesis might depend in part upon the local availability of postmitotic trophic support. In

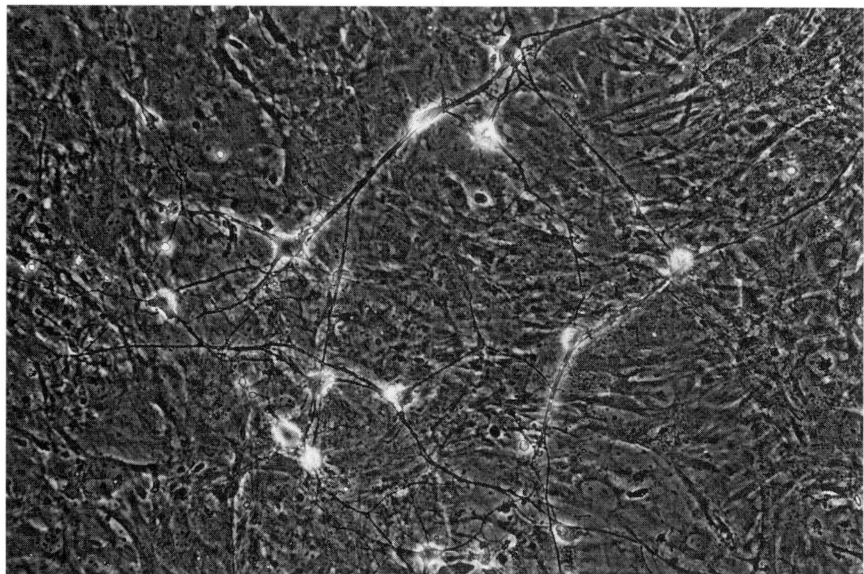

FIGURE 8. Sequential treatment with FGF2 and BDNF promotes neuronal outgrowth from the adult human SZ *in vitro*. This photomicrograph shows the outgrowth from an adult human temporal SZ explant, 7 weeks in culture. A field of mature neurons is seen lying upon a confluent layer of ependymal cells and astrocytes. This sample was raised for 1 week in the neuroectodermal mitogen FGF2 (20 ng/mL), followed by 6 weeks in BDNF (40 ng/mL). *Not shown here*: The neurons exhibited significant glutamate and depolarization-induced increments in cytosolic calcium, indicating their functional maturation; immunocytochemistry after confocal imaging confirmed their expression of neuronal MAP-2, while autoradiography of matched cultures exposed to [³H]thymidine during the first week *in vitro* confirmed the origin *in vitro* of many adult SZ-derived neurons.[38,46,47] Scale = 25 μm.

fetal rats, the production of BDNF has been noted by astrocytes as well as by neurons, but glial expression of BDNF had typically been described as abating in early ontogeny. We therefore asked whether *adult* human astrocytes could express BDNF. We further asked if adult glia could also express the neurotrophin (NT) family members NGF and NT-3. We used RT-PCR to detect their mRNAs in highly enriched, neuron-free cultures of adult human neocortical astrocytes, which we prepared from fresh temporal lobe resections. We found that mRNA for NGF, BDNF, and NT-3 was each expressed in these cultures, appearing as PCR products of 189, 296, and 176 base pairs, respectively.[50] GDNF mRNA was also detected, as possible splice variants of 197 and 272 bp, but at lower levels than the NTs. Treatment with 1 mM dibutyryl-cAMP up-regulated the mRNA of each NT, concurrent with astrocytic stellation. Thus, adult human astrocytes can express mRNAs for at least some of the neurotrophic agents—BDNF most notably—needed to support neuronal production by the adult SZ.[50,51]

We next found that adult human astrocytes were fully competent to translate and express BDNF protein, as well as mRNA. Immunocytochemistry and immunoblots revealed that adult cortical astrocytes expressed significant levels of BDNF protein,

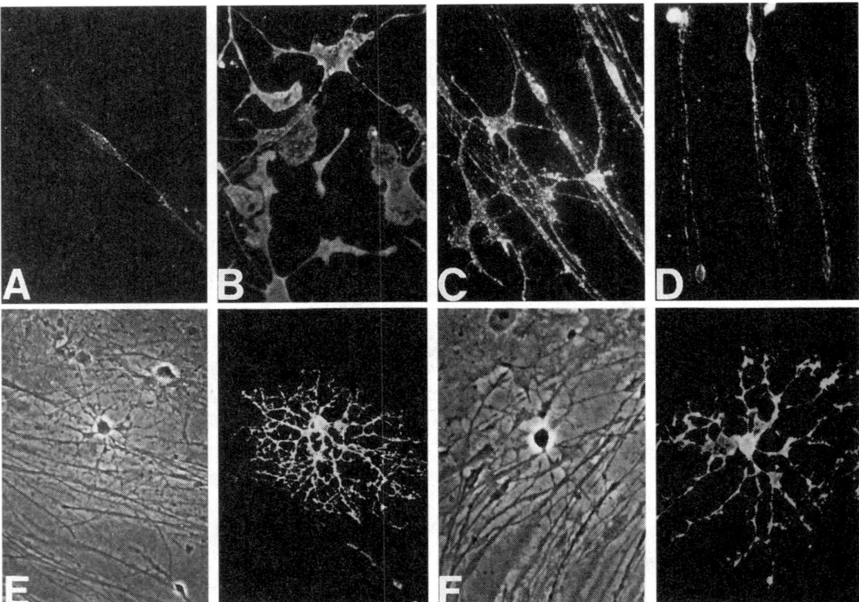

FIGURE 9. Oligodendrocytes as well as neurons arise from the adult mammalian SZ. Oligo-dendroglia arise from SZ explants taken from both adult rats and humans, suggesting the persistence of oligodendrocytic as well as neuronal progenitors in the adult mammalian ventricular lining. This plate shows the development of new oligodendrocytes arising from explants of the adult rat SZ. (**A**) Immature oligodendroglia initially emigrated as elongated bipolar cells, which expressed oligodendrocytic O4 upon initial departure from the SZ; 7 DIV. (**B**) The O4[+] migrants frequently spread into flat cells, morphologically indistinct but heavily O4 immunoreactive; 14 DIV. (**C**) By 14 days in culture, the young oligodendrocytes had developed bipolar and multipolar morphologies. (**D**) Initial oligodendrocytic migration frequently occurred upon other O4[+] fibers arising from the VZ border; 14 DIV. (**E–F**) By 28 DIV, the cells assumed complex oligodendroglial morphologies (phase and immunofluorescent views of O4[+] oligodendrocytes).

and ELISA established expression levels of >200 pg BDNF/mg in these cultures, with or without cAMP stimulation.[52] In addition, several inflammatory cytokines were causally associated with elevated levels of astrocytic BDNF, most notably TNFα and FGF2, each of which substantially raised BDNF expression levels, concurrent with their activation of astrocytic stellation.[52]

Adult Human Endothelial Cells, Like Astrocytes, Can Express BDNF

Using RT-PCR for NT family members, we found that human bone-marrow endothelial cultures produced BDNF mRNA (Leventhal, Rafii, Acheson, Shahar, and Goldman, manuscript submitted). ELISA revealed that BDNF protein was made by endothelial monolayers and secreted into the culture media to concentrations of >1 ng/mL. These levels of BDNF were sufficient to yield a significant increase in the outgrowth and survival of neurons arising from the adult rat SZ. Furthermore, the neurotrophic effect of endothelial cells could be replaced by adding BDNF to cultures deprived of endothelia, and was blocked by the addition of 5 μg/mL trkB-Fc to endothelial-explant co-cultures. Thus, vascular endothelial cells, like astroglial cells, may act as sources of endogenous BDNF, and as such may provide direct support for neuronal recruitment and survival. Taken together, these results suggest that the induction of endogenous endothelial and astrocytic production of BDNF may be a viable strategy for delivering it to a brain region in which one wishes to recruit new SZ-derived neurons.

IDENTIFICATION AND ENRICHMENT OF SZ PRECURSOR CELLS

Our ability to follow individual adult SZ precursor cells in any quantitatively meaningful manner has hitherto been limited by the low yields attending enzymatic dissociation of the adult SZ. The few such successful attempts, whether in avian, murine, or human brain, have all reported <1% survival of the dissociated sample, and experimental conclusions have been based upon these small, possibly misrepresentative samples. Furthermore, serum has proven antimitogenic and prodifferentiative for adult neuronal precursors, which has necessitated the use of serum-free media; this in turn has sharply limited the survival of newly dissociated adult SZ cells.

Serum-free Suspension Culture of Adult SVZ Microaggregates

To address the shortcomings of enzymatic dissociation of adult brain, we developed a method of raising small congregations of adult SZ cells in suspension. By preparing adult SZ cells as incompletely dissociated aggregates bound to charged cellulose microcarriers,[53] we can maintain cultures that remain viable and mitotically competent for weeks *in vitro*. In this procedure, very small SZ fragments of <0.01 mm^3, less than a tenth the volume of our described explants, are raised on cellulose carrier strips in serum-free media. The carrier strips adhere to the microexplants and continue to float in suspension; they can be centrifuged from the media both gently and in seconds, to allow decanting and media change without cell loss (a traditional problem with suspension culture). After experimenter-defined periods of mitogenic stimulation, the cell-bearing microcarriers can be replated onto a hyaluronic acid/laminin gel, to which they readily and quickly adhere. Microexplants raised in this manner can resume neuronal outgrowth after as long as two weeks in suspension, allowing ample time for exposure to mitogens or differentiation agents. This technique has allowed us to maintain small aggregates of <20 SZ cells in suspension, with [³H]thymidine-confirmed clonal expansion to added FGF2, for periods ranging from 4 to 14 days *in vitro*; propagation may well be feasible for substantially longer periods of time. The subsequent plating onto the HA/LMN gels has allowed us to recover cells within these aggregates readily and reliably, with little loss, and with preserved competence for neuronal differentiation and survival in added BDNF (FIG. 10; Shahar, Harrison and Goldman, unpublished data).

Green Fluorescent Protein, When Expressed Under the Control of Neural Regulatory Elements, Is an Effective Live Reporter of Neuronal Phenotype

Until recently, no technique was suitable for identifying live neuronal precursors as such; approaches for precursor identification and lineage analysis, such as nestin

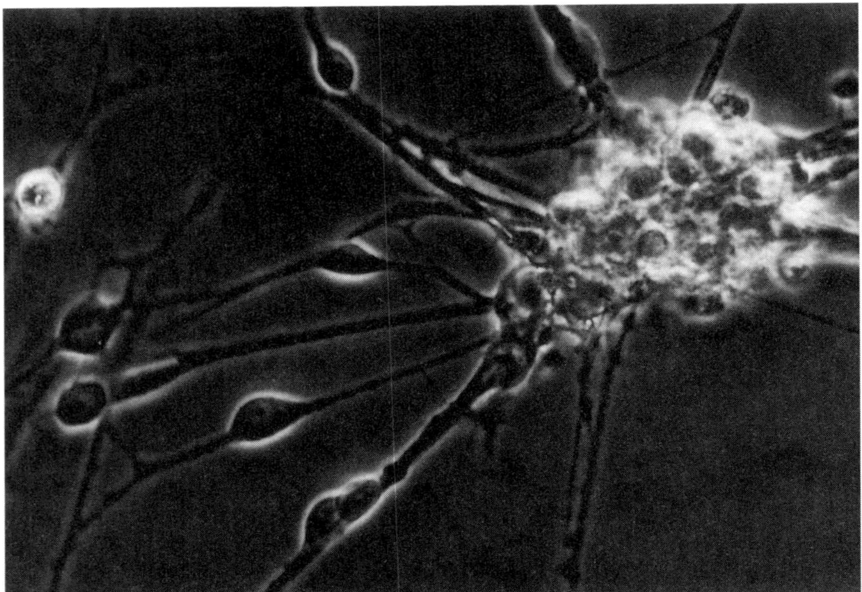

FIGURE 10. Charged cellulose carrier strips permit the long-term suspension culture and replating of adult SZ cells. This photomicrograph shows a cluster of neurons migrating from a microcarrier-borne aggregate of adult ventricular zone cells, after 2 weeks *in vitro*. This minced piece of adult SZ was maintained for its first week in suspension culture, during which it remained adherent to a charged cellulose microcarrier strip;[53] it was maintained throughout in 1% FBS and 20 ng/mL bFGF. During this period, cells derived from the SZ tissue fragment aggregated about the cellulose microcarrier. It was then plated onto a hyaluronic acid/laminin gel, in 10% FBS with 20 ng/mL BDNF, and photographed a week later. Typically, these carriers bridged the cell mass and the substrate layer, and thereby promoted adhesion and outgrowth. As a result, the carrier is subjacent to, and largely covered by, the spherical SZ cell mass in this photograph. Immunocytochemistry confirmed the neuronal antigenic phenotype (MAP-2$^+$/TuJ1$^+$/βIII-tubulin$^+$) of the fiber-bearing cells departing the SZ cell microaggregate.

localization and retroviral introduction of reporter genes, have been limited in that immunolabeled and reporter-labeled cells could only be identified after fixation. Clonal relationships could be ascertained, but not division-by-division family trees. To follow single cells in real-time requires a heritable reporter with detectable expression in live cells. The gene encoding green fluorescent protein (GFP)[54] fulfills these criteria: GFP fluoresces in live cells upon blue light excitation, with little toxicity. With the advent of mutated forms of strongly emitting GFP,[55] combined with improvements in optical imaging techniques and stronger transcriptional promoters, GFP has developed into an effective transcriptional reporter in live cells. In order to target GFP expression specifically to neuronal progenitors and young neurons, we developed constructs of the red-shifted, "humanized" mutant form of GFP, designated hGFP,[56] placed under the control of the early neuronal Tα1 tubulin promoter.[57,58] In accord with the neuronal specificity of Tα1 tubulin promoter expression (hereinafter referred to as Tα1),[58] Tα1:hGFP was strongly expressed by precursors and their neuronal progeny, but not by glia. In transfections of cultured embryonic VZ cells, Tα1:hGFP fluorescence quenched little, appeared specific to neurons and their precursors, was non-toxic, and remained bright up to 14 days after transfection. Most importantly, the expression of GFP allowed us for the first time to observe and follow, alive and in real-time, individual adult neuronal progenitor cells (FIG. 11).[59]

Fluorescence-activated Cell Sorting Based upon Tα1-driven GFP Expression Allows the Enrichment of Neuronal Precursor Cells

The use of neural stem cells has been hampered seriously by the difficulty of isolating adult progenitors in any sort of reasonable yield and purity. Contemporary approaches toward the study of these cells have therefore focused on preparing clonal lines derived from single progenitors (e.g., refs. 33, 34, 60, and 61). However, such lines can become progressively less representative of their parental precursors with time and passage *in vitro*. To circumvent these difficulties, we developed a strategy for the enrichment of native precursors and their neuronal daughter cells, by fluorescence-activated cell sorting (FACS) of forebrain cells transfected with the Tα1-driven hGFP. Having first established the effectiveness of the Tα1 promoter in driving specific neuronal expression of hGFP, we then combined its use with FACS to enrich neuronally committed embryonic SZ cells on the basis of their Tα1:GFP expression. By transfecting SZ cultures with pTα1:hGFP, then sorting the transfectants based upon their Tα1-driven GFP fluorescence, and culturing the harvested Tα1:hGFP transfectants, we identified and enriched both embryonic chick and rat brain neural precursors, under conditions that allowed their subsequent neuronal maturation (FIGS. 12 and 13).

Adenoviral Insertion of Fluorescent Transgenes into Adult SZ Cells

To improve the efficiency of our plasmid transfections, with an eye towards the high-yield enrichment of precursors from the adult SZ, we used adenoviral vectors to target pCMV:hGFP to SZ cells. In cultures of dissociated ventricular zone cells, the transfection efficiency of the AdCMV:hGFP virus rose from 12% at 10 pfu/cell to 52% at 100 pfu/cell. At this level of infection, most cells were likely infected with multiple episomal copies, vastly improving the duration of transgene expression (to over a month *in vitro*, on average) and the retention of transgene expression after multiple cell divisions. Most importantly, increasing the initial yield of SZ transfectants in this manner effectively increased, by over an order of magnitude, the number of cells that could be separated from an initial SZ dissociate.

Adenoviral Gene Transfer to Progenitor Populations in the Adult Rat Brain

Adenoviral vectors have additionally been shown to permit gene transfer to ependymal and subependymal cells *in vivo*.[62] On this basis, we employed intraventricular injection of AdCMV:hGFP into adult rats, with the intention of prelabeling the subependymal neuronal progenitor cells *in situ*, with fluorescent reporters that would allow their subsequent identification and isolation *in vitro*. We found that

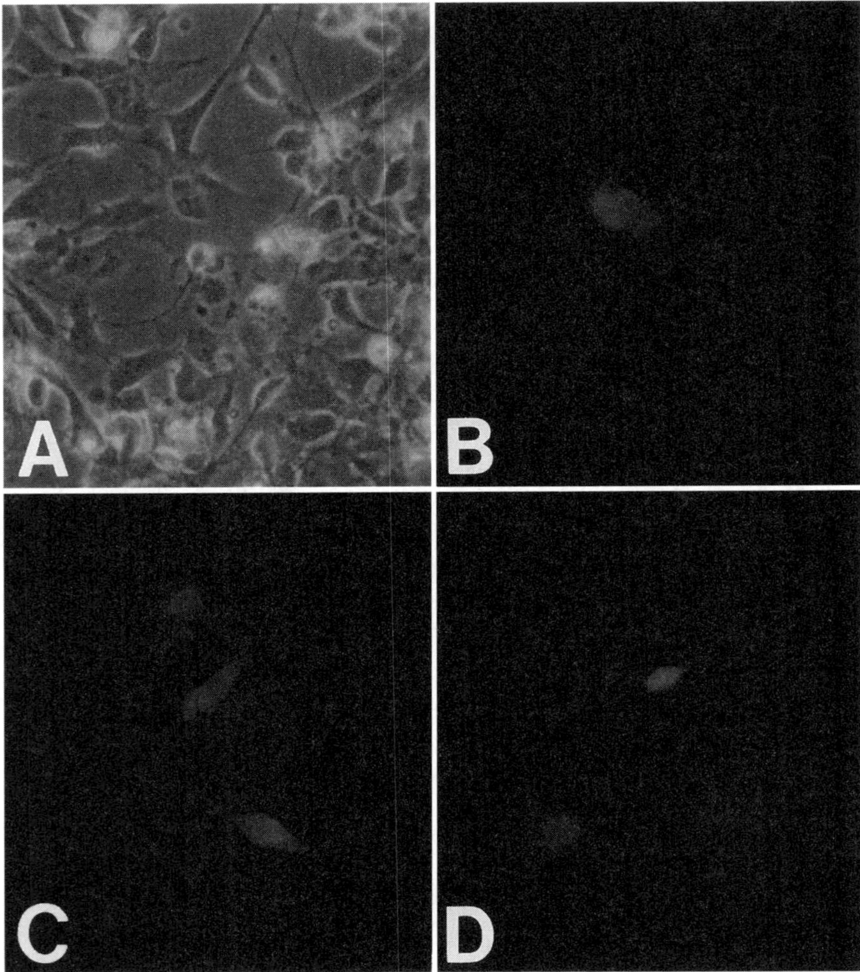

FIGURE 11. Live cell identification of neuronal precursor cells. Upon initial plating, cultured cells from the E6 chick telencephalic vesicle exhibited undistinguished morphologies. Within two days of transfection by Tα1:GFP, a minority of these flat cells were revealed to be neuronally committed cells, by virtue of their Tα1-driven GFP$^+$ expression. (**A** and **B**) show phase and fluorescent images of one such Tα1:GFP$^+$ cell, alone in a dense field of E6-derived neurons, glia, and ventricular zone cells. It was this cell type that Tα1:GFP-based FACS (see FIG. 12) was developed to isolate and enrich. (**C**) A cluster of these Tα1:GFP$^+$ cells, two days after transfection of a dissociated E6 forebrain vesicle. (**D**) By 5 DIV, some Tα1:GFP$^+$ cells developed neuronal morphology (*right-hand cell*), whereas others remained flat and morphologically undistinguished. Scale: **A** and **B**, 25 μm; **C** and **D**, 50 μm.

Preparation and Enrichment of
Neural Precursor Cells from the Embryonic Forebrain

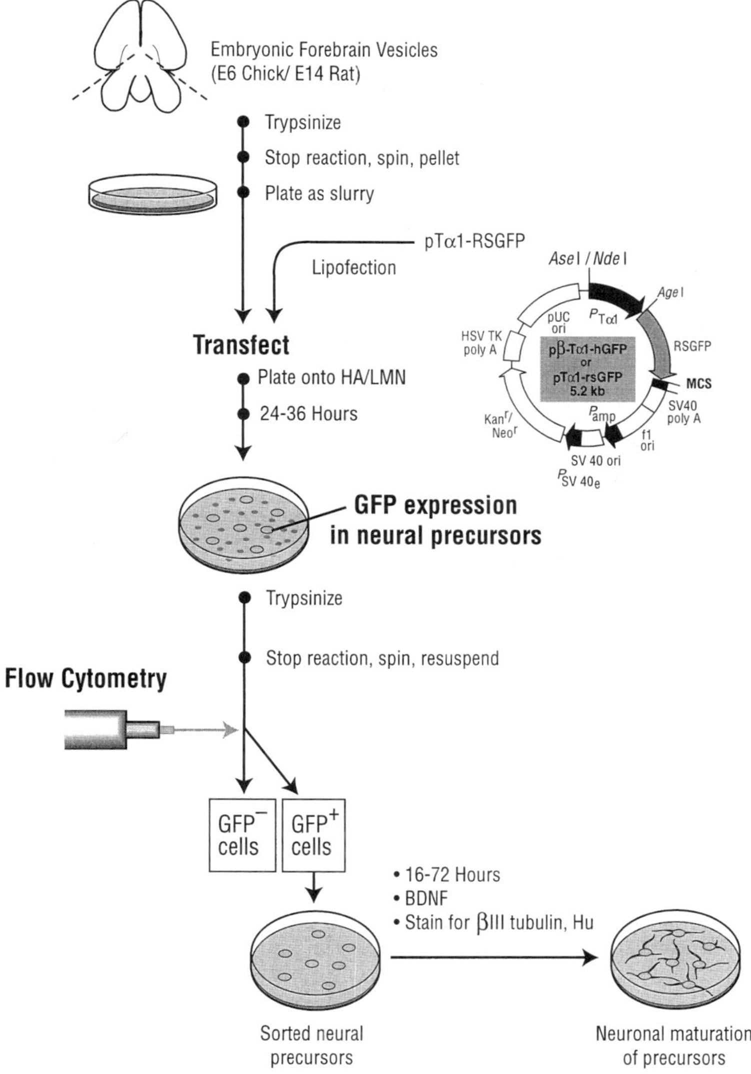

FIGURE 12. Technique: An overview of the strategy by which Tα1-hGFP-directed fluorescence-activated cell sorting was used to separate neuronal progenitors from late embryonic forebrain.

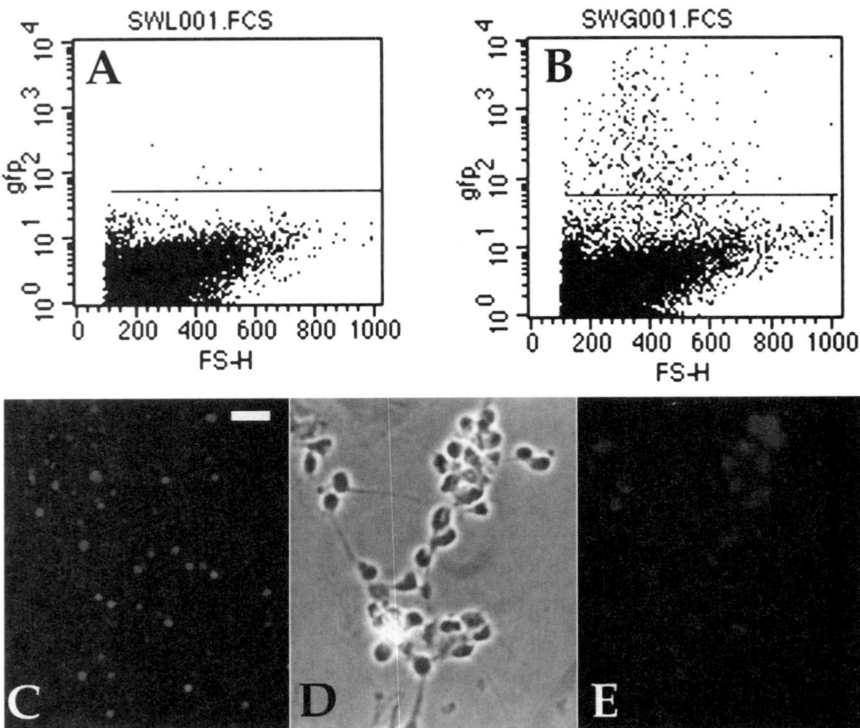

FIGURE 13. Fluorescence-activated sorting (FACS) enriched Tα1 : GFP⁺ neuronal progenitors. (**A** and **B**) illustrate the results of sorting E6 chick forebrain, transfected with either pTα1 : *lacZ*, a nonfluorescent control (**A**) or pTα1 : GFP (**B**). In both graphs, GFP fluorescence intensity is plotted against forward scatter, an index of cell size. Each graph shows 10,000 cells (sorting events). Among the pTα1 : GFP-transfected cells, 1.4% achieved an arbitrary threshold of fluorescence intensity, which was calibrated to correspond to that achieved by 0.1% of the control cells. The cells lying above the threshold line of the right-hand plot represent those separated from the remainder on the basis of their Tα1 : GFP. (These transfections utilized the red-shifted GFP reporter RSGFP-C1 [Clontech], rather than the hGFP[56] used in our transfections of rodent brain.) (**C**) A low-power micrograph of a field of pTα1 : RSGFP⁺ cells after sorting; most visibly expressed RSGFP. (**D** and **E**) Phase and fluorescent images of Tα1-GFP-sorted E6 chick cells, immunostained for the early neuronal protein Hu two days after FACS. Sorting enriched Hu⁺ neurons in cultures derived from the Tα1 : RSGFP⁺ cell pool, generally > fivefold, consistent with the Tα1 : GFP-based enrichment of neuronal progenitors. Scale: **C**, 50 μm; **D** and **E**, 25 μm.

intracerebroventricular injection of AdCMV : hGFP indeed led to the high efficiency transfection of SZ cells, with little transfection of other parenchymal cells (FIG. 14). We have now prepared an AdTα1 : hGFP vector that labeled neuronal precursors as specifically as its plasmid counterpart, and in higher yield; combined with FACS in the days after viral infection, this strategy may soon allow us to achieve the high-yield enrichment of viable neuronal progenitor cells from adult brain tissue.

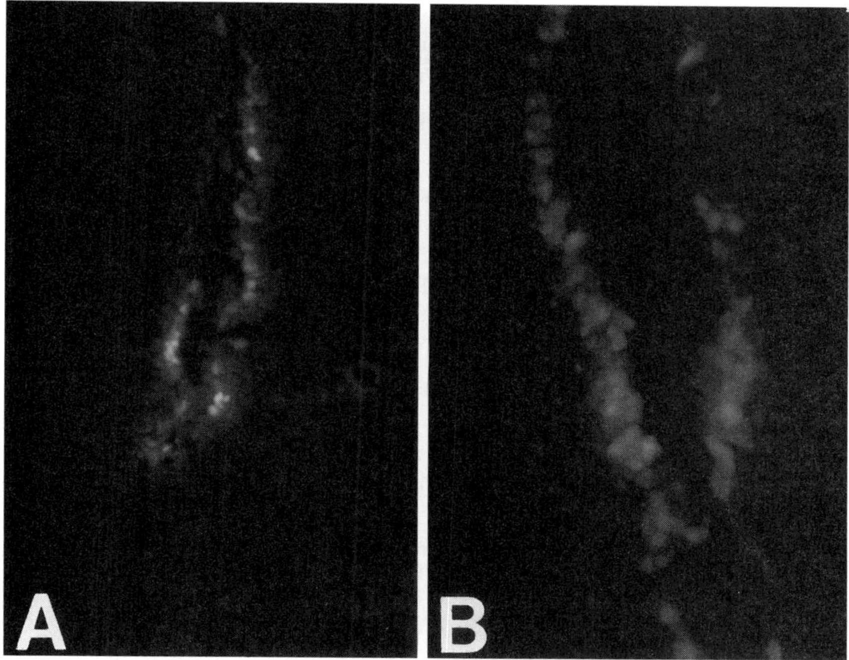

FIGURE 14. Expression of green fluorescent protein (hGFP) after intraventricular injection of AdCMV:hGFP. (**A**) A low-power view of AdCMV-GFP infected ependymal and sub-ependymal cells lining the lateral ventricular wall of an adult rat two weeks after intra-ventricular injection of AdCMV:hGFP. (**B**) A higher magnification view of another section taken from the same rat. Note the sustained high level of expression of the fluorescent transgene. This sample showed no evidence of significant local inflammation, necrosis or microglial invasion.

OVERVIEW: A GLIMPSE OF THE FUTURE

The enrichment of neural progenitors from the adult brain may allow novel strategies of brain repair by means of *in situ* neurogenesis to soon be attempted and evaluated. Yet this underlying strategy for cell separation, based upon fluorescent transgenes placed under the control of cell-specific promoters, may also prove amenable to the enrichment of defined non-neuronal progenitor phenotypes. These include oligodendrocyte progenitors competent for remyelination, and transmitter-specific neuronal phenotypes, such as dopaminergic neuroblasts for implantation in Parkinson's disease. As these strategies evolve, we will cross the threshold from basic studies of progenitor cell biology to their disease and repair-oriented application *in vivo*. This evolution may allow clinical trials of enriched neural progenitors for the treatment of structural brain disease to become relatively imminent. Indeed, the substantial progress in this field over the last five years provides us realistic hope that treatment strategies that include native progenitors, whether intended for structural repair or gene delivery,[68] may become integral to neurological therapeutics within the next decade.

The promise of these new approaches notwithstanding, a word of caution is in order: It is important to ask why examples of adult neurogenesis in the adult mammalian brain are so few and spatially restricted, given what we now understand to be the widespread persistence of competent neuronal progenitor cells. Our ability to employ these cells to replace cell populations lost to disease may hinge upon our understanding why evolution has selected against adding new neurons into adult brain, and to circumvent those considerations to permit the beneficial addition of new neurons to the adult human brain.

REFERENCES

1. GOLDMAN, S. A. 1995. Neuronal precursor cells and neurogenesis in the adult forebrain. Neuroscientist **1:** 338–350.
2. GOLDMAN, S. A. & F. NOTTEBOHM. 1983. Neuronal production, migration, and differentiation in a vocal control nucleus of the adult female canary brain. Proc. Natl. Acad. Sci. USA **80:** 2390–2394.
3. NOTTEBOHM, F. 1981. A brain for all seasons: Cyclical anatomical changes in song control nuclei of the canary brain. Science **214:** 1368–1370.
4. GOLDMAN, S. A. 1997. Comparative strategies of subependymal neurogenesis in the adult forebrain. *In* Isolation, Characterization and Utilization of CNS Stem Cells. F. Gage & Y. Christen, Eds.: 43–65. Springer-Verlag. New York
5. NOTTEBOHM, F. 1985. Neuronal replacement in adulthood. Ann. N. Y. Acad. Sci. **457:** 143–161.
6. ALVAREZ-BUYLLA, A. & C. LOIS. 1995. Neuronal stem cells in the brain of adult vertebrates. Stem Cells **13:** 263–272.
7. GOLDMAN, S. A. 1990. Neuronal development and migration in explant cultures of the adult canary forebrain. J. Neurosci. **10:** 2931–2939.
8. GOLDMAN, S. A. & M. NEDERGAARD. 1992. Newly generated neurons of the adult songbird brain become functionally active in long-term culture. Dev. Brain Res. **68:** 217–223.
9. GOLDMAN, S. A., A. ZAREMBA & D. NIEDZWIECKI. 1992. In vitro neurogenesis by neuronal precursor cells derived from the adult songbird brain. J. Neurosci. **12:** 2532–2541.
10. GOLDMAN, S. A., V. LEMMON & S. S. CHIN. 1993. Migration of newly generated neurons upon ependymally derived radial guide cells in explant cultures of the adult songbird forebrain. Glia **8:** 150–160.
11. GOLDMAN, S. A., A. ZUKHAR, K. BARAMI, T. MIKAWA & D. NIEDZWIECKI. 1996. Ependymal/subependymal cells of the postnatal and adult songbird brain generate both neurons and non-neuronal siblings, *in vitro* and *in vivo*. J. Neurobiol. **30:** 505–520.
12. BARAMI, K., K. IVERSEN, H. FURNEAUX & S. A. GOLDMAN. 1995. Hu protein as an early marker of neuronal phenotypic differentiation by subependymal zone cells of the adult songbird forebrain. J. Neurobiol. **28:** 82–101.
13. BARAMI, K., B. KIRSCHENBAUM, V. LEMMON & S. A. GOLDMAN. 1994. N-cadherin and Ng-CAM/8D9 are involved serially in the migration of newly generated neurons into the adult songbird brain. Neuron **13:** 567–582.
14. GOLDMAN, S. A., S. WILLIAMS, K. BARAMI, V. LEMMON & M. NEDERGAARD. 1996. Transient coupling of NgCAM expression to NgCAM-dependent calcium-signaling during migration of new neurons in the adult songbird forebrain. Mol. Cell. Neurosci. **7:** 29–45.
15. HIDALGO, A., K. BARAMI & S. A. GOLDMAN. 1995. Estrogens and non-estrogenic ovarian influences combine to promote the recruitment and decrease the turnover of new neurons in the adult female canary brain. J. Neurobiol. **27:** 470–487.
16. WILLIAMS, S., V. LEMMON, M. NEDERGAARD & S. GOLDMAN. 1996. Estrogen-dependent development of NgCAM-dependent calcium signaling by newly generated neurons in the adult songbird brain. Soc. Neurosci. Abstr. **216.11.**

17. JIANG, W., J. MCMURTRY & S. GOLDMAN. 1997. Insulin-like growth factor-1 is a radial cell-associated neutrophin that promotes neuronal recruitment from the adult songbird ventricular zone. J. Neurobiol. In press.

18. GOLDMAN, S. A. & M. B. LUSKIN. 1997. Strategies utilized by migrating neurons of the postnatal vertebrate forebrain. Trends Neurosci. In press.

19. ALTMAN, J. & G. D. DAS. 1965. Autoradiographic and histological evidence of postnatal hippocampal neurogenesis in rats. J. Comp. Neurol. **124:** 319–335.

20. KAPLAN, M. S., N. A. MCNELLY & J. W. HINDS. 1985. Population dynamics of adult-formed granule neurons of the rat olfactory bulb. J. Comp. Neurol. **239:** 117–125.

21. BAYER, S., J. YACKEL & P. PURI. 1982. Neurons in the rat dentate gyrus granular layer substantially increase during juvenile and adult life. Science **216:** 890–892.

22. LOIS, C. & A. ALVAREZ-BUYLLA. 1994. Long-distance neuronal migration in the adult mammalian brain. Science **264:** 1145–1148.

23. LUSKIN, M. B. 1993. Restricted proliferation and migration of postnatally generated neurons derived from the forebrain subventricular zone. Neuron **11:** 173–189.

24. COROTTO, F. S., J. A. HENEGAR & J. A. MARUNIAK. 1993. Neurogenesis persists in the subependymal layer of the adult mouse brain. Neurosci. Lett. **149:** 111–114.

25. SMART, I. 1961. The subependymal layer of the mouse brain and its cell production as shown by radioautography after thymidine injection. J. Comp. Neurol. **116:** 325–347.

26. MORSHEAD, C. & D. VAN DER KOOY. 1992. Postmitotic death is the fate of constitutively proliferating cells in the subependymal layer of the adult mouse brain. J. Neurosci. **12:** 249–256.

27. LOIS, C. & A. ALVAREZ-BUYLLA. 1993. Proliferating subventricular zone cells in the adult mammalian forebrain can differentiate into neurons and glia. Proc. Natl. Acad. Sci. USA **90:** 2074–2077.

28. KIRSCHENBAUM, B. & S. A. GOLDMAN. 1995. Brain-derived neurotrophic factor promotes the survival of neurons arising from the adult rat forebrain subependymal zone. Proc. Natl. Acad. Sci. USA **92:** 210–214.

29. REYNOLDS, B. A. & S. WEISS. 1992. Generation of neurons and astrocytes from isolated cells of the adult mammalian central nervous system [see comments]. Science **255:** 1707–1710.

30. RICHARDS, L. J., T. J. KILPATRICK & P. F. BARTLETT. 1992. De novo generation of neuronal cells from the adult mouse brain. Proc. Natl. Acad. Sci. USA **89:** 8591–8595.

31. GENSBURGER, C., G. LABOURDETTE & M. SENSENBRENNER. 1987. Brain basic fibroblast growth factor stimulates the proliferation of rat neuronal precursor cells in vitro. FEBS Lett. **217:** 1–5.

32. KILPATRICK, T. J. & P. F. BARTLETT. 1995. Cloned multipotential precursors from the mouse cerebrum require FGF-2, whereas glial restricted precursors are stimulated with either FGF-2 or EGF. J. Neurosci. **15:** 3653–3661.

33. GRITTI, A., E. A. PARATI, L. COVA, P. FROLICHSTHAL, R. GALLI, *et al.* 1996. Multipotential stem cells from the adult mouse brain proliferate and self-renew in response to basic fibroblast growth factor. J. Neurosci. **16:** 1091–1100.

34. PALMER, T. D., J. RAY & F. H. GAGE. 1995. FGF-2-responsive neuronal progenitors reside in proliferative and quiescent regions of the adult rodent brain. Mol. Cell. Neurosci. **6:** 474–486.

35. MORSHEAD, C. M., B. A. REYNOLDS, C. G. CRAIG, M. W. MCBURNEY, W. A. STAINES, D. MORASSUTTI, S. WEISS & D. VAN DER KOOY. 1994. Neural stem cells in the adult mammalian forebrain: A relatively quiescent subpopulation of subependymal cells. Neuron **13:** 1071–1082.

36. MENEZES, J. R. & M. B. LUSKIN. 1994. Expression of neuron-specific tubulin defines a novel population in the proliferative layers of the developing telencephalon. J. Neurosci. **14:** 5399–5416.

37. DOETSCH, F. & A. ALVAREZ-BUYLLA. 1996. Network of tangential pathways for neuronal migration in the adult mammalian brain. Proc. Natl. Acad. Sci. USA **93:** 14895–14900.

38. PINCUS, D. W., C. HARRISON, R. R. GOODMAN, M. EDGAR, H. KEYOUNG, R. A. R. FRASER, M. NEDERGAARD & S. A. GOLDMAN. 1997. BDNF-responsive neuronal progenitor cells in the adult human subependyma. Ann. Neurol. In press.

39. WEISS, S., C. DUNNE, J. HEWSON, C. WOHL, M. WHEATLEY, A. C. PETERSON & B. A. REYNOLDS. 1996. Multipotent CNS stem cells are present in the adult mammalian spinal cord and ventricular neuroaxis. J. Neurosci. **16:** 7599–7609.

40. LINDSAY, R. M. 1994. Neurotrophins and receptors. Prog. Brain Res. **103:** 3–14.

41. LINDSAY, R. M., S. J. WIEGAND, C. A. ALTAR & P. S. DISTEFANO. 1994. Neurotrophic factors: From molecule to man. Trends Neurosci. **17:** 182–190.

42. HOFER, M., S. PAGLIUSI, A. HOHN, J. LEIBROCK & Y. BARDE. 1990. Regional distribution of brain derived neurotrophic factor mRNA in adult mouse brain. EMBO J. **9:** 2459–2464.

43. GOLDMAN, S. A. & B. KIRSCHENBAUM. 1995. NT-4, like BDNF, supports the survival of new neurons arising from the adult rat subventricular zone. Soc. Neurosci. Abstr. **317.7.**

44. GOLDMAN, S., B. KIRCHENBAUM & C. HARRISON. 1997. Neuronal precursor cells of the adult rat ventricular zone persist into senescence, with no change in spatial extent or BDNF response. J. Neurobiol. **32:** 554–566.

45. KIRSCHENBAUM, B., M. NEDERGAARD, A. PREUSS, K. BARAMI, R. A. FRASER & S. A. GOLDMAN. 1994. In vitro neuronal production and differentiation by precursor cells derived from the adult human forebrain. Cerebr. Cortex **4:** 576–589.

46. PINCUS, D., C. HARRISON, R. GOODMAN, R. LABAR, R. FRASER, M. NEDERGAARD & S. GOLDMAN. 1996. Sequential treatment with FGF2 and BDNF permits the production of new neurons by precursors derived from the adult human epileptic temporal lobe. Ann. Neurol. **40:** 550.

47. PINCUS, D. W., C. HARRISON, J. BARRY, R. R. GOODMAN, D. LABAR, R. A. R. FRASER, M. NEDERGAARD & S. A. GOLDMAN. 1997. In vitro generation of precursor-derived neurons from adult human epileptic temporal neocortex. *In* Clinical Neurosurgery. Vol. 44. Williams & Wilkins. Baltimore, MD.

48. ARMSTRONG, R. C., H. H. DORN, C. V. KUFTA, E. FRIEDMAN & M. E. DUBOIS-DALCQ. 1992. Pre-oligodendrocytes from adult human CNS. J. Neurosci. **12:** 1538–1547.

49. SCOLDING, N. J., P. J. RAYNER, J. SUSSMAN, C. SHAW & D. A. COMPSTON. 1995. A proliferative adult human oligodendrocyte progenitor. Neuroreport **6:** 441–445.

50. MORETTO, G., B. KIRSCHENBAUM & S. A. GOLDMAN. 1995. Expression of mRNA for GDNF and the neurotrophins, NGF, BDNF and NT-3 by adult human astrocytes in culture. Soc. Neurosci. Abstr. **600.3.**

51. MORETTO, G., R. Y. XU, D. G. WALKER & S. U. KIM. 1994. Co-expression of mRNA for neurotrophic factors in human neurons and glial cells in culture. J. Neuropathol. & Exp. Neurol. **53:** 78–85.

52. PINCUS, D., C. LEVENTHAL, G. MORETTO & S. A. GOLDMAN. 1997. Induced expression of BDNF mRNA and protein by adult human astrocytes in vitro. Soc. Neurosci. Abstr. **23:** 27.18.

53. SHAHAR, A. 1990. Cultivation of nerve and muscle cells on microcarriers. *In* Methods in Neurosci. vol. 2.: Cell Culture. M. Conn, Ed.: 195–209. Academic Press. San Diego.

54. CHALFIE, M., Y. TU, G. EUSKIRCHEN, W. WARD & D. PRASHER. 1994. Green fluorescent protein as a marker for gene expression. Science **263:** 802–805.

55. HEIM, R. & R. TSEIN. 1996. Engineering green fluorescence protein for improved brightness, longer wavelengths and energy transfer. Curr. Biol. **6:** 178–183.

56. LEVY, J., R. MULDOON, S. ZOLOTUKHIN & C. LINK. 1996. Retroviral transfer and expression of a humanized, red-shifted green fluorescent protein gene into human tumor cells. Nature Biotechnol. **14:** 610–614.

57. MILLER, F., C. NAUS, M. DURAND, F. BLOOM & R. MILNER. 1987. Isotypes of α-tubulin are differentially regulated during neuronal maturation. J. Cell Biol. **105:** 3065–3073.

58. GLOSTER, A., W. WU, A. SPLEELMAN, S. WEISS, C. CAUSING, *et al.* 1994. The Tα1 α-tubulin promoter specifies gene expression as a function of neuronal growth and regeneration in transgenic mice. J. Neurosci. **14:** 7319–7330.

59. WANG, S., H. WU, W. JIANG, F. ISDELL, T. DELOHERY & S. GOLDMAN. 1997. Identification and enrichment of forebrain neuronal precursor cells by fluorescence-activated sorting of ventricular zone cells transfected with the green fluorescent driven by the Tα1 tubulin promoter. Nature Biotechnol. In press.

60. REYNOLDS, B. A. & S. WEISS. 1992. Generation of neurons and astrocytes from isolated cells of the adult mammalian central nervous system. Science **255:** 1707–1710.

61. REYNOLDS, B. A. & S. WEISS. 1996. Clonal and population analyses demonstrate that an EGF-responsive mammalian embryonic CNS precursor is a stem cell. Dev. Biol. **175:** 1–13.

62. BAJOCCHI, G., S. FELDMAN, R. CRYSTAL & A. MASTRANGELI. 1993. Direct in vivo gene transfer to ependymal cells in the central nervous system using recombinant adenovirus vectors. Nature Genet. **3:** 229–234.

63. LEMMON, V. 1985. Monoclonal antibodies specific for glia in the chick central nervous system. Dev. Brain Res. **23:** 111–120.

64. SAKAKIBARA, S., T. IMAI, K. HAMAGUCHI, M. OKABE, J. ARUGA, *et al.* 1996. Mouse-Musashi-1, a neural RNA-binding protein highly enriched in the mammalian CNS stem cell. Dev. Biol. **176:** 230–242.

65. MARUSICH, M. & J. WESTON. 1992. Identification of early neurogenic cells in the neural crest lineage. Dev. Biol. **149:** 295–306.

66. MARUSICH, M., H. FURNEAUX, P. HENION & J. WESTON. 1994. Hu neuronal proteins are expressed in proliferating neurogenic cells. J. Neurobiol. **25:** 143–155.

67. SZABO, A., J. DALMAU, G. MANLEY, M. ROSENFELD, J. POSNER & H. FURNEAUX. 1991. HuD, a paraneoplastic encephalomyelitis antigen, contains RNA binding domains and is homologous to elav and sex-lethal. Cell **67:** 325–333.

68. SNYDER, E. & M.-C. SENUT. 1997. The use of nonneural cells for gene delivery. Neurobiol. Dis. **4:** 69–102.

Central Regulation of Sympathetic Ganglia Development: Heterogeneous Response of Paravertebral, Prevertebral, and Terminal Ganglia[a]

ROBERT W. HAMILL

Department of Neurology
College of Medicine of the University of Vermont
Burlington, Vermont 05401

INTRODUCTION

The central nervous system is known to regulate the growth and development as well as the functional adaptation of the peripheral sympathetic nervous system (SNS). Previous studies in neonatal rodents (rat) revealed that interruption of descending pathways within the spinal cord altered the biochemical and morphological development of paravertebral ganglia (the sixth lumbar sympathetic ganglia, L-6).[1-3] Similarly, interruption of central pathways within the spinal cord in adult animals altered the functional adaptation of the L-6 as evidenced by the failure of reserpine to induce tryosine hydroxylase (T-OH).[4] In these experiments the L-6 was chosen for study because other paravertebral ganglia—the superior cervical ganglia (SCG)—had received extensive study, and many of the mechanisms governing neuronal maturation and regulation revealed in this model system should be applicable to the L-6. These investigations in the SCG indicated that preganglionic and postganglionic connections were important for maturational development, and that target organs were also instrumental in ensuring that maturation of sympathetic neuronal systems occurred normally (see ref. 5 for review). The SCG could not be used for studies of central control because interruption of pathways within the spinal cord would require lesions rostral to the first thoracic spinal cord level and injury at this level would be lethal to developing animals. Central pathways to the L-6, which is innervated by neuronal populations in the caudal thoracic and rostral lumbar cord, may be interrupted by a midthoracic spinal cord lesion, thus permitting examination of the role of the central nervous system in SNS development.

The current studies extend these observations and were directed at trying to understand whether central pathways exerted similar effects on other components of the peripheral SNS. That is, since the SNS is organized into three groups of ganglia (paravertebral, prevertebral, and terminal-short adrenergic) and since these ganglia have varying targets and are regulated differently, it seemed reasonable to ask whether central nervous system pathways would exert similar regulatory effects on these different sympathetic neuronal populations. Furthermore, the adrenal medulla was examined because this autonomic target organ also receives preganglionic innervation from sympathetic nerve cell populations in the spinal cord, but is regulated somewhat differently.

[a] This work was supported by NINDS Grant No. 22103-07.

Neurochemical markers exist to examine the maturation and functional adaptation of sympathetic neurons. In the present studies, postsynaptic T-OH, the rate-limiting enzyme in catecholamine biosynthesis and a well-described marker of noradrenergic neuronal development and function, was used to monitor noradrenergic neuron and adrenal medullary development following high spinal injury. The basic hypothesis is that peripheral ganglia will respond in a heterogeneous fashion following interruption of central pathways (spinal cord injury) and specifically that pelvic sympathetic ganglia (terminal ganglia-short adrenergic) will be less affected. These ganglia demonstrate resistance to various neurotoxins, exhibit substantial dependence on other regulatory events such as hormonal control, and may be less influenced by central mechanisms. Thus, depending on the ganglia of interest, a developmental hierarchy may exist wherein certain ganglia will be more or less susceptible to specific regulatory factors.

MATERIALS AND METHODS

Experimental Animals

Litters of Charles River Sprague-Dawley rats were housed with mothers, received traditional feed and water, exposed to similar lighting, and were standardized by assigning control and experimental animals to each mother. After weaning, spinal animals were kept in stainless steel cages and meticulous skin and bladder care maintained.

Surgical Procedures

Ganglion dissection. SCG, L-6, celiac, and hypogastric ganglia (HG) and adrenal medulla were identified and removed. The procedures required for removal of these structures are well described.[1,2,6]

Spinal transection. Spinal cord transection was performed rostral to the third thoracic level using methods previously described for midthoracic transections.[2] The more rostral transection was indicated because the innervation of the adrenal medulla and presumably the celiac ganglia arises from T-3 to L-1, and transection at a more caudal level would directly injure preganglionic spinal cord neurons that send cholinergic terminals to the adrenal gland and celiac ganglia.

Biochemical Procedures

T-OH activity was measured as previously described using tetrahydrobiopterin as cofactor.[6] Total protein was assayed by the method of Lowry *et al.* using bovine serum albumin as a standard.[7]

Statistical Analysis

The unpaired *t* test was used to analyze data from ganglia and adrenal studies at four weeks, whereas analysis of variance was employed to examine data from the longitudinal time points of the L-6 and HG ganglia.

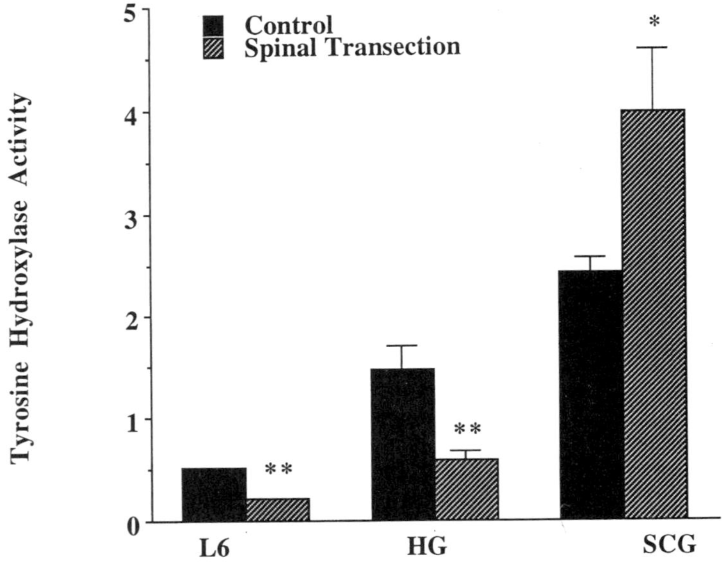

FIGURE 1. Effect of spinal cord transection on the maturation of tyrosine hydroxylase activity in peripheral sympathetic ganglia. Rats received spinal transection and littermates underwent sham-operation at 10–11 days of age. Groups of 6–8 animals were killed at four weeks following surgery. Tyrosine hydroxylase activity is expressed as nmoles/ganglion · h ± SEM. L6 refers to the sixth lumbar ganglion; HG, hypogastric ganglion; SCG, superior cervical ganglion. * Differs from respective control groups, $p < 0.005$; ** differs from respective control group, $p < 0.001$.

RESULTS

Paravertebral and Terminal Ganglia

In order to compare the role of central nervous system pathways in the regulation of biochemical maturation of these ganglia, animals were operated on at 10 days of age and ganglia were studied one month following spinal surgery. Previous studies indicated that by approximately 40 days of age these three ganglia have either completed the major developmental increase in transmitter biochemistry (SCG) or the early phase of neurochemical maturation has been accomplished (L-6 and HG). Studies of the L-6 mimicked previous observations that following spinal transection the normal biochemical maturation fails to occur and T-OH activity is approximately 42% of control (FIG. 1). These results confirmed the experimental paradigm. The HG, a terminal or short adrenergic ganglia, also failed to develop normally following interruption of spinal pathways: T-OH activity failed to increase normally and was 40% of control (FIG. 1). The SCG was studied in order to examine two questions: whether the paraplegic state created by a relatively high thoracic injury might alter neural development as a whole, and whether a more rostral spinal transection (T-3) might directly injure enough preganglionic neurons that SCG maturation would be altered. In contrast to what was expected (i.e., no significant alteration in enyzme activity), T-OH was increased significantly one month following the spinal lesion: enzyme activity increased 1.6-fold (FIG. 1).

Prevertebral Ganglia and Adrenal Medulla

Spinal injury early in development also resulted in a failure of T-OH activity to mature normally in the celiac ganglia—a prevertebral ganglia which receives its major innervation from cell populations caudal to the level of injury. T-OH activity was reduced to 68% of control at four weeks following spinal transection at T-3 (FIG. 2). In contrast to the ganglia, no change was found in the level of T-OH activity in the adrenal medulla following the spinal lesion. At one month following surgery, the enzyme activity in the control and experimental groups was 22.181 nmoles/h and 21.031 nmoles/h, respectively (FIG. 2). These experiments were repeated and the same results obtained. Of interest, protein maturation and wet weight within the adrenal were altered by transection (data not shown), but overall enzyme activity was unchanged.

Longitudinal Time Course of L-6 and HG Maturation

Previous studies of the L-6 indicated that the effects of spinal injury during neonatal life were long lasting. Since different regulatory events exist for the HG,

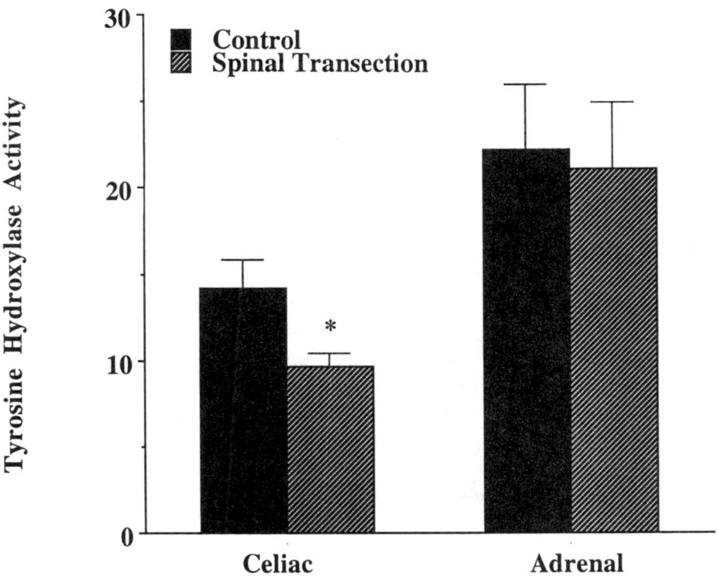

FIGURE 2. Effect of spinal cord transection on the maturation of tyrosine hydroxylase activity in the celiac ganglion and adrenal medulla. Rats received spinal transection and litter mates underwent sham-operation at 10–11 days of age. Groups of 6–8 animals were killed at four weeks following surgery. Tyrosine hydroxylase activity is expressed as nmoles/ganglion · h ± SEM. * Differs from respective control groups, $p < 0.05$.

it was of interest to characterize the longitudinal time course of the changes in HG transmitter enzyme development and to compare these results with studies of the L-6. Confirming previous studies of the L-6,[2] spinal transection permanently altered the maturation of T-OH: enzyme activity remained at approximately 200 pmoles/ h over a time period of approximately 13 weeks following spinal transection at 10 days of age (FIG. 3). In contrast, HG T-OH activity in experimental animals continued to increase gradually over the weeks following transection. Initially it remained less than control for approximately 8 weeks following transection, but then gradually increased so that by 13 weeks no significant difference existed between control and transected groups ($p < 0.10$), although the level of T-OH enzyme activity was still less in the experimental animals (FIG. 3).

DISCUSSION

Studies of neuronal maturation and development indicate that a broad array of events and factors influence the maturation of sympathetic neurons (see refs. 5, 8–10 for reviews); alterations of these regulatory processes may occur within the intrinsic and extrinsic environmental milieu and may impair sympathetic maturation. Examples of intrinsic mechanisms include genetic encoding and gene regulation-translation and posttranslational control, pattern formation (such as homeobox, PAX, POU genes), intra- and intercellular signaling, and transduction mechanism, converting extracellular signals to intracellular messages. Extrinsic influences are represented by adhesion systems (such as CAMs, SAMs, integrins, cadherins), hormonal regulation, and interneuronal influences, including peripheral and central regulation of autonomic development, target organ regulation, and neuronotrophic factors, to name a few. The present studies contribute to the idea that interneuronal influences are important for normal biochemical maturation and specifically examine the role of central pathways in the growth and development of four components of the peripheral sympathetic nervous system.

Previous investigations of interneuronal regulation indicate that injury of preganglionic and postganglionic neural processes that presumably alter anterograde or retrograde transsynaptic communication result in failed maturation of sympathetic ganglia.[5] Subsequently, studies in paravertebral ganglia demonstrated that central nervous system pathways regulate neuronal maturation.[2,3] The present results reveal that the effect of interruption of descending central pathways in the spinal cord does not affect the peripheral sympathetic nervous system in a uniform fashion. As indicated in FIG. 1, the L-6 ganglia failed to develop the normal complement of T-OH activity following spinal transection at T-3, confirming previous studies mentioned above, and at one month following spinal injury the terminal ganglia, HG, also exhibited delayed enzyme maturation. Central pathways also regulate the development of the celiac ganglia (FIG. 2), although the magnitude of the effects (68% of control) was slightly less than that observed for the paravertebral (33% of control) and prevertebral (37% of control) ganglia. In contrast, the development of T-OH activity in the adrenal medulla proceeded unimpaired by the central lesion. Thus, although during adulthood transsynaptic pathways influence the activation of adrenal T-OH activity following stressful stimuli,[11,14] these observations indicate that interruption of descending pathways to the preganglionic neurons within the spinal cord that innervate the adrenal gland does not alter the ontogeny of T-OH. Since the development of adrenal peptidergic and monoaminergic phenotypes within the adrenal medulla are under substantial influence of corticosteroids,

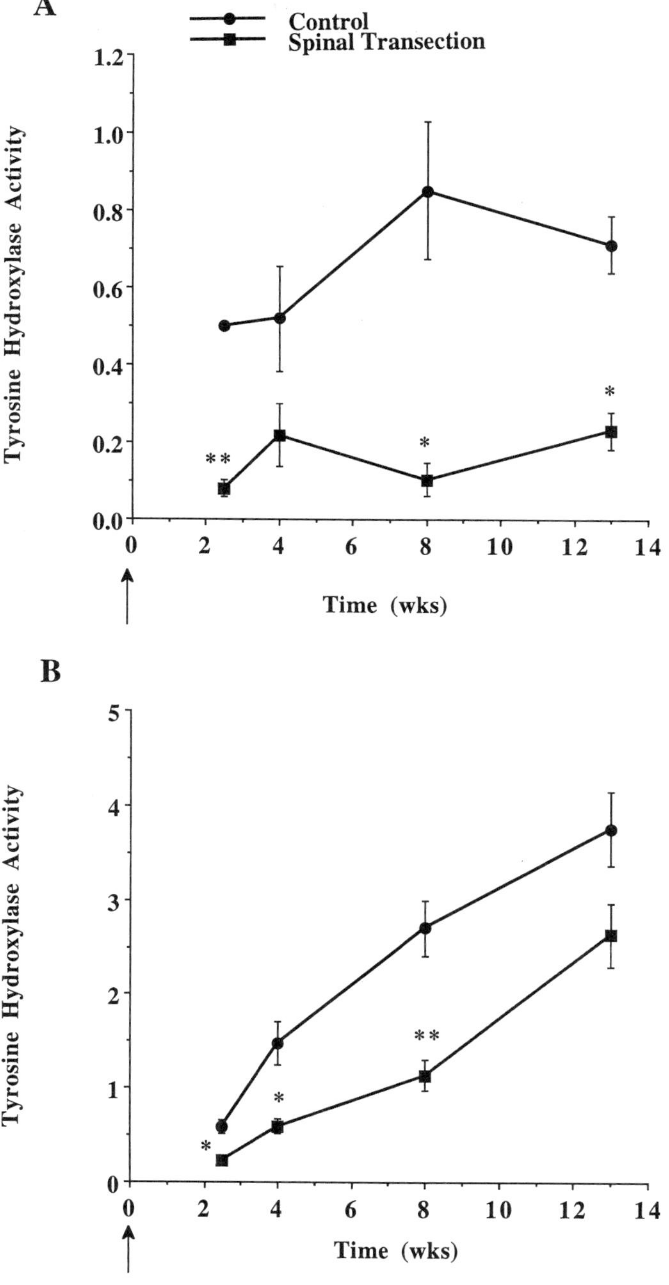

FIGURE 3. Comparison of the longitudinal effect of spinal cord transection on the maturation of tyrosine hydroxylase activity in the L-6 (**A**) and HG (**B**). Rats received spinal transection and littermates underwent sham-operation at 10–11 days of age. Groups of 6–8 animals were killed at the various times indicated. The arrow indicates the time point of surgery. Tyrosine hydroxylase activity is expressed as nmoles/ganglion · h ± SEM. * Differs from respective control groups, $p < 0.05$; ** differs from respective control group, $p < 0.01$.

compensatory events may occur to ensure normal T-OH maturation in the adrenal gland.[12] Another conceivable explanation is that the spinal lesion did not fully interrupt descending input to the preganglionic cells supplying the adrenal medulla because a small percentage of preganglionic neurons originate from the segments rostral to T-3. However, this innervation is minimal and the observation that the celiac, which is supplied from approximately the same spinal levels, does not mature normally following the same lesion mitigates this possibility.

The development of the SCG following the T-3 lesion was examined to determine whether the more rostral spinal lesion (previous studies of central regulation used a lesion at T-5) might have produced systemic effects that would have adversely influenced the development of the SNS. Alternatively, the T-3 lesion might have directly injured preganglionic neurons destined to innervate the SCG. Neurons as far caudal as T-7 have been identified to innervate the SCG, and their interruption would have altered preganglionic input and in turn impaired development. Surprisingly, T-OH activity was elevated in the SCG four weeks after transection (FIG. 1). These data may reflect a compensatory change in sympathetic activity secondary to the high thoracic lesion and sustained induction of enzyme molecules. Alternatively, a developmental regulatory change may have occurred resulting in an elevation in the ontogenic baseline level of T-OH.

Previous studies of the HG indicate that the developmental maturation of T-OH activity is quite delayed compared to other peripheral sympathetic ganglia with enzyme activity increasing up to 75 days of age before reaching a plateau.[6] This long maturational process coincides with hormonal events as the adult level of testosterone is not approached until approximately 60 days of age.[13] These ganglia are remarkably sensitive to gonadal steroids: castration at 10 days of age completely precludes normal maturation.[6] In order to determine whether the change in T-OH activity observed in the HG persisted over time, animals were studied up to three months post surgery, and these changes were compared with the L-6. The developmental profile of these two ganglia were clearly different following interruption of central pathways (FIG. 3). L-6 ganglia enzyme activity failed to develop following transection and remained at essentially the same level for 13 weeks (i.e., approximately 30% of control). In contrast, HG ganglia enzyme activity continued to increase throughout the postoperative period; the initial slope of the lines characterizing the two groups were somewhat parallel, but between 8 and 13 weeks the slope appeared to have changes so that the significant difference between groups was lost at week 13 (FIG. 3). The difference, expressed as percent reduction from control, between groups at 4 weeks was approximately 70%, but by 13 weeks this value was only 30%. This rather striking change clearly indicates that the role of central pathways in regulating development of the preterminal ganglia HG is clearly different from that observed for the L-6. On the one hand, the integrity of supraspinal input must be maintained for normal maturation of L-6, whereas the HG appears to be affected adversely only during the initial few months of postnatal growth and development. Subsequently, the absence of central input apparently does not preclude the later phase of T-OH maturation. Furthermore, because this later phase is believed to be androgen dependent, it might be reasoned that hormonal influences occur independent of central input.

SUMMARY

These studies expand previous observations regarding the central control of neuronal maturation and indicate that paravertebral, prevertebral, and terminal ganglia are all under central influences, but in varying degrees. These variations are probably related to the relative contributions that central pathways exert on specific peripheral neuronal populations during growth and development as well as the various roles of more peripheral developmental modulators such as target organs and hormones, especially in the case of the HG. It is apparent, therefore, that during development central injury may result in heterogeneous deficits depending on the unique intrinsic and extrinsic environment that each ganglion population shares.

REFERENCES

1. BLACK, I. B., E. M. BLOOM & R. W. HAMILL. 1976. Central regulation of sympathetic neuron development. Proc. Natl. Acad. Sci. USA **73:** 3575–3578.
2. HAMILL, R. W., P. COCHARD & I. B. BLACK. 1983. Long-term effects of spinal transection on the development and function of sympathetic ganglia. Brain Res. **266:** 21–27.
3. LAWRENCE, J. M., R. W. HAMILL, P. COCHARD, G. RAISMAN & I. B. BLACK. 1981. Effects of spinal cord transection on synapse numbers and biochemical maturation in rat lumbar sympathetic ganglia. Brain Res. **212:** 83–88.
4. BLOOM, E. M., R. W. HAMILL & I. B. BLACK. 1976. Elevation of tyrosine hydroxylase activity in sympathetic neurons after reserpine: The role of the central nervous system. Brain Res. **115:** 525–528.
5. BLACK, I. B. 1978. Regulation of autonomic development. Annu. Rev. Neurosci. **1:** 183–214.
6. MELVIN, J. E. & R. W. HAMILL. 1986. Gonadal hormone regulation of neurotransmitter synthesizing enzymes in the developing hypogastric ganglion. Brain Res. **383:** 38–46.
7. LOWRY, O. H., N. J. ROSEBOROUGH, A. L. FARR & R. J. RANDALL. 1951. Protein measurement with Folin phenol reagent. J. Biol. Chem. **193:** 265–275.
8. BLACK, I. B. 1982. Stages of neurotransmitter development in autonomic neurons. Science **215:** 1198–1204.
9. BUNGE, R., M. JOHNSON & C. D. ROSS. 1978. Nature and nurture in development of the autonomic neuron. Science **199:** 1409–1416.
10. HAMILL, R. W. & E. F. LAGAMMA. 1992. Autonomic nervous system development. *In* Autonomic Failure: A Textbook of Clinical Disorders of the Autonomic Nervous System, 3rd edit. R. Bannister & C. J. Mathias, Eds.: 15–35. Oxford University Press. New York.
11. KVETNANSKY, R. 1971. Trans-synaptic and humoral regulation of adrenal catecholamine synthesis in stress. Frontiers in Catecholamine Research. *In* E. Usdin & S. Snyders, Eds.: 223–229. Pergamon Press. New York.
12. LAGAMMA, E. F., J. D. DECRISTOFARO & G. WEISINGER. 1989. Ontogeny of the opiate phenotype: An approach to defining transsynaptic mechanisms at the molecular level in the rat adrenal medulla. Int. J. Dev. Neurosci. **7:** 499–511.
13. RESCO, J. A., H. H. FEDER & R. W. GOY. 1968. Androgen concentrations in plasma and testis of developing rats. J. Endocrinol. **40:** 485–491.
14. THOENEN, H., R. A. MUELLER & J. AXELROD. 1969. Increased tyrosine hydroxylase activity after drug induced alteration of sympathetic transmission. Nature **221:** 1264–1267.

Sodium Channel Regulation of Skeletal Muscle Membrane Excitability[a]

ROBERT L. RUFF[b]

Departments of Neurology and Neurosciences
Cleveland Veterans Administration Medical Center
Case Western Reserve University Medical School
Cleveland, Ohio 44106

INTRODUCTION

Membrane depolarization activates Na^+ channels via conformation changes from closed, nonconducting states to an open, current-conducting state. With continued depolarization Na^+ current (I_{Na}) declines due to fast inactivation.[1,2] The declining portion of I_{Na} elicited by a prolonged depolarization results from late openings of Na^+ channels and transition of open channels to a nonconducting fast-inactivated state.[2] Na^+ channels can also transit directly between closed and fast-inactivated states.[2] Inactivated channels do not open when the membrane is depolarized. The transition rate from the open to the fast-inactivated state is independent of voltage over part of its operative range,[3] and the transition rate increases for potentials more positive than about -30 mV.[2] The transition rate from the closed to the fast-inactivated state increases with depolarization.[4]

Mammalian skeletal muscle has two inactivation processes with different kinetics and voltage dependencies.[5-10] Fast inactivation closes channels on a millisecond time scale, whereas slow inactivation (SI) takes seconds to minutes. In rat and human skeletal muscle, fast inactivation helps to terminate the action potential (AP).[6] SI is too slow to affect AP termination. However, SI operates at more negative potentials than fast inactivation, so that the distribution of channels between the closed and slow-inactivated state regulates the number of excitable Na^+ channels as a function of the membrane potential.[2,5-9,11]

Fast inactivation and SI represent different conformations of the Na^+ channel.[2,12] Gating charge studies suggest that distinct conformation changes are associated with transition from the closed states of the Na^+ channel to states associated with fast inactivation or SI.[13-17] Protease treatment of the intracellular side of a cell membrane or other chemical treatments can selectively alter SI or fast inactivation.[18-22] SI represents the accumulation of Na^+ channels into an inexcitable state, the slow-inactivated state.[23] SI changes the number of excitable channels. SI does not change the single-channel conductance or single-channel open time.

[a] This work was supported by the Office of Research and Development, Medical Research Service of the Department of Veterans Affairs, and the Muscular Dystrophy Association.

[b] Address correspondence to Dr. R. L. Ruff, Chief, Neurology Service 127(W), Cleveland VAMC, 10701 East Boulevard, Cleveland, OH 44106.

Mammalian skeletal muscle fibers are characterized physiologically and histochemically as fast-twitch-glycolytic (type IIb), fast-oxidative-glycolytic (type IIa), or slow-oxidative (type I) fibers.[6–9,11,24,25] The quantity and composition of myofibrillar and soluble proteins vary among these three fiber types. The calcium-tension relationships of type I, IIa, and IIb fiber contractile proteins differ.[24,25] Myosin heavy chains differ among type I, IIa, and IIb fibers.[24] Motor units composed of type I, IIa or IIb fibers have different contractile properties and fatigue resistances.[26] Type IIb motor units function at higher firing frequencies and are more susceptible to fatigue than type I or type IIa motor units. Type I motor units operate at the lowest firing frequencies and are the least susceptible to fatigue.[26]

The density of Na^+ channels and the fraction of Na^+ channels that are excitable control the excitability of skeletal muscle membranes. The different firing patterns of type I, IIa, and IIb fibers create distinct demands on membrane excitability. Type IIb fibers need to fire at high rates, but do not have to sustain excitability for prolonged periods. Type I fibers have to remain excitable during prolonged low-frequency firing.[6–9]

In this paper, we examine how SI and Na^+ channel density and distribution vary among skeletal muscle fiber types. We will show that the characteristics of Na^+ channel voltage-dependent gating and distribution of Na^+ channels enable each type of skeletal muscle fiber to have a unique firing pattern.

METHODS

Muscle preparation. Intercostal muscle specimens with intact fibers came from patients undergoing a thoracotomy.[7,8,9,27] The patients gave informed consent according to a protocol approved by the Institutional Review Board of the Department of Veterans Affairs Medical Center in Cleveland. Soleus, adductor longus, extensor digitorum longus (EDL) and omohyoid muscles were obtained from male rats (290–320 g) according to a protocol approved by the Animal Subcommittee of the Institutional Review Board of the Department of Veterans Affairs Medical Center in Cleveland. Rats were anesthetized with intraperitoneal pentobarbital, selected muscles were removed, and the rats were killed by pentobarbital overdose. Dissection techniques and enzymatic treatment to remove the nerve terminal from the end plate have been previously described.[6–9] The bathing solution for the muscles contained (mM): 115 NaCl, 3.5 KCl, 25 $NaHCO_3$, 1 NaH_2PO_4, 1 $MgCl_2$, 6 $CaCl_2$, and 12 glucose. The solutions were continually gassed with 95% O_2, 5% CO_2, and were at pH 7.4. The dissections and experiments were performed at 23 ± 1 °C.

Fiber types were determined by histochemistry for rat and human fibers using previously described techniques.[7,8,9,24,25,28,29]

Loose-patch voltage clamp. The technical details of the loose-patch voltage clamp technique used to measure I_{Na} and membrane capacitance (C_m) were previously described.[6,11]

Measurement of membrane current. The muscle fibers were visualized with Nomarski optics using an inverted microscope with a fixed stage. The patch pipette was gently pressed against the muscle surface at an area of interest. Suction applied to the micropipette was monitored with a manometer and kept to <10 cm H_2O to avoid the formation of membrane blebs.[11] Even with the small amount of suction used, seal resistances were greater than 2 MΩ for all cells. A potential applied to the micropipette changed the transmembrane potential of the small patch of membrane under the pipette. Analogue and digital corrections compensated for the current that flowed across the seal between the pipette and the sarcolemma so that transmembrane potential was controlled and the transmembrane current measured.[6] The details of the stimulating pulse protocols used to measure I_{Na} have been previously described.[6,11]

$I_{Na,max}$ was measured at three different regions: (1) the end-plate border, (2) >200 μm from the end plate (extrajunctional membrane), and (3) on the end-plate postsynaptic membrane. Within each region current was measured at three or more different sites. I_{Na} amplitudes were normalized to the cross-sectional area of the patch pipette orifice or the capacitance of the patch of membrane from which currents were recorded. The membrane depolarization that produced the largest inward I_{Na}, $V_{I,Na,max}$, the potential associated with closure of 50% of the Na^+ channels due to fast inactivation, $V_{h,1/2}$, and the steepness of voltage dependence of fast inactivation, A_h, were measured repeatedly during an experiment to determine changes in the membrane potential throughout an experiment. Current measurements were terminated if the membrane depolarized by more than 5 mV. The intracellular microelectrode indicated that the membrane potential changed by less than 4 mV for the largest currents evoked.

SI of I_{Na} was studied by measuring the magnitude and time course of the change in the maximal inward I_{Na}, $I_{Na,max}$, after the holding potential was changed.[6-9] To remove fast inactivation at a given holding potential, each of the test pulses used to define $I_{Na,max}$ was preceded by a 20-ms duration 50-mV hyperpolarizing prepulse. The holding potential at which the maximum $I_{Na,max}$ was obtained and the relative value of $I_{Na,max}$ at other holding potentials for fibers within a given group were plotted together and fit with a Boltzmann distribution:

$$S_\infty = I_{Na,max}/\text{Maximum } I_{Na,max} = 1/[1 + \exp([V_m - V_{s,1/2}]A_s)] \tag{1}$$

where $I_{Na,max}/\text{Maximum}_{Na,max}$ is the steady state $I_{Na,max}$ obtained at a given holding potential relative to the maximum $I_{Na,max}$ that could be obtained when SI was completely removed, $V_{s,1/2}$ is the potential at which 50% of Na^+ channels are closed due to SI, and A_S describes the steepness of the voltage dependence of SI.

Resting potentials were measured in each cell after current recordings were completed using an intracellular microelectrode filled with 3M KCl and having a resistance of 10–20 mΩ. The intracellular pipette was located 0.1 to 0.15 mm from the patch electrode. $V_{I,Na,max}$ and V_h were measured before and after impalement with the voltage electrode to determine the depolarization produced by the impalement.[6,11] The actual resting potential was the potential measured by the voltage electrode minus the depolarization associated with the impalement, which was <5 mV.[6,11]

AP threshold and AP overshoot potentials of rat omohyoid fibers were measured *in vitro* as previously described.[10,30] Two microelectrodes, one for passing current and the other for recording membrane potential, were used to measure AP threshold and overshoot. The electrodes were positioned within 20 μm of each other and connected to a voltage-clamp amplifier (Axoclamp 2A, Axon Instruments, Foster City, CA). The AP amplitude and threshold were determined using depolarizing current pulses of gradually increasing amplitude.

Statistical analysis. Data were analyzed with analysis of variance (ANOVA) using two-tailed tests with alpha set at 0.05. When significant interactions were present post hoc comparisons between different groups were made using Tukey's Honestly Significant Difference Test.[31] Values are expressed as means ± SE.

RESULTS

SI Affects I_{Na} on Fast-Twitch Muscle Fibers More Than Slow-Twitch Muscle Fibers

SI was operative at more negative potentials than was true for fast inactivation (FIG. 1). For rat or human fibers, $V_{s,1/2}$ occurred at more negative potentials for fast-twitch than slow-twitch fibers (TABLE 1, $p < 0.001$). For rat and human fast-twitch muscle fibers, $V_{s,1/2}$ occurred at about the resting potential, whereas for rat and human slow-twitch fibers $V_{s,1/2}$ was 13 to 14 mV more positive than the resting potential (TABLE 1, FIG. 1). $V_{s,1/2}$ occurred at about the resting potential for both rat EDL, rat omohyoid, and human fast-twitch muscle fibers even though the resting potentials of EDL fibers were 14 mV more negative than the other fast-twitch fibers (TABLE 1, FIG. 1). Consequently, SI reduced I_{Na} at the resting potential by about 50% for rat and human fast-twitch fibers, but SI had little impact on I_{Na} at the resting potential for slow-twitch fibers (FIG. 1). At their resting potentials fast-twitch fibers were at the middle of the steep portion of the S_∞-membrane potential relationship and slow-twitch fibers operated on the upper knee of the S_∞-potential relationship (FIG. 1). Therefore, small changes in the resting membrane potentials of fast-twitch fibers produced larger changes in I_{Na} for fast-twitch fibers compared with slow-twitch fibers.

I_{Na} Was Larger on the End Plate and the End-Plate Border Than on Extrajunctional Membrane and Larger on Fast-Twitch Compared with Slow-Twitch Fibers

The maximum I_{Na} obtained from a region of membrane when fast inactivation and SI of I_{Na} were removed by membrane hyperpolarization, $I_{Na,max}$, differed among the three regions studied (TABLE 1, FIG. 2). $I_{Na,max}$ normalized to the area of the patch pipette (mA cm^{-2}) was largest at the end plate, intermediate at the end-plate border, and smallest on extrajunctional membrane. C_m is a measure of the actual membrane area with a smooth, unfolded membrane having a capacitance of 1 μF cm^{-2}.[32] C_m (μF cm^{-2}) was largest at the end plate, intermediate at the end-plate border, and smallest on extrajunctional membrane (FIG. 2). $I_{Na,max}$ normalized to C_m (mA μF^{-1}), which provides a measure of the number of channels per unit area of actual membrane, was similar at the end plate and the end-plate border and smallest on extrajunctional membrane (TABLE 1, FIG. 2).

Fast-twitch fibers had larger $I_{Na,max}$ on the end plate, the end-plate border and extrajunctional membrane compared with slow-twitch fibers (TABLE 1). $I_{Na,max}$ normalized to C_m was about fivefold larger on the end plate and the end-plate border membrane compared with extrajunctional membrane for fast-twitch fibers and about threefold larger on end plate and end-plate border membrane for slow-twitch fibers (TABLE 1; $p < 0.001$). On the end-plate border and the end plate, $I_{Na,max}$ was four- to fivefold larger on fast- compared to slow-twitch fibers (TABLE 1; $p < 0.001$). On extrajunctional membrane, $I_{Na,max}$ was about twofold larger on fast- compared to slow-twitch fibers (TABLE 1, FIG. 2; $p < 0.001$). For a given membrane region and fiber type, $I_{Na,max}$ was similar on rat and human skeletal muscle fibers. For a given membrane region, $I_{Na,max}$ was larger on type IIb compared to type IIa human skeletal muscle fibers (TABLE 1; $p < 0.01$ for the end plate, $p < 0.05$ for the end-plate border and extrajunctional membrane).

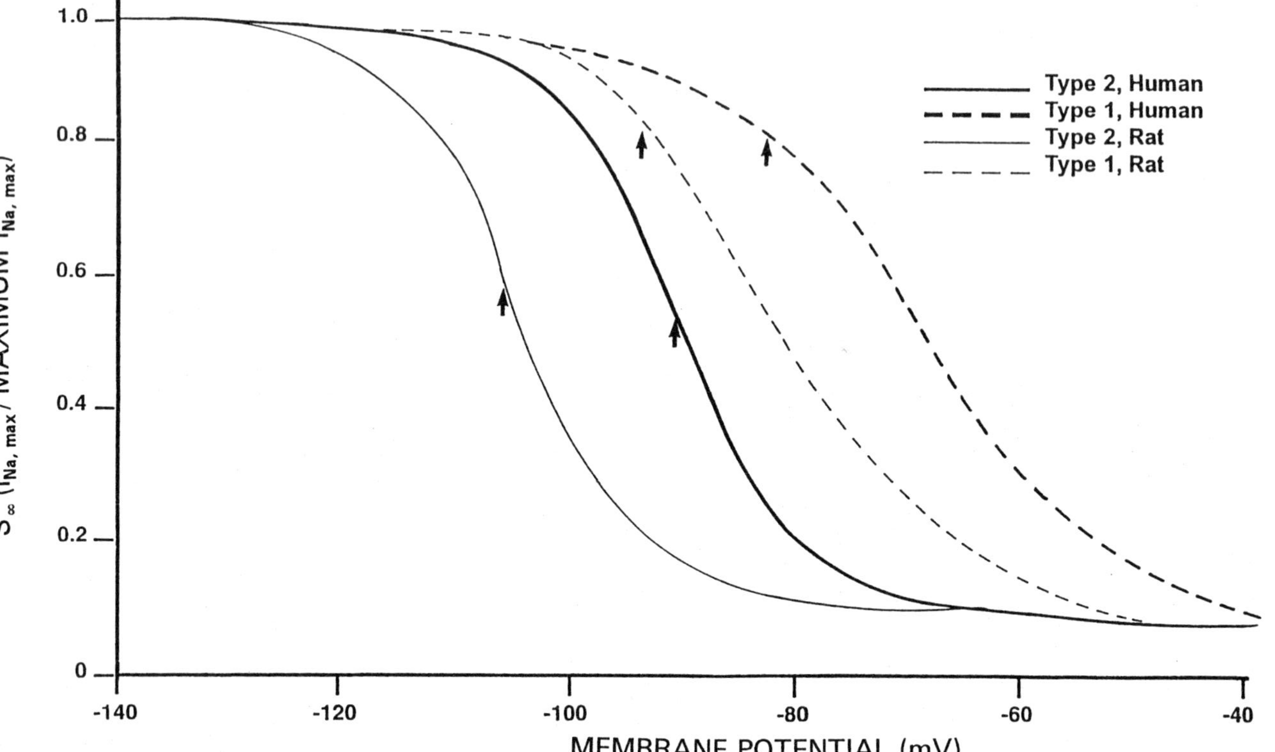

FIGURE 1. The voltage dependence of SI of $I_{Na,max}$ for human intercostal (*thick lines*) and rat (*thin*) fast (*thin, solid lines*) and slow (*thin, dashed lines*) twitch muscle fibers. The rat muscles studied were the fast-twitch EDL and the slow-twitch soleus muscles. The maximum value of $I_{Na,max}$ for each fiber was obtained by hyperpolarizing the membrane to a potential more negative than -140 mV. The curves are least squares fits of Eq. 1 to the data. $V_{s,1/2}$ was human fast-twitch fibers, -93.4 mV; human slow-twitch fibers, -71.5 mV; rat fast-twitch fibers, -108 mV; and rat slow-twitch fibers, -84.4 mV. A_s was human fast-twitch fibers, 5.6 mV; human slow-twitch fibers, 8.7 mV; rat fast-twitch fibers, 5.8 mV; and rat slow-twitch fibers 8.7 mV. The resting membrane potentials of the different types of fibers are indicated by arrows pointing to the membrane potential–S_∞ relationship of a given fiber type. The values of $V_{s,1/2}$, A_s, and resting potential were different among the four groups of fibers ($p < 0.001$ for A_s and $V_{s,1/2}$; $p < 0.05$ for resting potentials). (From Ruff.[10] Reprinted with permission from *Acta Physiologica Scandinavica*.)

TABLE 1. Comparison of I_{Na} Amplitude and Gating of Fast- and Slow-Twitch Rat and Human Skeletal Muscle Fibers

	Voltage-Dependent Gating of I_{Na}			
	RP (mV)	$V_{I,Na,max}$ (mV)	$V_{h,1/2}$ (mV)	$V_{s,1/2}$ (mV)
Rat				
Fast twitch (23 fibers)	-95.1 $\pm$ 1.6	-24.1 $\pm$ 1.5	-76.9 $\pm$ 0.6	-98.1 $\pm$ 1.9
Slow twitch (24 fibers)	-89.6 $\pm$ 1.1	-18.4 $\pm$ 0.5	-68.1 $\pm$ 0.8	-76.2 $\pm$ 1.8
Human				
Fast twitch (31 fibers)	-93.2 $\pm$ 0.8	-28.3 $\pm$ 0.6	-70.5 $\pm$ 0.8	-93.3 $\pm$ 1.9
Slow twitch (29 fibers)	-85.3 $\pm$ 0.8	-19.3 $\pm$ 0.7	-60.7 $\pm$ 0.7	-71.6 $\pm$ 1.8
Type IIa (10 fibers)	-94.5 $\pm$ 1.2	-28.3 $\pm$ 1.2	-68.0 $\pm$ 0.4	-93.4 $\pm$ 2.1
Type IIb (11 fibers)	-92.6 $\pm$ 1.3	-29.5 $\pm$ 1.4	-73.9 $\pm$ 0.8	-93.3 $\pm$ 2.0

I_{Na} Amplitude on the End Plate, End-Plate Border, and Extrajunctional Membrane		
E-$I_{Na,max}$ (mA μF^{-1})	EB-$I_{Na,max}$ (mA μF^{-1})	EJ-$I_{Na,max}$ (mA μF^{-1})
Rat		
Fast twitch (12 fibers): 26.5 $\pm$ 1.7	26.1 $\pm$ 1.2	4.33 $\pm$0.39
Slow twitch (12 fibers): 6.94 $\pm$ 0.59	6.75 $\pm$ 0.54	2.20 $\pm$0.31
Human		
Fast twitch (11 fibers): 23.5 $\pm$ 2.2	27.3 $\pm$ 2.5	4.87 $\pm$0.62
Slow twitch (10 fibers): 5.51 $\pm$ 0.67	6.18 $\pm$ 0.51	1.89 $\pm$0.29
Type IIa (10 fibers): 19.6 $\pm$ 1.4	23.7 $\pm$ 1.5	4.01 $\pm$ .41
Type IIb (11 fibers): 26.9 $\pm$ 1.5	30.3 $\pm$ 2.7	5.84 $\pm$0.38

RP, resting potential; E, end plate; EB, end-plate border; EJ, extrajunctional membrane. (Data is based upon Ruff.[10])

AP Rate of Rise Was Faster and the AP Threshold Was Lower on the End-Plate Border Compared with Extrajunctional Membrane for Fast-Twitch Fibers

We measured the AP threshold, rate of rise and overshoot at the end-plate border and on extrajunctional membrane of rat fast-twitch omohyoid muscle fibers (TABLE 2).[10] The resting potentials and AP overshoot potentials were similar. The

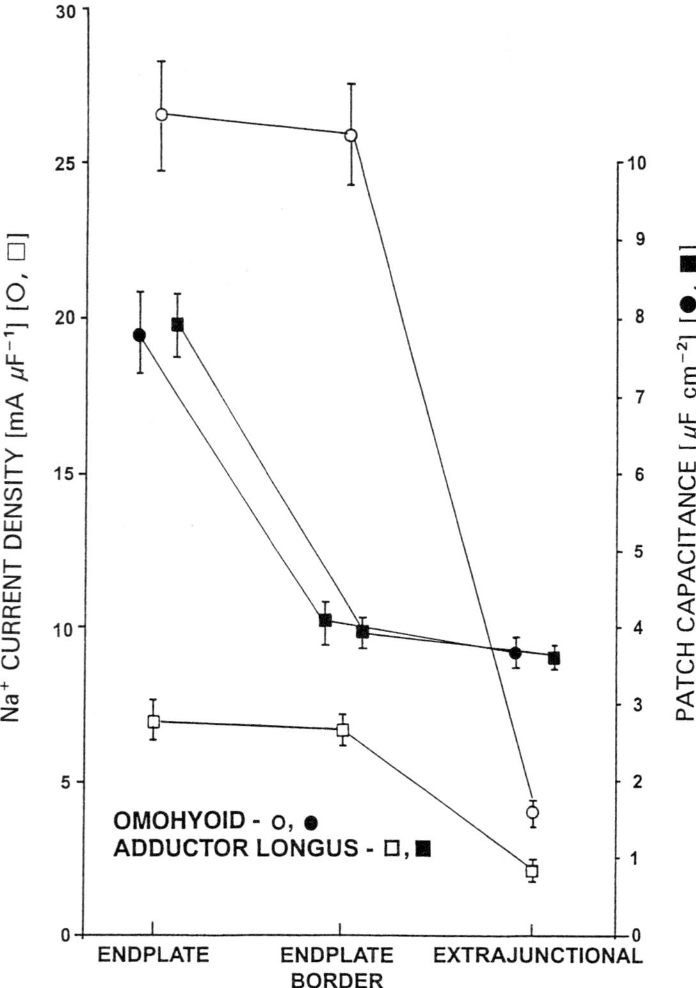

FIGURE 2. $I_{Na,max}$ amplitude (normalized to C_m; *unfilled symbols*) and C_m (*filled symbols*) on the end plate, the end-plate border, and extrajunctional membrane of fast-twitch omohyoid (*circles*) and slow-twitch adductor longus (*squares*) fibers. The symbols indicate mean ± SE for 39–45 measurements from 12 omohyoid and 12 adductor longus fibers. $I_{Na,max}$ on omohyoid fibers was greater than on adductor longus fibers for each of the three regions studied ($p <$ 0.001). The end plate or end-plate border current densities of either adductor longus or omohyoid fibers were greater than the extrajunctional current densities ($p < 0.001$). The end plate and end-plate border current densities were not different for adductor longus or omohyoid fibers. C_m on the end plate was significantly larger than on the end-plate border or on extrajunctional membrane for omohyoid or adductor longus fibers ($p < 0.001$). At each of the three regions, $I_{Na,max}$ was larger on omohyoid fibers ($p < 0.001$), but C_m values for adductor longus and omohyoid fibers for each region were similar. (From Ruff.[10] Reproduced with permission from *Acta Physiologica Scandinavica*.)

TABLE 2. Resting Membrane Potential and Action Potential Properties on the End-Plate Border Compared to Extrajunctional Membrane for 29 Rat Omohyoid Muscle Fibers[a]

	RP (mV)	AP Threshold (mV)	AP dV/dt (Vs^{-1})	AP Overshoot (mV)
End-plate border	−95.2 ± 1.9	25.6 ± 2.1	589 ± 24	34.4 ± 3.0
Extrajunctional	−95.5 ± 1.6	36.8 ± 2.0	347 ± 18	34.2 ± 2.9
		$p < 0.001$	$p < 0.001$	

[a] RP, resting potential; AP, action potential. AP properties: AP threshold is the depolarization from the RP required to trigger an AP. AP dV/dt is the maximum rate of rise of the AP. AP overshoot is the most positive membrane potential achieved by the AP.

(Data in the table is based upon Ruff.[10])

threshold depolarization required to trigger an AP was about 11 mV smaller on the end-plate border compared to extrajunctional membrane. The maximal rate of rise of the AP, dV/dt, was more than 1.5-fold larger on the end-plate border compared to extrajunctional membrane.

DISCUSSION

In this paper it was demonstrated that (1) slow-twitch fibers were resistant to SI, (2) I_{Na} was larger on fast-twitch fibers, (3) I_{Na} was larger near the end plate, (4) AP threshold was lower on the end-plate border compared to extrajunctional membrane, and (5) the rate of rise of the AP was faster on the end-plate border compared to extrajunctional membrane. The Na^+ channel gating and distribution may partially enable fast-twitch fibers to fire at high rates for brief periods and slow-twitch fibers to fire tonically at low rates.

SI Regulation of Membrane Excitability

I_{Na} amplitude in mammalian skeletal muscle is controlled by the density of excitable Na^+ channels in a given region. SI of I_{Na} regulates the fraction of Na^+ channels that are excitable based upon the membrane potential. The voltage dependence of SI varies with skeletal muscle fiber type.[6–10] Slow-twitch fibers had more positive values for resting potential, $V_{I,Na,max}$, $V_{h,1/2}$, and $V_{s,1/2}$ compared to fast-twitch fibers (TABLE 1, FIG. 1).[6–8] Type IIb fibers developed fast inactivation at more negative potentials than type IIa fibers (TABLE 1; $p < 0.005$). The steady-state voltage dependence of SI was similar for IIa and IIb fibers (TABLE 1).[9] The maximum I_{Na} away from the end plate on slow-twitch fibers was less than half of that found in fast-twitch fibers.[6–8] Because of the greater effect of SI on fast-twitch fibers, the I_{Na} available at the resting potential on extrajunctional membrane was similar for fast- and slow-twitch fibers. Consequently, SI regulates the excitability of skeletal muscle fibers based upon the resting potential.

A portion of the fatigue that develops in muscles stimulated or spontaneously contracting at >20 Hz comes from reduced muscle fiber excitability associated with muscle fiber depolarization.[9,33–35] The fatigue resistance of human muscle fibers to stimulation at frequencies >20 Hz[36] parallels the resistance of the fibers to fast inactivation and SI. Slow-twitch motor units in mammals are active *in vivo* at 10–20 Hz.[26] In contrast, motor units composed of type IIa fibers are phasically active at 40–90 Hz, and motor units composed of type IIb fibers are briefly active at rates exceeding 200 Hz.[26] At higher rates of stimulation, K^+ may accumulate in the muscle fiber extracellular space, resulting in membrane depolarization and Na^+ channel inactivation.[6–8] Type IIb muscle fibers may be more susceptible to use-related decrease in membrane excitability in part because fast inactivation and SI occur at more negative membrane potentials in IIb fibers compared with type I or IIa fibers (TABLE 1).[9] Na^+ channel inactivation may provide a peripheral mechanism that limits how long a fiber can fire at high rates to protect them from exhaustion or injury associated with prolonged high-frequency contraction.[37] Na^+ channel susceptibility to inactivation may enable fast-twitch fibers to operate only briefly at high rates and slow-twitch fibers to fire tonically at lower rates.

Fast-Twitch Muscle Fibers Have More Na^+ Channels on Extrajunctional Membrane Than Slow-Twitch Fibers

$I_{Na,max}$ and the natural AP firing frequency are closely correlated for each histochemical type of skeletal muscle fiber.[7–9,11] On extrajunctional membrane the $I_{Na,max}$ amplitudes are largest for type IIb fibers and smallest for type I fibers (TABLE 1; $p < 0.01$ for type IIb versus type IIa and $p < 0.001$ for fast- versus slow-twitch fibers).[6–9,11] The natural firing frequencies of motor units are arranged in the same order as the I_{Na} densities of the muscle fibers. Motor units made of type I fibers fire at the lowest rates and motor units composed of type IIb fibers fire at the highest rates.[26] Therefore, Na^+ channel distribution plays an important role in the way a muscle fiber adapts to its work load.[9] Fast-twitch fibers may also need higher densities of Na^+ channels than do slow-twitch fibers because fast-twitch fibers require larger depolarizations to initiate contraction compared with type I fibers.[38,39] Of interest, continuous activity, similar to the tonic firing of type I fibers, reduces the level of expression of the Na^+ channel α-subunit mRNA in developing muscle fibers so that a muscle fiber activity pattern may influence Na^+ channel production and perhaps distribution.[40]

Na^+ Channels Are Concentrated Near the End Plate More Prominently on Fast-Twitch Than Slow-Twitch Muscle Fibers

$I_{Na,max}$ and C_m were largest on the end plate and smallest on extrajunctional membrane, and $I_{Na,max}$, normalized to C_m, was the same on the end plate and on the end-plate border (TABLE 1, FIG. 2). Because $I_{Na,max}$ is a measure of the number of Na^+ channels and C_m is proportional to actual membrane area,[7,11] the Na^+ channel density normalized to actual membrane area is similar on the end plate and the end-plate border.[11] The data are consistent with morphological studies indicating that Na^+ channels are concentrated and immobilized in the end-plate region particularly in the depths of the synaptic folds and end-plate border membrane.[41–45] The voltage-dependent characteristics of Na^+ channel gating were the same at and away from the end plate. Consequently, it is likely that the increased I_{Na} on the end plate and the end-plate border results from an increase in Na^+ channel number and not a different population of channels in the end-plate region.

The density of Na^+ channels at the end plate depended upon fiber type (TABLE 1, FIG. 2).[8-11] Fast-twitch fibers had a higher density of Na^+ channels at all regions than did slow-twitch fibers (TABLE 1; $p < 0.001$),[8,11] and IIb fibers had more Na^+ channels than IIa fibers (TABLE 1; $p < 0.005$).[9,10]

The high firing rates of fast-twitch motor units makes them more susceptible to compromise of neuromuscular transmission due to depletion of readily releasable vesicles of transmitter from the nerve terminal.[11] A high concentration of Na^+ channels on the end plate and the end-plate border of fast-twitch fibers increases the safety factor for neuromuscular transmission of fast-twitch fibers by reducing the threshold for AP generation near the end plate of fast-twitch fibers (TABLE 2). The larger I_{Na} at the end plate and the end-plate border permits fast-twitch fibers to operate at high firing sequences.[7-11] Other studies also found that the rate of rise of the AP was faster near the end plate.[46-48]

Role of Fast Inactivation and SI in Hyperkalemic Periodic Paralysis with Myotonia

The primary periodic paralyses are autosomal dominant muscle diseases characterized by episodic attacks of muscle paralysis. They are classified according to changes in serum $[K^+]$ as hypokalemic, hyperkalemic or normokalemic periodic paralysis.[1,2,49-52] Hyperkalemic periodic paralysis can be subclassified based upon the presence of myotonia. In all forms of periodic paralysis, paralysis is associated with modest sarcolemmal depolarization and Na^+ channel inexcitability.[49,50] A persistent inward current produces the depolarization. In hyperkalemic periodic paralysis with myotonia, the inward current is completely blocked by tetrodotoxin and is clearly a noninactivating Na^+ current.[53] In several families, hyperkalemic periodic paralysis with or without myotonia is genetically tightly linked to SCN4A, the skeletal muscle Na^+ channel gene.[54] Several α-subunit point mutations have been identified in hyperkalemic periodic paralysis.[1,2,51,52]

Several mutations producing hyperkalemic periodic paralysis and myotonia showed persistent I_{Na} attributed to (1) disrupted fast inactivation[1,51,52] and (2) "window" currents created by shifting the voltage dependence of activation[12] or activation and inactivation,[55] resulting in a voltage range over which some channels will open and not fast inactivate. Inhibition of fast inactivation is sufficient to produce myotonia. However, SI must be inhibited in hyperkalemic periodic paralysis for persistent I_{Na} and hence paralysis lasting from minutes to hours (the typical duration of paralytic attacks).[56] SI was disrupted in the most common mutation associated with hyperkalemic periodic paralysis and myotonia.[12] The difference between Na^+ channel mutations that produce only myotonia and those that produce prolonged depolarization-induced paralysis and myotonia may be that SI must be disrupted to produce prolonged depolarization-induced paralysis.[2,56]

Importance of Na⁺ Channels at the End Plate in Myasthenia Gravis

Myasthenia gravis (MG) is an autoimmune disease in which antibodies are produced against the skeletal muscle AChR and possibly other elements in the muscle membrane portion of the end plate.[57] MG is characterized by weakness and fatigability with preferential involvement of extraocular muscles.[58] The number of

AChRs at the end plate is reduced due to complement-mediated membrane lysis and increased AChR turnover due to antibody cross-linking of AChRs.[57]

The safety factor (SF) for neuromuscular transmission can be defined as:

$$SF = EPP/(E_M - E_{AP}) \tag{2}$$

where EPP is the end-plate potential amplitude, E_M is the membrane potential, and E_{AP} is the action potential threshold.[57] The increased Na^+ channel density at and near the end plate raises the SF for neuromuscular transmission by lowering the threshold for AP generation at the end plate.[10,30]

Na^+ channels are lost from the end-plate region in MG.[59] The Na^+ channels are probably lost due to destruction of the synaptic folds caused by autoimmune attack at the end plate. The AP threshold at the end plate is increased in MG (Ruff, unpublished data). Therefore, the loss of end-plate Na^+ channels in MG contributes to the neuromuscular transmission defect by decreasing the SF for neuromuscular transmission. End-plate damage may also cause focal depolarization that will further reduce the available I_{Na} at the end plate because of depolarization-induced SI of I_{Na}.

REFERENCES

1. BARCHI, R. L. 1995. Molecular pathology of the skeletal muscle sodium channel. Annu. Rev. Physiol. **57:** 355–385.
2. RUFF, R. L. & M. H. MURAD. 1997. Voltage-gated sodium channels. *In* Encyclopedia of Neuroscience. G. Adelman & B. Smith, Eds. Elsevier Science B.V. Amsterdam. In press.
3. ALDRICH, R. W. & C. F. STEVENS. 1987. Voltage-dependent gating of single sodium channels from mammlian neuroblastoma cells. J. Neurosci. **7:** 418–431.
4. RAYNER, M. D., J. G. STARKUS, P. C. RUBEN & D. A. ALICATA. 1992. Voltage-sensitive and solvent-sensitive processes in ion channel gating. Kinetic effects of hyperosmolar media on activation and deactivation of sodium channels. Biophys. J. **61:** 96–108.
5. RUFF, R. L., L. SIMONCINI & W. STÜHMER. 1987. Comparison between slow sodium channel inactivation in rat slow and fast twitch muscle. J. Physiol. (Lond.) **383:** 339–348.
6. RUFF, R. L., L. SIMONCINI & W. STÜHMER. 1988. Slow sodium channel inactivation in mammalian muscle: A possible role in regulating excitability. Muscle Nerve **11:** 502–510.
7. RUFF, R. L. & D. WHITTLESEY. 1992. Na^+ current densities and voltage dependence in human intercostal muscle fibers. J. Physiol. (Lond.) **458:** 85–97.
8. RUFF, R. L. & D. WHITTLESEY. 1993. Na^+ currents near and away from endplates on human fast and slow twitch muscle fibers. Muscle Nerve **16:** 922–929.
9. RUFF, R. L. & D. WHITTLESEY. 1993. Comparison of Na^+ currents from type IIa and IIb human intercostal muscle fibers. Am. J. Physiol. **265** (Cell Physiol. **34**): C171–C177.
10. RUFF, R. L. 1996. Sodium channel slow inactivation and the distribution of sodium channels on skeletal muscle fibres enable the performance properties of different skeletal muscle fibre types. Acta Physiol. Scand. **156:** 159–168.
11. RUFF, R. L. 1992. Na current density at and away from end plates on rat fast- and slow-twitch skeletal muscle fibers. Am. J. Physiol. **262** (Cell Physiol. **31**): C229–C234.
12. CUMMINS, T. R. & F. J. SIGWORTH. 1996. Impaired slow inactivation in mutant sodium channels. Biophys. J. **71:** 227–236.
13. BEKKERS, J. M., I. C. FORSTER & N. G. GREEFF. 1990. Gating current associated with inactivated states of the squid axon sodium channel. Proc. Natl. Acad. Sci. USA **87:** 8311–8315.
14. RUBEN, P. C., J. G. STARKUS & M. D. RAYNER. 1990. Holding potential affects the apparent voltage-sensitivity of sodium channel activation in crayfish giant axons. Biophys. J. **58:** 1169–1181.
15. RUBEN, P. C., J. G. STARKUS & M. D. RAYNOR. 1992. Steady-state availability of sodium

channels. Interactions between activation and slow inactivation. Biophys. J. **61:** 941–946.

16. BEZANILLA, F., R. E. TAYLOR & J. M. FERNANDEZ. 1982. Distribution and kinetics of membrane dielectric polarization. I. Long-term inactivation of gating currents. J. Gen. Physiol. **79:** 21–40.
17. MEVES, H. & W. VOGEL. 1977. Slow recovery of sodium current and "gating current" from inactivation. J. Physiol. **267:** 395–410.
18. STARKUS, J. G. & P. SHRAGER. 1978. Modification of slow sodium inactivation in nerve after internal perfusion with trypsin. Am. J. Physiol. **235:** C238–C244.
19. ARMSTRONG, C. M. 1981. Sodium channels and gating currents. Physiol. Rev. **61:** 644–683.
20. OXFORD, G. S. 1981. Some kinetic and steady-state properties of sodium channels after removal of inactivation. J. Gen. Physiol. **77:** 1–22.
21. QUANDT, F. N. 1988. Modification of slow inactivation of single sodium channels by phenytoin in neuroblastoma cells. Mol. Pharmacol. **34:** 557–565.
22. RUDY, B. 1981. Inactivation in *Myxicola* giant axons responsible for slow and accumulative adaptation phenomenon. J. Physiol. (Lond.) **283:** 1–21.
23. RUFF, R. L. 1997. The single channel basis of slow inactivation of Na$^+$ channels in rat skeletal muscle. Am. J. Physiol. (Cell Physiol. 40) **271:** C971–C981.
24. LASZEWSKI-WILLIAMS, B., R. L. RUFF & A. M. GORDON. 1989. Influence of fiber type and muscle source on the Ca^{2+} sensitivity of rat fibers. Am. J. Physiol. **256:** (Cell Physiol. **25**): C420–C427.
25. RUFF, R. L. & D. WHITTLESEY. 1991. Ca-, Sr-tension relationships and contraction velocities of human muscle fibers. Muscle Nerve **14:** 1219–1226.
26. HENNIG, R. & T. LØMO. 1985. Firing patterns of motor units in normal rats. Nature **314:** 164–166.
27. ALMERS, W., W. M. ROBERTS & R. L. RUFF. 1984. Voltage clamp of rat and human skeletal muscle: Measurements with an improved loose-patch clamp technique. J. Physiol. (Lond.) **347:** 751–768.
28. RUFF, R. L. 1989. Calcium sensitivity of fast and slow twitch human muscle fibers. Muscle Nerve **12:** 32–37.
29. RUFF, R. L. 1991. Ca-tension relationships of muscle fibers from patients with periodic paralysis. Muscle Nerve **14:** 838–844.
30. RUFF, R. L. 1997. Effects of length changes on Na$^+$ current amplitude and excitability near and far from the end-plate. Muscle Nerve **19:** 1084–1092.
31. KIRK, R. E. 1968. Experimental Design: Procedures for the Behavioral Sciences.: 68–79. Cole Publishing Co. Belmont, CA.
32. FALK, G. & P. FATT. 1964. Linear electrical properties of striated muscle fibres observed with intracellular electrodes. Proc. R. Soc. Lond. B. **160:** 69–158.
33. JUEL, C. 1986. Potassium and sodium shifts during in vitro isometric muscle contraction and the time course of the ion-gradient recovery. Pflügers Arch. **406:** 458–463.
34. JUEL, C. 1988. Muscle action potential propagation velocity changes during activity. Muscle Nerve **11:** 714–719.
35. BIGLAND-RITCHIE, B., D. A. JONES & J. J. WOODS. 1979. Excitation frequency and muscle fatigue: Electrical responses during human voluntary and stimulated contractions. Exp. Neurol. **64:** 414–427.
36. JONES, D. A. 1981. Muscle fatigue due to changes beyond the neuromuscular junction. *In* Human Muscle Fatigue: Physiological Mechanisms. R. Porter & J. Whelan, Eds.: 178–196. Ciba Foundation Symposium 82. Pitman Medical Press. London.
37. GRIMBY, L., J. HANNERZ & B. HEDMAN. 1981. The fatigue and voluntary discharge properties of single motor units in man. J. Physiol. (Lond.) **316:** 545–554.
38. DULHUNTY, A. F. 1980. Potassium contractures and mechanical aviation in mammalian skeletal muscles. J. Membr. Biol. **57:** 223–233.
39. LASZEWSKI, B. & R. L. RUFF. 1985. The effects of glucocorticoid treatment on excitation-contraction coupling. Am. J. Physiol. **248** (Endocrinol. Metab. **11**): E363–E369.
40. OFFORD, J. & W. A. CATTERALL. 1989. Electrical activity, cAMP and cytosolic calcium regulate mRNA encoding sodium channel α subunits in rat muscle cells. Neuron **2:** 1447–1452.

41. ANGELIDES, K. J. 1986. Fluorescently labeled Na$^+$ channels are localized and immobilized to synapses of innervated muscle fibres. Nature **321:** 63–66.
42. HAIMOVICH, B., D. L. SCHOTLAND, W. E. FIELES & R. L. BARCHI. 1987. Localization of sodium channel subtypes in rat skeletal muscle using channel-specific monoclonal antibodies. J. Neurosci. **7:** 2957–2966.
43. FLUCHER, B. E. & M. P. DANIELS. 1989. Distribution of Na$^+$ channels and ankyrin in neuromuscular junctions is complementary to that of acetylcholine receptors and the 43 kD protein. Neuron **3:** 163–175.
44. LE TEUT, T., J.-L. BOUDIER, E. JOVER & P. CAU. 1990. Localization of voltage-sensitive sodium channels on the extrasynaptic membrane surface of mouse skeletal muscle by autoradiography of scorpion toxin binding sites. J. Neurocytol. **19:** 408–420.
45. BOUDIER, J. L., T. LE TEUT & E. JOVER. 1992. Autoradiographic localization of voltage-dependent sodium channels on the mouse neuromuscular junction using ^{125}I-alpha scorpion toxin. II. Sodium channel distribution on postsynaptic membranes. J. Neurosci. **12:** 454–466.
46. BETZ, W. J., J. H. CALDWELL & S. C. KINNAMON. 1984. Increased sodium conductance in the synaptic region of rat skeletal muscle fibres. J. Physiol. (Lond.) **352:** 189–202.
47. THESLEFF, S., F. VYSKOCIL & M. R. WARD. 1974. The action potential in end-plate and extrajunctional regions of rat skeletal muscle. Acta Physiol. Scand. **91:** 196–202.
48. WOOD, S. J. & C. R. SLATER. 1995. Action potential generation in rat slow- and fast-twitch muscles. J. Physiol. (Lond.) **486:** 401–410.
49. RUFF, R. L. & A. M. GORDON. 1986. Disorders of muscle: The periodic paralyses. *In* Physiology of Membrane Disorders. T. E. Andreoli, D. D. Fanestil, J. F. Hoffman & S. G. Schultz, Eds.: 59–73. Plenum Medical Book Company. New York.
50. RÜDEL, R. & K. RICKER. 1985. The primary periodic paralyses. Trends Neurosci. **8:** 407–410.
51. CANNON, S. C. 1996. Ion channel defects and aberrant excitability in myotonia and periodic paralysis. Trends Neurosci. **19:** 3–10.
52. CANNON, S. C. 1996. Sodium channel defects in myotonia and periodic paralysis. Annu. Rev. Neurosci. **19:** 141–164.
53. RICKER, K., L. CAMACHO, P. GRAFE, F. LEHMAN-HORN & R. RÜDEL. 1989. Adynamia episodica hereditaria: What causes the weakness. Muscle Nerve **12:** 883–891.
54. MCCLATCHEY, A. I., J. TROFATTER, D. M. YASEK, W. RASKIND, T. BIRD, M. P. VANCE, J. GILCHRIST, K. ARAHATA, D. RADOSAVLJEVIC, H. G. WORTHEN, P. VAN DEN BERGH, J. L. HAINES, J. F. GUSELLA & R. H. BROWN. 1992. Dinucleotide repeat polymorphisms at the SCN4A locus suggest allelic heterogeneity of hyperkalemic periodic paralysis and paramyotonia congenita. Am. J. Hum. Genet. **50:** 896–901.
55. YANG, N., S. JI, M. ZHOU, L. J. PTACEK, R. L. BARCHI, R. HORN & A. L. GEORGE. 1994. Sodium channel mutations in paramyotonia congenita exhibit similar biophysical phenotypes *in vitro*. Proc. Natl. Acad. Sci. USA **91:** 12785–12789.
56. RUFF, R. L. 1994. Slow Na$^+$ channel inactivation must be disrupted to evoke prolonged depolarization-induced paralysis. Biophys. J. **66:** 542–545.
57. KAMINSKI, H. J. & R. L. RUFF. 1996. The myasthenic syndromes. *In* Physiology of Membrane Disorders. S. G. Schultz. T. E. Andreoli, A. M. Brown, D. Fambrough, J. F. HOFFMAN & M. Welsh, Eds. Plenum Publishing Co. New York.
58. KAMINSKI, H. J., E. MAAS, P. SPIEGEL & R. L. RUFF. 1990. Why are eye muscles frequently involved by myasthenia gravis? Neurology **40:** 1663–1669.
59. RUFF, R. L. & L. CORSILLO. 1994. Sodium channels near the endplate are lost in myasthenia gravis. Neurology **44:** A189.

The Effectiveness of Distal Synaptic Inputs on Neurons[a]

WAYNE E. CRILL[b]

Departments of Physiology and Biophysics, and Neurology
University of Washington
Seattle, Washington

Neurons serve as the fundamental units for information transfer in the brain. One characteristic of neurons, recognized for over a century, is their complex and variable structure. Unlike parenchymal cells in other organs, the physical shape of neurons shows great systematic diversity although neurons with similar input and projection have a comparable structure. Most neurons have extensive spatial dendritic fields, arranged in a spherical (stellate interneurons), radial (cortical pyramidal neurons) or planar pattern (cerebellar Purkinje cells). Although neurons have a wide variety of shapes, a few generalizations can be made relating their complex structures to information transfer. Nearly all of the synaptic input from many different neurons converges on the soma and dendrites. The spike-generating region of many neuron types is on the axon side of the soma. This allows the dendrites to provide a mechanism for spatially and temporally summing the synaptic input. This conceptual model, however, requires the effective transmission of current from distal dendritic synapses to the spike-generating region.

The cable model of electrical transmission is used to understand the flow of synaptic or impulse current along the cylindrical structures of the dendrites or axon.[1] This model was developed by Lord Kelvin to describe the flow of signals along undersea telegraph cables. For example, when depolarizing current flows into a dendrite through channels activated by synaptic transmitters, the current spreads in both directions along the cytoplasm of the dendritic cable. A fraction of the intradendritic current is lost at each point along the cable depending upon the relative resistance to current flow out through the membrane compared to flow down the dendrite. High membrane resistance favors transmission with a small loss of axial current, whereas low membrane resistance allows intracellular current to escape through the membrane, and synaptic current does not spread far. The capacitative properties of the membrane also filter rapidly changing synaptic inputs.[2] Based on this physical model, it was proposed in the 1950s[3] that much of the synaptic current from distal dendrites might not reach the spike-generating region in the proximal axon.[4] Rall's quantitative analysis of dendritic cable properties[1] showed that, on the average, synapses were not as electrically far from the soma as assumed by earlier researchers. Nonetheless, distal synapses would be much less effective than synapses close to the soma.

Spencer and Kandel[5] first described small dendritic all-or-none responses recorded in the soma. In the succeeding 35 years many experiments have provided

[a] This work was supported by National Institutes of Health Grant NS-16792 and the Keck Foundation.

[b] Address correspondence to Wayne E. Crill, M.D., Department Physiology and Biophysics, University of Washington, Seattle, WA 98195.

indirect and direct evidence for spikes generated by voltage-dependent conductances in the dendrites.[3] Investigators immediately realized that dendritic spikes could boost synaptic signals but this property would also complicate analysis of dendritic signaling. Action potentials generated at far sites and propagated to the soma and axon would remove the integrative benefits of a single summing site. However, voltage-dependent conductances in the dendrites need not generate all-or-nothing responses. Jack, Noble and Tsien[6] first called our attention to the amplification of signals in cable-like structures by graded voltage-dependent currents. For example, if the dendrite contains voltage-dependent potassium channels, depolarization of the dendrites will increase membrane conductance, and a larger fraction of the synaptic current will be lost before it can depolarize the spike-generating region of the neuron. On the other hand, voltage-dependent channels conducting inward current flow into the dendrite would add with the synaptic current flowing down the dendrite. Depending upon the type of voltage-dependent channels in the dendrites, the effectiveness of dendritic synapses compared to the passive dendrite can be either increased or decreased without the necessity of generating dendritic action potentials. It is likely that both hyperpolarizing potassium channels and depolarizing channels are present in the dendrites. Whether or not the synaptic current is attenuated or amplified depends on which dendritic conductance mechanism dominates.

Candidate conductance mechanisms for amplification of dendritic synaptic signals are the inward calcium and sodium currents. Stuart and Sakmann[7] directly measured transient sodium channel activity in dendrites and also demonstrated the retrograde propagation of action potentials from the soma after spike initiation. Transient sodium currents responsible for the action potential are inactivated rapidly and would not be expected to amplify tonic synaptic activity. Some authors have suggested that all-or-nothing responses in the dendrites might amplify synaptic signals, but the Stuart and Sakmann analysis[7] found that dendritic spikes only occur after activation of the spike-generating region on the axon side of the neuron. The precise effect of retrograde propagation of action potentials on synaptic efficacy during repetitive firing remains to be determined.

In our laboratory we had measured a tonic voltage-dependent inward current in neocortical pyramidal neuron.[8,9] It is tetrodotoxin (TTX) sensitive and is carried by sodium ions. The noninactivating sodium current (I_{NaP}) is responsible for depolarizing inward rectification[10] in hippocampal neurons and the plateau responses recorded in cerebellar Purkinje neurons.[11] Most investigators assumed the I_{NaP} flowed through a subtype of sodium channels with altered inactivation properties.[9,11–13] However, Alzheimer et al.[30] found no channels that consistently failed to inactivate. Rather, on-cell patches from neocortical neurons revealed that rare failures of inactivation occur in all sodium channels which is best explained by modal changes in sodium inactivation properties. That is, the transient and persistent sodium currents are carried by a single type of sodium channel. More than 99% of the depolarizations are associated with transient sodium channel opening, but in less than 1% of the depolarizations a channel continues to open during the entire depolarizing pulse. If one considers the large number of channels responding to a single depolarization, less than 1% of the sodium channels fail to inactivate, but even this small number of noninactivating channels produces a significant noninactivating depolarizing current.[14] This type of intermittent change in channel behavior is called modal gating. It is not a new idea because noninactivating sodium channels occur in skeletal[15] and cardiac muscle.[16] Because activation and inactivation of sodium channels are sequential[17] and are not independent properties of sodium channels, the I_{NaP} is first activated about 10 mV negative to resting potential.[18] The input resistance of the neuron is high at subthreshold potentials and relatively small currents, like I_{NaP}, flowing through the membrane resistance can cause appreciable voltage changes. It is at subthreshold voltages where summation of excitatory synaptic input brings the membrane potential to threshold.

These observations: the electrical remoteness of distal dendritic synapses, the theoretical support for potential amplification of excitatory synaptic currents by even, graded inward rectification, the demonstration of transient sodium channels in dendrites, and the putative identification of I_{NaP} as a modal change in transient channel gating led us to hypothesize that the dendrites of neocortical neurons (and probably other neuron types) have a noninactivating sodium conductance. If I_{NaP} dominates the voltage-dependent properties of dendrites, they would cause significant amplification of toxic excitatory inputs.

We tested the hypothesis that dendritic noninactivating sodium currents amplify synaptic current by iontophoresing glutamate at different distal sites on the dendrites of neocortical pyramidal neurons (FIG. 1A) to mimic synaptic activity. Iontophoresis was necessary because the test for sodium channel involvement is the application of TTX, which could alter synaptically evoked responses by affecting the number of active presynaptic fibers. The soma of the neuron receiving iontophoresed glutamate on the dendrite was voltage clamped with another electrode (FIG. 1A). With a voltage clamp an electronic circuit keeps the soma potential constant at a value determined by the experimenter and measures the amount of injected soma current that is needed to oppose the membrane current generated by the neuron. With spatially extensive dendrites a soma voltage clamp cannot keep the entire neuron at a known constant voltage. Only the soma and possibly the proximal dendrite are under voltage-clamp control, that is, isopotential. The voltage-clamp potential fades along the dendrites with distance from the soma. Glutamate applied to dendrite evokes an inward current that flows toward the soma. If it is not voltage clamped, the spike-generating region is depolarized and generates action potentials if threshold is reached. When the soma is voltage clamped the current from the iontophoretic site flows into the soma but membrane potential does not change because of the voltage clamp. The glutamate current is exactly counteracted by current injected through the voltage-clamp electrode. This prevents the glutamate current from depolarizing the spike-generating region and allows a direct measure of the current flowing into the voltage-clamp region, that is, the transmitted current from the dendrite to the soma.

FIGURE 1 shows the results of this type of experiment. FIGURE 1A is the experimental setup. Iontophoretic electrodes were located 145–555 μm from the soma. When the soma potential was held at -76 mV (resting potential) as in FIGURE 1B, the inward depolarizing current flowing during the iontophoresis did not change after application of TTX. There was no TTX-sensitive increase in transmitted current at resting potential. If the apical dendrite had voltage-sensitive sodium channels, the dendrite was not depolarized sufficiently to activate them. When the soma was depolarized to -61 mV, which also depolarized the dendrite between the soma and iontophoretic site, the glutamate current increased in magnitude. Since depolarization is moving the membrane potential toward the equilibrium potential for glutamate current (about zero potential), we would expect current flowing through glutamate-gated channels to actually decrease. The increase in magnitude with depolarization means there must be dendritic voltage-dependent amplification. Because that amplification is largely abolished by TTX and it occurs throughout a one-second iontophoresis, the increased current must be caused by noninactivating TTX-sensitive sodium channels. This TTX-sensitive amplification was present in all cells. In many cells adding the NMDA glutamate receptor blocker APV reduced the amplification somewhat.[19]

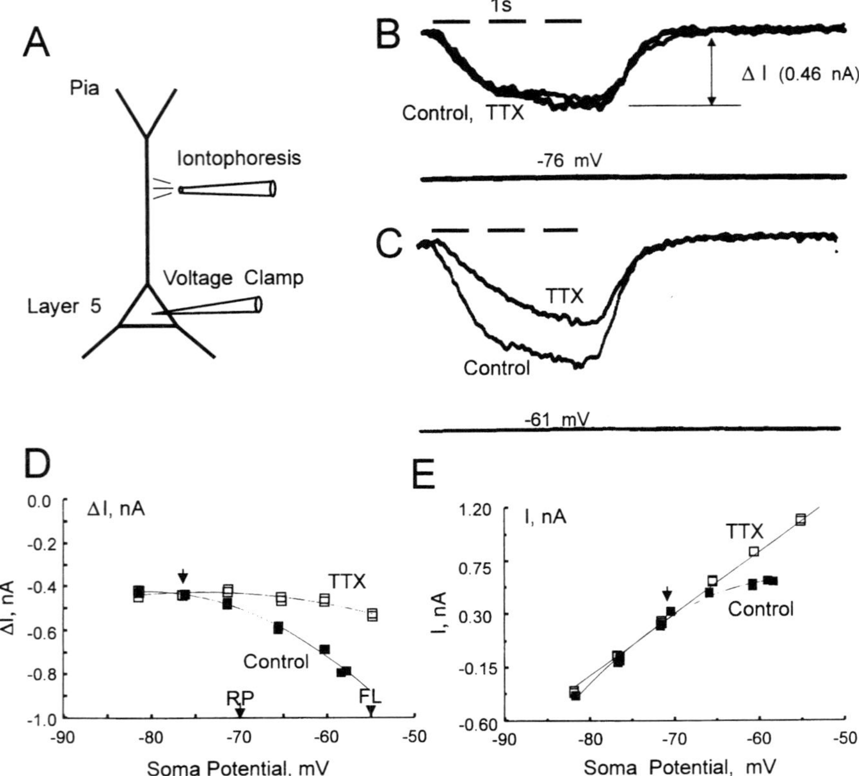

FIGURE 1. Voltage-dependent amplification of dendritic glutamate current. (**A**) Experimental setup. Glutamate is iontophoresed onto the dendrite of a voltage-clamped layer 5 pyramidal neuron in a rat neocortical slice. (**B**) *Top trace* is current measured at soma during dendritic glutamate iontophoresis with and without tetrodotoxin (TTX) while soma is voltage clamped at −76 mV (*bottom trace*). ΔI is inward current evoked by iontophoresis of glutamate during dashed line. (**C**) Same as **B** but soma is voltage clamped at −61 mV. Transmitted current (ΔI is larger and reduced by application of TTX). (**D**) Plot of ΔI as function of soma voltage clamp to different potentials. FL, firing level; *solid boxes* show transmitted current in control; *open boxes* show transmitted current after application of TTX. (**E**) Steady current measured at soma without glutamate dendritic iontophoresis. Arrow shows resting potential. (From Schwindt and Crill.[19] Reprinted with permission of the *Journal of Neurophysiology*.)

We conclude that the balance of voltage-dependent currents in the dendrites causes a significant amplification of tonic distal dendritic synaptic activity. Most of the inward current responsible for this amplification is mediated by sodium ions flowing through noninactivating sodium channels. Some amplification is caused by voltage-dependent glutamate receptor channels of the NMDA type (this observation indicates that the soma potential actually spreads to the site of iontophoresis where ligand-gated channels are activated). The role of voltage-gated calcium channels in the dendrites remains to be determined.

A number of potassium channel types, particularly those mediated by calcium influx, and sodium channels are modulated by various transmitter systems.[20] This provides the nervous system with a mechanism to alter the effectiveness of synaptic input. Decreasing dendritic potassium currents or increasing I_{NaP} will markedly amplify an input. The reverse could make synaptic transmission less effective. Thus, the electrical distance of a particular set of synapses from the soma may be dynamic. Pathological conditions like epilepsy might be sustained by increased synaptic effectiveness. Recent experiments have shown that anticonvulsants such as phenytoin selectively decrease I_{NaP},[21] which is one mechanism for decreasing the spread of abnormal neuron firing that occurs in epilepsy.

REFERENCES

1. RALL, W. 1977. Core conductor theory and cable properties of neurons. *In* Handbook of Physiology. The Nervous System. E. R. Kandel, Ed.: 39–97. American Physiological Society. Bethesda, MD.
2. SPRUSTON, N., D. B. JAFFE & D. JOHNSTON. 1994. Dendritic attenuation of synaptic potentials and currents: The role of passive membrane properties. Trends Neurosci. **17:** 161–166.
3. JOHNSTON, D., J. C. MAGEE, C. M. COLBERT & B. M. CHRISTIE. 1996. Active properties of neuronal dendrites. Annu. Rev. Neurosci. **19:** 165–186.
4. ECCLES, J. C. 1957. The Physiology of Nerve Cells. Johns Hopkins Press. Baltimore, MD.
5. SPENCER, W. A. & E. R. KANDEL. 1961. Electrophysiology of hippocampal neurons. IV. Fast prepotentials. J. Neurophysiol. **24:** 272–285.
6. JACK, J. J. B., D. NOBLE & R. W. TSIEN. 1975. Electric current flow in excitable cells. Oxford University Press.
7. STUART, G. J. & B. SAKMANN. 1994. Active propagation of sodium action potentials into neocortical pyramidal cell dendrites. Nature **367:** 69–72.
8. STAFSTROM, C. E., P. C. SCHWINDT & W. E. CRILL. 1982. Negative slope conductance due to a persistent subthreshold sodium current in cat neocortical neurons in vitro. Brain Res. **236:** 221–226.
9. STAFSTROM, C. E., P. C. SCHWINDT, J. A. FLATMAN & W. E. CRILL. 1984. Properties of subthreshold response and action potential recorded in layer V neurons from cat sensorimotor cortex in vitro. J. Neurophysiol. **52:** 244–263.
10. HOTSON, J. R., D. A. PRINCE & P. A. SCHWARTZKROIN. 1979. Anomalous inward rectification in hippocampal neurons. J. Neurophysiol. **42:** 889–895.
11. LLINÁS, R. & M. SUGIMORI. 1980. Electrophysiological properties of in vitro Purkinje cell somata in mammalian cerebellar slices. J. Physiol. **305:** 171–195.
12. CONNORS, B. W., M. J. GUTNICK & D. A. PRINCE. 1982. Electrophysiological properties of neocortical neurons in vitro. J. Neurophysiol. **48:** 1302–1320.
13. FRENCH, C. R., P. SAH, K. J. BUCKETT & P. W. GAGE. 1990. A voltage-dependent persistent sodium current in mammalian hippocampal neuron. J. Gen. Physiol. **95:** 1139–1157.
14. ALZHEIMER, C., P. C. SCHWINDT & W. E. CRILL. 1993. Modal gating of Na^+ channels as a mechanism of persistent Na^+ currents in pyramidal neurons from rat and cat sensorimotor cortex. J. Neurosci. **13:** 660–673.
15. PATLAK, J. B. & M. ORTIZ. 1986. Two modes of gating during late Na+ channel currents in frog sartorius muscle. J. Gen. Physiol. **87:** 305–326.
16. NILIUS, B. 1988. Modal gating behavior of cardiac sodium channels in cell-free membrane patches. Biophys. J. **5:** 857–862.
17. ALDRICH, R. W., D. P. COREY & C. F. STEVENS. 1983. A reinterpretation of mammalian sodium channel gating based on single channel recording. Nature **306:** 436–441.
18. GONOI, T. & B. HILLE. 1987. Gating of sodium channels: Inactivation modifiers discriminate among models. J. Gen. Physiol. **89:** 253–274.
19. SCHWINDT, P. C. & W. E. CRILL. 1995. Amplification of synaptic current by persistent

sodium conductance in apical dendrite of neocortical neurons. J. Neurophysiol. **74:** 2220–2224.

20. DUNLAP, K. & G. D. FISCHBACH. 1978. Neurotransmitters decrease the Ca component of sensory neurone action potentials. Nature **276:** 837–838.

21. CHAO, T. I. & C. ALZHEIMER. 1995. Effects of phenytoin on the persistent Na^+ current of mammalian CNS neurons. Neuroreport **6:** 1778–1780.

Paraneoplastic Syndromes:
A Brief Review

JEROME B. POSNER

Department of Neurology
Memorial Sloan-Kettering Cancer Center
1275 York Avenue
New York, New York 10021

It is a great pleasure to participate in this symposium in honor of Dr. Fred Plum. Forty-two years ago, when I first began to work for Dr. Plum for what I assumed was a 2½-month summer medical student job, I little suspected that the ideas he introduced me to would determine my career and, indeed, the rest of my life. Before Dr. Plum's arrival to head the Department of Neurology at the University of Washington, we medical students were taught that neurology was an interesting intellectual specialty but of little practical use. We were taught that academic neurology as a specialty was reserved for those who wanted to teach others the names of nineteenth century French and German neurologists that served as eponyms for a bewildering number of clinical syndromes, none of which was understood at a biochemical or physiological level. Practitioners of neurology, we believed, would of necessity have to also practice general internal medicine or psychiatry in order to make a living. The best any neurologist could offer our neurological patients, we believed, was to put a name on their disorder and tell them that little could be done. Furthermore, neurologists, we believed, were concerned only with disorders in which abnormalities of the brain affected the body. We knew about diseases of the nervous system that could paralyze limbs, cause muscles to waste away, and cause the respiratory and cardiovascular system to fail. What I learned from Dr. Plum that summer, and in the ensuing years, was that not only could brain dysfunction affect the rest of the body, but that disorders of bodily function could affect the brain. Furthermore, I learned from him that it was not enough to recognize what was happening to the patient, but one also had to try to understand how it was happening as well as the pathophysiology of the patient's symptoms and signs.

The first paper I published with Dr. Plum demonstrated those themes.[1] We tried to discover how abnormalities of the liver affected the brain and, in particular, whether patients with liver disease overbreathe as a compensatory mechanism to protect the brain. I continued to study with Dr. Plum the effects of other systemic diseases on the brain after we came to Cornell in 1963.[2,3] When he sent me to Memorial Sloan-Kettering Cancer Center in 1967 as a neurologist, my implied charge was to study how cancer affected the brain. My 30 years at Memorial have been an attempt, with varying success, to carry out that charge. To paraphrase the wise words of one of our former presidents of Memorial Sloan-Kettering, "Plum must accept responsibility for that work but he needn't accept the blame."

What I want to discuss here is one of the ways in which a systemic illness, namely cancer, can affect the brain. It has been known for over 50 years that very small numbers of patients with cancer could develop rather striking abnormalities of brain function, which were not caused by metastases or by destruction of vital organs, but by conditions termed paraneoplastic syndromes.[4,5] FIGURE 1 illustrates a photomicrograph of one such patient showing a generally normal cerebellum save

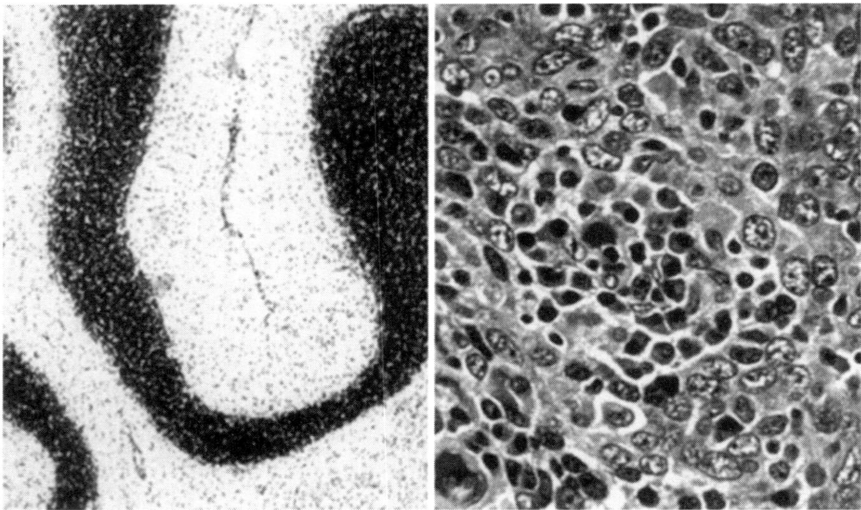

FIGURE 1. Pathology of antibody positive paraneoplastic cerebellar degeneration. On the left is a photomicrograph of the cerebellum demonstrating normal architecture except for total absence of Purkinje cells. The rest of the brain was grossly and histologically normal. On the right is a photomicrograph of the ovary demonstrating a cancer that had not been visible grossly, but was identified only on microscopic examination.

for the complete loss of Purkinje cells. Serial sections of cerebellum from this and other patients frequently fail to reveal a single Purkinje cell remaining in the entire cerebellum.[6] The histologic sections of the remainder of the brain often reveal no other abnormality. The figure also illustrates that the cause of this cerebellar disorder was a microscopic tumor found in the ovary.

While such patients are still alive but suffering cerebellar symptoms, a search should be made for a systemic cancer. At times, the cancer encountered may be apparent only microscopically. What the Purkinje cells and the ovarian cancer of the patient illustrated in FIGURE 1 had in common is that they both expressed a protein antigen that is normally expressed only in Purkinje cells of the cerebellum but is aberrantly expressed in the patient's cancer. Furthermore, her serum contained high titers of an antibody that reacted with this protein antigen both by immunohistochemistry and by Western blot.[7,8] The antibody, called anti-Yo, is seen almost exclusively in women who have paraneoplastic cerebellar degeneration caused by breast or gynecologic cancers.

Let us now consider another patient. A middle-aged woman who was a heavy smoker presented to medical attention with the subacute development of memory loss, complex partial seizures, and a sensory neuropathy. On magnetic resonance imaging of the brain, both medial temporal lobes were hyperintense on the T2 weighted images, and a small area of contrast enhancement was found in the left medial temporal lobe on T1 weighted image. A chest CT scan revealed a slightly enlarged mediastinal lymph node but two biopsies performed by mediastinoscopy showed only inflammatory cells. During the course of her workup, she suffered an acute cardiovascular collapse and died. At autopsy she was found to have inflammatory infiltrates in the brain, particularly the hippocampus and medulla, and also in dorsal root ganglia. A dramatic loss of neurons was also evident in her dorsal root ganglia. A microscopic small cell lung cancer was found in one mediastinal lymph node. As with the woman with paraneoplastic cerebellar degeneration illustrated in FIGURE 1, the neurons of the central nervous system and the small cell lung cancer of this woman contained an antigen normally expressed only in neurons of the central and peripheral nervous system. Furthermore, her serum contained high titers of an antibody that reacted both with the small cell lung cancer and neurons including those of the hippocampus, amygdala, and dorsal root ganglia. The antibody, called anti-Hu, is usually found in patients with paraneoplastic encephalomyelitis and/or sensory neuropathy associated with small cell lung cancer (FIG. 2).[9]

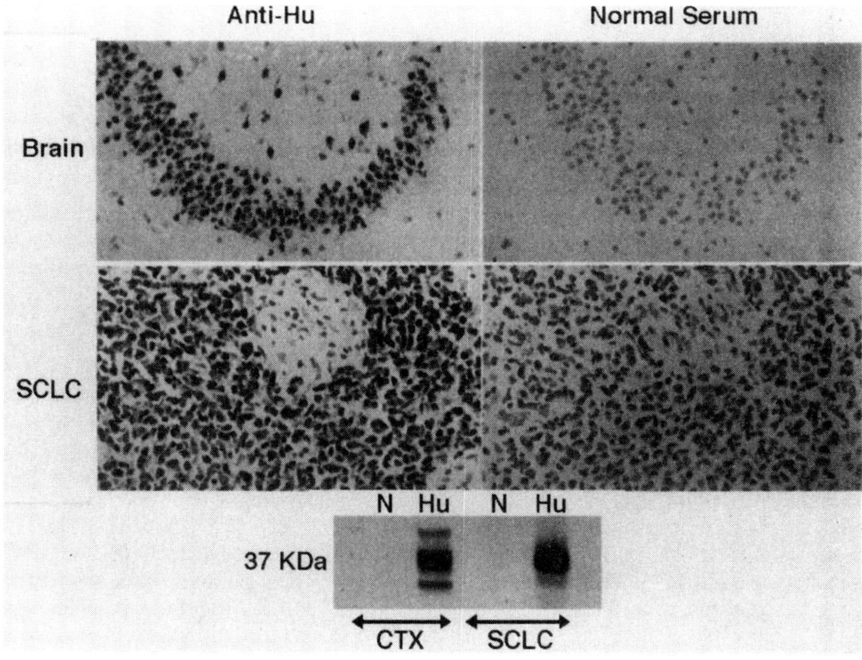

FIGURE 2. Anti-Hu antibody. The two **upper panels** are photomicrographs of sections of human hippocampus taken at autopsy from a patient who had been neurologically intact during life. **Left panel** is reacted with the serum of the patient with anti-Hu antibody positive encephalomyelitis (see text). **Right panel** shows the reaction of the hippocampus with normal human serum. The patient's serum contains an antibody that reacts with the nuclei of all neurons in this section as well as all neurons in the central and peripheral nervous system. No such reaction is seen with normal human serum. The **lower panels** are from a small cell lung cancer in a mediastinal lymph node. On the left the section is reacted with the patient's serum, on the right with normal human serum. The patient's serum reacts with an antigen present in small cell lung cancer, but not in the lymphocytes (*arrow*). Normal human serum does not react. Below is a Western blot using cortex neurons (*left*) and small cell lung cancer (*right*) as the antigen and the patient's serum as the antibody. Bands between 35 and 40 kD are seen when the patient's serum is reacted with cortical neurons. One band is seen when small cell lung cancer is reacted. Normal human serum gives no reaction.

TABLE 1. Paraneoplastic Syndromes: Some Unresolved Questions

- How common are paraneoplastic syndromes?
- Does the immune response affect growth of the cancer?
- Do paraneoplastic antibodies assist the neurologist?
- Why do only a few patients mount an immune response?
- What do "onconeural" antigens do?

These findings, as well as many others investigated in laboratories throughout the world, have led to the concept that, in certain cancers, protein antigens normally restricted to the nervous system are aberrantly expressed in the cancer, and some but not all patients have the capacity to mount an immune response to these aberrantly expressed but otherwise normal protein antigens. The immune response attacks both the cancer and the nervous system. The clinical results are twofold: (1) A paraneoplastic syndrome usually characterized by severe neurologic deficits develops and (2) tumor growth appears to be more indolent than would have occurred had the immune reaction not been present.

What I would like to discuss now are some recent data, much of which are as yet unpublished, addressing several currently unresolved questions concerning paraneoplastic syndromes (TABLE 1). This presentation is by no means inclusive as there are many unresolved questions concerning paraneoplastic syndromes, the discussions of which would require much more space than is available here.

The first question is, How common are paraneoplastic syndromes? The American Cancer Society has estimated the incidence of new cancers of the ovary and small cell cancers of the lung in the United States in 1996.[10] The numbers are fairly large, with predicted incidence of ovarian cancer being almost 27,000 and that of small cell lung cancer 35,000. It is generally conceded that paraneoplastic syndromes are rare, particularly if one insists on the florid symptomatology in the patients alluded to in the previous slides. However, some years ago Erlington and his colleagues[11] examined 150 patients with small cell lung cancer. They discovered that almost half of these patients had symptoms and signs that could be considered neurologic. Symptoms included anorexia in 53%, weight loss in 51%, erectile impotence in 44%, dry mouth in 41%, weakness in 31%, sphincter disturbances in 24%, sweating in 21%, and visual abnormalities in 6%. Signs included difficulty rising from a squatting position in 21%, sensory changes in 16%, hyperactive reflexes in 13%, diminished reflexes in 10%, motor weakness (excluding inability to rise from a squatting position) in 8%, ataxia or nystagmus in 5%. Only three patients had an unequivocal paraneoplastic syndrome, including Lambert-Eaton myasthenic syndrome in two and a subacute sensory neuropathy in one. Dalmau and colleagues at Memorial Sloan-Kettering have begun a prospective analysis of all patients with small cell lung cancer who come to the pulmonary clinic. So far, 33 patients have been entered into the study. On entry, an astounding 66% had symptoms or signs that could be caused by nervous system dysfunction. As TABLE 2 shows, 18 patients had symptoms including dry mouth, headache, motor weakness, confusion, and seizures. Twenty-two patients had signs, including three patients with an unequivocal paraneoplastic syndrome, one cerebellar degeneration, one encephalomyelitis, and one Lambert-Eaton myasthenic syndrome. Seven additional patients had ataxia on examination, 1 confusion, 9 cranial nerve abnormalities, 10 motor abnormalities, 9 sensory abnormalities, and 11 abnormalities of deep tendon reflexes. Brain metastases were found at entry in 9 of the 33 patients; many of the other symptoms

TABLE 2. Neurologic Findings in 33 Patients with Small Cell Lung Cancer

Symptoms (n = 8)		Signs (n = 22)	
Dry mouth	5	Paraneoplastic	3
Headache	3	Ataxia	7
Monoparesis	2	Confusion	1
Insomnia	2	Cranial nerve	9
Ataxia	1	Motor	10
Itch	1	Sensory	9
Tremor	1	DTR's	11
Confusion	1	Brain metastases	9
Seizure	1		

appeared not to be related to structural disease of the nervous system but could be considered paraneoplastic.

The import of this and the Erlington study is that, at least in small cell lung cancer, paraneoplastic neurologic symptoms and signs mild enough to be overlooked by oncologists but severe enough to impact negatively on the quality of the patient's life may be much more common than we had heretofore believed. A similar prospective analysis is under way in patients with ovarian cancer.

The next question is, Does the immune reaction have any effect on the growth of the cancer? I suggested above that the immune reaction might inhibit the growth of the cancer, but that conclusion held by many neurologists was based on their clinical impression that patients who suffered paraneoplastic syndromes seemed to have a slow-growing cancer. Because in patients with paraneoplastic syndromes neurologic signs usually precede evidence of the cancer, the paraneoplastic disorder may lead to an earlier diagnosis of the cancer. This early detection gives the false impression of a smaller and slower-growing cancer. Drs. Francesc Graus in Barcelona and Josep Dalmau took advantage of the fact that although florid paraneoplastic syndromes are rare in patients with small cell lung cancer, approximately 20% of patients with small cell lung cancer harbor very low titers of the anti-Hu antibody even though they do not have clear-cut paraneoplastic syndromes.[12,13] In a prospective analysis of 170 patients, those with low titers of paraneoplastic antibodies, but without neurologic disease, that led them to prematurely seek medical advice were (1) more likely to have localized disease, (2) were more likely to have a complete response to conventional therapy, and (3) survived longer (TABLE 3). That this is

TABLE 3. Clinical Characteristics of 170 Patients with Small Cell Lung Cancer

Clinical State (*n* = 170)	Anti-Hu Pos (*n* = 27)	Anti-Hu Neg (*n* = 143)	*p* Value
Age (years)	60.4 ± 10.2	61.6 ± 9.6	0.572
Sex = male	26 (96%)	128 (90%)	1.000
ECOG = 0–2	25 (93%)	128 (90%)	1.000
Weight ↓ < 5%	20 (74%)	91 (65%)	0.361
Stage = limit	16 (59%)	54 (39%)	0.046
CR	15 (56%)	28 (20%)	<0.001
Survival	14.9 months	10.2 months	0.018
Survival >36 months	26%	6%	
Anti-p53 pos	2 (7.4%)	25 (17.4%)	

Pos, positive; neg, negative.

not a nonspecific response to production of any autoantibody was shown by Dr. Myrna Rosenfeld who found that anti-p53 antibodies do not confer a similar survival benefit on patients with small cell lung cancer; however, anti-p53 antibodies also occur in about 20% of patients with small cell lung cancer, but they are not the same patients.[14] Thus, the prolonged survival appears to be associated with a specific immune response against the Hu onconeural antigen.

The next question I wish to address is, Does measurement of antibodies in patients with neurologic disease assist the neurologist in diagnosis and treatment? (TABLE 1). Because the antibodies do not occur in normal individuals and do not usually occur at high titer except in patients with paraneoplastic syndromes, they are obviously helpful in informing the neurologist that his patient's neurologic symptoms are probably caused by cancer. The presence of a specific antibody is also helpful in informing the oncologist what specific cancer may be present. This is because specific autoantibodies are associated with specific cancers. However, not every patient with a paraneoplastic syndrome has a measurable antibody. More importantly, not every patient with a paraneoplastic syndrome associated with a specific cancer, such as small cell lung cancer, has the anti-Hu antibody in his or her serum. An interesting new finding is that the presence or absence of the anti-Hu antibody in a patient with small cell lung cancer and a given paraneoplastic syndrome supplies useful information to the neurologist. Dr. Warren Mason and colleagues looked at 57 patients with small cell lung cancer and paraneoplastic cerebellar degeneration.[15] Only half of those patients had high titer anti-Hu antibodies in their serum. Fifty-six percent either had other antibodies or no identifiable antibody. The finding of anti-Hu antibodies in serum defined a subset of patients who differed from the seronegative or non-anti-Hu patients in that they were more likely (1) to be women, (2) to have evidence of multifocal neurologic disease, with brainstem encephalopathy and sensory neuropathy being the common extracerebellar manifestations, and (3) to be severely disabled. Interestingly, in both groups of patients, 16% had electrophysiologically confirmed Lambert-Eaton myasthenic syndrome, another paraneoplastic syndrome associated with small cell lung cancer. When voltage-gated calcium channel antibodies were examined by Dr. John Newsom-Davis and his colleagues, they were present in 40% of patients with anti-Hu negative antibody, but in only 16% of those with anti-Hu antibody. Because the Lambert-Eaton symptoms may be masked by the cerebellar degeneration, and because the Lambert-Eaton syndrome responds to treatment whereas cerebellar degeneration usually does not,[16] a careful search for Lambert-Eaton syndrome in patients with antibody negative cerebellar degeneration is indicated. Appropriate treatment may ameliorate some of the symptoms.

Although low titers of the anti-Hu antibody appear to protect patients against their cancer, leading to a longer survival, patients with high titer anti-Hu antibodies do not live as long as patients who are anti-Hu negative and do not have paraneoplastic syndromes. Their life span is shorter but their death is due to the neurologic disease and not to the growth of the cancer.

A fourth question is, Why does only a subset of patients with cancer, whose tumor aberrantly expresses a neuronal antigen, raise antibodies against that antigen? (TABLE 1). The answer is unknown but preliminary data from Dalmau suggest that it may be a result of expression of Class I major histocompatibility antigens (MHC) on the surface of tumor cells. Many tumors do not express Class I MHC. Dalmau's data show that the small cell lung cancers of patients with paraneoplastic syndromes expressed Class I MHC, whereas tumors of patients without paraneoplastic syndromes did not.[17]

A final unresolved question is, Why are antigens normally restricted to the nervous system expressed in cancers and what does their expression have to do, if anything, with the growth of the cancer? (TABLE 1). It is not surprising that voltage-gated calcium channels and the Hu antigens would be expressed in small cell lung cancer. Small cell lung cancers are neuroendocrine tumors that are believed to arise from cells that originated in the neural crest. The preservation of neural antigens in such tumors should not be surprising, but why they appear to be so strongly preserved, even as the tumors substantially dedifferentiate, is not clear. The Hu antigens are actually a family, only one antigen of which, HuD, appears to be expressed in small cell lung cancer. Cloning of the gene that encodes for that antigen demonstrates a high homology to a protein (ELAV) present in drosophila and necessary for the growth and maintenance of the nervous system.[18] It is possible but not proved that the protein may also be necessary for the continued growth of the small cell lung cancer.

More intriguing is why a protein normally expressed in Purkinje cells is aberrantly expressed in ovarian or breast adenocarcinoma, but not neuroendocrine tumors. The function of the Yo antigen—like Hu, also a family of antigens, more than one of which may be expressed in ovarian cancer—is not known. Its role in the growth and development of the Purkinje cell, if any, has not been established nor is its role in the cancer established.

This short tour through paraneoplastic syndromes suggests that in the last decade we have raised more questions than we have answered. Those questions which have been answered have been answered with the encouragement, support, and teaching of Fred Plum. All of us at Memorial Sloan-Kettering—and particularly me—thank him.

REFERENCES

1. POSNER, J. B. & F. PLUM. 1960. The toxic effects of carbon dioxide and acetazolamide in hepatic encephalopathy. J. Clin. Invest. **39:** 1246.
2. POSNER, J. B. & F. PLUM. 1967. Spinal fluid pH and neurologic symptoms in systemic acidosis. N. Engl. J. Med. **277:** 605–613.
3. RAICHLE, M. E., J. B. POSNER & F. PLUM. 1970. Cerebral blood flow during and after hyperventilation. Arch. Neurol. **23:** 394–403.
4. BRAIN, W. R., P. M. DANIEL & J. G. GREENFIELD. 1951. Subacute cortical cerebellar degeneration and its relation to carcinoma. J. Neurol. Neurosurg. Psychiatry **14:** 59–75.
5. BROUWER, B. & A. BIEMOND. 1938. Les affections parenchymateuses du cervelet et leur signification du point de vue de l'anatomie et la physiologie de cet organe. J. Belge Neurol. Psychiatrie **38:** 691–757.
6. VERSCHUUREN, J., L. CHUANG, M. K. ROSENBLUM, F. LIEBERMAN, A. PRYOR, J. B. POSNER & J. DALMAU. 1996. Inflammatory infiltrates and complete absence of Purkinje cells in anti-Yo-associated paraneoplastic cerebellar degeneration. Acta Neuropathol. (Berl.) **91:** 519–525.
7. FURNEAUX, H. M., M. K. ROSENBLUM, J. DALMAU, *et al.* 1990. Selective expression of Purkinje-cell antigens in tumor tissue from patients with paraneoplastic cerebellar degeneration. N. Engl. J. Med. **322:** 1844–1851.
8. DALMAU, J. & J. B. POSNER. 1994. Neurologic paraneoplastic antibodies (anti-Yo; anti-Hu; anti-Ri): The case for a nomenclature based on antibody and antigen specificity. Neurology **44:** 2241–2246.
9. DALMAU, J., F. GRAUS, M. K. ROSENBLUM, *et al.* 1992. Anti-Hu-associated paraneoplastic encephalomyelitis/sensory neuropathy. A clinical study of 71 patients. Medicine **71:** 59–72.
10. PARKER, S. L., T. TONG, S. BOLDEN & P. A. WINGO. Cancer statistics, 1996. Ca Cancer J. Clin. **65:** 5–27.

11. ERLINGTON, G. M., N. M. MURRAY, S. G. SPIRO, *et al.* 1991. Neurological paraneoplastic syndromes in patients with small cell lung cancer. A prospective survey of 150 patients. J. Neurol. Neurosurg. Psychiatry **54:** 764–767.

12. DALMAU, J., H. M. FURNEAUX, R. J. GRALLA, *et al.* 1990. Detection of the anti-Hu antibody in the serum of patients with small cell lung cancer—A quantitative western blot analysis. Ann. Neurol. **27:** 544–552.

13. GRAUS, F., J. DALMAU, R. RENÉ, M. TORÀ, N. MALATS, J. J. VERSCHUUREN, F. CARDENAL, N. VIÑOLAS, J. G. DEL MURO, C. VADELL, W. P. MASON, R. ROSELL, J. B. POSNER & F. X. REAL. 1997. Anti-Hu antibodies in patients with small cell lung cancer: Association with complete response to therapy and improved survival. J. Clin. Oncol. **15:** 2866–2872.

14. ROSENFELD, M. R., N. MALATS, L. SCHRAMM, F. GRAUS, F. CARDENAL, N. VIÑOLAS, R. ROSELL, M. TORÀ, F. X. REAL, J. B. POSNER & J. DALMAU. 1997. Serum anti-p53 antibodies and prognosis of patients with small cell lung cancer. J. Natl. Cancer Inst. **89:** 381–385.

15. MASON, W. P., F. GRAUS, B. LANG, J. HONNORAT, J. Y. DELATTRE, F. VALLDEORIOLA, J. C. ANTOINE, M. K. ROSENBLUM, M. R. ROSENFELD, J. NEWSOM-DAVIS, J. B. POSNER & J. DALMAU. 1977. Small-cell lung cancer, paraneoplastic cerebellar degeneration and the Lambert-Eaton myasthenic syndrome. Brain **120(8):** 1279–1300.

16. UCHUYA, M., F. GRAUS, F. VEGA, R. RENÉ & J.-Y. DELATTRE. 1996. Intravenous immunoglobulin treatment in paraneoplastic neurological syndromes with antineural autoantibodies. J. Neurol. Neurosurg. Psychiatry **60:** 388–392.

17. DALMAU, J., F. GRAUS, N.-K.V. CHEUNG, M. K. ROSENBLUM, A. HO, A. CANETE, J.-Y. DELATTRE, S. J. THOMPSON & J. B. POSNER. 1995. Major histocompatibility proteins, anti-Hu antibodies, and paraneoplastic encephalomyelitis in neuroblastoma and small cell lung cancer. Cancer **75:** 99–109.

18. SZABO, A., J. DALMAU, G. MANLEY, *et al.* 1991. HuD, a paraneoplastic encephalomyelitis antigen, contains RNA-binding domains and is homologous to Elav and Sex-lethal. Cell **67:** 325–333.

Immune Responses and Dementia[a]

DANA GIULIAN

Department of Neurology
Baylor College of Medicine
Houston, Texas 77031

OVERVIEW

Microglia, mononuclear phagocytes endogenous to the central nervous system (CNS), serve as the principal immune cells of the brain.[1] Although normally found in quiescent state, microglia are activated by a variety of signals. When stimulated, this class of brain glia releases a variety of cytokines and cytotoxins. These factors, in turn, promote gliotic reactions or induce neuron injury.[1] Various stimuli, including amyloid plaques and human immunodeficiency virus-1 (HIV-1), drive microglia to damage neurons and impair cognitive function. It is proposed that chronic reactive microgliosis contributes to the neuronal loss found in Alzheimer's disease and HIV-1 infection of the brain. Strategies to block neurotoxic microgliosis may slow cognitive decline in some chronic brain disorders.

PROPERTIES OF MICROGLIA

Rio-Hortega first described microglia as argentophilic cells with "wavy, branched processes beset with spines."[2] Presently, most investigators agree that microglia arise during early embryonic development from precursor elements common with those of blood, but later proliferate within the CNS.[3] Bone-marrow chimera studies of Hickey and co-workers[4,5] indicate that perivascular CNS mononuclear phagocytes, but not parenchymal microglia, exchange with blood monocytes throughout normal adult life. During CNS injury, ramified microglia retract processes, take on ameboid shapes, and transform into dynamic secretory cells, referred to as reactive and microglia.

In vitro studies have been used to compare the growth and structure of ameboid microglia with other classes of mononuclear phagocytes such as peritoneal macrophages, splenic macrophages, blood monocytes, and bone marrow progenitor cells.[6,7] When grown under identical conditions in chemically defined culture medium, all mononuclear phagocytes possess scavenger receptors. Spontaneous proliferation occurs with microglia whereas marrow cells proliferate only in the presence of colony-stimulating factors. Ameboid microglia develop long, thin projections (up to several hundred microns in length) that resemble ramified cells in tissue, but appear differently from cultures of short, stubby macrophages or of round, oval marrow cells. Microglia and macrophages are active phagocytes of yeast and bacteria with very little engulfment among marrow cells. Kettenmann and co-workers[8] have shown that inward rectifying K^+ currents of microglia can be distinguished from those in macrophages and blood monocytes. In addition, scanning electron micros-

[a] This work was supported by funding from the National Institutes of Health.

91

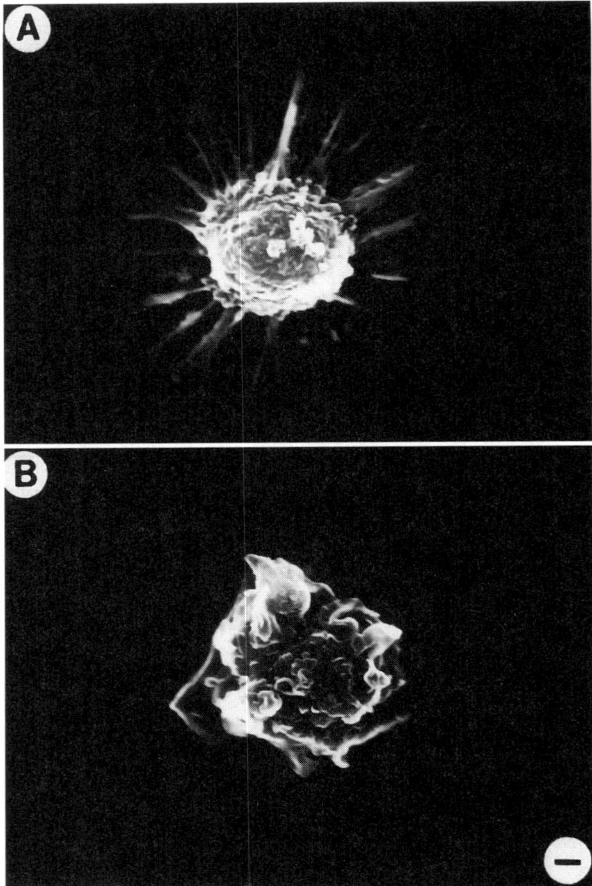

FIGURE 1. Scanning electron micrographs of microglia (**A**) and liver macrophage (**B**) isolated from adult rat and placed in culture. Microglia show a characteristic spine-bearing surface which is readily distinguished from the ruffled appearance of mononuclear phagocytes isolated from tissues outside the CNS.

copy (SEM) shows that the surfaces of microglia bristle with spines whereas tissue macrophages show a "ruffled" appearance (FIG. 1; refs. 6 and 7). These differences in surface morphology, moreover, persist despite prolonged growth in culture, differentiation of microglia, or exposure to various immunostimulants.[7] About 30% of inflammatory cells at lesions with disrupted blood–brain barrier (such as in stroke or trauma) involve invading macrophages whereas injury without such breakdown (such as distal axotomy) recruits >98% reactive microglia.[7]

Further evidence that microglia are distinct from macrophages comes from co-culture experiments with astroglia. Contacts between microglia and astroglia stimulate maturation of microglia transforming ameboid to ramified forms typical of adult CNS.[7] The ramified microglia persist as quiescent cells without apparent phagocytic or secretory activity until driven into a reactive state. Because macrophage do not differentiate when in contact with astroglia, it is likely that specific microglial interactions with the CNS environment suppress immunoreactivity, thereby limiting microglial disruption of normal brain function. The overall pattern suggests that microglia possess a unique set of qualities that may have arisen during adaptation to neural tissues.[1,6,7] As noted below, activation of ramified microglia unleashes a deluge of factors that help to control wound healing and neuronal survival during CNS injury.

ACTIONS OF SECRETORY MICROGLIA

It is now well established that microglia release cytokines including interleukin 1 (IL-1), tumor necrosis factor α (TNFα), and granulocyte macrophage colony stimulating factor (GM-CSF; refs. 9–11). One way to study cytokine mediation of cell–cell interactions is to culture highly enriched populations of microglia with other target cells. For example, microglia can be placed in filtered chambers to allow diffusion of soluble factors onto coverslips containing specific populations of neurons or glia. Under these conditions, GM-CSF is identified as a microglial mitogen that does not alter the growth or survival of neurons or astroglia.[10] In contrast, TNFα has no effect upon either cultured neurons or glia. Astroglia incubated for only 24 h with 5 units of IL-1α markedly proliferate. This effect can be blocked by IL-1 receptor antagonist as well as a neutralizing antibody.[11] Although IL-1 has no direct growth or toxic effects upon cultured neurons,[11] IL-1-stimulated astroglia do enhance neuron survival *in vitro*. Moreover, direct infusion of IL-1 into rat neocortex elicits both reactive astroglia and new capillary growth.[10] Gage and co-workers[12] have suggested that IL-1 from microglia stimulates astroglial production of nerve growth factor *in vivo*. In this way, reactive microglia control neighboring would healing (astrogliosis and neovascularization) during brain injury through the release of factors including IL-1.[13] Such microglia-dependent healing, in turn, helps to preserve neurons after CNS injury.

Reactive microglia also produce toxic molecules in response to such CNS insults as ischemia or trauma.[14] These factors include short-lived substances such as free radicals and nitric oxide which have *nonspecific cytotoxic* effects. *In vitro* experiments also uncovered a class of microglia-derived molecules which has *neuron-specific* toxicity (FIG. 2). This neurotoxic activity, referred to as NTox, is long-lived and appears by gel filtration chromatography to be <1000 Da. Other cytotoxic molecules with low molecular masses (<1 kDa) such as hydrogen peroxide, nitric oxide, leukotrienes, lipoxins, and superoxide anion are highly reactive and, in contrast to NTox, would not be recovered in culture media or retain activity after boiling.[15] NTox has no apparent COOH groups (resistant to butyl esterification), but shows a lipophilic quality that is pH sensitive (binding to reverse phase resins; extraction into ethyl acetate at basic pH). Inactivation studies also determine that NTox loses activity under strong reducing conditions, suggesting such double bond structures as phenols or pyridines; the phenolic ring is more likely because of inactivation by polyphenol oxidase. Moreover, the presence of a terminal -NH$_3$ group is shown by inactivation with acetic anhydride and plasma amine oxidase. Importantly, NTox resists acid hydrolysis ruling out potential molecules such as free radicals, excitatory amino acids, quinolinic acid, and all peptides or proteins as the microglia-derived poison. NTox appears to be a phenolic amine with lipophilic properties (FIG. 3).

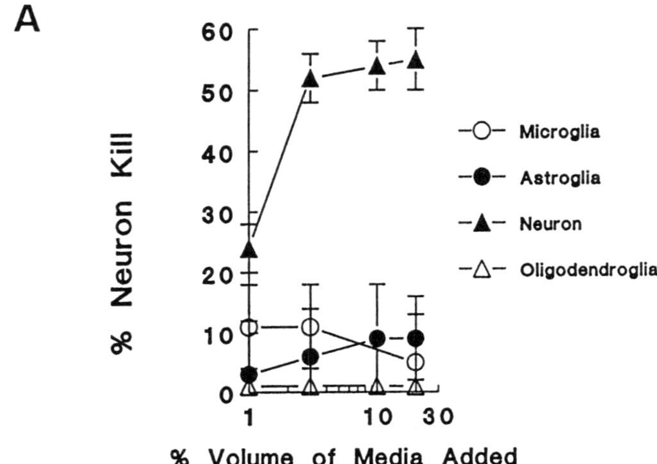

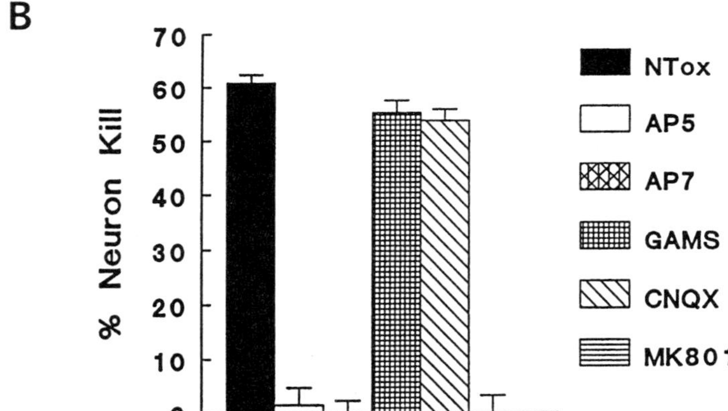

FIGURE 2. Actions of neurotoxin released by activated microglia. **(A)** Conditioned media from activated microglia show a dose-dependent killing effect upon neurons but not other cell populations of the CNS. **(B)** The action of the toxin isolated from microglia, NTox, was sensitive to such NMDA receptor blocking agents as AP5, AP7, and MK-801, but was unaffected by non-NMDA receptor antagonists including GAMS and CNQX.

Further investigation demonstrates that NTox destroys neurons by actions involving the N-methyl-D-aspartate (NMDA) class of glutamate receptor.[14,15] For example, selective NMDA antagonists protected against NTox whereas the antagonists to non-NMDA type excitatory amino acid receptors did not (FIG. 2). Similar results obtained with rat hippocampal, cortical, and spinal cord neurons as well as with chick ciliary neurons indicate that microglia secrete a single factor toxic to

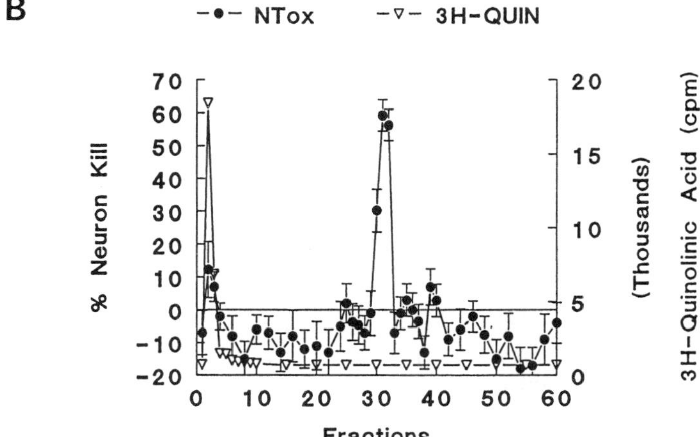

FIGURE 3. (A) Putative structure of NTox which appears as a phenolic amine. Both the phenolic group and terminal amine are necessary for biological action. Orb spider venoms show similar structural features but contain a peptide bond lacking in NTox. Quinolinic acid contains two carboxyl groups not found in NTox. **(B)** Reverse-phase HPLC showing separation of NTox, a lipophilic structure, from [³H]quinolinic acid (³H-QUIN). Such separation methods allow study of microglial production levels for these two classes of NMDA-like neurotoxins.

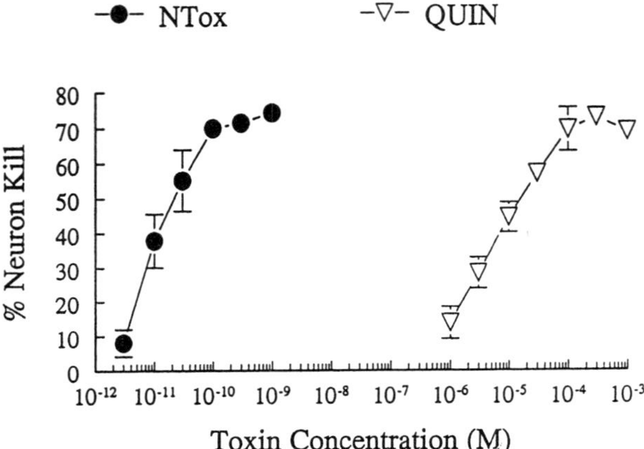

FIGURE 4. Neuron-killing activity for NTox and quinolinic acid (QUIN) in rat hippocampal cultures. Dose-response curves show NTox to be >100,000-fold more potent than QUIN. Similar patterns of toxicity are found after hippocampal infusions *in vivo*.

NMDA receptor-bearing neurons. Because perturbations in NMDA receptor-dependent transmission (particularly within such limbic structures as the hippocampus) are thought to disrupt cognitive function,[16] it follows that neurotoxic microglia could damage pathways resulting in cognitive decline. Two types of dementia, HIV-1 infection of the brain and Alzheimer's disease, display chronic microgliosis and are, therefore, likely to involve microglia-dependent neuronal pathology.

MICROGLIAL NEUROTOXINS AND HIV-1 DAMAGE TO THE CNS

Clinical studies indicate that nearly 60% of adult patients and more than 75% of pediatric patients with acquired immune deficiency syndrome (AIDS) have some degree of cognitive dysfunction.[17,18] Patients with AIDS often show apathy or severe depression and nearly 50% have bouts of delirium. Eventually the cognitive dysfunction progresses to global dementia. At autopsy, the brains of patients with AIDS show atrophy, gliosis, and loss of neurons.[17-19] Cellular changes include diffuse invasion of macrophages, clusters of reactive microglia (the microglial nodules), and giant cell formation. HIV-1 has been isolated from several classes of mononuclear phagocytes including resident microglia, invading macrophages, or multinucleated macrophage-like cells. Although loss of neurons and synapses are features of AIDS dementia, the retrovirus does not directly infect neurons. Two agents thought to contribute to the neuronal pathology observed during HIV-1 infection have been quinolinate, a dicarboxylic acid, and NTox, a neurotoxic amine (FIG. 3; refs. 19–23). Both these factors readily destroy neurons *in vitro*; killing by quinolinate of hippocampal neurons (grown atop a feeder layer of astroglia) requires micromolar concentrations (ED$_{50}$ = 10 μM), whereas NTox readily destroys hippocampal cells in the low pM range (ED$_{50}$ = 50 pM; FIG. 4). The cytotoxic actions of both quinolinic acid and NTox are blocked by antagonists to the NMDA receptor channel complex[21] such as AP5, AP7, and MK-801.

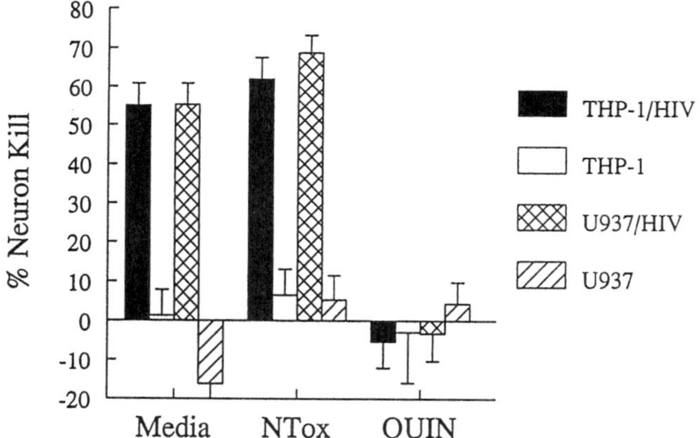

FIGURE 5. Release of neurotoxins from human monocytic cell lines infected with HIV-1. Condition media (Media) from either THP-1 or U937 cells release neuron-killing activity following infection. Separation of NTox from QUIN by ion-exchange chromatography shows that all cytotoxic activity recovered from the cells was NTox. Additional experiments showed that HIV-1 infection did not induce synthesis or release of quinolinic acid.

Although human monocytic cell lines infected with HIV-1 release NTox (FIG. 5), no significant quinolinate is detected in conditioned media from HIV-1(+) infected THP-1 or U937 cells.[21] Furthermore, no correlation exists between the presence of neurotoxic activity in culture media and the measured levels of quinolinic acid (FIG. 5). Second, chemical analyses using strong anionic exchangers to isolate quinolinate[21] show that all neurotoxic activity in culture media is attributable to NTox. Although mononuclear cells infected with HIV-1 produce little quinolinate, it is possible that alternative culture conditions could boost biosynthetic capacity by infected cells. An initial step in the quinolinate pathway involves the flavin-dependent enzyme indoleamine 2,3-dioxygenase (IDO), which converts tryptophan to N-formylkynurenine. Because the cytokine interferon γ (IFNγ) can induce IDO,[23] it may also accelerate production of quinolinic acid. Although concentrations of IFNγ in the physiological range (<100 units/mL) do not alter cultured THP-1 or U937 cells to produce quinolinic acid, very high cytokine concentrations (≥200 units/mL of IFN-γ) stimulate a release of quinolinate, but not in HIV-1 infected cells. Increasing amounts of the substrate 3-hydroxyanthranlic acid (3-HANA), the immediate biosynthetic precursor of quinolinic acid, do not alter the ability of cells to convert 3-HANA to quinolinate. Moreover, various concentrations of the precursors tryptophan or kynurenine reveal no differences in quinolinic acid release between infected and uninfected cells. Such experiments demonstrate that production of quinolinic acid by mononuclear phagocytes remains low despite IFNγ induction of IDO or very high concentrations of biosynthetic precursors. Importantly, HIV-1 infection of mononuclear phagocytes does not stimulate quinolinate production or release.

Although cultured monocytic cell lines release neuron poisons after exposure to HIV-1 *in vitro*, it remains uncertain whether mononuclear cells within HIV-1 infected individuals actually produce neuron-killing agents. To address this question, freshly isolated blood cells collected from volunteers with and without HIV-1 infec-

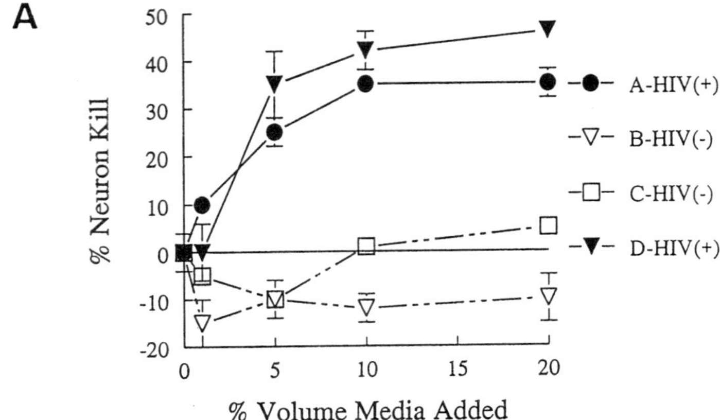

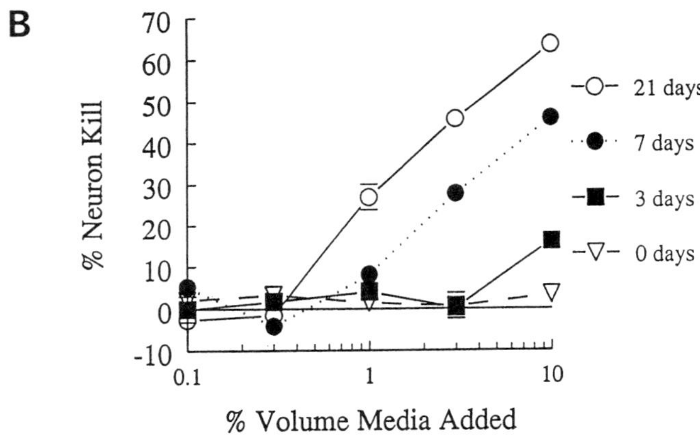

FIGURE 6. (A) Media conditioned by blood monocytes isolated from volunteers showed the presence of neurotoxic activity from individuals infected with HIV-1. Secretion products from uninfected control [HIV-1(−)] cells had no effect upon neuron survival. **(B)** Human microglia isolated from HIV-1(+) brain showed a time-dependent release of NTox.

tion are monitored for secretion of toxins. Monocytes from the blood of HIV-1 infected adults produce neuron-killing activity which is dose dependent and not found among blood cells of normal adult volunteers (FIG. 6A) or in lymphocyte cultures of HIV-1 infected individuals. Although human microglia isolated from normal brain do not release neuron poisons, these cells became neurotoxic within three days after infection with HIV-1 *in vitro* (FIG. 6B). Ultrafiltrates of gray matter show that NTox exists within virally infected brain tissues, but not normal brain tissues (FIG. 7; ref. 21). Biochemical study of the neurotoxic activities released by

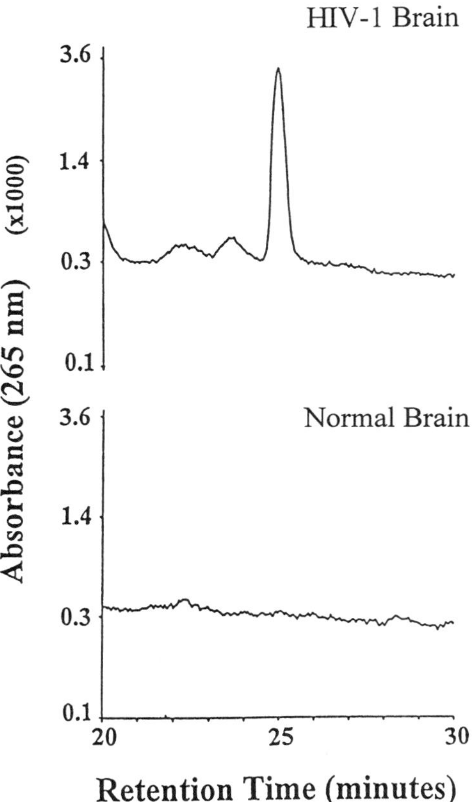

FIGURE 7. Direct extraction of NTox from HIV-1 infected human brain showed the presence of a biologically active phenolic compound that could be separated by reverse-phase HPLC. In contrast, normal brain lacked both cytotoxic activity or the phenol-containing agent detected by UV spectrometry.

cells stimulated *in vitro* and recovered from brain extracts (including acid hydrolysis, binding to cationic exchange resins, pH-dependent extraction into ethyl acetate, and elution on RP-HPLC) confirm that NTox released by cells *in vitro* is indistinguishable from the toxin found in HIV-1 infected brain.[21]

As noted, HIV-1 infected human cell lines, blood monocytes, or brain microglia do not release significant amounts of quinolinic acid. Moreover, brain tissue levels of quinolinic acid are nearly identical among samples recovered from infected brain ultrafiltrates (30 ± 5 nM quinolinate) and normal brain ultrafiltrates (25 ± 4 nM; ref. 21). Such results are puzzling in view of reports describing an association between quinolinate and AIDS dementia.[22,23] To address this problem, my laboratory returned to the original observation that HIV-1 infection brought about quinolinate elevations in cerebrospinal fluid (CSF). Significantly higher mean concentrations of CSF quinolinate (208 ± 31 nM; n = 66) are recovered from HIV-1(+) donors when compared to donors with multiple sclerosis (MS; 73 ± 6 nM quinolinate;

$n = 20$; Student's $t = 2.31$; df $= 84$; $p = 0.023$; FIG. 8A). In a similar way, plasma of donors infected with HIV-1 contain levels of quinolinate (1406 ± 127 nM; $n = 63$) that are significantly higher than those found in MS donors (677 ± 89; $n = 20$; Student's $t = 3.14$; df $= 81$; $p = 0.002$; FIG. 8B). Importantly, there is a striking correlation between CSF elevations of quinolinate and CSF elevations of albumin (FIG. 8C; $r = 0.722$; $n = 63$; $p < 0.0001$), which indicates that the highest concentrations of CSF quinolinate are found in those HIV-1 infected individuals with the greatest CSF concentrations of a serum protein. The abnormally high levels of CSF albumin found in HIV-1(+) donors indicate defects in the blood–brain barrier as noted by other investigators.[24] It is likely therefore, that quinolinate elevations in CSF are the result of leakage across the blood–brain barrier, and are not due to enhanced production by HIV-1 infected mononuclear phagocytes.

If NTox, in fact, plays some role in the pathogenesis of HIV-1 associated brain injury, this agent should also demonstrate biological action when infused into the brain. The rationale for hippocampal injections into rats is based upon observations that NMDA receptor(+) hippocampal neurons are particularly sensitive to NTox *in vitro*. Following infusion of NTox (derived from stimulated THP-1 cells), large numbers of pyknotic and dying pyramidal neurons are apparent five days later (FIG. 9). Little cell damage in the hippocampus is produced by injection of an identical, highly purified fraction from unstimulated THP-1 cells (FIG. 9). NTox (100 pmoles) shows a uniform pattern of pyknotic neurons within 150 μm (rostral to caudal) to either side of the injection site. Damage occurs primarily among pyramidal neurons in the CA3 and CA4 regions with sparing of the dentate granule cells and CA2. No seizure activity is noted after NTox infusion, and the toxin-induced cell loss does not match patterns of selective CA1 destruction found after global ischemia or prolonged seizures. Thus, several lines of evidence suggest that NTox produced by reactive microglia help to drive neuron injury during HIV-1 infection. Recovery of NTox from peripheral blood mononuclear cells of volunteers with infection and its production by microglia isolated from infected brains all point to the importance of this inflammatory neurotoxin. Moreover, both *in vitro* and *in vivo* experiments show NTox to be >500-fold more potent than quinolinic acid and suggest this inflammatory cell-derived neuron poison disrupts cognition during retroviral infections.

MICROGLIA AND ALZHEIMER'S DISEASE

Alzheimer's disease is a neurodegenerative dementia associated with loss of neurons and reactive gliosis.[25] The neuropathological hallmarks of this disorder

→

FIGURE 8. Measurement of quinolinic acid in donors with HIV-1 infection or multiple sclerosis (MS). **(A)** Individual concentrations of QUIN found in cerebrospinal fluid (CSF) of HIV-1(+) donors with [neuro(+)] or without [neuro(−)] neurological abnormalities. As shown, higher values are noted in both categories of infected donors when compared to MS controls. Mean CSF QUIN concentrations in HIV-1 groups were 126 ± 26 nM for neuro(−) and 268 ± 50 nM for neuro(+) compared with 74 ± 6 nM for the MS group. **(B)** Mean serum QUIN concentrations are higher for HIV-1 infected donors than for those measured in the MS group. [Mean scores for serum QUIN were 1249 ± 170 nM for neuro(−); 1530 ± 180 for neuro(+), and 677 ± 90 nM for MS.] **(C)** Correlation of mean CSF albumin concentration with mean QUIN concentrations found in HIV-1 infected donors. As shown, increasing amounts of QUIN correspond to increasing amounts of albumin ($r = 0.722$; $n = 63$; $p < 0.0001$). Such data suggest that defects in blood–brain barrier account for elevations of both QUIN and a serum protein. (From ref. 21.)

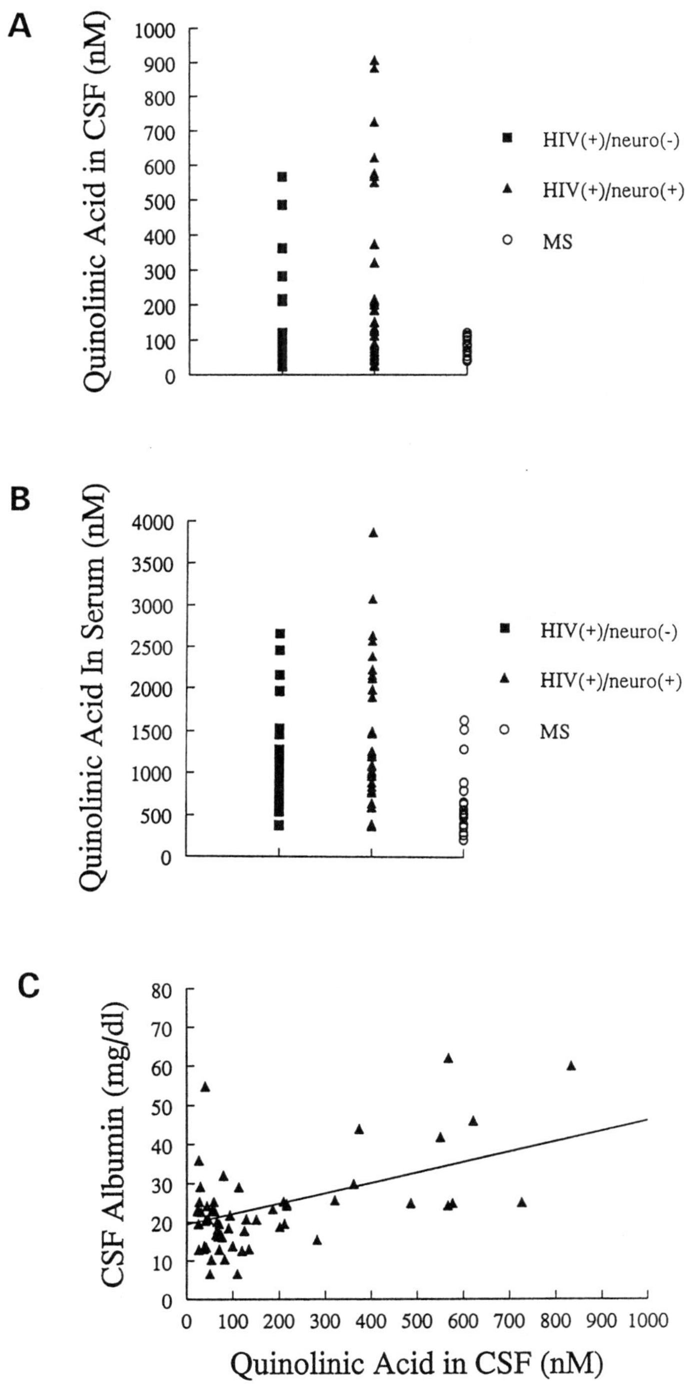

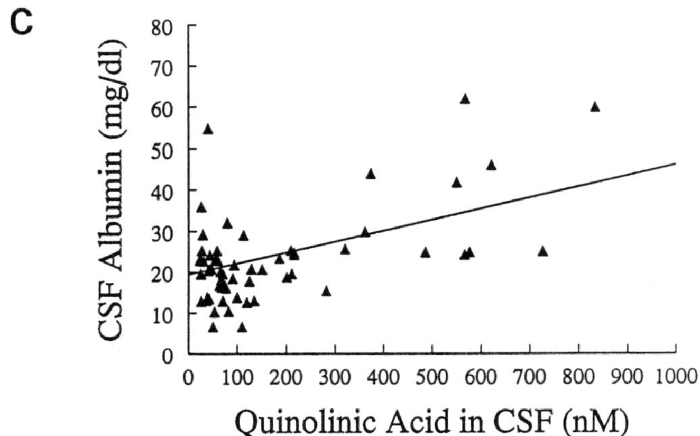
A
Quinolinic Acid in CSF (nM)
1000
900
800
700
600
500
400
300
200
100
0
HIV(+)/neuro(-)
HIV(+)/neuro(+)
MS

B
Quinolinic Acid In Serum (nM)
4000
3500
3000
2500
2000
1500
1000
500
0
HIV(+)/neuro(-)
HIV(+)/neuro(+)
MS

C
CSF Albumin (mg/dl)
80
70
60
50
40
30
20
10
0
0 100 200 300 400 500 600 700 800 900 1000
Quinolinic Acid in CSF (nM)

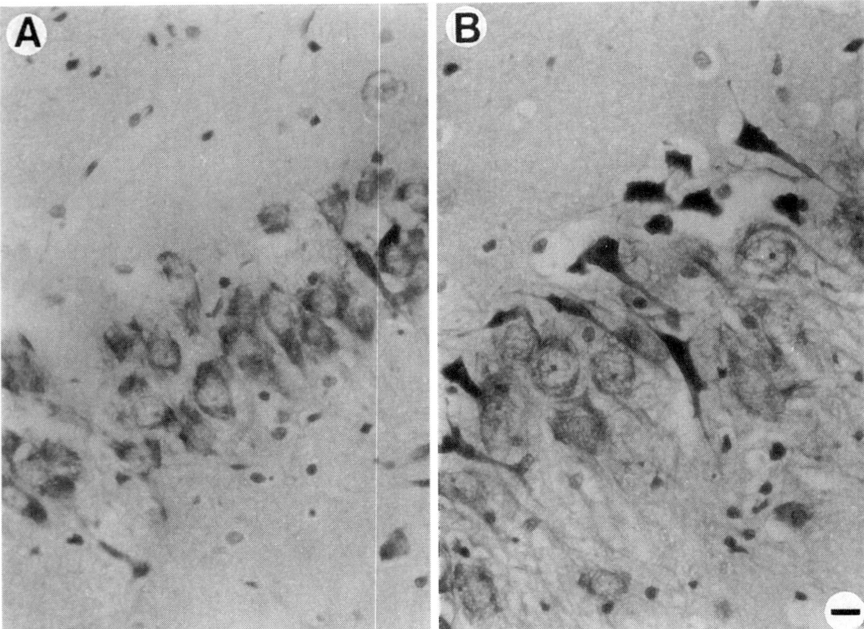

FIGURE 9. NTox infused directly into rat hippocampus kills neurons *in vivo*. Five days after injections neurons most sensitive to NTox included the pyramidal cells of the CA1 and CA3 regions. **(A)** Fink Heimer degeneration stain of CA1 neurons after infusion with a nontoxic control fraction (recovered from media conditioned by unstimulated THP-1 cells) showed little cell damage. **(B)** In contrast, contralateral hippocampus after NTox infusion (purified from media conditioned by gp120 stimulated THP-1 cells) demonstrated significant neuronal degeneration. In these experiments, 1 μL of artificial CSF with or without NTox (about 100 pmoles) was injected over a 4-min period at 2.9 mm from the brain's surface, at a distance of 4.5 mm caudal to bregma, 3.0 mm lateral to the midline into the hippocampus.

$\rightarrow$

FIGURE 10. **(A)** Effects of co-culture of human microglia, grown in chambers, with neurons grown atop coverslips. Microglia in contact with isolated senile plaques (microglia + plaque) released toxic activity that destroyed neurons. In contrast, when plaques are placed directly atop neurons (neuron + plaque) no cell loss occurred, indicating microglia, not plaques, were responsible for the neuron-killing activity. Brain fractions free of plaques from Alzheimer's disease (AD) tissue (microglia + AD fraction) obtained from the same preparation in which the plaques were isolated or amyotrophic lateral sclerosis (ALS) tissues (microglia + ALS fraction) also free of plaques did not stimulate microglia to release toxins. No toxic effect is noted for microglia placed alone in chambers. **(B)** Size-exclusion chromatography of neuritic/core plaque proteins using two Superose 12 columns in tandem (300 nm $\times$ 10 mm $\times$ 2). The approximate molecular masses of the fractions were S1, 200 kDa; S2, 45 kDa; S3, 15 kDa; S4, 10 kDa; and S5, 5 kDa. **(C)** Fractions of solubilized neuritic/core plaques were applied to hippocampal cultures in the presence or absence of microglia. No neuron killing was detected in cultures free of microglia. Neuron loss appeared, however, in microglia containing cultures exposed to peaks S3, S4, and S5, all which contain Aβ. (From refs. 28 and 36.)

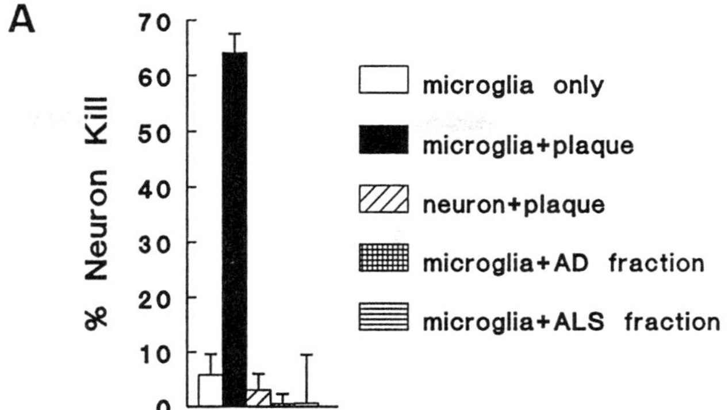
A
% Neuron Kill
70
60
50
40
30
20
10
0
microglia only
microglia+plaque
neuron+plaque
microglia+AD fraction
microglia+ALS fraction

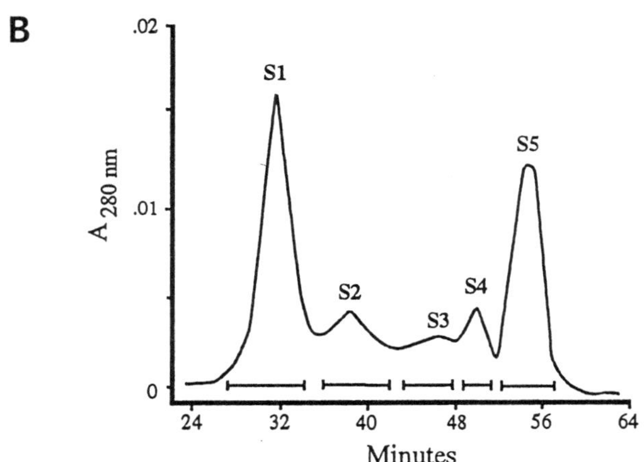
B
.02
.01
0
$A_{280\ nm}$
S1
S2
S3
S4
S5
24
32
40
48
56
64
Minutes

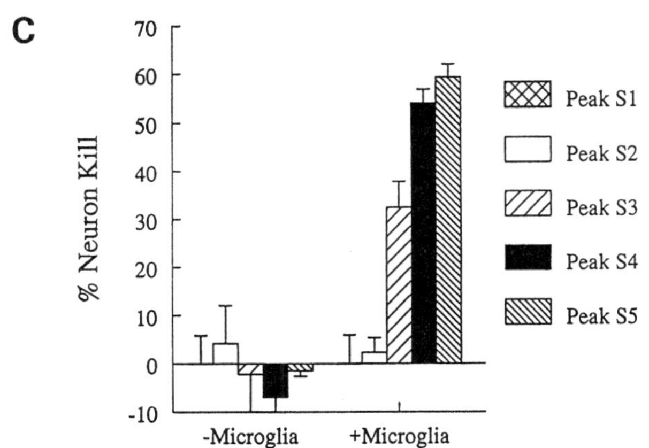
C
% Neuron Kill
70
60
50
40
30
20
10
0
-10
-Microglia
+Microglia
Peak S1
Peak S2
Peak S3
Peak S4
Peak S5

include neuritic and core senile plaques,[25] which are complex aggregations of proteins composed largely of a 42-residue peptide, β-amyloid (Aβ1–42). It is generally believed that Aβ is in some way responsible for the synaptic and neuronal loss associated with dementia. Two principal hypotheses have been advanced: (1) that Aβ acts as a potent and direct neurotoxic agent[26] or (2) that neuritic/core plaques elicit a cascade of cellular events which lead to neuronal pathology.[27,28] Support for the first hypothesis comes from *in vitro* observations in which synthetic Aβ peptides appear to poison enriched cultures of neurons[29] or various nonneuronal cell lines.[30] Support for the second hypothesis comes from evidence that neuritic/core plaques are not directly neurotoxic, as shown by the fact that neurons can be grown successfully atop Aβ peptides,[31,32] that neuritic/core plaques added directly to neurons do not cause neuronal damage,[28] and that Aβ peptides infused into the brain do not cause tissue injury.[33] One pathway for Aβ-induced neuronal damage may involve inflammatory cells, because it has long been recognized that reactive microglia are closely associated with neuritic or core plaques.[34,35] Quantitative histopathology reveals that >80% of core plaques are associated with clusters of reactive microglia whereas fewer than 2% of diffuse Aβ deposits show such an association.[28] Moreover, cultured microglia incubated with neuritic/core plaque fragments release NTox (FIG. 10A; ref. 28). These observations suggest that brain inflammatory responses may be directed specifically against the constituents of neuritic and core plaques.

To determine which plaque components activate microglia, solubilized neuritic/core plaque material is fractionated into five major peaks by sizing chromatography (FIG. 10B; ref. 36). Dominant constituents found in these plaque fractions include glycoproteins and α-1 antichymotrypsin in peak S1, apolipoprotein E in S2, and significant amounts of Aβ-amyloid (predominantly Aβ1–42) in peaks S3, S4, and S5, as trimers, dimers, and monomers, respectively.[36] The addition of plaque fractions S3, S4, and S5 to hippocampal cultures causes severe loss of neurons, but only in the presence of microglia (FIG. 10C). These data suggest that plaque-derived fractions S3, S4, and S5 contained factors capable of inducing neurotoxic microglia. Aβ1–40 or Aβ1–42 peptides, common to these three fractions, are, therefore, likely candidates as microglial activators.[36] When applied in 10 μM concentrations, Aβ1–42 had no damaging effects upon neurons grown in microglia-free rat hippocampal cultures (FIG. 11A). However, addition of microglia to this culture system in the presence of either human Aβ1–40 or Aβ1–42 produces widespread neuronal loss (FIG. 11A). In the presence of 1 μmole/L Aβ1–42, the microglial density required for maximum neuron killing was about 150 cells per mm^2 (microglia : neuron ratio of 0.8:1), although neuron killing can occur in the presence of <50 microglia per mm^2. Clearly, depletion of microglia from mixed neuron-glia cultures is necessary to demonstrate killing by inflammatory cells brought about by Aβ. The neurotoxic activity recovered from Aβ1–42 stimulated human microglia or extracted directly from Alzheimer disease brain is co-purified with NTox found in HIV-1 infected brain.

Because adherence to plaques serves as an important first step in eliciting brain inflammation, Aβ on plaque surfaces may act as anchoring sites for microglia. Covalent coupling of synthetic Aβ peptides or native plaque-derived proteins to 90 μm Sepharose beads allows testing of this hypothesis.[36] Within six hours, the number of microglia adhering to plaque-protein-coated beads increased by fivefold when compared to cells adhering to control beads coupled to glycine or albumin. Interestingly, Aβ peptides that contained N-terminal residues, such as Aβ1–28, promote cell binding, while the C-terminal portion (Aβ17–42) does not. Phagocytosis assays involving 1-μm microspheres linked to synthetic peptides yield a similar result. For example, microglial binding to Aβ1–42, Aβ1–40, Aβ1–16, or Aβ12–28

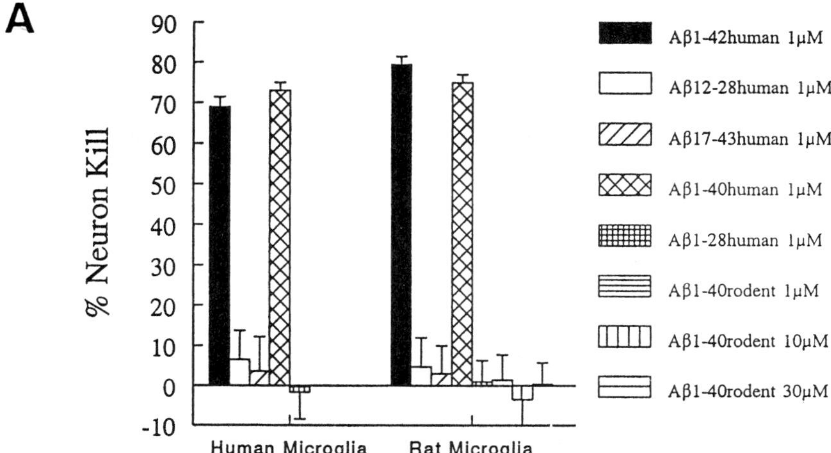

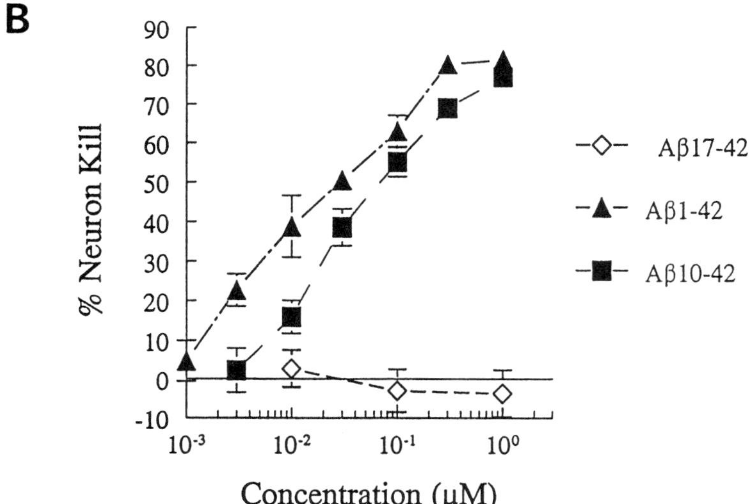

FIGURE 11. Toxic actions of synthetic Aβ peptides upon neurons. **(A)** In the absence of microglia, none of the Aβ peptides (at 1 μmole/L) destroyed neurons. When either human or rat microglia were added to neuronal cultures, however, Aβ1–40 and Aβ1–42 brought about neuron killing. Other Aβ peptides including the N-terminal (Aβ1–28) or C-terminal (Aβ17–43) did not. Importantly, rodent Aβ1–40 was ineffective in activating neurotoxic microglia. Further structural studies identified residues 13–16 (HHQK domain) found in human Aβ as necessary for microglial stimulation. **(B)** Dose-response curves showed that Aβ1–42 was a potent stimulus for microglia-dependent neuron killing whereas Aβ17–42 was not. Additional residues found in Aβ10–42 (including the HHQK domain) produced a peptide capable of stimulating microglia which confirmed the required structure to interact with microglia.

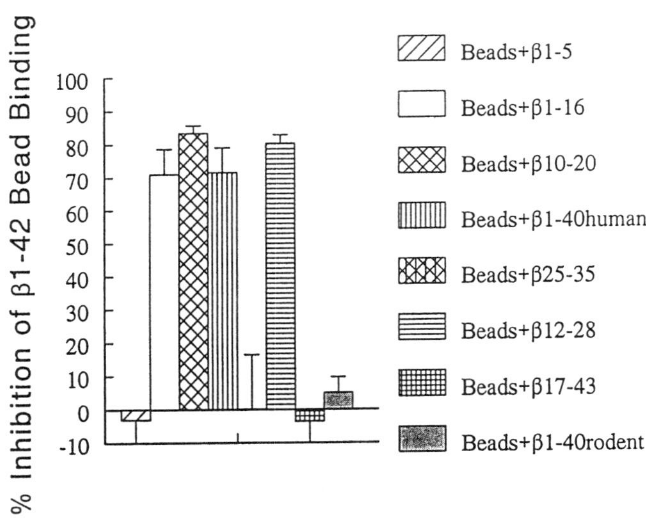

FIGURE 12. Inhibition of Aβ binding to microglia. Aβ1–42 was coupled to fluorescent microspheres and the beads monitored for binding to microglia after 4 h at 37 °C in the presence of peptides (all at 10 μmoles/L). Only peptides containing residues 13–16 (HHQK domain) were able to competitively block sphere binding.

readily occurs (FIG. 12), whereas little cell-microsphere interaction is apparent using Aβ17–43, Aβ25–35, or Aβ36–42. Importantly, the lack of microglial binding to rodent Aβ1–40 (^{5}Arg → Gly, ^{10}Tyr → Phe, ^{13}His → Arg) suggests that the primary structure of human Aβ, the N-terminus, is essential for immune activation. Subsequent experiments determined the microglial binding site to exist between residues 13 to 16 (the HHKQ domain). The importance of this N-terminal cell binding domain is supported by the fact that neither Aβ17–42 nor Aβ1–40$_{rodent}$ induces neurotoxic cells despite test concentrations 100-fold above that required for human Aβ1–40. The patterns of binding and toxicity predict that the 10 to 16 binding domain would be a necessary component for activation of neuron-killing microglia.

→

FIGURE 13. (A) The HHQK domain of Aβ blocks neurotoxic microglia activated by plaques. Suspensions of neuritic/core plaque fragments were incubated with microglia placed in cell chambers (each containing 250,000 cells) atop rat hippocampal cultures. Despite 72 h of exposure to plaque material, microglia did not become neurotoxic if Aβ peptides containing HHQK domain were present. All peptides were tested at 10 μM. **(B)** Immune-inhibiting concentrations of test agents (range from 10 nM to 10 μM) showed that only chloroquine was effective in blocking Aβ-induced neurotoxic microglia. **(C)** The *in vivo* action of NTox can be blocked by preinfusion of 1 nmole of AP5 prepared in 1 μL artificial CSF prior to NTox injection. In contrast, a control preinfusion with 1 μL artificial CSF did not block hippocampal injury. Quantitative measure of CA3 neuronal damage showed a 60 to 70% cell loss after NTox infusion with about a 10% pyramidal cell loss seen in control injections (Student's t test; $p < 0.0001$). Blockade with AP5 reduces cell loss to control levels. Cell counts were obtained at 100 μm rostral and caudal to the site of injection. (From ref. 36.)

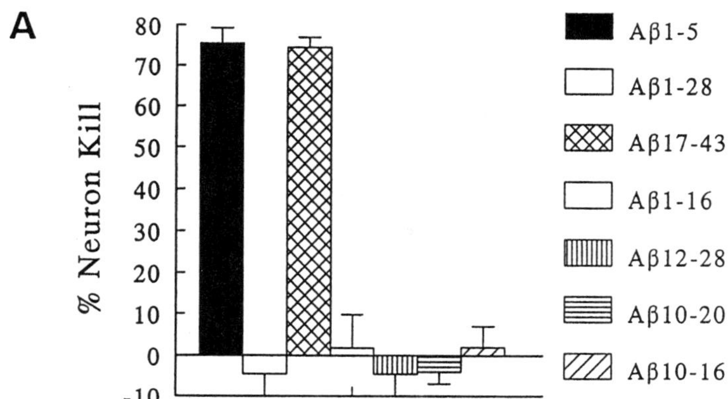
A
% Neuron Kill
80
70
60
50
40
30
20
10
0
-10
Aβ1-5
Aβ1-28
Aβ17-43
Aβ1-16
Aβ12-28
Aβ10-20
Aβ10-16

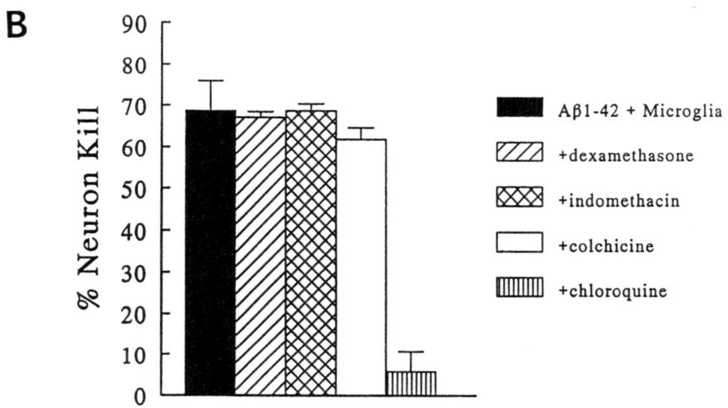
B
% Neuron Kill
90
80
70
60
50
40
30
20
10
0
Aβ1-42 + Microglia
+dexamethasone
+indomethacin
+colchicine
+chloroquine

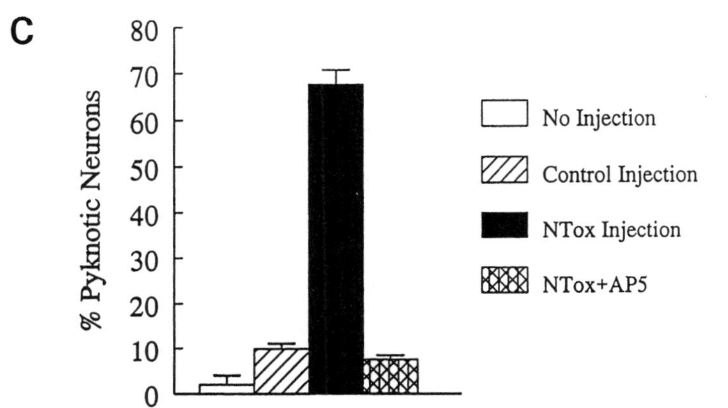
C
% Pyknotic Neurons
80
70
60
50
40
30
20
10
0
No Injection
Control Injection
NTox Injection
NTox+AP5

Aβ10–42 at increasing concentrations is as potent as Aβ1–42 in eliciting microglia-dependent killing of cells (FIG. 11B). However, the Aβ10–16 binding domain or the Aβ17–42 region by themselves does not injure neurons. Thus, the N-terminus of human Aβ (particularly residues 13–16) is necessary, though not sufficient, for eliciting neurotoxic microglia. Such observations point to novel strategies for impairing plaque induction of brain inflammation.

SUPPRESSION OF NEUROTOXIC MICROGLIA AS TREATMENT FOR DEMENTIA

Strategies to reduce CNS pathology stemming from neurotoxic microglia include (1) the suppression of signals (i.e., infection by HIV or contact with neuritic/core plaques in Alzheimer's disease), which transform quiescent microglia into neurotoxic ones, (2) the inhibition of microglial synthesis and secretion of neurotoxins, including NTox, and (3) the blockade of microglial neuron poisons. Examples for each of these strategies are given below.

Peptides that contain the HHQK domain block Aβ1–42 adherence to microglia and thus may also prevent Aβ1–42 induction of neurotoxic glia. To test this possibility, various peptides (each at 10 μmoles/L) are added together with human Aβ1–42 (1 μmole/L) to neuron cultures containing microglia. Only peptides with residues 13 to 16, namely, Aβ1–28, Aβ1–16, Aβ10–20, Aβ10–16, and Aβ13–16, block neurotoxin production whereas peptides Aβ1–5, Aβ1–11, Aβ17–43, and Aβ36-42 (lacking HHKQ) do not (FIG. 13A). In contrast to Aβ1–40 and Aβ1–42, none of the blocking peptides elicits neuron killing. Although HHQK-containing peptides prevent Aβ1–42 activation of microglia, these experiments do not determine whether such agents would also inhibit plaque-microglia interactions. Aβ1–16, Aβ13–20, Aβ10–16, and Aβ13–16 all suppress neurotoxic activity of either rat or human microglia exposed to plaques. Perhaps HHKQ-like agents will reduce plaque activation of microglia *in situ* and thus provide a selective treatment to slow Alzheimer's disease pathology secondary to inflammation.

Treatments encompassing a second microglia suppression strategy are reflected in several retrospective studies which suggest anti-inflammatory drugs as beneficial for Alzheimer's disease.[37,38] However, commonly used immunosuppressants (including glucocorticoids) often do not reduce neurotoxic activities of brain mononuclear phagocytes.[1,39] As shown in FIGURE 13B, chloroquine, but not indomethacin, dexamethasone, or colchicine, prevents Aβ-activation of neurotoxic microglia. Because chloroquine also reduces neuron killing in rodents during trauma or stroke,[13,39] its use as a microglial suppressant in clinical trials is warranted.

A third therapeutic approach involves blockade of NTox by antagonists of the NMDA receptor. In addition to *in vitro* experiments, such a strategy shows promise *in vivo*. For example, one nmole of AP5 infused into the brain protects CA3 neurons against damage by NTox (FIG. 13C). Interestingly, Masliah *et al.*[40] find that the CA3 region had the greatest level of hippocampal pathology among a group of encephalopathic patients infected with HIV-1. Perhaps NMDA receptor antagonists now in clinical trials for stroke, trauma, and epilepsy may offer benefit to patients with neurotoxic microgliosis due to HIV-1 infection or senile plaques.

CONCLUSIONS

Although signaling mechanisms vary among neuropathic conditions, the activation of microglia is a response common to all inflammatory and necrotizing processes in the brain. As suggested by histopathology, microglia are scavengers that clear debris from sites of CNS injury. *In vitro* studies, however, show that reactive microglia are also a source of cytotoxic agents. Neuron-killing microglial reactions are common to chronic brain disorders which produce dementia. These reactive microglia appear responsible for neuronal injury and subsequent cognitive impairment. Novel therapeutic interventions to suppress neurotoxic microglia may offer ways to slow neuronal loss in HIV-1 encephalopathy or Alzheimer's disease.

REFERENCES

1. GIULIAN, D. 1992. Microglia and diseases of the nervous system. *In* Current Neurology, Vol. 12. S. H. Appel, Ed.: 23–54. Mosby Year Book. St. Louis, MO.
2. RIO-HORTEGA, P. 1932. Microglia. *In* Cytology and Cellular Pathology of the Nervous System. W. Penfield, Ed.: 481–584. Hocker, Inc. New York.
3. GIULIAN, D. 1987. Ameboid microglia as effectors of inflammation in the central nervous system. J. Neurosci. Res. **18:** 155–171.
4. HICKEY, W. F. & H. KIMURA. 1988. Perivascular microglial cells of the CNS are bone marrow-derived and present antigen in vivo. Science **239:** 290–292.
5. FLARIS, N. A., T. L. DENSMORE, M. C. MOLLESTON & W. F. HICKEY. 1993. Characterization of microglia and macrophages in the central nervous system of rats: Definition of the differential expression of molecules using standard and novel monoclonal antibodies in normal CNS and in four models of parenchymal reaction. Glia **7:** 34–40.
6. GIULIAN, D. & T. J. BAKER. 1986. Characterization of ameboid microglia isolated from developing mammalian brain. J. Neurosci. **6:** 2163–2178.
7. GIULIAN, D., J. LI, S. BARTEL, J. BROKER, X. LI & J. B. KIRKPATRICK. 1995. Cell surface morphology identifies microglia as a distinct class of mononuclear phagocyte. J. Neurosci. **15:** 7712–7726.
8. KETTENMANN, H., D. HOPPE, K. GOTTMANN, R. BANATI & G. KREUTZBERG. 1990. Cultured microglial cells have a distinct pattern of membrane channels different from peritoneal macrophages. J. Neurosci. Res. **26:** 278–287.
9. GIULIAN, D. & L. B. LACHMAN. 1985. Interleukin-1 stimulates astroglial proliferation after brain injury. Science **228:** 497–499.
10. GIULIAN, D., J. WOODWARD, D. G. YOUNG, J. F. KREBS & L. B. LACHMAN. 1988. Interleukin-1 injected into mammalian brain stimulates astrogliosis and neovascularization. J. Neurosci. **8:** 2485–2490.
11. GIULIAN, D., J. LI, X. LI, J. GEORGE & P. A. RUTECKI. 1994. The impact of microglia-derived cytokines upon gliosis in the CNS. Dev. Neurosci. **16:** 128–136.
12. FAGAN, A. M. & F. H. GAGE. 1990. Cholinergic sprouting in the hippocampus: A proposed role for IL-1. Exp. Neurol. **100:** 105–120.
13. GIULIAN, D., J. CHEN, J. E. INGEMAN, J. K. GEORGE & M. NOPONEN. 1989. The role of mononuclear phagocytes in wound healing after traumatic injury to adult mammalian brain. J. Neurosci. **9:** 4416–4429.
14. GIULIAN, D., M. CORPUZ, S. CHAPMAN, M. MANSOURI & C. ROBERTSON. 1993. Reactive mononuclear phagocytes release neurotoxins after ischemic and traumatic injury to the central nervous system. J. Neurosci. Res. **36:** 681–693.
15. GIULIAN, D., K. VACA & M. CORPUZ. 1993. Brain glia release factors with opposing actions upon neuronal survival. J. Neurosci. **13:** 29–37.
16. ROBERTS, P. & S. DAVIES. 1987. Excitatory receptors and their role in excitotoxicity. Biochem. Soc. Trans. **15:** 218–219.
17. SNIDER, W. D., D. M. SIMPSON, *et al.* 1983. Neurological complications of AIDS: Analysis of 50 patients. Ann. Neurol. **14:** 403–418.
18. NAVIA, B. A., B. D. JORDAN & R. W. PRICE. 1986. The AIDS dementia complex: I. Clinical features. Ann. Neurol. **19:** 517–524.
19. GIULIAN, D., K. VACA & C. A. NOONAN. 1990. Secretion of neurotoxins by mononuclear phagocytes infected with HIV-1. Science **250:** 1593–1596.

20. GIULIAN, D., E. WENDT, K. VACA & C. A. NOONAN. 1993. The envelope glycoprotein of human immunodeficiency virus type 1 stimulates release of neurotoxins from monocytes. Proc. Natl. Acad. Sci. USA **90:** 2769–2773.

21. GIULIAN, D., J. H. YU, X. LI, D. TOM, J. LI, E. WENDT, S. N. LIN, R. SCHWARCZ & C. NOONAN. 1996. Study of receptor-mediated neurotoxins released by HIV-1 infected mononuclear phagocytes found in human brain. J. Neurosci. **16:** 3139–3153.

22. HEYES, M. P., D. RUBINOW, C. LANE & S. P. MARKEY. 1989. Cerebrospinal fluid quinolinic acid concentrations are increased in acquired immune deficiency syndrome. Ann. Neurol. **26(2):** 275–277.

23. SAITO, K., C. Y. CHEN, M. MASANA, J. S. CROWLEY & M. P. HEYES. 1993. 4-Chloro-3-hydroxyanthranilate, 6-chlorotryptophan, and norhamane attentuate quinolinic acid formation by interferon gamma-stimulated monocytes (THP-1 cells). Biochem. J. **291:** 11–14.

24. PETITO, C. K. & K. S. CASH. 1992. Blood-brain barrier abnormalities in the acquired immunodeficiency syndrome: Immunohistochemical localization of serum proteins in postmortem brain. Ann. Neurol. **32:** 658–666.

25. TERRY, R. D., R. KATZMAN & K. L. BICK, Eds. 1994. Alzheimer's Disease. Raven Press. New York.

26. YANKER, B. A., L. K. DUFFY & D. A. KIRSCHNER. 1990. Neurotrophic and neurotoxic effects of amyloid β protein: Reversal by tachykinin neuropeptides. Science **250:** 279–282.

27. DAVIES, P. 1994. Neuronal abnormalities, not amyloid, are the cause of dementia in Alzheimer's disease. *In* Alzheimer's Disease. R. D. Terry, R. Katzman & K. L. Bick, Eds.: 327–333. Raven Press. New York.

28. GIULIAN, D., L. J. HAVERKAMP, J. LI, W. L. KARSHIN, J. YU, D. TOM, X. LI & J. B. KIRKPATRICK. 1995. Senile plaques stimulate microglia to release a neurotoxin found in Alzheimer brain. Neurochem. Int. **27:** 119–137.

29. PIKE, C. J., A. J. WALENCEWICZ, C. G. GLABE & C. W. COTMAN. 1991. Aggregation-related toxicity of synthetic β-amyloid protein in hippocampal cultures. Eur. J. Pharmacol. **207:** 367–368.

30. BEHL, C., J. B. DAVIS, R. LESLEY & D. SCHUBERT. 1994. Hydrogen peroxide mediates amyloid β protein toxicity. Cell **7:** 817–827.

31. KOO, E. H., L. PARK & D. J. SELKOE. 1993. Amyloid β-protein as a substrate interacts with extracellular matrix to promote neurite outgrowth. Proc. Natl. Acad. Sci. USA **90:** 4748–4752.

32. WUJEK, J. R., M. D. DORITY, R. C. A. FREDRICKSON & K. R. BRUDENT. 1996. Deposits of Aβ fibrils are not toxic to cortical and hippocampal neurons in vitro. Neurobiol. Aging **17:** 107–113.

33. GAMES, D., K. M. KHAN, F. G. SORIANO, P. S. KEIM, D. L. DAVIS, K. BRYANT & I. LIEBERBURG. 1992. Lack of Alzheimer pathology after β-amyloid protein injections in rat brain. Neurobiol. Aging **13:** 569–576.

34. BOLSI, D. 1927. Placche senile e microglia. Riv. di Patol. Nerv. Ment. **32:** 65–72.

35. MCGEER, P. L., S. ITAGAKI, B. E. BOYES & E. G. MCGEER. 1988. Reactive microglia are positive for HLA-DR in the substantia nigra of Parkinson's and Alzheimer's disease brains. Neurology **38:** 1285–1291.

36. GIULIAN, D., L. J. HAVERKAMP, J. H. YU, W. KARSHIN, D. TOM, J. LI, J. KIRKPATRICK, Y. M. KUO & A. E. ROHER. 1996. Specific domains of β-amyloid from Alzheimer plaque elicit neuron killing in human microglia. J. Neurosci. **16:** 6021–6037.

37. MCGEER, P. L., E. MCGEER, J. ROGERS & J. SIBLEY. 1990. Anti-inflammatory drugs and Alzheimer disease. Lancet **335:** 1037.

38. EIKELENBOOM, P., S-S. ZHAN, W. A. VAN GOOL & D. ALLSOP. 1994. Inflammatory mechanisms in Alzheimer's disease. TIPS **15:** 447–450.

39. GIULIAN, D. & C. ROBERTSON. 1990. Inhibition of mononuclear phagocytes reduces ischemic injury in the spinal cord. Ann. Neurol. **27:** 33–42.

40. MASLIAH, E., N. GE, C. L. ACHIM, L. A. HANSEN & C. A. WILEY. 1992. Selective neuronal vulnerability in HIV encephalitis. J. Neuropathol. Exp. Neurol. **51:** 585–593.

Autoimmune Neuromyotonia (Isaacs' Syndrome): An Antibody-mediated Potassium Channelopathy

JOHN NEWSOM-DAVIS[a]

Neurosciences Group
Institute of Molecular Medicine
University of Oxford
John Radcliffe Hospital
Oxford OX3 9DU, United Kingdom

INTRODUCTION

The concept of an autoimmune antibody-mediated channelopathy stems from the seminal experimental and clinical studies in myasthenia gravis (MG). Crucial for these advances was the availability of purified neurotoxins (α-bungarotoxin) that, with high specificity and affinity, labeled the target acetylcholine receptor (AChR; a muscle cation channel). Evidence for an antibody-mediated etiology included induction of experimental autoimmune MG by immunization with affinity-purified AChR,[1] detection of serum anti-AChR antibodies in patients with MG,[2] passive transfer of MG to mice by injection of IgG from patients with MG,[3] and demonstration of clinical improvement following plasmapheresis.[4] Criteria for defining a disease as autoimmune, modified for an antibody-mediated effector mechanism, can thus be restated as follows: (1) Evidence for a circulating antibody to a defined antigen; (2) passive transfer of the physiological and morphological characteristics to experimental animals by injection of patients' immunoglobulins; and (3) induction of the disease in experimental animals by immunization with purified antigen, and passive transfer of their immunoglobulins as in (2).

Additional clinical features that may be found in an antibody-mediated disorder are a response to plasmapheresis, association with other autoimmune diseases, or with particular neoplasms. In MG, the response to plasmapheresis occurs within a few days because AChRs have a rapid turnover and new channels are generated free of antibody. Where the antibody-mediated process has destroyed the target cell, such a response would not be seen. The association with other autoimmune diseases is conferred by shared immune response genes. Thymoma, an epithelial cell tumor,[5] is known to associate with immune-mediated disorders and is present in 10% of MG cases.

The second channelopathy to be recognized as antibody-mediated was the Lambert-Eaton myasthenic syndrome (LEMS).[6] Here the target is principally the P/Q-type voltage-gated calcium channel (VGCC) at motor nerve terminals, on which quantal release of transmitter depends. Serum anti-VGCC antibodies can be detected in 90% of patients using $[^{125}I]\omega$-conotoxin MVIIC,[7] a neurotoxin purified from a species of marine fish-eating snail. Weakness improves following plasmapheresis,[6] although the response is less immediate than in MG. The principal neurophysiologi-

[a] E-mail: neurosciences@imm.ox.ac.uk

cal abnormality in LEMS is a reduction in the quantal content of the end-plate potential (i.e., the number of quanta released by each nerve impulse), as first recognized by Lambert and Elmqvist.[8] These changes can be passively transferred to mice by injection of LEMS IgG,[6,9] and are consistent with a decrease in the number of functional VGCCs, leading to a reduction in the number of quanta of acetylcholine released by each nerve impulse. The morphological changes in LEMS that are characterized by a disorganization and reduction in the number of active-zone particles (believed to represent VGCCs) at motor nerve terminals[10] can also be transferred to mice by LEMS IgG.[11] In addition, there is an increased association of LEMS with other autoimmune diseases, especially vitiligo, and about 60% of patients have associated small cell lung cancer.[12] Clinical and experimental evidence now exists for a third antibody-mediated channelopathy, namely, acquired neuromyotonia (Isaacs' syndrome), in which voltage-gated potassium channels (VGKCs) are targeted. These data will be reviewed in this paper.

CLINICAL FEATURES

Autoimmune neuromyotonia (ANMT) is characterized by widespread myokymia (muscle twitching) and cramps.[13] It may be associated with muscle hypertrophy, muscle weakness or stiffness, pseudomyotonia, increased sweating, and sometimes also with central nervous system (CNS) symptoms including insomnia and hallucinations. Some patients experience transient parasthesiae. ANMT needs to be distinguished from the myokymia that can occur in patients with hereditary disorders such as episodic ataxia with myokymia and hereditary neuropathies, in which immune mechanisms are not implicated.

The syndrome has been given several different names over the years. Morvan,[14] who first recognized neuromyotonia in association with CNS changes, named the condition *chorée fibrillaire*. Denny-Brown and Foley[15] described the condition as "undulating myokymia," and Isaacs[16] termed it a syndrome of "continuous muscle fiber activity." After the publication of Isaacs' paper, however, the disorder often became known as Isaacs' syndrome. The term *neuromyotonie* was coined by Mertens and Zschocke.[17,18] Autoimmune neuromyotonia will be used here to specify the antibody-mediated disorder.

ELECTROMYOGRAPHIC FEATURES

The hallmark of ANMT is the spontaneous burst discharge of single motor units, occurring as doublets, triplets or multiplets (FIG. 1A).[13] The bursts themselves occur irregularly, and may be provoked by voluntary muscle activation. The intraburst frequency can range from 40 to >300 Hz. These electromyographic (EMG) abnormalities were first recognized by Denny-Brown and Foley[15] in two young men, one a 37-year-old physician. These authors illustrated irregular burst discharges in one of these patients, recording an intraburst frequency of about 50/s. The above definition of an EMG discharge as "neuromyotonic" does not fully accord with the AAEE Glossary of Terms in Clinical Electromyography[18] which, arbitrarily, requires the intraburst frequency to be 150–300 Hz. However, the discharge that illustrates this definition also clearly shows doublet and triplet discharges from the same motor unit at intraburst frequencies as slow as 40–50 Hz, emphasizing that such low burst frequencies are also characteristic of neuromyotonia.

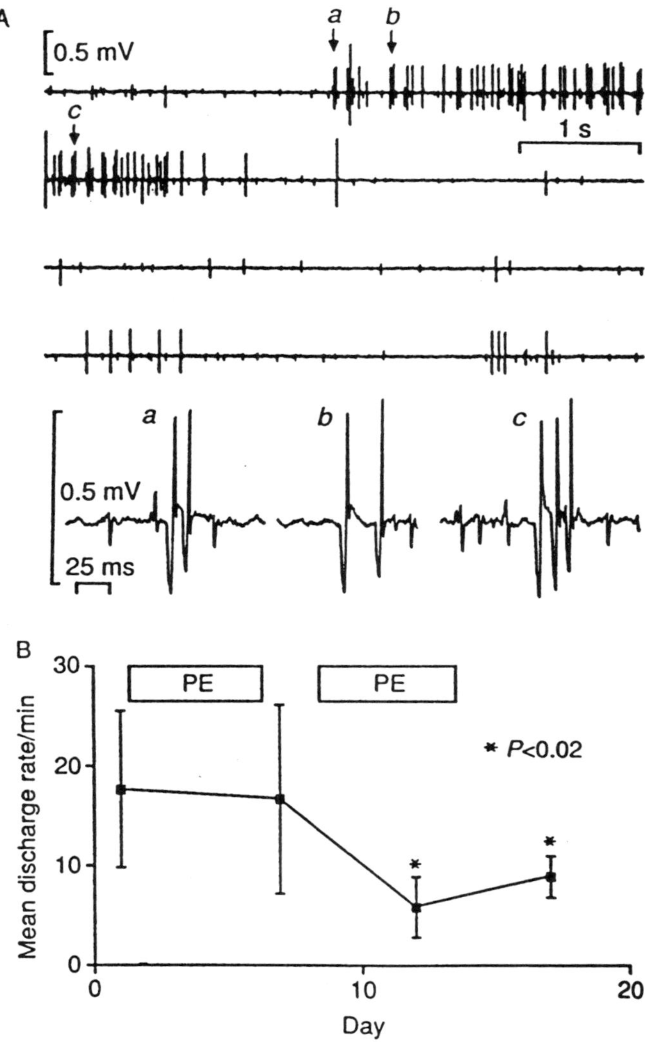

FIGURE 1. (**A**) Needle recording from the first dorsal interosseous muscle of a 43-year-old man with autoimmune neuromyotonia. The upper four traces are continuous and show a neuromyotonic discharge lasting some 4 s. Within the discharge, single motor units fire as doublets (at *a* and *b*, *see below*) or triplets (at *c*, *see below*). (**B**) The effect of plasma exchange on the mean (±SD) discharge frequency in serial surface EMG recordings made from the medial gastrocnemius muscle. The second course of exchange leads to a significant ($p <$ 0.02) but transient reduction in the frequency of discharge. (Reproduced from ref. 12, with permission of Oxford University Press.)

EMG may also reveal occasional fasciculations and fibrillation potentials. In some patients, changes indicating a mild axonal or demyelinating neuropathy may be present. "After-discharges" following nerve stimulation may occur.

SITE OF ORIGIN OF ABNORMAL DISCHARGES

Isaacs[16] established unequivocally that the discharges originated in peripheral motor nerves by demonstrating that muscle activity continued after proximal peripheral nerve block with local anesthetic, but was abolished by curare (thereby excluding an end-plate origin). In Isaacs' cases, the site of origin was in the "distal arborization of motor nerve terminals" as in many reported cases including those described by Wallis, van Poznak, and Plum.[19] However, other cases have been documented (reviewed in ref. 13) in which complete distal motor nerve block did not abolish the discharges, indicating that they may arise partly or exclusively from more proximal sites, possibly even including the anterior horn cell itself. Further supporting evidence for a lower motor neuron origin is the continued neuromyotonic activity during sleep or general anesthesia, distinguishing the disorder from the Stiffman syndrome.

AUTOIMMUNE ASSOCIATIONS

A number of clinical clues suggest an autoimmune disease process. First, autoimmune diseases tend to cluster within individuals or families, and ANMT shows an increased association with MG. Second, thymoma is known to occur in 10% of MG cases, and also associates with other autoimmune diseases. We have observed thymoma in about 20% of our ANMT cases. Third, the cerebrospinal fluid (CSF) may contain oligoclonal bands in occasional cases.[13] Finally, intensive plasma exchange can be followed by clinical improvement.[20] This is illustrated in FIGURE 1B, which shows a significant reduction in the quantified neuromyotonic discharges in a resting muscle, recorded with surface electrodes for a 50-min period from the same site before and after two 5-day courses of plasma exchange in a 22-year-old man with an eight-year history of ANMT. This patient also had a high titer of anti-thyroid antibodies.

INITIAL EXPERIMENTAL STUDIES

Hyperexcitability of peripheral nerve could be due either to a reduction in the number of VGKCs, or to a prolonged open time of the voltage-gated sodium channels. The reduction in neuromyotonic discharges following plasmapheresis suggested that an antibody-mediated process might underlie the disorder. Down-regulation of VGKCs seemed the most attractive hypothesis because other anti-channel autoantibodies (e.g., anti-AChR in MG) are known to reduce the number of functional channels.

We argued that such an antibody-mediated reduction in functional VGKCs would not only result in membrane hyperexcitability (by interfering with repolarization), but would also prolong the action potential at the nerve terminal. This would result in nerve terminal VGCCs being open for a longer period, thereby increasing the number of quanta released by each nerve impulse. The antibodies would thus be acting similarly to 4-aminopyridine.

In our first 'passive transfer' experiments, mice were intraperitoneally injected for several days with ANMT or control plasma or immunoglobulins, and neuromuscular transmission was then studied *ex vivo* in the peripheral nerve–diaphragm preparation.[20] Resistance to d-tubocurarine (d-Tc) was then evaluated. The experiments showed that diaphragms from mice injected with ANMT plasma or immunoglobulins required significantly larger doses of d-TC to block transmission than was the case in control-injected mice. The results were therefore consistent with the hypothesis that ANMT plasma or immunoglobulins contained antibodies that increased resistance to d-Tc by down-regulating VGKCs.

DIRECT MEASUREMENTS OF QUANTAL CONTENT

In a further set of passive transfer experiments, the quantal content of the end-plate potential was measured directly using microelectrodes to record miniature end-plate potentials (MEPP) and end-plate (EPP) amplitudes.[21] ANMT IgG was prepared from the plasma of five patients with clinical and electromyographic evidence of ANMT. Mice were injected intraperitoneally with 1 mg IgG for 10–12 days, and the phrenic nerve–diaphragm then studied *ex vivo*. Results were compared with those in mice injected with control human IgG. Similar studies were undertaken by Dr. Peter Molenaar and colleagues at the University of Leiden in another patient with ANMT.[21] The results showed a highly significant increase (21%; $p = 0.005$) in the quantal content in ANMT-injected mice compared with control mice. The Leiden group also demonstrated repetitive firing in dorsal root ganglion cells exposed for 24 h to IgG from their ANMT patient.[21] Further studies showed that the addition of 4-aminopyridine (which blocks VGKCs) to the phrenic nerve–diaphragm preparation increased the quantal content in a similar manner to ANMT IgG.

These physiological studies thus strongly suggested that ANMT sera contained IgG antibodies that were underlying the pathophysiological effects. The likely target for these would be VGKCs with A-type or delayed rectifier electrophysiological properties that would be of the *Shaker*-related potassium channel family.

VOLTAGE-GATED POTASSIUM CHANNELS

A functional VGKC comprises four transmembrane α-subunits that combine as homomultimeric or heteromultimeric tetramers, and associate with four intracellular β-subunits. At least six *Shaker*-related VGKC α-subunit genes have been isolated from human brain.[22] TABLE 1 indicates their terminology, sites of expression, and whether they bind the potassium channel blocker α-dendrotoxin. The activation characteristics of the channels are influenced by β-subunit association.[23]

DETECTION OF ANTI-VGKC ANTIBODIES BY RADIOIMMUNOASSAY

The improvement following plasmapheresis and the pathophysiological effects in mice of injected ANMT IgG are consistent with the presence of circulating anti-

TABLE 1. *Shaker*-related Human Voltage-gated K$^+$ Channel Gene Family

Property	Chromosome	Human Gene Nomenclature	Dendrotoxin Binding
Kv1.1	12	KCNA1.HBK1	+
kV1.1A	n/a	KCNA1a/	−
Kv1.2	1	KCNA2/HBK5	+
Kv1.3	13	KCNA3/	−
KV1.4	11	KCNA4/HBK4	−
Kv1.5	12	KCNA5/	−
Kv1.6	12	KCNA6/HBK2	+

VGKC antibodies in patients with ANMT. These anti-VGKC antibodies were first looked for by radioimmunoassay, using [^{125}I]α-dendrotoxin-labeled VGKCs as antigen.[21] Raised titers were detected in about one-half the patients studied, but the titers were generally quite low. However, in a patient with a relatively high initial titer, decline in antibody level in response to plasmapheresis and immunosuppressive drug treatment correlated with clinical and electromyographic improvement.[21]

Because α-dendrotoxin does not label all *Shaker*-related VGKCs (see TABLE 1), it was possible that some antibodies were not being detected in this assay. To try to overcome this, an alternative approach was used in which a molecular-immunohistochemical assay was developed.

MOLECULAR-IMMUNOHISTOCHEMICAL AUTOANTIBODY ASSAY

In this assay, *Xenopus* oocytes were injected with cRNAs for individual *Shaker*-related VGKC α-subunits.[24] Serum at various dilutions was applied to fixed sections, and binding to the α-subunit polypeptide expressed in the *Xenopus* cytoplasm was detected by a biotin-conjugated anti-human IgG and streptavidin/horseradish peroxidase. Controls included a rabbit polyserum raised against a known VGKC polypeptide, serum from other neurological diseases, and *Xenopus* oocytes injected with the AChR α-subunit. All results were evaluated on coded material.

Immunoreactivity at serum dilutions of 1:128 to 1:2,500 was found for all 12 ANMT sera studied to at least one of the three expressed human VGKC α-subunits.[24] As TABLE 2 shows, four ANMT sera reacted with all three subtypes, whereas only two of these were positive in the radioimmunoassay. The staining pattern of the positives showed the same characteristics as the rabbit polyclonal serum raised against a known VGKC peptide that served as a positive control. ANMT sera did

TABLE 2. Immunoreactivity of 12 Autoimmune Neuromyotonia Sera

	Subtype			
	Kv1.1a Kv1.2 Kv1.6	Kv1.2 Kv1.6	Kv1.1a Kv1.2	Kv1.6
Molecular-immunohistochemical assay	4	5	1	2
α-Dendrotoxin radioimmunoassay	2	3	0	1

not react with the expressed AChR subunit except in patients who also had MG and had detectable serum anti-AChR antibodies. Other disease control sera (LEMS, Guillain-Barré syndrome) were also negative.

These results demonstrate the heterogeneity of anti-VGKC antibodies in that at least three different *Shaker*-related VGKCs can be targeted. It will be interesting to test reactivity to other α-subunits of the Kv1 family. Heterogeneity has been seen before in human antibody-mediated disorders. In LEMS, for example, autoantibodies from individual patients can react with P-type, Q-type, N-type, and L-type voltage-gated calcium channels.[25]

These results also suggest that the assay used in this study should provide a novel means of identifying and characterizing the target antibodies in other autoimmune diseases where the genes for the putative antigens are available.

CENTRAL NERVOUS SYSTEM EFFECTS

Although the ANMT manifests itself primarily as a peripheral motor disorder, CNS symptomatology can occur, and the CSF sometimes contains oligoclonal bands as mentioned above. Moreover, preliminary experiments suggest that CSF can stain neurons in the dentate nucleus of the human cerebellum.[24] Neurons and glial cells are known to express VGKCs. The absence of central effects in many ANMT patients may depend upon whether there is synthesis of these autoantibodies within the CNS.

RESPONSE TO TREATMENT

Isaacs[16,26] showed that phenytoin and carbamazepine can reduce the spontaneous neuromyotonic discharges. They appear to do so by reducing voltage-gated sodium channel function, thereby diminishing the hyperexcitability brought about by loss of functional VGKCs. In some patients, use of these agents alone may be sufficient to control symptoms fully. In resistant cases, it is worth considering the use of immunosuppressive drugs in addition. No randomized control trial data are available, but the author has observed individual patients who have responded to combination therapy with prednisolone and azathioprine or prednisolone and methotrexate. In severe cases, plasmapheresis may produce short-term relief. Intravenous immunoglobulin has not yet been adequately evaluated.

COMPARISON OF AUTOIMMUNE AND HEREDITARY MYOKYMIA

It is of special interest that five of the ANMT sera reacted with Kv1.1a. Mutations at different sites in the VGKC α-subunit gene Kv.1.1 have recently been identified in several families with the syndrome of episodic ataxia with myokymia.[27,28] Kv1.1 differs by only two nucleotides from Kv1.1a. In affected individuals, the myokymia is persistent, in contrast to the ataxia. Electromyography shows that the neuromyotonic burst discharges occur regularly, rather than irregularly as in ANMT. Thus, the genetic findings are broadly in accord with anti-VGKC antibody specificity.

CONCLUSIONS

These experimental studies in ANMT satisfy two of the three main criteria for an antibody-mediated autoimmune disease and directly implicate anti-VGKC antibodies in its etiology. The clinical features are also in accord with this conclusion. Thus, ANMT joins MG and the LEMS as examples of autoantibody-mediated channelopathies. The association of ANMT with thymoma and with MG is intriguing, but the reason for this is not clear. Its occasional association with small cell lung cancer suggests that human VGKCs may trigger the disorder in such cases, in the same manner in which tumor VGCCs appear to provoke anti-calcium channel antibodies in the LEMS.[25] In this context it may be relevant that Kv1.1a was derived from a cDNA library obtained from a small cell lung cancer cell-line.[24] Finally, the discovery of an antibody-mediated mechanism for ANMT provides a new focus for therapy.

REFERENCES

1. PATRICK, J. & J. LINDSTROM. 1973. Autoimmune response to acetylcholine receptor. Science **180:** 871–872.
2. LINDSTROM, J. M., M. E. SEYBOLD, V. A. LENNON, S. WHITTINGHAM & D. D. DUANE. 1976. Antibody to acetylcholine receptor in myasthenia gravis. Prevalence, clinical correlates and diagnostic value. Neurology **26:** 1054–1059.
3. TOYKA, K. V., D. B. DRACHMAN, D. E. GRIFFIN, A. PESTRONK, J. A. WINKELSTEIN, K. H. FISCHBECK & I. KAO. 1977. Myasthenia gravis: Study of humoral immune mechanisms by passive transfer to mice. N. Engl. J. Med. **296:** 125–131.
4. PINCHING, A. J., D. K. PETERS & J. NEWSOM-DAVIS. 1976. Remission of myasthenia gravis following plasma exchange. Lancet **2:** 1373–1376.
5. WILLCOX, N., M. SCHLUEP, M. A. RITTER, H. J. SCHUURMAN, J. NEWSOM-DAVIS & B. CHRISTENSSON. 1987. Myasthenic and nonmyasthenic thymoma. An expansion of a minor cortical epithelial cell subset? Am. J. Pathol. **127:** 447–460.
6. LANG, B., J. NEWSOM-DAVIS, D. WRAY, A. VINCENT & N. M. F. MURRAY. 1981. Autoimmune aetiology for myasthenic (Eaton-Lambert) syndrome. Lancet **2:** 224–226.
7. MOTOMURA, M., I. JOHNSTON, B. LANG, A. VINCENT & J. NEWSOM-DAVIS. 1995. An improved diagnostic assay for Lambert-Eaton myasthenic syndrome. J. Neurol. Neurosurg. Psychiatry **58:** 85–87.
8. LAMBERT, E. H. & D. ELMQVIST. 1971. Quantal components of end-plate potentials in the myasthenic syndrome. Ann. N. Y. Acad. Sci. **183:** 183–199.
9. LANG, B., J. NEWSOM-DAVIS, C. PRIOR & D. WRAY. 1983. Antibodies to motor nerve terminals: An electrophysiological study of a human myasthenic syndrome transferred to mouse. J. Physiol. (Lond.) **344:** 335–345.
10. FUKUNAGA, H., A. G. ENGEL, M. OSAME & E. H. LAMBERT. 1982. Paucity and disorganisation of presynaptic membrane active zones in the Lambert-Eaton myasthenic syndrome. Muscle Nerve **5:** 686–697.
11. FUKUNAGA, H., A. G. ENGEL, B. LANG, J. NEWSOM-DAVIS & A. VINCENT. 1983. Passive transfer of Lambert-Eaton myasthenic syndrome with IgG from man to mouse depletes the presynaptic membrane active zones. Proc. Natl. Acad. Sci. USA **80:** 7636–7640.
12. O'NEILL, J. H., N. M. MURRAY & J. NEWSOM-DAVIS. 1988. The Lambert-Eaton myasthenic syndrome. A review of 50 cases. Brain **111:** 577–596.
13. NEWSOM-DAVIS, J. & K. R. MILLS. 1993. Immunological associations of acquired neuromyotonia (Isaacs' syndrome): Report of 5 cases and literature review. Brain **116:** 453–469.
14. MORVAN, A. 1890. De la chorée fibrillaire. Gaz. Hebd. Med. Chir. **27:** 173–200.
15. DENNY-BROWN, D. & J. M. FOLEY. 1948. Myokymia and the benign fasciculation of muscular cramps. Trans. Assoc. Am. Physicians **61:** 88–96.

16. ISAACS, H. 1961. A syndrome of continuous muscle-fibre activity. J. Neurol. Neurosurg. Psychiatry **24:** 319–325.
17. MERTENS, H. G. & S. ZSCHOCKE. 1965. Neuromyotonie. Klin. Wocehenschr. **43:** 917–925.
18. AAEE. Glossary of terms in clinical electromyography. 1987. Muscle Nerve **10:** G47.
19. WALLIS, W. E., A. VAN POZNAK & F. PLUM. 1970. Generalized muscular stiffness, fasciculations, and myokymia of peripheral nerve origin. Arch. Neurol. **22:** 430–439.
20. SINHA, S., J. NEWSOM-DAVIS, K. MILLS, N. BYRNE, B. LANG & A. VINCENT. 1991. Autoimmune aetiology for acquired neuromyotonia (Isaacs' syndrome). Lancet **338:** 75–77.
21. SHILLITO, P., P. C. MOLENAAR, A. VINCENT, K. LEYS, W. ZHENG, R. J. VAN DEN BERG, J. J. PLOMP, G. TH. H. VAN KEMPEN, G. CHAUPLANNAZ, A. R. WINTZEN, G. VAN DIJK & J. NEWSOM-DAVIS. 1995. Acquired neuromyotonia: Evidence for autoantibodies directed against K$^+$ channels of peripheral nerves. Ann. Neurol. **38:** 714–722.
22. JAN, L. Y. & Y. N. JAN. 1994. Potassium channels and their evolving gates. Nature **371:** 119–122.
23. RETTIG, J., S. H. HEINEMANN, F. WUNDER, C. LORRA, D. N. PARCEJ, J. O. DOLLY & O. PONGS. 1994. Inactivation properties of voltage-gated K$^+$ channels altered by presence of β-subunit. Nature **369:** 289–294.
24. HART, I. K., C. WATERS, A. VINCENT, C. NEWLAND, D. BEESON, O. PONGS, C. MORRIS & J. NEWSOM-DAVIS. 1997. Autoantibodies detected to expressed K$^+$ channels are implicated in neuromyotonia. Ann. Neurol. **41:** 238–246.
25. LANG, B. & J. NEWSOM-DAVIS. 1995. Immunopathology of the Lambert-Eaton myasthenic syndrome. Springer Semin. Immunopathol. **17:** 3–15.
26. ISAACS, H. 1967. Continuous muscle fibre activity in an Indian male with additional evidence of terminal motor fibre abnormality. J. Neurol. Neurosurg. Psychiatry **30:** 126–133.
27. BROWNE, D., S. T. GANCHER, J. G. NUTT, E. R. P. BRUNT, D. ROOT, T. PHROMCHOTIKUL, C. J. DUBAY & J. NUTT. 1994. Episodic ataxia/myokymia syndrome is associated with point mutations in the human potassium channel gene KCNA1. Nat. Genet. **8:** 136–140.
28. BROWNE, D., E. R. P. BRUNT, R. C. GRIGGS, J. G. NUTT, S. T. GANCHER, E. A. SMITH & M. LITT. 1995. Identification of two new KCNA1 mutations in episodic ataxia/myokymia families. Hum. Mol. Genet. **4:** 1671–1672.

Oral Administration of Myelin Induces Antigen-specific TGF-β1 Secreting T Cells in Patients with Multiple Sclerosis[a]

DAVID A. HAFLER,[b] SALLY C. KENT,
MATTHEW J. PIETRUSEWICZ, SAMIA J. KHOURY,
HOWARD L. WEINER, AND HIKOAKI FUKAURA

Center for Neurologic Diseases
Brigham and Women's Hospital
and Harvard Medical School
Boston, Massachusetts

INTRODUCTION

Multiple sclerosis (MS) is a chronic inflammatory disease characterized by lymphocytic infiltration and demyelination in the central nervous system (CNS), which thought to be initiated by Th1 type T cells recognizing myelin components of the CNS.[1,2] Alterations in regulation of immune responses are found in patients with the disease, although these defects are not well defined.[1,2] Experimental autoimmune encephalomyelitis (EAE), a model for a cell-mediated Th1 type autoimmune CNS disease, shows pathologic similarities to MS and is induced by activated T cells recognizing myelin basic protein (MBP),[3] proteolipid protein (PLP),[4] or myelin-oligodendrocyte glycoprotein (MOG).[5] In the EAE model, activated CD4$^+$ myelin-reactive T cells secreting the cytokines interleukin-2 (IL-2), interferon-γ (IFN-γ), tumor necrosis factor-α, and lymphotoxin migrate into the CNS and initiate a cascade of events that can lead to clinical paralysis in the animals. Spontaneous recovery is associated with secretion of IL-4, IL-10, and transforming growth factor-β1 (TGF-β1).[6]

The oral administration of antigen is a long-recognized method of inducing tolerance by suppressing systemic T cell mediated immune responses.[7,8] More recently, oral tolerance has been used to suppress experimental autoimmune diseases, including EAE,[9,10] collagen-[11,12] and adjuvant-induced arthritis,[13] uveitis,[14] and spontaneous diabetes in the nonobese mouse.[15] Investigations in experimental models of autoimmune diseases have led to a series of phase I/II double-blind clinical trials of oral tolerance in subjects with MS, rheumatoid arthritis, and uveitis. We reported previously no adverse toxicity or side effects in a pilot double-blind trial involving 30

[a] This work was supported by National Institutes of Health Grants RO1-NS24247 (D.A.H.), RO1-NS-29352 (H.L.W.), and Program Project Grant AR 43220 (D.A.H., H.L.W.), and grants from The National Multiple Sclerosis Society (H.L.W., D.A.H.) and AutoImmune Inc., Lexington, Massachusetts.
[b] Address correspondence to David A. Hafler, M.D., Center for Neurologic Diseases, Department of Neurology, 77 Avenue Louis Pasteur, Boston, MA 02115. E-mail: hafler@CND.BWH.Harvard.edu

relapsing-remitting MS patients receiving daily capsules of bovine myelin containing both MBP and PLP proteins for one year. The frequency of T cells reactive with MBP from myelin-treated individuals with MS was reduced as compared to non-myelin-treated control individuals with MS. Clinically, there was a tendency for the treated group to have fewer exacerbations, especially in the subgroup of DR2-males.[16] A statistically significant clinical effect following oral administration of type II collagen has been shown in the subjects with rheumatoid arthritis.[17] The clinical efficacy of oral myelin tolerization in subjects with MS is presently under phase III investigation in a multicenter, 504-patient randomized double-blind clinical trial.[18]

Based on the identification of antigen-reactive TGF-β1 secreting T cells in mice that were orally tolerized to MBP,[19–21] we wished to determine the effect of oral administration of myelin to patients with MS in terms of induction of cytokine secretion by antigen-specific MBP- or PLP-reactive T cells. It was important to determine whether the prolonged oral administration of myelin autoantigens would result in TGF-β1 secreting cells or rather whether such treatment would elicit Th1 type response to the orally administered myelin antigens. Despite numerous studies of oral tolerance in animals, such questions can only be addressed in patients with the disease who are given oral autoantigens over prolonged periods of time. Our results demonstrate no Th1 sensitization after prolonged oral antigen administration in MS patients; instead, MBP- and PLP-reactive TGF-β1 secreting cells were induced.

MATERIALS AND METHODS

Patients

Seventeen relapsing-remitting patients with MS from the continuation study of the phase I/II oral myelin trial were examined. These patients had been orally dosed with 300 mg bovine myelin (Myloral™) daily for at least two years. The preparation contained approximately 7.5 mg of MBP and 15 mg of PLP, and was supplied to patients by AutoImmune, Inc. (Lexington, MA). The open-label clinical results of the continuation study have been reported separately. Seventeen relapsing-remitting patients with MS who did not receive bovine myelin were examined as controls. The average disease duration for oral myelin-treated group was 11.8 ± 4.3 years (age, 37.8 ± 4.8) and for controls was 11.6 ± 8.7 years (age, 37.1 ± 5.7). MS patients were not treated with immunosuppressive drugs or Betaseron™ in the past or with steroids within three months of blood sampling. These investigations were approved by the human subjects committee of the Brigham and Women's Hospital.

Antigens

Human MBP was purified from the white matter of the human brain by the method previously described and was provided by AutoImmune, Inc.[22] Bovine PLP was purified as previously described.[23] Tetanus toxoid (TT) was obtained in purified form from the Massachusetts Public Health Laboratory (Boston, MA).

Antigen-specific T Cell Lines

Peripheral blood mononuclear cells (PBMC) were isolated from heparinized venous blood by Ficoll-Hypaque density gradient, washed twice with Hanks balanced salts solution, counted, and resuspended in media containing 10% autologous serum (collected from each patient and heat inactivated; this serum was used throughout the experiment for each patient) in RPMI 1640, 10 mM Hepes buffer, 2 mM L-glutamine, and 100 U/100 μg per mL penicillin/streptomycin. All media and components were purchased from BioWhittaker (Walkersville, MD). PBMC from each patient were frozen in 10% dimethyl sulfoxide/fetal bovine serum (from Sigma Co., St. Louis, MO and BioWhittaker, respectively) at -70 °C and were used as antigen presenting cells for the remainder of the assay. PBMC from each patient were pulsed with antigen; 1.2×10^7 PBMC in 1.2 mL were pulsed with either MBP (50 μg/mL), bovine PLP (50 μg/mL) or TT (12 Lf/mL) for 2 h at 37 °C, washed in media twice with 10% autologous serum and then seeded in 96-well U-bottom plates (CoStar, Cambridge, MA) at 2×10^5 cells/well (with total volume of 200 μL/well). On day 7, each well was restimulated with the primary antigen as used at day 0. Autologous PBMC were pulsed with antigen by incubating 10^7 PBMC in 1 mL of media with antigen at a concentration of 100 μg/mL (MBP or PLP) or 10 Lf/mL (TT) for 2 h at 37 °C, washed twice in media and then irradiated with 5000 rad; 2×10^5 antigen-pulsed PBMC were added to each well. On day 9, 100 μL media were removed from each well and 100 μL of media with IL-2 (T cell supernatant derived from phytohemagglutinin-P stimulated human PBMC, final concentration per well, 5% v/v; Collaborative Biomedical Products, Bedford, MA) and rIL-4 (2.5 U/mL, final concentration/well; Boehringer Mannheim, GmbH, Mannheim, Germany) were added to the wells.

On day 14, a split-well assay was performed. Each well was split into four wells: two received 1×10^5 autologous, antigen pulsed, washed, and irradiated cells each and two received 1×10^5 autologous, non-antigen pulsed, washed, and irradiated cells each. All antigen pulsing, washing, and irradiation were performed as described above for the day 7 antigen pulse. Final well volume was 200 μL. Supernatants were collected after 24 h for cytokine measurements of IL-4 and IFN-γ by ELISA. The lines were cultured for an additional 72 h in 150 μL/well of serum-free media (X-Vivo 20, BioWhittaker) and supernatants were then collected for measurement of TGF-β1. Each cell line was pulsed with 1 μCi/well of [^{3}H]thymidine during the last 18 h of culture and subsequently harvested by an automated cell harvester (Beta plate 1295-004, Wallac, Gaithersburg, MD). [^{3}H]thymidine uptake was measured in a beta scintillation counter (Beta plate 1205, Wallac). As previously described, antigen-reactive lines were defined by exhibiting both a stimulation index of greater than 3 and a ΔCPM of greater than 500. The relative frequency of antigen-reactive lines was calculated by dividing the numbers of wells positive for reactivity, as defined above, by the total number of lines generated after stimulation with that antigen.[16] Each well in the 96-well plate yielded a growth positive well under these culture conditions that could be examined for antigen reactivity.

Cytokine Assays

Cytokines produced by T cell lines were assayed by ELISA. To measure IL-4, a capture ELISA method was employed as follows: Immulon 4 microtiter plates (Dynatech, Chantilly, VA) were coated with capture monoclonal antibody (Pharmingen, San Diego, CA) at 1 μg/mL diluted in 0.1 M NaHCO$_3$ (pH 8.2), and incubated at 4 °C overnight. Plates were then blocked with 3% BSA (Kirkegaard and Perry Labs [KPL], Gaithersburg, MD) in PBS for 2 h at room temperature (RT), washed and supernatant (100 μL of culture supernatant) and standards of IL-4 (R&D Systems, Minneapolis, MN) (21–1667 pg/mL) were then added and incubated at 4 °C overnight. Plates were washed and detecting biotinylated monoclonal antibody (Pharmingen) was added to plates at 0.5 μg/mL and incubated for 1 h at RT. After washing, the plates were incubated for 45 min with avidin-peroxidase (Sigma) at a 1:2000 dilution. After washing, plates were developed with TMB one component peroxidase substrate (KPL), and reactions were stopped by TMB one component stop solution (KPL). Absorbance was measured using ELISA reader (Bio-Rad, Melville, NY) at 450 nm, and standard curve for each assay was generated and cytokine production from each line calculated. IFN-γ was measured employing a mouse monoclonal anti-human IFN-γ at 1 μg/mL as coating antibody, a rabbit anti-human IFN-γ polyclonal antibody at 1 μg/mL for secondary antibody (both from Endogen, Cambridge, MA), followed by a goat anti-rabbit-immunoglobulin-horseradish peroxidase labeled antibody at 1:20,000 (Biosource International, Camarillo, CA). The IFN-γ standard was purchased from Gibco BRL (Gaithersburg, MD). Human TGF-β1 was measured by a TGF-β1 ELISA kit (Promega, Madison, WI). Cytokine production from each line, performed in duplicate, was calculated by substracting antigen-negative cytokine production from antigen-positive cytokine production. A line was considered positive if the antigen-specific cytokine secretion was >50 pg/mL of IL-4 and >100 pg/mL of IFN-γ or TGF-β1. The lowest measurable concentration for each assay was 5 pg/mL for IL-4, 10 pg/mL for IGN-γ, and 16 pg/mL for TGF-β1.

Statistical Analyses

A non-paired two-tailed Student's *t* test was used to perform the statistical analyses. Linear regression analysis was used to correlate cytokine secretion between PLP- and MBP-reactive T cells from each patient.

RESULTS

Frequency of Antigen-specific T Cell Lines

The frequency of antigen-reactive T cell lines from PBMCs from myelin-treated and non-myelin-treated patients with MS was determined by [³H]thymidine incorporation. A T cell line was considered positive when the stimulation index was greater than 3.0 and the ΔCPM was greater than 500. A comparison of the frequencies in responses of the two groups to individual antigens is shown in TABLE 1. Although there was a lower frequency of MBP- and PLP-reactive T cells in the myelin-treated group as compared to the non-treated group in response to MBP and PLP, this difference did not reach statistical significance in this cross-sectional analysis. The frequency of TT reactive lines was similar in both myelin-treated and non-treated groups.

Reactivity of human T cells is usually measured by [³H]thymidine incorporation. Therefore it was important to know if this measure of T cell proliferation correlated with cytokine secretion. This was examined by screening several hundred lines (both negative and positive for antigen-induced [³H]thymidine incorporation) for secretion of IL-4, IFN-γ, and TGF-β1 by ELISA. Although a correlation between thymidine uptake and IFN-γ secretion was found (correlation coefficient $r = 0.60$, $p = 0.0004$), no correlation was found between stimulation index and cytokine secretion for IL-4 and TGF-β1. Thus, we measured cytokine secretion from all wells whether or not there was antigen-specific [³H]thymidine incorporation.

TABLE 1. Relative Frequency of Antigen-reactive T Cell Lines in Patients with Multiple Sclerosis[a]

	MBP-reactive Lines(n)/Total Lines (n)	Mean Frequency of MBP-reactive Wells (%)	PLP-Reactive Lines(n)/Total Lines (n)	Mean Frequency of PLP-reactive Wells (%)	TT-reactive Lines(n)/Total Lines (n)	Mean Frequency of TT-reactive Wells (%)
Myelin, orally administered	14/1020	1.3 ± 0.5[b] ($n = 17$)	37/1020	3.7 ± 1.0 ($n = 17$)	112/480	23.3 ± 9.0 ($n = 8$)
Control	34/1020	3.4 ± 2.5 ($n = 17$)	65/1020	7.6 ± 3.6 ($n = 17$)	57/300	19.0 ± 8.9 ($n = 5$)

[a] PBMC were plated directly into 96-well plates and stimulated with antigens as described in MATERIALS AND METHODS. Each well was restimulated in the presence of antigen with APC on day 7 and for reactivity by a split-well assay on day 14. Antigen-reactive lines were defined as stimulation index > 3 and ΔCPM > 500. Each well in the 96-well plate yielded a growth-positive well under these culture conditions that could be examined for antigen reactivity.

[b] The percentage of antigen-reactive lines out of the total number of lines generated was calculated for each subject. The values represent the mean percentage of antigen-reactive lines for each group. The results are expressed as the mean ± SE.

(From Fukaura *et al.*[24] Reprinted with permission from *The Journal of Clinical Investigation*.)

Relative Frequency of Cytokine-secreting Lines

The relative frequency of cytokine-secreting lines in response to MBP, PLP, and TT in T cell lines from oral myelin-treated and non-treated patients was calculated for individual subjects, and the mean relative frequency for each group was calculated (FIG. 1). An increase was found in TGF-β1 secreting lines recognizing MBP in the oral myelin-treated as compared to non-treated patients (myelin-treated, 9.9 ± 2; non-treated, 1.3 ± 0.5; $p < 0.001$) (FIG. 1A). We also observed an increase in the relative frequency of IL-4 secreting lines reactive to MBP in the oral myelin-treated MS patients, but this did not reach statistical significance (myelin-treated, 6.5 ± 2.7; non-treated, 1.3 ± 0.7; $p < 0.099$). No difference in the relative frequency of IFN-γ secreting lines was observed (myelin-treated, 5.0 ± 2.5; non-treated, 6.4 ± 1.8). In response to PLP, a significant increase was also found in the relative frequency of TGF-β1 secreting T cell lines in the myelin-treated group (myelin-treated, 9.5 ± 2.2; non-treated 1.1 ± 0.7; $p < 0.003$), whereas no difference was observed for IL-4 secreting lines (myelin-treated, 3.1 ± 1.9; non-treated, 2 ± 1.6) (FIG. 1B). There was a trend for lower IFN-γ secretion from the oral myelin-treated group in response to PLP, but this did not achieve statistical significance (myelin-treated, 6.1 ± 2.5; non-treated, 13.7 ± 7.4; $p < 0.264$).

To examine whether the frequency of TGF-β1 secreting lines from the oral myelin-treated group was specific for myelin antigens, we measured cytokine secretion from T cell lines using TT as a control antigen. Both oral myelin-treated and non-myelin-treated groups showed similar relative frequencies of TGF-β1, IL-4, and IFN-γ cell lines in response to TT (TGF-β1: myelin-treated, 1.9 ± 1.2; non-treated, 2.0 ± 1.2; IL-4: myelin-treated, 1.0 ± 0.5; non-treated, 0; IFN-γ: myelin-treated, 39.8 ± 12.1; non-treated, 65.8 ± 6.3) (FIG. 1C).

Correlation between the Relative Frequencies of MBP vs. PLP TGF-β1 Secreting T Cells

The frequency of both MBP- and PLP-reactive TGF-β1 secreting T cells varied among MS patients orally treated with myelin. This led us to examine whether a correlation existed between the relative frequencies of MBP vs. PLP TGF-β1 secreting T cells among individual subjects. As shown in FIGURE 2, a highly significant correlation was found between the frequency of MBP vs. PLP TGF-β1 secreting T cells in individual patients.

DISCUSSION

The present study was carried out to determine whether the prolonged oral administration of myelin in patients with MS alters the frequency or cytokine secretion patterns of MBP- or PLP-reactive T cells. We demonstrate an increase in the frequency of MBP- and PLP-, but not TT-, reactive TGF-β1 secreting T cell lines in myelin-treated MS patients as compared to non-myelin-treated MS patients; these data are presented in greater detail elsewhere.[24] These studies, showing cytokine deviation with antigen-specific immunotherapy in subjects with autoimmune disease, are consistent with our observation that there is an increase in MBP-specific TGF-β1 secreting T cells in mice receiving oral MBP.[21]

A number of studies have defined mechanisms by which oral tolerization occurs

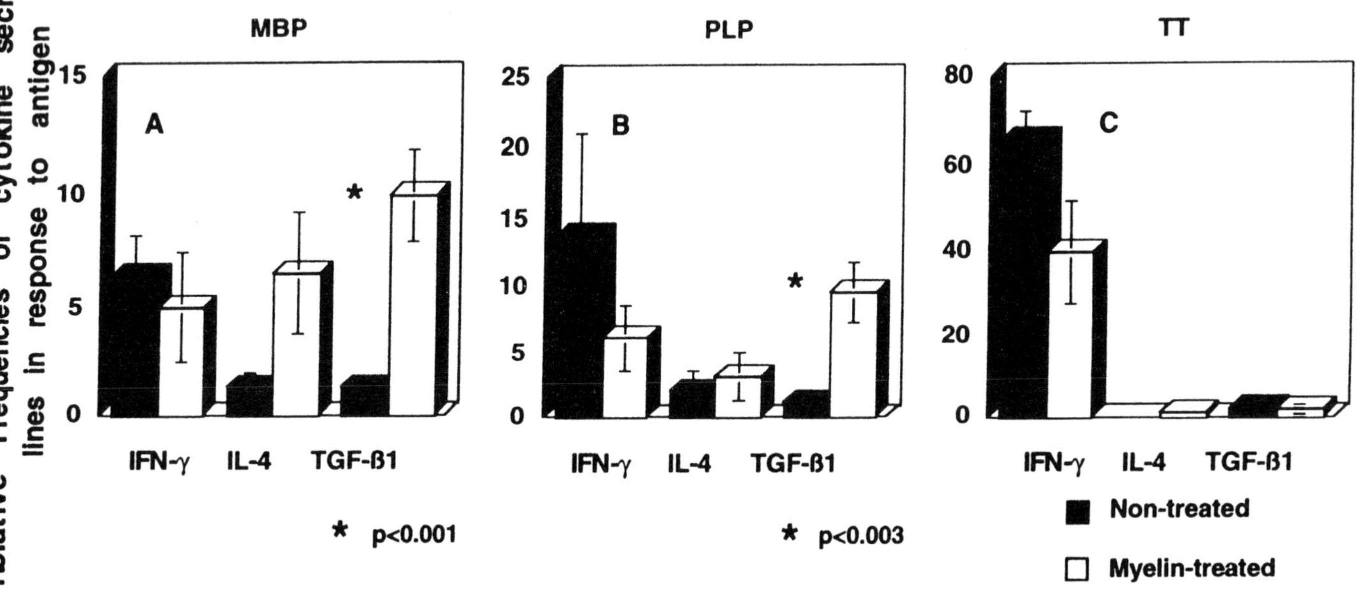

FIGURE 1. Relative frequency of antigen-reactive T cell lines secreting IL-4, IFN-γ, or TGF-β1 from either MS patients receiving myelin orally or controls. The differences in cytokine secretion on day 14 of T cell lines stimulated by antigen-pulsed APCs were compared to T cell lines stimulated with APCs alone, as described in MATERIALS AND METHODS. Culture supernatants were collected 24 h after antigenic stimulation for IL-4 and IFN-γ ELISA. Serum-free media were added to each well and after an additional 72 h, culture supernatant was collected for TGF-β1 ELISA. A line was considered positive if the antigen-specific cytokine secretion was >50 pg/mL of IL-4 and >100 pg/mL of IFN-γ or TGF-β1. The relative frequencies of cytokine-secreting lines with antigenic stimulation were calculated for each patient, 17 myelin-treated and 17 non-treated patients, and the average values ± SE are shown. Significant p values for TGF-β1 secretion are in boldface. (**A**) MCP stimulation. TGF-β1: Myelin-treated, 9.9 ± 2; non-treated, 1.3 ± 0.5; **p < 0.001;** IL-4: Myelin-treated, 6.5 ± 2.7; non-treated, 1.3 ± 0.7; p < 0.099; IFN-γ: Myelin-treated, 5.0 ± 2.5; non-treated, 6.4 ± 1.8. (**B**) PLP stimulation. TGF-β1: Myelin-treated, 9.5 ± 2.2; non-treated, 1.1 ± 0.7; **p < 0.003;** IL-4: Myelin-treated, 3.1 ± 1.9; non-treated, 2 ± 1.6; IFN-γ: Myelin-treated, 6.1 ± 2.5; non-treated, 13.7 ± 7.4; p < 0.264. (**C**) TT stimulation. TGF-β1: Myelin-treated, 1.9 ± 1.2; non-treated, 2.0 ± 1.2; IL-4: Myelin-treated, 1.0 ± 0.5; non-treated, 0; IFN-γ: Myelin-treated, 39.8 ± 12.1; non-treated, 65.8 ± 6.3; no values significantly different. (From Fukaura et al.[24] Reprinted by permission from The Journal of Clinical Investigation.)

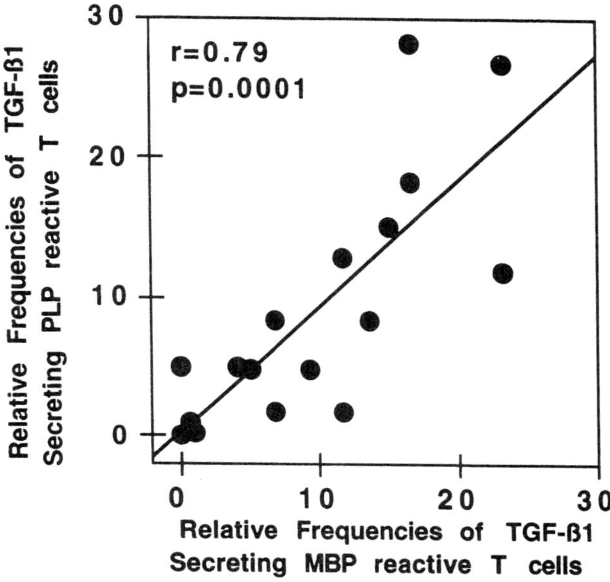

FIGURE 2. Correlation between the relative frequencies of MBP vs. PLP TGF-β1 secreting T cells. The relative frequencies of MBP vs. PLP TGF-β1 secreting T cells among individual subjects were correlated by a linear-regression analysis. A significant correlation ($r = 0.79$, $p = 0.0001$) was found in individual patients between the relative frequency of MBP vs. PLP TGF-β1 secreting T cells. (From Fukaura *et al.*[24] Reprinted with permission from *The Journal of Clinical Investigation.*)

in rodents. In the EAE model, one of the primary mechanisms involves the generation of active suppression, and this is mediated by T cells that secrete TGF-β1 and suppress the immune response.[25] Furthermore, T cell clones isolated from the mesenteric lymph nodes of mice orally tolerized with MBP secreting IL-4, IL-10, and TGF-β1 suppressed ongoing EAE induced by either MBP or PLP.[20] The regulatory properties of these T cell clones were abrogated when mice were given anti-TGFβ1 antibodies, suggesting a critical role for local secretion of TGF-β1 in suppressing the immune response. The importance of cytokines in regulating the inflammatory CNS response in EAE has also been suggested by immunopathologic examination of cytokine secretion in the CNS. Animals with acute EAE exhibit perivascular infiltration with activated mononuclear cells secreting the inflammatory cytokines IL-1, IL-2, TNF-α, IFN-γ, IL-6, and IL-8. In contrast, animals with EAE that had been orally tolerized with MBP exhibit a marked reduction of the perivascular infiltrate, with down-regulation of inflammatory cytokines and increased amounts of TGF-β1 and IL-4.[6] These results suggest that the suppression of EAE, by oral tolerization and natural recovery, is related to regulatory cells that secrete inhibitory cytokines at the target organ.

TGF-β1 has a number of properties consistent with a role in regulating the immune response. It is potent in inhibiting T and B cell entry into S/G$_2$/M cell cycle and thus inhibiting proliferation. Paradoxically, TGF-β1 also can attract macrophages to sites of inflammation while inducing up-regulation of IgA secretion by activated B lymphocytes.[26,27] In addition, T cells grown in the presence of TGF-β1 secrete more IL-2 than those responding to CD2 and CD28 stimulation. These T cells also expressed an increased amount of $\alpha^E\beta$ integrin, a human mucosal epithelium adhesion molecule.[28] TGF-β1 also can induce fibrin deposition and is involved in scar formation.[29] Thus, a combined physiologic action of TGF-β1 may be to down-regulate inflammatory T cell responses while inducing tissue repair as well as inducing T cells primed in the gut.

There are few investigations in humans regarding the mechanism of oral tolerization. The immune responses in normal individuals orally administered with keyhole limpet hemocyanin (KLH) decreased subsequent cell-mediated immune responses when subjects were injected with KLH, although antibody responses were not affected.[30] The mechanism for this suppression has not been elucidated. Myelin antigens have also been given by other routes in an attempt to tolerize human T cell responses. These studies showed that with parenteral administration of MBP, subsequent delayed type hypersensitivity responses were observed, presumably representing a Th1 type response.[31]

We previously reported that the frequency of MBP-reactive T cells was significantly decreased in a longitudinal study investigating frequencies prior to and after initiating oral administration of myelin in patients with MS.[16] Although a similar trend was observed in the present study, the data did not reach statistical significance. We believe the lack of statistical significance in the present cross-sectional study is related to the variability in the frequency of MBP-reactive T cells among different patients with MS as compared to the serial measurements we performed in our first investigation. We attempted to determine whether a correlation existed between frequency of TGF-β1 secreting cells and response to therapy by arbitrarily dividing patients into responders and nonresponders and performing a chi-square statistical analysis. No correlation was found in the small number of patients studied. As mentioned above, this will be examined in a larger study powered to address this experimental question.

As expected from treating an outbred group of patients with MS, there was a distribution in the range of both MBP- and PLP-reactive TGF-β1 secreting T cells. This may have been due to differences among individual patients in their ability to recognize these myelin antigens or, alternatively, individual patients may have differential abilities to generate TGF-β1 secreting T cells. This question was addressed by determining whether a correlation existed among individual patients in the frequencies of MBP- vs. PLP-reactive TGF-β1 secreting T cells. Indeed, we found a highly significant correlation in individual MS patients between the frequency of these two myelin-reactive T cell populations. Since MBP- and PLP-reactive TGF-β1 secreting T cells were found in the same patients, these data suggest the latter hypothesis that individual patients, as with different strains of mice, may have a differential ability to generate different cytokine-secreting populations of T cells.

Taken together, these data suggest that T cells generated in the gut, primed with whole myelin, may have the ability to migrate into the CNS and nonspecifically suppress ongoing autoimmune responses at the target organ by secreting TGF-β1. This represents an antigen-specific immunotherapy capable of suppressing autoimmune responses to multiple self-antigens at the target organ. Moreover, these data show that autoantigen-specific T cells secreting TGF-β1 can be generated in humans with autoimmune disease.

In summary, oral administration of myelin to patients with MS generated an increased frequency of MBP- and PLP-specific TGF-1 secreting T cells. These results are consistent with the cytokine profile of regulatory T cells observed in animals following oral tolerization with MBP.[19–21,25] Such antigen-specific regulatory T cells upon homing to the CNS would be predicted to suppress ongoing autoimmune responses in an antigen nonspecific fashion by the secretion of TGF-β1, a mechanism that has been termed bystander suppression. T cells induced by mucosal stimulation with antigen that secrete TGF-β1 appear to represent a distinct lineage of T cells (Th3 type).[32] Our data demonstrate that oral tolerization with self-antigens in a human autoimmune disease may provide a therapeutic approach to the treatment of autoimmune disease which does not depend upon knowledge of the antigen specificity of the original T cell clone triggering the autoimmune cascade.

SUMMARY

Oral administration of antigen is a long-recognized method of inducing systemic immune tolerance. In animals with experimental autoimmune disease, a major mechanism of oral tolerance involves the induction of regulatory T cells that mediate active suppression by secreting the cytokine TGF-β1. Multiple sclerosis (MS) is a presumed T cell-mediated Th1 type autoimmune disease. In this paper we investigated, in patients with MS, whether oral myelin treatment (myelin containing both MBP and PLP) induced antigen-specific MBP- or PLP-reactive T cells that were either Th2-like (secreted IL-4 or TGF-β1), or alternatively whether Th1 type sensitization occurred as measured by IFN-γ secretion. Specifically, 4,860 short-term T cell lines were generated to either MBP, PLP or TT from 34 relapsing-remitting patients with MS; 17 were orally treated with bovine myelin daily for a minimum of two years as compared to 17 non-treated patients. We found a marked increase in the relative frequencies of both MBP- and PLP-specific TGF-β1 secreting T cell lines in the myelin-treated MS patients as compared to non-treated MS patients (MBP, $p < 0.001$; PLP, $p < 0.003$). In contrast, no changes in the frequency of MBP- or PLP-specific IFN-γ or TT-specific TGF-β1 secreting T cells were observed. These results suggest that the oral administration of antigens generates antigen-specific TGF-β1 secreting T cells of presumed mucosal origin that may represent a distinct cytokine-secreting lineage of T cells (Th3). Since, in animal models, antigen-specific TGF-β1 secreting cells localize to the target organ and then suppress inflammation in the local microenvironment, oral tolerization with self-antigens may provide a therapeutic approach for the treatment of cell-mediated autoimmune disease which does not depend upon knowledge of the antigen specificity of the original T cell clone triggering the autoimmune cascade.

REFERENCES

1. McFARLIN, D. E. & H. F. McFARLAND. 1982. Multiple sclerosis. N. Engl. J. Med. **307:** 1183–1188.
2. HAFLER, D. A. & H. L. WEINER. 1995. Immunologic mechanisms and therapy in multiple sclerosis. Immunol. Rev. **144:** 75–107.
3. ZAMVIL, S., P. NELSON, J. TROTTER, D. MITCHELL, R. KNOBLER, R. FRITZ & L. STEINMAN. 1985. T cell clones specific for myelin basic protein induce chronic relapsing paralysis and demyelination. Nature **317:** 355–358.
4. TUOHY, V. K., R. A. SOBEL & M. B. LEES. 1988. Myelin proteolipid protein-induced experimental allergic encephalomyelitis. Variations of disease expression in different strains of mice. J. Immunol. **140:** 1868–1873.
5. LININGTON, C., T. BERGER, L. PERRY, S. WEERTH, D. HINZE-SELCH, Y. ZHANG, H. C. LU, H. LASSMANN & H. WEKERLE. 1993. T cells specific for the myelin oligodendrocyte

glycoprotein mediate an unusual autoimmune inflammatory response in the central nervous system. Eur. J. Immunol. **23:** 1364–1372.

6. KHOURY, S. J., W. W. HANCOCK & H. L. WEINER. 1992. Oral tolerance to myelin basic protein and natural recovery from experimental autoimmune encephalomyelitis are associated with downregulation of inflammatory cytokines and differential upregulation of transforming growth factor-β, interleukin-4, and prostaglandin E expression in the brain. J. Exp. Med. **176:** 1355–1364.

7. CHASE, M. W. 1946. Inhibition of experimental drug allergy by prior feeding of the sensitizing agent. Proc. Soc. Exp. Biol. Med. **61:** 257–259.

8. MOWAT, A. M. 1987. The regulation of immune responses to dietary protein antigens. Immunol. Today **8:** 93–98.

9. HIGGINS, P. J. & H. L. WEINER. 1988. Suppression of experimental autoimmune encephalomyelitis by oral administration of myelin basic protein and its fragments. J. Immunol. **140:** 440–445.

10. BITAR, D. M. & C. C. WHITACRE. 1988. Suppression of experimental autoimmune encephalomyelitis by the oral administration of myelin basic protein. Cell. Immunol. **112:** 364–370.

11. THOMPSON, H. S. & N. A. STAINES. 1986. Gastric administration of type II collagen delays the onset and severity of collagen-induced arthritis in rats. Clin. Exp. Immunol. **64:** 581–586.

12. NAGLER-ANDERSON, C., L. A. BOBER, M. E. ROBINSON, G. W. SISKIND & G. J. THORBECKE. 1986. Suppression of type II collagen-induced arthritis by intragastric administration of soluble type II collagen. Proc. Natl. Acad. Sci. USA **83:** 7443–7446.

13. ZHANG, Z. J., C. S. Y. LEE, O. LIDER & H. L. WEINER. 1990. Suppression of adjuvant arthritis in Lewis rats by oral administration of type II collagen. J. Immunol. **145:** 2489–2493.

14. NUSSENBLATT, R. B., R. R. CASPI, R. MAHDI, C.-C. CHAN, F. ROBERGE, O. LIDER & H. L. WEINER. 1990. Inhibition of S-antigen induced experimental autoimmune uveoretinitis by oral induction of tolerance with S-antigen. J. Immunol. **144:** 1689–1695.

15. ZHANG, Z. J., L. DAVIDSON, G. EISENBARTH & H. L. WEINER. 1991. Suppression of diabetes in nonobese diabetic mice by oral administration of porcine insulin. Proc. Natl. Acad. Sci. USA **88:** 10252–10256.

16. WEINER, H. L., G. A. MACKLIN, M. MATSUI, E. J. ORAV, S. J. KHOURY, D. M. DAWSON & D. A. HAFLER. 1993. Double-blind pilot trial of oral tolerization with myelin antigens in multiple sclerosis. Science **259:** 1321–1324.

17. TRENTHAM, D. E., R. A. DYNESIUS-TRENTHAM, E. J. ORAV, D. COMBITCHI, C. LORENZO, K. L. SEWELL, D. A. HAFLER & H. L. WEINER. 1993. Effects of oral administration of type II collagen on rheumatoid arthritis. Science **261:** 1727–1730.

18. HOHOL, M. J., S. J. KHOURY, S. L. COOK, E. J. ORAV, D. A. HAFLER & H. L. WEINER. 1996. Three year open protocol continuation study of oral tolerization with myelin antigens in multiple sclerosis and design of a phase III pivotal trial. Ann. N. Y. Acad. Sci. **778:** 243–250.

19. MILLER, A., O. LIDER & H. L. WEINER. 1991. Antigen-driven bystander suppression following oral administration of antigens. J. Exp. Med. **174:** 791–798.

20. CHEN, Y., V. K. KUCHROO, J.-I. INOBE, D. A. HAFLER & H. L. WEINER. 1994. Regulatory T cell clones induced by oral tolerance: Suppression of autoimmune encephalomyelitis. Science **265:** 1237–1240.

21. CHEN, Y., J.-I. INOBE, V. K. KUCHROO, J. L. BARON, C. A. JANEWAY, JR. & H. L. WEINER. 1996. Oral tolerance in myelin basic protein T-cell receptor transgenic mice: Suppression of autoimmune encephalomyelitis and dose-dependent induction of regulatory cells. Proc. Natl. Acad. Sci. USA **93:** 388–391.

22. CHOU, F. C.-H., C.-H. J. CHOU, R. SHAPIRA & R. F. KIBLER. 1976. Basis of microheterogeneity of myelin basic protein. J. Biol. Chem. **251:** 2671–2679.

23. BIZZOZERO, O. A., G. ZUNIGA & M. B. LEES. 1991. Fatty acid composition of human myelin proteolipid protein in peroxisomal disorders. J. Neurochem. **56:** 872–878.

24. FUKAURA, H., S. C. KENT, M. J. PIETRUSEWICZ, S. J. KHOURY, H. L. WEINER & D. A. HAFLER. 1996. Induction of circulating myelin basic protein and proteolipid protein-

specific transforming growth factor-β1-secreting Th3 T cells by oral administration of myelin in multiple sclerosis patients. J. Clin. Invest. **98:** 70–77.

25. MILLER, A., O. LIDER, A. B. ROBERTS, M. B. SPORN & H. L. WEINER. 1992. Suppressor T cells generated by oral tolerization to myelin basic protein suppress both in vitro and in vivo immune responses by the release of transforming growth factor β after antigen-specific triggering. Proc. Natl. Acad. Sci. USA **89:** 421–425.

26. LEBMAN, D. A., F. D. LEE & R. L. COFFMAN. 1990. Mechanism for transforming growth factor β and IL-2 enhancement of IgA expression in lipopolysaccharide-stimulated B cell cultures. J. Immunol. **144:** 952–959.

27. KAGNOFF, M. F. & P. H. KIM. 1991. Effects of transforming growth factor beta-1 and interleukin-5 on IgA isotype switching at the clonal level. Immunol. Res. **10:** 396–399.

28. CERWENKA, A., D. BEVEC, O. MAJDIC, W. KNAPP & W. HOLTER. 1994. TGF-β1 is a potent inducer of human effector T cells. J. Immunol. **153:** 4367–4377.

29. WAHL, S. M., N. MCCARTHY-FRANCIS & S. E. MERGENHAGEN. 1989. Inflammatory and immunomodulatory roles of TGFβ. Immunol. Today **10:** 258–261.

30. HUSBY, S., J. MESTECKY, Z. MOLDOVEANU, S. HOLLAND & C. O. ELSON. 1994. Oral tolerance in humans: T cell but not B cell tolerance after antigen feeding. J. Immunol. **152:** 4663–4670.

31. SALK, R. J. S. 1983. A study of myelin basic protein as a therapeutic probe in patients with multiple sclerosis. *In* Multiple Sclerosis. J. F. Hallpike, C. W. M. Adams & W. W. Tourtellotte, Eds.: 621–630. Chapman and Hall. London.

32. MOSMANN, T. R. & S. SAD. 1996. The expanding universe of T-cell subsets: Th1, Th2 and more. Immunol. Today **17:** 138–146.

Management of Primary Brain Tumors—1996

WILLIAM R. SHAPIRO[a]

Division of Neurology
Barrow Neurological Institute
Phoenix, Arizona

MALIGNANT GLIOMA

Multimodality therapy for malignant glioma—cytoreductive surgery, radiation therapy, chemotherapy—has been used in one form or another for the past 25 years.[1] Much of this experience was directly a product of clinical research by individual institutions and in cooperative group trials. We shall briefly review each of the modalities, concentrating on recent results and controversies.

Surgery

The role of surgical resection in the treatment of malignant gliomas remains controversial even after 75 years of experience with primary malignant gliomas.[2] Surgery permits a pathological diagnosis to be established during life. However, many physicians consider that current methods of radiological diagnosis, including the CT scan and MRI, permit a diagnosis of malignant brain tumor without the necessity for attempted tumor resection, thus avoiding the risks of surgery. Although stereotactic biopsy usually provides enough tissue to make a diagnosis of primary glioma, the amount of tissue may be inadequate to grade the tumors.[3]

Stereotactic biopsy alone, or even small open craniotomy biopsy, denies a role for surgery as "cancer" therapy. There is evidence that surgical reduction of tumor to very small residual amounts can prolong survival and permit patients to return to active lives. In one Brain Tumor Cooperative Group (BTCG) study, CT scans from patients with brain tumors were studied at several times in their courses and compared to ultimate outcome.[4] This study found no significant relationship between preoperative tumor size and prognosis. On the other hand, a very strong relationship was found between postoperative size and survival. This was especially noticeable for patients with minimal or no residual enhancement. There was a statistically significant ordering of tumor size, such that those patients with very little residual enhancement (<1 cm^2 in length $\times$ width area) had the longest survival, followed by those with tumors of 1–4 cm^2, and then by patients with tumors >4 cm^2 ($p = 0.0001$). When the difference between preoperative and postoperative tumor size was evaluated, no significant relationship was found between percentage of tumor removed and survival, although a trend toward longer survival was seen in patients whose tumors were reduced by 75% or more. Thus, the most beneficial effect of

[a] Address for correspondence: Division of Neurology, Barrow Neurological Institute, St. Joseph's Hospital and Medical Center, 350 West Thomas Road, Phoenix, AZ 85013. E-mail: wshapir@mha.chw.edu

surgery is less the result of debulking than of leaving the least residual tumor possible.

In another similar study using postoperative MRI (days 1–3), a significant ordering of survival was associated with removal of more tumor.[5] Patients with postoperative residual contrast-enhanced tumor had nearly a sevenfold higher risk of death in comparison to patients without residual tumor. Postoperative MRI was three times more accurate in defining the extent of surgical resection than was the surgeon's estimate. Of note, 80% of the tumor "recurrences" emerged from contrast-enhanced remnants.

The relationship between extent of surgical resection and survival for glioblastoma was reviewed in three consecutive Radiation Therapy Oncology Group (RTOG) trials.[6] Surgical resection was defined as total in 19%, partial in 64%, and biopsy only in 17%. Greater surgical resection was associated with statistically significant longer survival; median survival of patients with total resection was 11.3 months, for biopsy only, 6.6 months.

Kelly and Hunt argue that there is little benefit to attempting major resection in elderly patients, although the survival advantage in their study was always to the patients undergoing resection over those whose tumors were merely biopsied.[7]

All such retrospective studies are subject to the criticism that the extent of attempted resection depends on the conditions of the patient at the time of surgery (age, tumor location, clinical state), and that favorable conditions usually lead the surgeon to attempt a greater resection. Therefore, in such studies is is not clear whether the *extent of surgery* was important to survival, or rather the more *favorable prognostic variables.* Nevertheless, these results support the surgical removal of the largest possible volume of tumor that safe operation allows. There is little justification in performing only biopsy or limited resection of accessible tumors. If the surgeon confines his resection to the tumor itself, he rarely induces a major new neurological defect. On the contrary, patients are frequently able to return to a full, active life without the need for large doses of corticosteroid hormones to ameliorate incapacitating symptoms.

Radiation Therapy

The proper portals and doses of radiation therapy in the treatment of brain tumor have changed with the advent of better imaging techniques. The Brain Tumor Study Group (BTSG) first reported in controlled studies that whole-brain radiation therapy increases the survival of patients over that which follows surgery alone.[8,9] Other data showed that patients receiving 5500–6000 cGy live significantly longer than those receiving 5000 cGy or less.[10] In the above-cited BTCG CT scan study, patients with no tumor enhancement after radiation therapy had better survival than those with residual tumor.[4] Patients with larger tumors that shrank by more than 50% survived longer than those whose tumors shrank less than 50% or those whose tumors actually increased in size. One BTCG study compared entirely whole-brain radiation therapy for malignant glioma with whole-brain plus partial coned-down radiation.[11] No statistical difference in survival was found among any of the groups, indicating that reduction of part of the radiotherapy to the tumor volume is as effective as full whole-brain irradiation. Neither increased fractionation of radiotherapy (twice daily) nor addition of the radiosensitizer misonidazole confers any survival advantage over conventional postoperative whole brain radiotherapy and chemotherapy with BCNU [1,3-bis(2-chloroethyl)-1-nitrosourea, carmustine].[12]

Focal radiotherapy techniques include interstitial implantation of radioactive seeds (brachytherapy) and radiosurgery. Prolonged survival has been reported in patients with recurrent malignant gliomas treated with temporarily implanted iodine-125 sources.[13] BTCG phase III trial 87-01 randomized newly diagnosed patients to receive (1) postoperative temporary [^{125}I] seed implantation in the residual tumor bed, followed by standard external beam radiotherapy plus intravenous (i.v.) BCNU, or (2) external radiotherapy plus BCNU, without the seed implantation. The purpose of this controlled trial was to test in newly diagnosed patients the potential survival value of adding an additional 60 Gy in the form of brachytherapy to the 60 Gy delivered by external irradiation. Accrual to the study reached 299 patients by April 1994, and the study was closed on May 1, 1994. Preliminary review of the results demonstrated that patients who received [^{125}I] seeds lived significantly longer than those who did not receive seeds ($p < 0.05$). This was specifically true for patients with glioblastoma multiforme, but not for those with anaplastic astrocytoma, although the latter group was small. About 50% of the patients underwent reoperation in both the implanted and the nonimplanted groups. Patients with recurrent tumor lived longer after resection if the recurrence was due to radiation necrosis (mostly from seeds) than if tumor was present at recurrence ($p = 0.001$). The incidence of biopsy versus tumor resection was approximately equal in the two groups, thus indicating that the difference in survival was *not* related to the extent of tumor resection at the time of failure.

The other technique for delivering local radiation therapy is radiosurgery. Radiosurgery, either by gamma knife or by linear accelerator, has been shown to be effective in the treatment of arteriovenous malformations, small primary and metastatic brain tumors, and benign brain tumors such as meningiomas and acoustic neuromas. Its use in the treatment of gliomas has been addressed in several reports. One trial used adjuvant radiosurgery as part of the initial management of malignant glioma.[14] Thirty-seven patients received radiosurgery to residual contrast-enhancing tumor after treatment with conventional external beam radiation therapy. The minimum radiosurgical dose was 1,000 to 2,000 cGy. Local recurrence still occurred, but overall survival time may have been longer. Seven (19%) patients required reoperation at a median time of 5 months after radiosurgery to remove necrotic tumor. A major problem in radiosurgery (as was true for brachytherapy) is selection bias in choosing patients to be treated. Curran *et al.* pointed out that patients eligible for radiosurgery live longer than patients ineligible for radiosurgery, when neither group actually receives radiosurgery.[15] One study of the value of radiosurgery for malignant gliomas revealed little additional survival benefit over that of reported external beam radiotherapy.[16] Radiosurgery may be of benefit for a small group of good-prognosis patients with small tumors.[17] The RTOG is performing a randomized trial that is similar to that of the BTCG interstitial radiotherapy study. RTOG 9305 randomizes patients with supratentorial malignant gliomas with Karofsky performance status (KPS) $\geq$60 and postoperative residual disease $\leq$4 cm in greatest diameter to radiosurgery followed by radiotherapy (60 Gy) and BCNU compared to radiotherapy and BCNU alone.

Chemotherapy

Chemotherapy completes the technique of multimodality treatment of malignant gliomas. The BTSG reported in 1983 that surgery plus radiation therapy and chemotherapy with BCNU significantly added to the survival of patients harboring malignant glioma in comparison to surgery plus radiaton therapy without chemotherapy.[18]

High-dose methyl prednisolone does not lead to longer survival.[18] Procarbazine and streptozotocin have each demonstrated effectiveness similar to that of BCNU.[12,18] BCNU alone is as effective as BCNU sequencing with procarbazine, or BCNU plus hydroxyurea sequencing with procarbazine plus VM-26.[11] Intraarterial (i.a.) BCNU is no more effective than i.v. BCNU, and substantially more toxic.[19] Serious toxicity was observed from i.a. BNCU, including irreversible encephalopathy and/or visual loss ipsilateral to the infused carotid artery. In the same study 5-FU did not influence survival. Neuropathologically, i.a. BCNU produced white matter necrosis.[20] i.a. BCNU as used in this protocol is neither safe nor effective. i.a. cisplatin is safer than i.a. BCNU, but no more effective than another nitro-sourea, PCNU.[21]

Over the past several years, there has been increasing interest in the use of targeted interstitial drug delivery using biodegradable microspheres and wafers. A controlled trial of such wafers in patients with recurrent malignant gliomas was conducted among a number of centers.[22] Two hundred twenty-two patients requiring reoperation were randomly assigned to receive surgically implanted biodegradable polymer discs with or without 3.85% BCNU. The median survival of the 110 patients who received BCNU-polymers was 31 weeks, significantly longer than the 23-week median survival of the 112 patients who underwent reoperation but received placebo polymers. Because BCNU is readily administered i.v., a comparative study between BCNU-containing wafers and i.v. BCNU would help define the role for wafers with this drug. However, studies of wafers containing other agents that do not readily enter brain tumors would be of greater interest.

In addition to these controlled survival-based clinical trials, a large number of agents has also been tested in response-based studies in glioma patients.[23] To date, however, no drug has been found to be more effective than the nitrosoureas. A combination of procarbazine (matulane), CCNU and vincristine (PCV) has become a popular chemotherapeutic regimen for malignant glioma and may be more effective than BCNU alone. Of the malignant gliomas, glioblastoma multiforme responds least well to chemotherapy, anaplastic astrocytoma better, and, according to recent studies, oligodendrogliomas may be most sensitive.[24]

LOW-GRADE GLIOMA

The advent of CT and MRI has had substantial impact on our ability to diagnose and follow brain tumors. Patients with low-grade gliomas may present only with a seizure, but the tumor is readily seen as a T2 mass on MRI. However, with earlier diagnosis, unresolved therapy questions have arisen, some of which are discussed below.

Low-grade astrocytomas of the cerebral hemisphere occurring in adults generally have a good prognosis, with expected survival of 3–7 years. Increasingly, patients with low-grade astrocytomas present with a single seizure, and the tumor is found on MRI. However, CT and MRI are not accurate enough to diagnose or grade such tumors.[25] Of 20 patients diagnosed by image studies who underwent stereotactic biopsy, only 10 (50%) had low-grade astrocytomas, whereas nine (45%) had anaplastic astrocytomas, and one (5%) had encephalitis. Thus, surgical biopsy is necessary to diagnose the tumor, and especially its grade.

Therapy includes resection, irradiation, and chemotherapy, but there has been controversy as to when to treat and with which of these modalities. Removal may be curative, but when residual tumor is present after attempted resection, the patient may benefit from radiation therapy. Laws *et al.* analyzed 461 cases of supratentorial low-grade astrocytomas.[26] Age was the most important prognostic indicator; 83% of patients under 20, but only 12% of patients 50 and over, survived 5 years. Other important prognostic variables included postoperative neurological deficit, altered consciousness, type of surgery (actually extent of resection), date of treatment (worse before 1949), and tumor site (frontal/temporal worse). The authors considered resection as the best hope for cure, or at the least associated with longest survival. Radiation therapy appeared to be valuable primarily in patients over age 40 with more extensive tumors.

Berger *et al.* also found that the extent of surgical resection impacts on outcome.[27] They reviewed 221 patients at the University of Washington. When the tumors were totally resected, there was no recurrence (mean follow-up 54 months). Postoperative residual tumor of <10 cm^3 was associated with a 14.8% recurrence at 50 months, whereas larger residual tumor was associated with a 46% recurrence at 30 months ($p = 0.002$). Furthermore, 46% of patients with residual tumors >10 cm^3 had histologically higher grade at recurrence. Radiotherapy, age, and histological subtype were not prognostic with respect to recurrence.

The role of radiation therapy in the treatment of low-grade astrocytoma remains controversial. Shaw *et al.*[28] updated the Mayo Clinic experience of Laws, dividing the cases into those between 1960 and 1974, and those between 1975 and 1982, and using the newer Daumas-Duport classification.[29] The new classification allowed those patients originally considered to be Kernohan grade I-II, who had the same prognosis, to be divided into four grades, with different prognoses. Four variables were identified on multivariate analysis. Of these, the most important was the classification into pilocytic versus "ordinary astrocytoma." The former had 5- and 10-year survival rates of 85% and 79%, respectively, whereas the ordinary astrocytomas had 5- and 10-year survival rates of 51% and 23%, respectively. Ordinary astrocytomas included astrocytoma and mixed-oligoastrocytoma. Review of the postoperative status of the ordinary astrocytoma groups revealed that those receiving at least 53 Gy of radiotherapy had 5- and 10-year survival rates of 68% and 39%, respectively, whereas corresponding figures for those receiving less than 53 Gy were 47% and 21%; for those undergoing resection without radiation therapy the figures were 32% and 11%, respectively. It is not possible to draw definitive conclusions from these data because of the retrospective nature of the study, although the authors' data support the notion that patients with incompletely resected ordinary astrocytomas should receive radiation therapy. Soffietti *et al.* noted that in 85 well-differentiated astrocytomas, total removal produced a 5-year survival of 51.3%, whereas subtotal resection yielded 23.5% alive at 5 years; no patient with partial resection survived longer than five years.[30] Vertosick *et al.* reviewed their experience with 25 patients, concluding that such patients live longer than they used to, in part because of the earlier diagnosis possible with modern imaging; they questioned the need for surgical resection.[31] In Paris, one study failed to document a decisive role for radiation therapy.[32] Eighty percent of patients with total tumor removal survived five years, compared with 50% with incomplete removal and 45% with biopsy. Sixty-five percent were alive at 5 years without radiotherapy, compared with 55% with radiotherapy.

Recht *et al.* found that the overall survival of a group of 26 patients who were not operated on for a newly diagnosed supratentorial nonenhancing mass lesion on CT or MRI was similar to that of another group of 20 patients in whom the decision was made to treat immediately.[33] The overall median survival of both groups was 84 months. Winger *et al.* addressed the issue of malignant transformation of low-grade glioma and its relationship to overall survival.[34] In their study of 285 patients with malignant gliomas, they noted that those with a prior history of low-grade glioma lived significantly longer after the diagnosis of anaplastic gliomas than when anaplastic glioma arose *de novo*. Thus, radiating low-grade gliomas early might extend overall survival. One concern about radiating the brains of patients with low-grade gliomas is the potential for radiation damage in a population expected to live long enough to experience such damage. One report suggests that radiation damage is uncommon in that specific cognitive deficits were not encountered in patients so treated.[35]

Oligodendrogliomas occur mostly in middle-aged adults, although a small peak of incidence is also found in children. The most common clinical manifestation is seizures, and many of the tumors demonstrate calcification on routine skull films or CT scans. Several reports have related survival to grading of oligodendrogliomas. Grading was histologically related to number of mitoses and degree of necrosis in one study,[36] and to endothelial proliferation, necrosis, maximal nuclear/cytoplasmic ratios, maximal cell density and pleomorphism, in another study.[37,38] In the latter study, tumor grades ranged from lower grade A to highly malignant grade D. Sixty-eight percent of grade A patients were under age 40, and 83% of grade D patients were over age 40. Median survival in months were grade A, 94; grade B, 51; grade C, 45; and grade D, 17.

The role of radiation therapy in treating oligodendroglioma is not established. Lindegaard *et al.* found that 108 irradiated patients had a significantly better median postoperative survival time (38 months) than did 62 patients not receiving radiotherapy (26.5 months, $p = 0.039$).[39] Radiation therapy was most beneficial in patients undergoing subtotal resection; it was less clearly valuable in those patients whose tumors were thought to have been totally resected. This was also true for the series of Shaw *et al.* in which patients receiving subtotal resection plus radiotherapy lived longer than those undergoing resection alone, although this was a retrospective series and patients often were not treated with radiation.[40] Similarly, Bullard *et al.* found no statistical difference in survival between patients treated with radiation therapy (37 patients) and those operated on but without radiation therapy (34 patients).[41] Recently, Shaw *et al.* reviewed their experience with mixed oligoastrocytomas, noting in 71 patients that tumor grade (Kernohan) was most strongly associated with survival.[42] The 60 patients with tumors grades 1 and 2 had a median survival of 6.3 years and 5- and 10-year survival rates of 58% and 32%, respectively, compared with 2.8 years (36% and 9%, respectively) for 11 patients with tumors grades 3 and 4. Age <37 years, gross total resection, partial brain radiation, and radiation dose $\geq 5,000$ cGy were associated with improved survival. However, a large series of patients reported by Celli *et al.* yielded slightly different results.[43] Three variables (only) correlated positively with survival: benign histology, recent operative period, and postoperative radiation therapy. Subgroup analysis found that radiotherapy prolonged survival only in patients with neurological deficits, but not in patients who presented with seizures and negative neurological status. They suggested that different clinical presentations corresponded to different stages in the natural history of the disease, and that radiation results varied with the tumor type.

Finally, there is increasing evidence that oligodendrogliomas may be sensitive to chemotherapy.[24,44,45] Several controlled trials of chemotherapy are currently under way.

PRIMARY CENTRAL NERVOUS SYSTEM LYMPHOMA

Previously thought to be rare, lymphoma arising primarily in the brain is now recognized to be much more frequent.[46] This increased incidence includes patients at special risk—transplant recipients, patients with acquired immunodeficiency syndrome (AIDS), and those with congenital immunodeficiencies—but also nonimmunosuppressed individuals, especially in the elderly. The tumor usually presents as solitary or multifocal parenchymal brain masses, but may also occur as meningeal lymphoma or uveal or vitreous deposits or localized intradural spinal masses. Pathologically, most of the tumors are B-cell lymphomas, frequently of the immunoblastic type.[47] Epstein-Barr virus (EBV) genome/protein is expressed in lymphomatous tumor from two-thirds of HIV-related primary central nervous system lymphoma (PCNSL), but in only 15% of immunocompetent individuals.[48] In contrast to PCNSL, metastatic lymphoma from systemic primaries tends more often to be spinal epidural or meningeal in location. Clinically, PCNSL resembles glioblastoma multiforme. Diagnosis is suggested by MRI and/or CT, but pathological confirmation is required. Cerebrospinal fluid examination may reveal evidence of leptomeningeal tumor. In patients with AIDS the major differential is cerebral toxoplasmosis.

Until recently, treatment of PCNSL consisted of corticosteroids, surgical resection if possible, plus radiation therapy. Such treatment produces a dramatic initial improvement, but early relapse is the rule. Indeed, it is surprising, given the radiosensitivity of systemic lymphoma, that radiotherapy by itself is so ineffective. The RTOG treated 41 patients with PCNSL with combined whole-brain and focal irradiation; overall median survival was only 11.6 months.[49] Chemotherapy with several regimens has been reported to be effective.[50] Regimens initially included combination chemotherapy with cyclophosphamide, doxorubicin, vincristine, and prednisone, usually with radiation therapy. Methotrexate-containing regimens, delivered as high-dose intravenous infusions, intrathecally, or in association with blood–brain barrier modification, have been tested most extensively. Today, most chemotherapy regimens include radiotherapy, usually delivered after the course (12–16 weeks) of chemotherapy, but some authors have held off radiation therapy until recurrence after chemotherapy in order to reduce radiotoxicity. There has also been increasing interest in treating PCNSL in patients with AIDS, although the long-term results are dismal because the patients are at risk for other complications.

REFERENCES

1. SHAPIRO, W. R. 1986. Therapy of adult malignant brain tumors: What have the clinical trials taught us? Semin. Oncol. **13:** 38–45.
2. NAZZARO, J. M. & E. A. NEUWELT. 1990. The role of surgery in the management of supratentorial intermediate and high-grade astrocytomas in adults. J. Neurosurg. **73:** 331–344.
3. GLANTZ, M. J., P. C. BURGER, J. E. HERNDON, A. H. FRIEDMAN, J. G. CAIRNCROSS, N. A. VICK & S. C. SCHOLD, JR. 1991. Influence of the type of surgery on the histologic diagnosis in patients with anaplastic gliomas. Neurology **41:** 1741–1744.
4. WOOD, J. R., S. B. GREEN & W. R. SHAPIRO. 1988. The prognostic importance of tumor size in malignant gliomas: A computed tomographic scan study by the Brain Tumor Cooperative Group. J. Clin. Oncol. **6:** 338–343.
5. ALBERT, F. K., M. FORSTING, K. SARTOR, H. P. ADAMS & S. KUNZE. 1994. Early postoperative magnetic resonance imaging after resection of malignant glioma: Objective evaluation of residual tumor and its influence on regrowth and prognosis. Neurosurgery **34:** 45–61.
6. SIMPSON, J. R., J. HORTON, C. SCOTT, W. J. CURRAN, P. RUBIN, J. FISCHBACH, S. ISAACSON, M. ROTMAN, S. O. ASBELL, J. S. NELSON, A. S. WEINSTEIN & D. F. NELSON. 1993. Influence of location and extent of surgical resection on survival of patients with glioblastoma multiforme: Results of three consecutive Radiation Therapy Oncology Group (RTOG) clinical trials. Int. J. Radiat. Oncol. Biol. Phys. **26:** 239–244.

7. KELLY, P. J. & C. HUNT. 1994. The limited value of cytoreductive surgery in elderly patients with malignant gliomas. Neurosurgery **34:** 62–67.

8. WALKER, M. D., E. ALEXANDER, W. E. HUNT, C. S. MACCARTY, M. S. MAHALEY, JR., J. MEALEY, JR., H. A. NORRELL, G. OWENS, J. RANSOHOFF, C. B. WILSON, E. A. GEHAN & T. A. STRIKE. 1978. Evaluation of BCNU and/or radiotherapy in the treatment of anaplastic gliomas: A cooperative clinical trial. J. Neurosurg. **49:** 333–343.

9. WALKER, M. D., S. B. GREEN, D. P. BYAR, E. ALEXANDER, JR., U. BATZDORF, W. H. BROOKS, W. E. HUNT, C. S. MACCARTY, M. S. MAHALEY, J. MEALEY, JR., G. OWENS, J. RANSOHOFF, J. T. ROBERTSON, W. R. SHAPIRO, K. R. SMITH, C. B. WILSON & T. A. STRIKE. 1980. Randomized comparisons of radiotherapy and nitrosoureas for the treatment of malignant glioma after surgery. N. Engl. J. Med. **303:** 1323–1329.

10. WALKER, M. D., T. A. STRIKE & G. E. SHELINE. 1979. an analysis of dose-effect relationship in the radiotherapy of malignant gliomas. Int. J. Radiat. Oncol. Biol. Phys. **5:** 1725–1731.

11. SHAPIRO, W. R., S. B. GREEN, P. C. BURGER, M. S. J. MAHALEY, R. G. SELKER, J. C. VANGILDER, J. T. ROBERTSON, J. RANSOHOFF, J. J. MEALEY, T. A. STRIKE & D. A. PISTENMAA. 1989. Randomized trial of three chemotherapy regimens and two radiotherapy regimens in postoperative treatment of malignant glioma: Brain Tumor Cooperative Group Trial 8001. J. Neurosurg. **71:** 1–9.

12. DEUTSCH, M., S. B. GREEN, T. A. STRIKE, P. C. BURGER, J. T. ROBERTSON, R. G. SELKER, W. R. SHAPIRO, J. J. MEALEY, J. RANSOHOFF, P. PAOLETTI, K. R. J. SMITH, G. L. ODOM, W. E. HUNT, B. YOUNG, E. ALEXANDER, M. D. WALKER & D. A. PISTENMAA. 1989. Results of a randomized trial comparing BCNU plus radiotherapy, streptozotocin plus radiotherapy, BCNU plus hyperfractionated radiotherapy, and BCNU following misonidazole plus radiotherapy in the postoperative treatment of malignant glioma. Int. J. Radiat. Oncol. Biol. Phys. **16:** 1389–1396.

13. GUTIN, P. H., S. A. LEIBEL, W. M. WARA, A. CHOUCAIR, V. A. LEVIN, T. L. PHILIPS, P. SILVER, V. DA SILVA, M. S. B. EDWARDS, R. L. DAVIS, K. A. WEAVER & S. LAMB. 1987. Recurrent malignant gliomas: Survival following interstitial brachytherapy with high-activity iodine-125 sources. J. Neurosurg. **67:** 864–873.

14. LOEFFLER, J. S., E. ALEXANDER III, W. M. SHEA, P. Y. WEN, H. A. FINE, H. M. KOOY & P. M. BLACK. 1992. Radiosurgery as part of the initial management of patients with malignant gliomas. J. Clin. Oncol. **10:** 1379–1385.

15. CURRAN, W. J., JR., C. B. SCOTT, A. S. WEINSTEIN, L. A. MARTIN, J. S. NELSON, T. L. PHILLIPS, K. MURRAY, A. J. FISCHBACH, D. YAKAR, J. G. SCHWADE, B. CORN & D. F. NELSON. 1993. Survival comparison of radiosurgery-eligible and -ineligible malignant glioma patients treated with hyperfractionated radiation therapy and carmustine: A report of Radiation Therapy Oncology Group 83-02. J. Clin. Oncol. **11:** 857–862.

16. MEHTA, M. P., J. MASCIOPINTO, J. ROZENTAL, A. LEVIN, R. CHAPPELL, K. BASTIN, J. MILES, P. TURSKI, S. KUBSAD, T. MACKIE & T. KINSELLA. 1994. Stereotactic radiosurgery for glioblastoma multiforme: Report of a prospective study evaluating prognostic factors and analyzing long-term survival advantage. Int. J. Radiat. Oncol. Biol. Phys. **30:** 541–549.

17. LOEFFLER, J. S., D. C. SHRIEVE & E. ALEXANDER III. 1994. Radiosurgery for glioblastoma multiforme: The importance of selection criteria. Int. J. Radiat. Oncol. Biol. Phys. **30:** 731–733.

18. GREEN, S. B., D. P. BYAR, M. D. WALKER, D. A. PISTENMAA, E. ALEXANDER, JR., U. BATZDORF, W. H. BROOKS, W. E. HUNT, J. MEALEY, JR., G. L. ODOM, P. PAOLETTI, J. RANSOHOFF, J. T. ROBERTSON, R. G. SELKER, W. R. SHAPIRO, K. R. SMITH, JR., C. B. WILSON & T. A. STRIKE. 1983. Comparisons of carmustine, procarbazine and high-dose methylprednisolone as additions to surgery and radiotherapy for the treatment of malignant glioma. Cancer Treat. Rep. **67:** 121–132.

19. SHAPIRO, W. R., S. B. GREEN, P. C. BURGER, R. G. SELKER, J. C. VANGILDER, J. T. ROBERTSON, J. MEALEY, JR., J. RANSOHOFF & M. S. MAHALEY, JR. 1992. A randomized comparison of intra-arterial versus intravenous BCNU, with or without intravenous 5-fluorouracil, for newly diagnosed patients with malignant glioma. J. Neurosurg. **76:** 772–781.

20. ROSENBLUM, M. K., J. Y. DELATTRE, R. W. WALKER & W. R. SHAPIRO. 1989. Fatal necrotizing encephalopathy complicating treatment of malignant gliomas with intra-arterial BCNU and irradiation: A pathological study. J. Neuro-Oncol. **7:** 269–281.

21. HIESIGER, E. M., S. B. GREEN, W. R. SHAPIRO, P. C. BURGER, R. G. SELKER, M. S. MAHALEY, JR., J. RANSOHOFF II, J. C. VANGILDER, J. MEALEY, JR., J. T. ROBERTSON, F. H. HOCHBERG & R. F. YOUNG. 1995. Results of a randomized trial comparing intra-arterial cisplatin and intravenous PCNU for the treatment of primary brain tumors in adults: Brain tumor cooperative group trial 8420A. J. Neuro-Oncol. **25:** 143–154.

22. BREM, H., S. PIANTADOSI, P. C. BURGER, M. WALKER, R. SELKER, N. A. VICK, K. BLACK, M. SISTI, S. BREM, G. MOHR, P. MULLER, R. MORAWETZ & S. C. SCHOLD. 1995. Placebo-controlled trial of safety and efficacy of intraoperative controlled delivery by biodegradable polymers of chemotherapy for recurrent gliomas. Lancet **345:** 1008–1012.

23. MAHALEY, M. S. 1991. Neuro-oncology index and review (adult primary brain tumors). Radiotherapy, chemotherapy, immunotherapy, photodynamic therapy. J. Neuro-Oncol. **11:** 85–147.

24. CAIRNCROSS, J. G., D. R. MACDONALD & D. A. RAMSAY. 1992. Aggressive oligodendroglioma: A chemosensitive tumor. Neurosurgery **31:** 78–82.

25. KONDZIOLKA, D., L. D. LUNSFORD & A. J. MARTINEZ. 1993. Unreliability of contemporary neurodiagnostic imaging in evaluating suspected adult supratentorial (low-grade) astrocytoma. J. Neurosurg. **79:** 533–536.

26. LAWS, E. R., W. F. TAYLOR, M. CLIFTON & H. OKAZAKI. 1984. Neurosurgical management of low-grade astrocytoma of the cerebral hemispheres. J. Neurosurg. **61:** 665–673.

27. BERGER, M. S., A. V. DELIGANIS, J. DOBBINS & G. E. KELES. 1994. The effect of extent of resection on recurrence in patients with low grade cerebral hemisphere gliomas. Cancer **74:** 1784–1791.

28. SHAW, E. G., C. DAUMAS-DUPORT, B. W. SCHEITHAUER, D. T. GILBERTSON, J. R. O'FALLON, J. D. EARLE, E. R. J. LAWS & H. OKAZAKI. 1989. Radiation therapy in the management of low-grade supratentorial astrocytomas. J. Neurosurg. **70:** 853–861.

29. DAUMAS-DUPORT, C. 1992. Histological grading of gliomas. Curr. Opin. Neurol. Neurosurg. **5:** 924–931.

30. SOFFIETTI, R., A. CHIO, M. T. GIORDANA, E. VASARIO & D. SCHIFFER. 1989. Prognostic factors in well-differentiated cerebral astrocytomas in the adult. Neurosurgery **24:** 686–692.

31. VERTOSICK, F. T., R. G. SELKER & V. C. ARENA. 1991. Survival of patients with well-differentiated astrocytomas diagnosed in the era of computed tomography. Neurosurgery **28:** 496–501.

32. PHILIPPON, J. H., S. H. CLEMENCEAU, F. H. FAUCHON & J. F. FONCIN. 1993. Supratentorial low-grade astrocytomas in adults. Neurosurgery **32:** 554–559.

33. RECHT, L. D., R. LEW & T. W. SMITH. 1992. Suspected low-grade glioma: Is deferring treatment safe? Ann. Neurol. **31:** 431–436.

34. WINGER, M. J., D. R. MACDONALD & J. G. CAIRNCROSS. 1989. Supratentorial anaplastic gliomas in adults. The prognostic importance of extent of resection and prior low-grade glioma. J. Neurosurg. **71:** 487–493.

35. TAPHOORN, M. J. B., A. KLEIN SCHIPHORST, F. J. SNOEK, J. LINDEBOOM, J. G. WOLBERS, A. B. M. F. KARIM, P. C. HUIJGENS & J. J. HEIMANS. 1994. Cognitive functions and quality of life in patients with low-grade gliomas: The impact of radiotherapy. Ann. Neurol. **36:** 48–54.

36. BURGER, P. C., C. E. RAWLINGS, E. B. COX, R. E. MCLENDON & S. C. SCHOLD, JR. 1987. Clinicopathological correlations in the oligodendroglioma. Cancer **59:** 1345–1352.

37. SMITH, M. T., C. L. LUDWIG, A. D. GODFREY & V. W. ARMBRUSTMACHER. 1983. Grading of oligodendrogliomas. Cancer **52:** 2107–2114.

38. LUDWIG, C. L., M. T. SMITH, A. D. GODFREY & V. W. ARMBRUSTMACHER. 1986. A clinicopathological study of 323 patients with oligodendrogliomas. Ann. Neurol. **19:** 15–21.

39. LINDEGAARD, K., S. J. MØRK, G. E. EIDE, T. B. HALVORSEN, R. HATLEVOLL,

T. SOLGAARD, O. DAHL & J. GANZ. 1987. Statistical analysis of clinicopathological features, radiotherapy, and survival in 170 cases of oligodendroglioma. J. Neurosurg. **67:** 224–230.

40. SHAW, E. G., B. W. SCHEITHAUER, J. R. O'FALLON, H. D. TAZELAAR & D. H. DAVIS. 1992. Oligodendrogliomas: The Mayo Clinic experience. J. Neurosurg. **76:** 428–434.

41. BULLARD, D. E., C. E. RAWLINGS III, B. PHILLIPS, E. B. COX, S. C. SCHOLD, P. BURGER & E. H. HALPERIN. 1987. Oligodendroglioma: An analysis of the value of radiation therapy. Cancer **60:** 2179–2188.

42. SHAW, E. G., B. W. SCHEITHAUER, J. R. O'FALLON & D. H. DAVIS. 1994. Mixed oligoastrocytomas: A survival and prognostic factor analysis. Neurosurgery **34:** 577–582.

43. CELLI, P., I. NOFRONE, L. PALMA, G. CANTORE & A. FORTUNA. 1994. Cerebral oligodendroglioma: Prognostic factors and life history. Neurosurgery **35:** 1018–1035.

44. CAIRNCROSS, J. G. & D. R. MACDONALD. 1991. Chemotherapy for oligodendroglioma: Progress report. Arch. Neurol. **48:** 225–227.

45. CAIRNCROSS, G., D. MACDONALD, S. LUDWIN, D. LEE, T. CASCINO, J. BUCKNER, D. FULTON, E. DROPCHO, D. STEWART, C. SCHOLD, JR., N. WAINMAN & E. EISENHAUER. 1994. Chemotherapy for anaplastic oligodendroglioma. J. Clin. Oncol. **12:** 2013–2021.

46. HOCHBERG, F. H. & D. C. MILLER. 1988. Primary central nervous system lymphoma. J. Neurosurg. **68:** 835–853.

47. MILLER, D. C., F. H. HOCHBERG, N. L. HARRIS, M. L. GRUBER, D. N. LOUIS & H. COHEN. 1994. Pathology with clinical correlations of primary central nervous system non-Hodgkin's lymphoma: The Massachusetts General Hospital experience 1958–1989. Cancer **74:** 1383–1397.

48. JELLINGER, K. A. & W. PAULUS. 1995. Primary central nervous system lymphomas—New pathological developments. J. Neuro-Oncol. **24:** 33–36.

49. NELSON, D. F., K. L. MARTZ, H. BONNER, J. S. NELSON, J. NEWALL, H. D. KERMAN, J. W. THOMSON & K. J. MURRAY. 1992. Non-Hodgkin's lymphoma of the brain: Can high dose, large volume radiation therapy improve survival? Report on a prospective trial by the Radiation Therapy Oncology Group (RTOG): RTOG 8315. Int. J. Radiat. Oncol. Biol. Phys. **23:** 9–17.

50. DEANGELIS, L. 1995. Current management of primary central nervous system lymphoma. Oncology **9:** 63–71.

Cellular and Humoral Immune Responses Associated with HTLV-I Associated Myelopathy/Tropical Spastic Paraparesis

MICHAEL C. LEVIN[a] AND STEVEN JACOBSON

Viral Immunology Section, Neuroimmunology Branch
National Institute of Neurological Disorders and Stroke
National Institutes of Health
Bethesda, Maryland 20892

To F.P., a good friend and superb mentor.
Thank you for so many lessons learned.
Yours, M.C.L.

Human T-cell lymphotropic virus type I (HTLV-I), a virus endemic in the Caribbean, Japan, Africa, South America, and the southern United States, is associated with HTLV-I associated myelopathy/tropical spastic paraparesis (HAM/TSP).[1-3] How patients infected with HTLV-I develop HAM/TSP, a chronic progressive disorder of the central nervous system (CNS) is unknown. However, there is evidence that HAM/TSP does not exclusively result from direct infection with retrovirus, but rather infection associated with an autoimmune or immunopathogenic mechanism. Patients with HAM/TSP develop a chronic myelopathy and have an activated immune response in the peripheral blood, cerebrospinal fluid (CSF), and CNS parenchyma. How CNS infection with HTLV-I and the immune response to HTLV-I result in the CNS damage in HAM/TSP patients is an area of intense investigation. The focus of this paper is to describe the humoral and cellular immune responses in HAM/TSP patients that may participate in an immunopathogenic mechanism of HTLV-I associated CNS injury.

CORRELATION OF CLINICAL DISEASE WITH CNS PATHOLOGY

Patients with HAM/TSP develop chronic myelopathy characterized clinically by paraparesis associated with spasticity, hyperreflexia, and Babinski signs of the lower extremities.[3] Patients may also have mild sensory symptoms. Diagnosis is made on clinical criteria in association with a positive serum antibody titer to HTLV-I by ELISA assay.[3] Because the ELISA assay also screens for HTLV-II and

[a] Current address: Department of Neurology, University of Tennessee-Memphis, Link Building #415, 855 Monroe Avenue, Memphis, TN 38163.

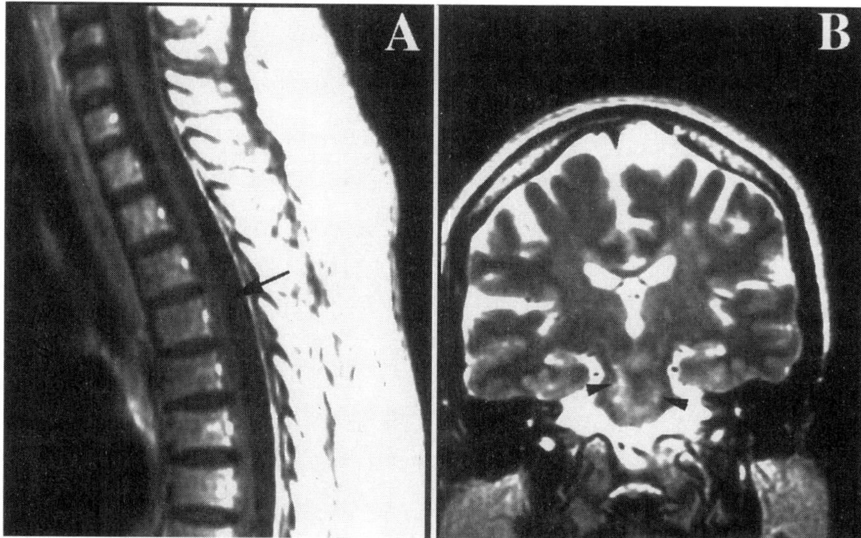

FIGURE 1. MRI of the spinal cord and brain of a patient with HAM/TSP in which neurologic signs and symptoms of the corticospinal tract predominate. (**A**) T1 weighted sagittal view of the spinal cord reveals thoracic cord atrophy (*arrow*). (**B**) T2 weighted coronal section of the brain reveals corticospinal tract damage in the brain stem (bright areas within the brain-stem parenchyma outlined by *arrowheads*).

other retroviral proteins, HTLV-I positive tests are confirmed by western blot analyses, which are designed to discriminate between HTLV types. CSF analysis typically reveals a mild lymphocytic pleocytosis, mild protein elevation, elevated IgG synthesis and IgG index, and oligoclonal bands.[4–6] Some of the oligoclonal bands are directed to HTLV-I proteins.[7] MRI of the spinal cord may reveal atrophy, and MRI of the brain shows periventricular white matter lesions in as many as 50% of patients.[8] An example of an MRI from one patient who presented with neurologic signs referable to the corticospinal tracts including paraplegia, upper extremity weakness with hyperreflexia, and dysphagia is shown in FIGURE 1. Consistent with the neuropathology, there is spinal cord atrophy (FIG. 1A, arrow) and evidence of corticospinal tract degeneration throughout the brain stem (FIG. 1B, arrowheads).[9]

The neuropathology of CNS autopsy specimens from patients with HAM/TSP has been carefully investigated and provides a model for the study of retroviral associated immune mediated damage to CNS tissues. Importantly, the clinical and neuroradiological information from patients with HAM/TSP correlates with the neuropathological findings. FIGURE 2 depicts a review of the neuropathological damage and immune cell infiltration of CNS autopsy specimens from patients with HAM/TSP in relation to duration of disease.[10–22] A robust immune response occurs in the spinal cord of patients with HAM/TSP (FIGURE 2). Leptomeninges and blood vessels are infiltrated with mononuclear cells that penetrate the surrounding parenchyma.[10–14] The phenotype of infiltrating immune cells is dependent upon the length of time the patient has neurologic disease. Early in disease (less than 2 to 5 years), there are greater numbers of inflammatory cells made up of almost equal

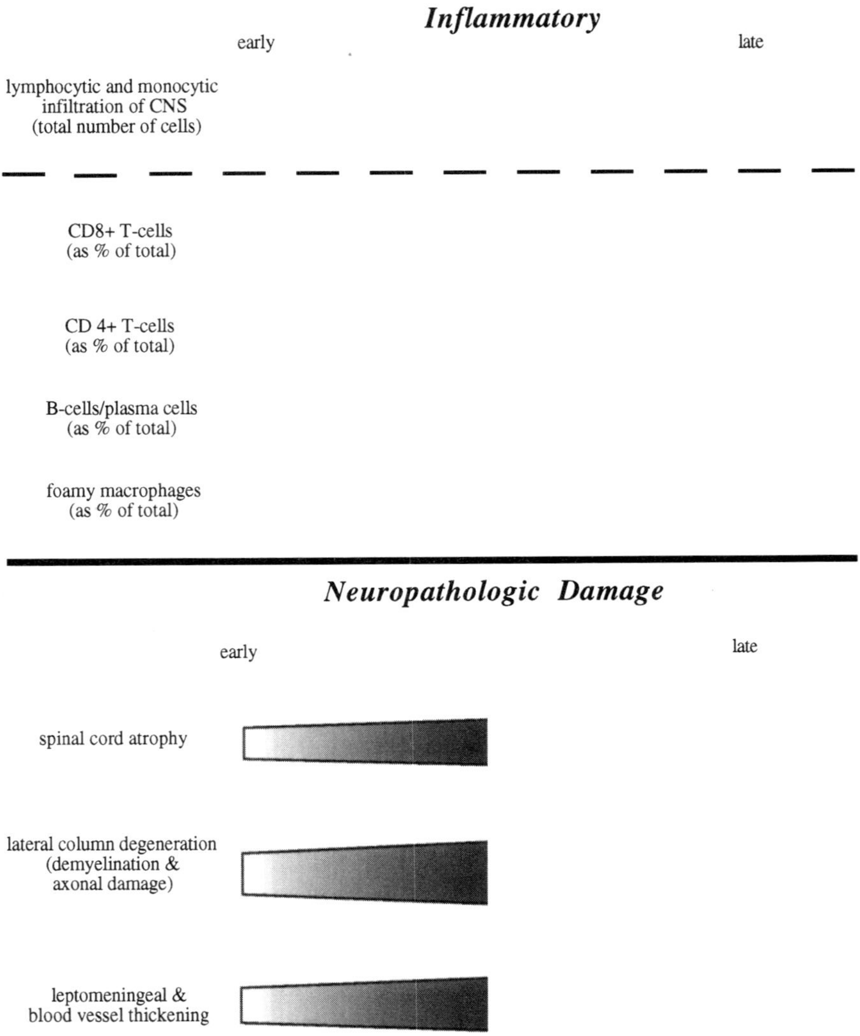

FIGURE 2. Summary of inflammatory infiltrates and neuropathologic damage found in CNS autopsy specimens of patients with HAM/TSP. Early in disease (typically less than two years), there is a robust infiltration of lymphocytes and monocytes. Phenotypically, there are similar numbers of CD8[+] cells, CD4[+] cells, and B-cells. Over time, the immune cell response decreases. B-cells essentially disappear, CD4[+] cells are sparse, and CD8[+] cells persist and become the predominant immune cell infiltrate. Foamy macrophages persist late in disease. Lateral column damage, predominantly secondary to corticospinal tract damage, is present early in disease and continues to progress significantly over the course of the disease. Spinal cord atrophy along with leptomeningeal and blood vessel thickening parallels the lateral column damage. Posterior column damage is also typically present, but this is mild in relation to the changes described.

amounts of CD8[+] T-lymphocytes, CD4[+] T-lymphocytes, and B-lymphocytes (FIG. 2).[14,15,17] Foamy macrophages are also present in damaged areas of spinal cord parenchyma (FIG. 2).[14,17] In chronic HAM/TSP (patients with disease greater than 5 years), inflammatory cells are less frequent, and almost exclusively CD8[+] T cells and macrophages (FIG. 2).[11,18,22]

Associated with this immune cell infiltration, there is extensive damage to the spinal cord predominantly, but not exclusively, at the thoracic level[10–13] (FIG. 2). The spinal cord is atrophic, and fibrosis of the leptomeninges and blood vessels increase proportionately to the duration of disease (FIG. 2).[11,14] There is symmetrical, widespread loss of myelin[11,17] and axonal dystrophy[18] of the lateral columns (FIG. 2), particularly of the corticospinal tracts of the spinal cord. Damage is most severe in thoracic and lumbar regions; however, corticospinal damage has been clearly described ascending to the cervical spinal cord[14,20–22] and brain stem.[22] These findings may be secondary to Wallerian degeneration.[11]

Since the inflammatory response in the CNS may be directed against HTLV-I proteins, many studies have attempted to localize HTLV-I in the CNS of patients with HAM/TSP. By electron microscopy, HTLV-I-like viral particles were found in the spinal cord of a HAM/TSP patient.[23] Also, HTLV-I DNA sequences were localized to the thoracic spinal cord of a HAM/TSP patient.[24] By quantitative polymerase chain reaction (PCR), HTLV-I DNA sequences were found to be increased in the thoracic cord in areas where CD4[+] cells were predominate.[25] In contrast, HTLV-I DNA sequences were localized to the spinal cord, but did not correlate with areas of lymphocyte infiltration.[26] Interestingly, *in situ* hybridization studies have more accurately localized HTLV-I RNA in CNS specimens to infiltrating CD4[+] T-lymphocytes in acute HAM/TSP[27] and to astrocytes in chronic HAM/TSP.[28]

PATIENTS WITH HAM/TSP HAVE AN ACTIVATED IMMUNE RESPONSE

Further evidence that the immune response may play a role in pathogenesis of HAM/TSP comes from the study of the humoral and cellular response in these patients. A number of studies have described both cellular and humoral immune responses in patients with HAM/TSP and compared these to HTLV-I seropositive asymptomatic individuals and normal HTLV-I seronegative controls.

An immunological profile from patients with HAM/TSP is shown in TABLE 1. HAM/TSP patients have elevated antibody titers to HTLV-I in sera and CSF, which are diagnostic criteria for this disorder.[1,2] Patients may have hypergammaglobulinemia, oligoclonal bands in their CSF, and elevated levels of lymphokines such as interleukin-6 (IL6) and soluble interleukin (IL2) in sera and CSF.[3,4,29] Neopterin and β microglobulin levels (markers of inflammation) have been reported to be elevated in CSF of patients with HAM/TSP.[8,30] Also, patients with HAM/TSP have increased levels of soluble vascular adhesion molecule type 1 (VCAM-1) in sera and CSF[31] and elevated levels of complements in sera.[32] In addition, abnormal cellular immune responses include decreased natural killer cell activity and natural killer subsets as well as decreased antibody-dependent cellular cytotoxicity (ADCC).[33,34] In the peripheral blood and CSF of HAM/TSP patients, activated T lymphocytes are present, and T cell activation can also be demonstrated by the capacity of peripheral blood lymphocytes (PBL) of HAM/TSP patients to proliferate spontaneously *in vitro* in the absence of exogenously added antigen.[29,35] Patients

TABLE 1. Immune Response in Patients with HAM/TSP

Immune Response	SERA	CSF
High antibody titer to HTLV-I	X	X
Elevated levels of IgG	X	X
Elevated IgG index		X
Oligoclonal bands to HTLV-I		X
Elevated levels of cytokines	X	X
Increased activated T-cells	X	X
Spontaneous lymphoproliferation	X	
Increased HTLV-I proviral DNA load	X	
Decreased natural killer cell subsets and activity	X	
Decreased ADCC activity	X	
Elevated $\beta2$ microglobulin		X
Oligoclonal expansion of TcR of CD8$^+$ cells	X	
Elevated neopterin levels		X
Elevated levels of complement	X	
Increased levels of VCAM-1	X	X
Increased HTLV-I specific, HLA class I-restricted CTL	X	X

with HAM/TSP may have up to 50 times more HTLV-I proviral DNA in PBL compared to asymptomatic carriers which may be related to many of the immunologic responses discussed above.[36,37]

Patients with HAM/TSP Have a Highly Specific Cellular Response to HTLV-I

Patients with HAM/TSP, in contrast to HTLV-I seropositive asymptomatic individuals and normal HTLV-I seronegative controls, develop a CD8$^+$ HLA class I restricted cytotoxic T-lymphocyte (CTL) response specific for immunodominant HTLV-I viral peptides that can be detected directly from mononuclear cells isolated from PBL and CSF cells.[38,39] Moreover, it was shown that the frequency of this HTLV-I specific CTL from HAM/TSP patients in both the peripheral blood and CSF was exceptionally high (1 in 86 and 1 in 60, respectively).[38,39] This extraordinarily high frequency of HTLV-I specific CD8$^+$ CTL should be kept in perspective because CTL play an important role in the normal immunologically mediated recovery from infectious disease. Precursor frequencies of CTL to more common viruses such as measles, mumps or influenza are typically in the range of 1 per 10^5 to 10^6 total lymphocytes. In contrast to the high frequency of CD8$^+$ HTLV-I specific CTL from patients with HAM/TSP, it has been shown that HTLV-I seropositive, asymptomatic individuals had no or significantly lower CTL responses. In addition, HTLV-I specific CTL from circulating PBL were not detected from two ATL patients (an HTLV-I associated leukemia).[38,39] Collectively, these results suggest that the presence of circulating CD8$^+$ HTLV-I specific CTL is a major immunologic feature of patients with HAM/TSP. The predominance of CD8$^+$ T cells in the subarachnoid space and parenchyma of CNS autopsy specimens of HAM/TSP patients suggests that the CD8$^+$ CTL plays a significant role in immune-mediated damage to the CNS.

IgG from Patients with HAM/TSP Recognizes Neurons in CNS Tissues

In addition to the highly specific CTL response to HLTV-I immunodominant peptides found in patients with HAM/TSP, we have begun to study a target-specific humoral response in HAM/TSP patients. Specifically, IgG was isolated from sera of HAM/TSP and control patients and used for immunohistochemistry of CNS tissues and cell lines. Preliminary data shows that IgG from patients with HAM/TSP reacted with neurons in CNS sections from HAM/TSP patients and normal human autopsy specimens, but not adjacent nonneuronal cells (FIG. 3A and B). HAM/TSP IgG reacted with the neuroblastoma cell line CHP-126, but not with astroglial cell lines or normal, uninfected lymphocytes. No neuronal activity was observed with IgG from an HTLV-I seropositive asymptomatic individual, an HTLV-I seronegative patient with chronic myelopathy or from uninfected normal controls (FIG. 3C).

Considering the many cell phenotypes in the CNS, an antibody response to a specified cell type localized to the target organ of the disease may have significant implications for immunopathogenesis. This strategy has been used to define target antigens recognized by the immune system in autoimmune diseases such as diabetes and paraneoplastic neurologic syndromes.[40,41] In diabetes, in which patients suffer from the effects of hypoinsulinemia, sera from diabetic patients localized target antigens in the insulin-secreting pancreatic islet cells.[40] Similarly, in the anti-Hu paraneoplastic neurologic syndrome, in which patients with cancer suffer from the clinical effects of neuronal damage, an antibody response recognizes an autoantigen (named Hu) found only on neurons, but not in other cells of the CNS.[41] Since the phenotype of the target cell(s) recognized by the CTL or other immune responses in the CNS of HAM/TSP patients is unclear, a humoral response specific for neurons may lend insight into the pathogenesis of the disease.

IMMUNOPATHOGENESIS OF HTLV-I ASSOCIATED NEUROLOGIC DISEASE

It has been over a decade since infection with HTLV-I was clearly associated with the development of HAM/TSP, and a definitive immunopathogenic mechanism describing how infection with a retrovirus results in a chronic progressive neurologic disease remains elusive. However, a number of hypothetical models have emerged based on an HLTV-I induced immune response that either (1) directly recognizes viral antigens or cross-reactive self-peptides on the surface of a target cell in the CNS leading to damaged tissue, or (2) indirectly causes CNS damage by developing an immune response to these peptides resulting in cytokine production, which in turn leads to damaged tissue (bystander mechanism).

Models on the pathogenesis of HTLV-I associated neurologic disease reflect two major experimental observations. First, a pathological hallmark of HAM/TSP is inflammatory T cells in affected spinal cord areas;[10–22] these are CD8[+] lymphocytes which dominate the inflammatory response as the disease progresses.[15,16] Second, an extraordinarily high frequency of CD8[+] HTLV-I specific CTL restricted to immunodominant epitopes of HTLV-I gene products has been demonstrated in both PBL and CSF of patients with HAM/TSP.[38,39] It is compelling to ask whether these CD8[+] T cells present in HAM/TSP lesions are HTLV-I specific CTL and what is the target for these cells.

A number of potential target cells are present in the CNS for the HLTV-I specific CTL and other components of the HTLV-I induced immune response. These include infiltrating immune cells as well as resident CNS cells such as endothelial cells, oligodendrocytes, astrocytes, microglia or neurons. Infection and subsequent expression of HTLV-I gene product(s) with a concomitant induction of HLA molecules could

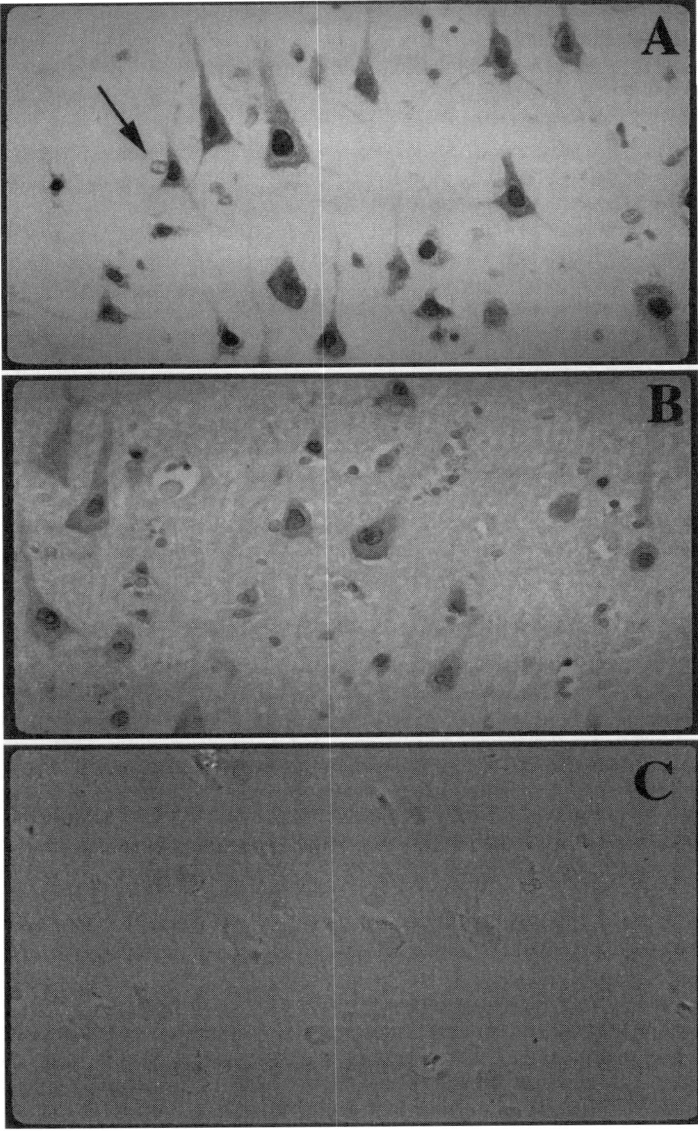

FIGURE 3. Immunohistochemistry of CNS tissues using IgG from HAM/TSP and control patients. All figures are 400×. (**A**) Immunohistochemistry of normal, uninfected CNS tissue using IgG from a patient with HAM/TSP. There is intense staining of neurons (both the nucleus and cytoplasm). The arrow shows an adjacent nonneuronal cell that is negative (methyl green counterstain which in this black-and-white photomicrograph is light gray). (**B**) Immunohistochemistry of HTLV-I infected (HAM/TSP) CNS tissue using IgG from a patient with HAM/TSP. There is intense staining of neurons (both the nucleus and cytoplasm) in a distribution identical to that in **A**. (**C**) Immunohistochemistry of normal, uninfected CNS tissue using IgG from a control, uninfected normal individual. There is no staining of neurons.

make these cells targets for cytotoxic $CD8^+$ cells that may be present at lesion sites. In support of this argument, class I expression was demonstrated in CNS autopsy specimens from patients with HAM/TSP where $CD8^+$ cells predominate.[18] Also, HTLV-I DNA sequences in the CNS of patients with HAM/TSP have been reported by solution phase PCR,[24,25] and *in situ* hybridization studies more accurately localized HTLV-I RNA to both infiltrating $CD4^+$ T-lymphocytes[27] and to astrocytes.[28]

The demonstration of both HTLV-I infected $CD4^+$ lymphocytes and HTLV-I infected neuroglial cells in the CNS may not be mutually exclusive events. Early in disease, when $CD4^+$ cells are numerous in HAM/TSP lesions (FIG. 2),[10–22] an HTLV-I infected $CD4^+$ cell from the peripheral blood may act as an antigen-presenting cell, stimulating an HTLV-I specific CTL. This same infected $CD4^+$ cell in periphery may traffic through the CNS, where it may trigger the CTL response locally, and upon the secretion of toxic levels of cytokines, indirectly damage CNS tissue. Alternatively, HTLV-I infected $CD4^+$ cells may infect resident CNS cells such as astrocytes and neurons. Viral peptides may be expressed in the setting of appropriate HLA conditions, and lead to CNS damage by inflammatory HTLV-I specific T-cells. Finally, a purely autoimmune phenomenon such as molecular mimicry may occur, in which the HTLV-I induced CTL response may recognize cross-reactive self-antigens in the CNS with similar structure and binding motifs as viral peptides, resulting in an immune response targeted against CNS tissue leading to CNS damage. Similarly, because patients with HAM/TSP develop an IgG response that reacts with neurons in the CNS, and neuronal tract degeneration is a predominant feature in the pathology of HAM/TSP, this humoral response may also play a role in immune-mediated CNS damage. Future studies are required to clarify which mechanism predominates in the immunopathogenesis of HTLV-I associated neurologic disease so that specific therapies for this and similar chronic progressive neurologic diseases, such as multiple sclerosis, can be designed.

REFERENCES

1. GESSAIN, A., J. C. VERNANT, L. MAURS, F. BARIN, O. GOUT, A. CALENDER & G. DE THE. 1985. Antibodies to human T-lymphotropic virus I in patients with tropical spastic paraparesis. Lancet **2:** 407–410.

2. OSAME, M., K. USUKU, S. IZUMO, N. IJICHI, H. AMITANI, A. IGATA, M. MATSUMOTO & M. TARA. 1986. HTLV-I associated myelopathy: A new clinical entity. Lancet **1:** 1031–1032.

3. HOLLSBERG, P. & D. A. HAFLER. 1993. Pathogenesis of diseases induced by human lymphotropic virus type I infection. N. Engl. J. Med. **328:** 1173–1182.

4. JACOBSON, S., A. GUPTA, D. MATTSON, E. MINGIOLI & D. E. MCFARLIN. 1990. Immunological studies in tropical spastic paraparesis. Ann. Neurol. **27:** 149–156.

5. CERONI, M., P. PICCARDO, P. RODGERS-JOHNSON, P. MORA, D. M. ASHER, D. C. GADJUSEK & C. J. GIBBS. 1988. Intrathecal synthesis of IgG antibodies to HTLV-I supports an etiological role for HTLV-I in tropical spastic paraparesis. Ann. Neurol. **23(Suppl.):** S188–S191.

6. LINK, H., M. CRUZ, A. GESSAIN, O. GOUT, G. DE THE & S. KAM-HANSEN. 1989. Chronic progressive myelopathy associated with HTLV-I: Oligoclonal IgG and anti-HTLV-I IgG antibodies in the cerebrospinal fluid and serum. Neurology **39:** 1566–1572.

7. KITZE, B., M. PUCCIONI-SOHLER, J. SCHAFFNER, P. RIECKMANN, T. WEBER, K. FELGENHAUER & W. BODEMER. 1995. Specificity of intrathecal IgG synthesis for HTLV-I cor and envelope proteins in HAM/TSP. Acta Neurol. Scand. **92(3):** 213–217.

8. NAKAGAWA, M., S. IZUMO, S. IJICHI, J. KUBOTA, K. ARIMURA, M. KAWABATA & M. OSAME. 1995. HTLV-I associated myelopathy: Analysis of 213 patients on clinical features and laboratory findings. J. Neurovirol. **1(1):** 50–61.

9. LEVIN, M. C. & S. JACOBSON. 1996. HTLV-I associated myelopathy/tropical spastic paraparesis (HAM/TSP): A chronic progressive neurologic disease associated with immunologically mediated damage to the central nervous system. J. Neurovirol. In press.

10. PICCARDO, P., M. CERONI, P. RODGERS-JOHNSON, C. MORA, D. M. ASHER, G. CHAR, C. J. GIBBS, JR. & D. C. GAJDUSEK. 1988. Pathological and immunological observations on tropical spastic paraparesis in patients from Jamaica. Ann. Neurol. **23(Suppl.):** S156–S160.

11. MOORE, G. R. W., U. TRAUGOTT, L. C. SCHEINBERG & C. S. RAINE. 1989. Tropical spastic paraparesis: A model of virus-induced cytotoxic T-cell mediated demyelination? Ann. Neurol. **26:** 523–530.

12. IWASAKI, I. 1990. Pathology of chronic myelopathy associated with HTLV-I infection (HAM/TSP). J. Neurol. Sci. **96:** 103–123.

13. YOSHIOKA, A., G. HIROSE, Y. UEDA, Y. NISHIMURA & K. SAKAI. 1993. Neuropathological studies of the spinal cord in early stage HTLV-I-associated myelopathy (HAM). J. Neurol. Neurosurg. Psychiatry **56:** 1004–1007.

14. AKIZUKI, S. 1989. The first autopsy case of HAM. *In* Neuropathology of HAM/TSP in Japan. Proceedings of the First Workshop on Neuropathology of Retrovirus Infections. Y. Iwasaki, Ed.: 1–6. Sendai, Japan.

15. UMEHARA, F., S. IZUMO, M. NAKAGA, A. T. RONQUILL, K. TAKASHI, K. MATSUMURO, E. SATO & M. OSAME. 1993. Immunocytochemical analysis of the cellular infiltrates in the spinal cord lesions in HTLV-I associated myelopathy. J. Neuropathol. Exp. Neurol. **52:** 424–430.

16. UMEHARA, F., A. NAKAMURA, S. IZUMO, R. KUBOTA, S. IJICHI, N. KASHIO, K. HASHIMOTO, K. USUKU, E. SATO & M. OSAME. 1994. Apoptosis of T lymphocytes in the spinal cord lesions of HTLV-I associated myelopathy: A possible mechanism to control viral infection in the central nervous system. J. Neuropathol. Exp. Neurol. **53:** 617–624.

17. IZUMO, S., I. HIGUCHI, T. IJICHI, A. TASHIRO, M. OSAME, K. YOSHIMI, F. MOTOKURA & A. OKUMURA. 1989. Neuropathological study in two autopsy cases of HTLV-I associated myelopathy (HAM). *In* Neuropathology of HAM/TSP in Japan. Proceedings of the First Workshop on Neuropathology of Retrovirus Infections. Y. Iwasaki, Ed.: 7–17. Tohuku University School of Medicine. Sendai, Japan.

18. WU, E., D. W. DICKSON, S. JACOBSON & C. S. RAINE. 1993. Neuroaxonal dystrophy in HTLV-I associated myelopathy/tropical spastic paraparesis: Neuropathologic and neuroimmunologic correlations. Acta Neuropathol. **86:** 224–235.

19. HARA, M., J. SANO, R. WATANABE & M. HONDA. 1989. An autopsy case of HAM with a history of blood transfusions. *In* Neuropathology of HAM/TSP in Japan. Proceedings of the First Workshop on Neuropathology of Retrovirus Infections. Y. Iwasaki, Ed.: 75–82. Tohuku University School of Medicine. Sendai, Japan.

20. AKIZUKI, S. 1989. An autopsy case of HAM with prolonged steroid therapy. *In* Neuropathology of HAM/TSP in Japan. Proceedings of the First Workshop on Neuropathology of Retrovirus Infections. Y. Iwasaki, Ed.: 25–32. Tohuku University School of Medicine. Sendai, Japan.

21. KOBAYASHI, I., K. OTA, K. YAMAMOTO, H. MURAKAMI, S. MARUYAMA, T. KASAZIMA & A. MASUDA. 1989. Clinical and pathological observations in HTLV-I associated myelopathy. *In* Neuropathology of HAM/TSP in Japan. Proceedings of the First Workshop on Neuropathology of Retrovirus Infections. Y. Iwasaki, Ed.: 33–46. Tohuku University School of Medicine. Sendai, Japan.

22. KISHIKAWA, M., K. KURIHARA, K. KITAI & T. KONDO. 1989. An autopsy case of HTLV-I associated myelopathy (HAM) caused by blood transfusions for uterine adenocarcinoma. *In* Neuropathology of HAM/TSP in Japan. Proceedings of the First Workshop on Neuropathology of Retrovirus Infections. Y. Iwasaki, Ed.: 18–24. Tohuku University School of Medicine. Sendai, Japan.

23. LIBERSKI, P. P., P. RODGERS-JOHNSON, G. CHAR, P. PICCARDO, C. J. GIBBS, JR. & D. C. GAJDUSEK. 1988. HTLV-I-like viral particles in spinal cord cells in Jamaican tropical spastic paraparesis. Ann. Neurol. **23(Suppl.):** S185–S187.

24. BHIGJEE, A. I., C. A. WILEY, W. WACHSMAN, T. AMENOMORI, D. PIRIE, P. L. A. BILL & I. WINDSOR. 1991. HTLV-I associated myelopathy: Clinicopathologic correlation with localization of provirus to the spinal cord. Neurology **41:** 1990–1992.

25. KUBOTA, R., F. UMEHARA, S. IZUMO, S. IJICHI, K. MATSUMURO, S. YASHIKI, T. FUJIYOSHI, S. SONODA & M. OSAME. 1994. HTLV-1 proviral DNA correlates with infiltrating CD4$^+$ lymphocytes in the spinal cord from patients with HTLV-I associated myelopathy. J. Neuroimmunol. **53:** 23–29.

26. KIRA, J., Y. ITOHAMA, Y. KOYANAGI, J. TATEISHI, M. KISHIKAWA, S. AKIZUKI, I. KOBAYASHI, N. TOKI, K. SUEISHI, H. SATO, Y. SAKAKI, N. YAMAMOTO & I. GOTO. 1992. Presence of HTLV-I proviral DNA in central nervous system of patients with HTLV-I-associated myelopathy. Ann. Neurol. **31:** 39–45.

27. MORITOYO, T., T. A. REINHART, H. MORITOYO, E. SATO, S. ISUMO, M. OSAME & A. T. HAASE. 1996. Human T-lymphocyte virus type I associated myelopathy and tax gene expression in CD4+ T lymphocytes. Ann. Neurol. **40:** 84–90.

28. LEHKY, T. J., C. H. FOX, S. KOENIG, M. C. LEVIN, N. FLERLAGE, S. IZUMO, E. SATO, C. S. RAINE, M. OSAME & S. JACOBSON. 1995. Detection of human T lymphotropic virus type I (HTLV-I) tax RNA in the central nervous system of HTLV-I associated myelopathy/tropical spastic paraparesis by in situ hybridization. Ann. Neurol. **37:** 246–254.

29. JACOBSON, S. 1992. Immune response to retroviruses in the central nervous system: Role in the neuropathology of HTLV-I associated neurologic disease. Semin. Neurosci. **4:** 285–290.

30. MATSUI, M., F. NAGUMO, J. TADANO & Y. KURODA. 1995. Characterization of humoral and cellular immunity in the central nervous system of HAM/TSP. J. Neurol. Sci. **130(2):** 183–189.

31. MATSUDA, M., N. TSUKADA, K. MIYAGI & N. YANAGISAWA. 1995. Increased levels of soluble vascular cell adhesion molecule-1 (VCAM-1) in the cerebrospinal fluid and sera of patients with multiple sclerosis and human T lymphotropic virus type 1 associated myelopathy. J. Neuroimmunol. **59(1–2):** 35–40.

32. SAARLOOS, M. N., R. E. KOENIG & G. T. SPEAR. 1995. Elevated levels of iC3b and C4d, but not Bb, complement fragments from plasma of persons infected with human T-cell leukemia virus (HTLV) with HTLV-I associated myelopathy/tropical spastic paraparesis. J. Infect. Dis. **172(4):** 1095–1097.

33. MORIMOTO, C., T. MATSUYAMA, C. OSHIGE, H. TANAKA, T. HERCEND, E. L. REINHERZ & S. F. SCHLOSSMAN. 1985. Functional and phenotypic studies of Japanese adult T cell leukemia cells. J. Clin. Invest. **75:** 836–843.

34. KITAJIMA, I., M. OSAME, S. IZUMO & A. IGATA. 1988. Immunological studies of HTLV-I associated myelopathy. Autoimmunity **1:** 125–131.

35. S. JACOBSON, V. ZANINOVIC, C. MORA, P. RODGERS-JOHNSON, W. A. SHERAMATA, C. J. GIBBS, D. C. GAJDUSEK & D. E. MCFARLIN. 1988. Immunological findings in neurological diseases: Activated lymphocytes in tropical spastic paraparesis. Ann. Neurol. **23:** 196–200.

36. GESSAIN, A., F. SAAL, O. GOUT, M. T. DANIEL, G. FLANDRIN, G. DE THE, G. PERIES & F. SIGAUX. 1989. High human T cell lymphotropic virus type I proviral DNA load with polyclonal integration in peripheral blood mononuclear cells from French West Indian patients with tropical spastic paraparesis. Int. J. Can. **43:** 327–333.

37. KIRA, J., Y. KOYANAGI, T. YAMADA, Y. ITOYAMA, I. GOTO, N. YAMAMOTO, H. SASAKI & Y. SAKAKI. 1991. Increased HTLV-I proviral DNA in HTLV-I associated myelopathy: A quantitative polymerase chain reaction study. Ann. Neurol. **29:** 194–201.

38. JACOBSON, S., H. SHIDA, D. E. MCFARLIN, A. S. FAUCI & S. KOENIG. 1990. Circulating CD8$^+$ cytotoxic lymphocytes specific for HTLV-I in patients with HTLV-I associated neurological disease. Nature **348** 245–248.

39. JACOBSON, S., D. MCFARLIN, S. ROBINSON, R. VOSKUHL, R. MARTIN, A. BREWAH, A. J. NEWELL & S. KOENIG. 1992. Demonstration of HTLV-I specific cytotoxic T lymphocytes in the cerebrospinal fluid of patients with HTLV-I associated neurologic disease. Ann. Neurol. **32:** 651–657.

40. ATKINSON, M. A. & N. K. MACLAREN. 1994. The pathogenesis of insulin-dependent diabetes mellitus. N. Engl. J. Med. **331(21):** 1428–1436.
41. MANLEY, G. T., P. S. SMITT, J. DALMAU & J. B. POSNER. 1995. Hu antigens: Reactivity with Hu antibodies, tumor expression and major immunogenic sites. Ann. Neurol. **38(1):** 102–110.

Functional Anatomical and Behavioral Consequences of Dopamine Receptor Stimulation

G. F. WOOTEN

Department of Neurology
Box 394
University of Virginia Health Sciences Center
Charlottesville, Virginia 22908

BASAL GANGLIA ANATOMY AND DOPAMINE RECEPTOR LOCALIZATION

The pharmacological effects of dopamine (DA) are mediated by cell surface receptors. At least five different dopamine receptors have been cloned and sequenced. Each of these receptor subtypes is a member of one of the two superfamilies of dopamine receptors designated D1 and D2. D1 dopamine receptors are positively linked to adenylate cyclase whereas D2 receptors are negatively linked to adenylate cyclase. Numerous agonist and antagonist drugs selective for one of these two families of DA receptors have been identified and characterized. The highest concentration of these two receptors in the brain is in the striatum (caudate and putamen). The striatum receives virtually all of the afferent input to the basal ganglia: from neocortex (glutamatergic), from centromedian parafascicular thalamus, and from substantia nigra pars compacta (SNPC; dopaminergic). Efferents from the basal ganglia arise from cell bodies in the internal segment of globus pallidus (GPI) and substantia nigra pars reticulata (SNPR). The striatum influences these output nuclei through both direct and indirect pathways. Striatopallidal and striatonigral neurons (both GABAergic) constitute the direct pathway. Striatal neurons projecting to the external segment of the GP (GPE), which in turn project to the subthalamic nucleus (STN), innervating the output neurons, constitute the indirect pathway (i.e., striato-GPE-STN-GPI/SNPR circuit). Striato-GPE and GPE-STN projections are inhibitory (GABAergic), whereas STN neurons are glutamatergic and provide excitatory influence on the GPI and SNPR.

Receptor autoradiographic studies demonstrated that in rats, monkeys, and humans both D1 and D2 dopamine receptors are present in high concentrations in the caudate and putamen; D1 receptors only are found in the GPI and SNPR. Studies of preparations with excitotoxic lesions of the striatum showed that D1 receptors in the GPI and SNPR were located on the terminals of afferents from the striatum.[1] More recently, intranigral injections of the retrogradely transported neurotoxin volkensin resulted in a selective reduction of D1 but not D2 receptors in the striatum,[2] whereas injections of the retrogradely transported neurotoxin OX7-saporin into the GPE resulted in a selective reduction in D2 but not D1 dopamine receptors in the striatum.[3] These findings strongly suggest that D1 receptors are preferentially expressed by striatal efferents to the GPI and SNPR (director pathways), whereas D2 dopamine receptors are preferentially expressed by striatal projections to the GPE (indirect pathway). Subsequent *in situ* hybridization studies revealed that enkephalin-expressing neurons in the striatum (project to GPE) also contained D2 dopamine receptor mRNA and substance P-expressing neurons (project to SNPR) also contained D1 DA receptor mRNA.[4]

EFFECTS OF DA RECEPTOR STIMULATION

Nearly 30 years after its introduction into clinical practice, levodopa (L-dopa) remains the treatment of choice in Parkinson's disease (PD). More rational and effective use of L-dopa and DA agonist drugs has resulted from a better understanding of the neuronal mechanisms that mediate their therapeutic effects; furthermore, the recurring problems associated with the currently available drugs such as clinical fluctuations and dyskinesias are better controlled with a fuller understanding of the mechanism of action of these drugs. Experimental approaches for understanding these mechanisms have included analysis of behavior, regulation of neurotransmitter synthesis, receptor regulation, electrophysiology, and regional brain metabolism. In the best studied animal model of striatal DA depletion, the rat unilateral nigral 6-hydroxydopamine lesion, selective D1 and D2 DA agonists are each capable of eliciting the classical direct dopamine agonist response of contralateral rotation. At least under some circumstances, the effects of D1 and D2 selective agonists may be synergistic. Since the elicitation of rotation is analogous in virtually every instance to the DA-stimulated motor response in PD, these data suggest that combined D1 and D2 receptor stimulation would be more efficacious than selective receptor stimulation in the therapy of PD. Certainly clinical experience is consistent with this suggestion.

To pursue the mechanism of action of antiparkinson drugs, we have studied the effects of dopaminergic drugs on regional cerebral glucose utilization (RCGU) and behavior. The autoradiographic measures of RCGU provide a functional map of brain physiological activity because glucose is the principal substrate for oxidative metabolism in the brain, and the major brain energy expenditure is in maintaining electrochemical gradients.[5] A major advantage of this method is the capacity to survey simultaneously the effects of dopaminergic drugs on all the major nuclei of the basal ganglia. Experimental evidence has suggested that under stimulated conditions, RCGU predominantly reflects the metabolic activity in nerve terminals as opposed cell bodies. Glucose utilization is therefore considered to be an index of synaptic activity. Accurate interpretation, however, always benefits from correlation with neurochemical anatomy and electrophysiology.

In rats with unilateral 6-hydrodopamine lesions of substantia nigra, systemically administered L-dopa elicits contralateral rotation identical to that seen with direct-acting dopamine agonists. In this model system, tracer doses of $[^{14}C]$-2-deoxyglucose given intravenously shortly after L-dopa result in an autoradiographic map of its physiological effects.[6] L-dopa markedly increased RCGU in the entopenduncular nucleus (EP, homologue of the primate GPI) and SNPR (approximately 100–200% increase), and moderately increased RCGU in the STN (approximately 30% increase). Other consistent effects included decreased RCGU in the lateral habenula (a target of the neurons of the EP), and increased RCGU in the deeper layers of the superior colliculus (a target of the output neurons of the SNPR). L-Dopa produced similar changes in monkeys with hemiparkinsonism. Given the massive direct projection of striatal neurons to the EP and SNPR, as well as the evidence that RCGU often reflects activity in nerve terminals, it was hypothesized that the increased RCGU in the EP and SNPR represents enhanced metabolism in the axon terminals of the striatoentopeduncular and striatonigral neurons. Similarly, increased RCGU in the STN was proposed to represent metabolic activity primarily in the axon terminals of its major afferent, the GPE. These results suggest that systemically administered L-dopa, after conversion to dopamine in the brain, activates striato-EP (striato-GPI), striato-SNPR, and GPE-STN pathways.

The motor effects of L-dopa are known to be dependent on the enzymatic conversion of L-dopa to dopamine in the striatum. Recent studies examined the contribution of D1 and D2 receptor stimulation to the effects of L-dopa, and considered other potential sites of action, particularly the D1 receptors in the output nuclei. To determine the functional consequences of selective D1 and D2 receptor stimulation, the metabolic effects of the D1 agonist SKF-38393 and the D2 agonist quinpirole were examined in rats with unilateral nigral lesions.[7] Both SKF-38393 and the quinpirole produce indistinguishable behavioral responses, including a vigorous contralateral rotation. Treatment with each drug similarly and dose dependently increased RCGU in the STN and the deep layers of the superior colliculus, whereas RCGU decreased in the lateral habenula. In contrast, D1 and D2 agonists differentially altered RCGU in the EP and SNPR: D1 stimulation markedly increased RCGU in these two nuclei, mimicking the effects of L-dopa, whereas D2 stimulation did not. These data are most straightforwardly interpreted in the context of the receptor localization studies already reviewed, suggesting that D1 receptors are selectively expressed on striato-EP and striato-SNPR neurons. These RCGU data are consistent with the hypothesis that, upon systemic administration, SKF-38393 and L-dopa selectively activate striato-EP and striato-SNPR neurons, an effect mediated by direct stimulation of D1 receptors on the cells.

Other clinically used dopamine agonists have been studied using this model.[8] Bromocriptine and (+)-4-propyl-9-hydroxynaphoxazine (PHNO), two agonists known to be D2 selective (based on ligand binding and biochemical studies), resulted in a D2 metabolic pattern similar to that seen with quinpirole. In contrast, pergolide (0.4 mg/kg) markedly increased RCGU in the EP and SNPR, consistent with D1 receptor stimulation. This finding is in accordance with electrophysiological studies demonstrating mixed D1/D2 actions of pergolide *in vivo*. Pretreatment with a selective D1 antagonist (SCH-23390; 0.5 mg/kg) completely blocked the RCGU increase elicited by pergolide, whereas pretreatment with a selective D2 antagonist (eticlopride; 1.0 mg/kg) only mildly attenuated this increase. These results demonstrate that the metabolic activation of the striato-EP and striato-SNPR pathways by a mixed D1/D2 agonist is critically dependent on D1 receptor stimulation.

The contributions of D1 and D2 receptor stimulation to the metabolic effects of L-dopa were studied using the same strategy of selective antagonist pretreatment.[9] As with pergolide, the major RCGU increases elicited by L-dopa in the EP and SNPR were completely blocked by D1 antagonist pretreatment, but only partially attenuated by D2 antagonist pretreatment. In contrast, the RCGU increase in the STN was not attenuated by either D1 or D2 antagonists alone, but was completely blocked by both antagonists in combination.

SUMMARY AND CONCLUSIONS

Taken together with electrophysiological data, these results suggest that in states of DA deficiency, systemically administered L-dopa or DA agonist drugs inhibit cell firing in the major output nuclei of the basal ganglia (GPI and SNPR). We propose that DA produces this net effect by a direct influence on the striato-GPI and striato-SNPR neurons, as well as indirectly via the striato-GPE-STN-GPI/

SNPR circuit. The RCGU data suggest that DA activates the direct pathway by stimulating D1 receptor-bearing striatal GABAergic neurons projecting to GPI and SNPR. Supportive evidence includes the ability of D1 agonists to facilitate GABA release in the striatum and to increase the firing rates of striatonigral neurons. The RCGU data also support a net stimulatory action of DA on the GPE output on STN, consistent with the excitatory effects of DA on GPE neuronal firing rates. This effect may be mediated by both D1 and D2 receptors. Stimulation of this pathway should physiologically inhibit the STN resulting in dysfacilitation of the GPI and SNPR. According to this scheme, DA exerts complementary actions via both direct and indirect anatomical pathways to decrease tonic firing rates of intrinsic neurons in the major output nuclei of the basal ganglia (i.e., GPI and SNPR).[10]

REFERENCES

1. ALTAR, C. A. & K. HAUSER. 1987. Topography of substantia nigra innervation by D1 receptor containing striatal neurons. Brain Res. **410:** 1–11.
2. HARRISON, M. B., R. G. WILEY & G. F. WOOTEN. 1990. Selective localization of striatal D1 receptors to striatonigral neurons. Brain Res. **528:** 317–322.
3. HARRISON, M. B., R. G. WILEY & G. F. WOOTEN. 1992. Changes in D2 but not D1 receptor binding in the striatum following a selective lesion of striatopallidal neurons. Brain Res. **590:** 305–310.
4. LeMOINE, C., E. NORMAND, A. F. GUITTENY, B. FOUQUE, R. TEOULE & B. BLOCH. 1990. Dopamine receptor gene expression by enkephalin neurons in rat forebrain. Proc. Natl. Acad. Sci. USA **87:** 230–234.
5. SKOLOFF, L. 1977. Relation between physiological function and energy metabolism in the central neurons systems. J. Neurochem. **29:** 13–26.
6. TRUGMAN, J. M. & G. F. WOOTEN. 1986. The effects of L-dopa on regional cerebral glucose utilization in rats with unilateral lesions of the substantia nigra. Brain Res. **379:** 264–274.
7. TRUGMAN, J. M. & G. F. WOOTEN. 1987. Selective D1 and D2 dopamine agonists differentially alter basal ganglia glucose utilization in rats with unilateral 6-hydroxydopamine substantia nigra lesions. J. Neurosci. **7:** 2927–2935.
8. TRUGMAN, J., W. S. ARNOLD, N. TOUCHET & G. F. WOOTEN. 1989. D1 dopamine receptor effects assessed *in vivo* with [14C]-2-deoxyglucose autoradiography. J. Pharmacol. Exp. Ther. **250:** 1156–1160.
9. TRUGMAN, J. M., C. L. JAMES & G. F. WOOTEN. 1991. D1/D2 dopamine receptor stimulation by L-dopa. Brain **114:** 1429–1440.
10. TRUGMAN, J. M. & G. F. WOOTEN. 1990. Functional consequences of dopamine receptor stimulation. Curr. Opin. Neurol. Neurosurg. **3:** 548–551.

Heat Shock or Stress Proteins and Their Role As Autoantigens in Multiple Sclerosis

GARY BIRNBAUM[a] AND LINDA KOTILINEK

Multiple Sclerosis Research and Treatment Center
Department of Neurology
University of Minnesota
School of Medicine
Minneapolis, Minnesota 55455

INTRODUCTION

Heat shock proteins (hsp), also called stress proteins, are families of proteins present in almost all prokaryotic and eukaryotic cells. They are classified according to their molecular weight and range in size from 17 kDa to more than 100 kDa. Hsp are required for a variety of critical cell functions ranging from protein synthesis to protein transport to protein degradation.[1] Because of these functions, many hsp are expressed constitutively. One of the major functions of certain hsp is to transport peptides from one intracellular compartment to another. These hsp do this by binding to newly synthesized peptides, preventing their aggregation into a denatured state and moving them across membranes into different cellular compartments. The hsp that perform these functions are primarily of molecular mass 60 kDa and are called "chaperones."

At times of stress, cells synthesize large quantities of new isoforms of hsp. Many different stresses can cause increases in hsp expression. Some examples are heat, viral infections, anoxia, and exposure to inflammatory cytokines, such as tumor necrosis factor and interferon-γ. There are several excellent reviews on hsp.[1–5]

STRESS PROTEINS AS TARGETS OF IMMUNE RESPONSES

Certain characteristics of hsp increase their potential to act as antigens in the development of autoimmune diseases.[6] First, hsp are phylogenetically conserved. Thus, there is greater than 50% sequence homology between certain prokaryotic hsp and those of mammalian cells.[6–9] Second, hsp are the immunodominant antigens for many infectious agents, including bacteria, mycobacteria, and parasites.[2,3,10] Third, hsp are expressed at sites of acute and chronic inflammation.[11,12] Thus, exposure to an infectious agent, in a genetically susceptible host, at the appropriate time during the host's development, may result in an immune response to the infecting agent's hsp that either cross-reacts with normal host hsp, or cross-reacts with organ-specific proteins, resulting in an autoimmune disease.

[a] Address for correspondence: Box 295, UMHC, Minneapolis, MN 55455. E-mail: birnb001@tc.umn.edu

Immune responses to hsp are implicated in the development of a number of human autoimmune diseases, including several inflammatory arthritides and Type I diabetes mellitus.[6,8,13,14] Their possible roles in autoimmune diseases of the central nervous system (CNS) will be discussed in this paper.

HEAT SHOCK PROTEINS AND MULTIPLE SCLEROSIS

The evidence that multiple sclerosis (MS) is an autoimmune disease or, for that matter, an immunologically mediated disease is circumstantial. Numerous laboratories have attempted to find immune responses to unique antigens in persons with MS or to find immune responses to myelin and other antigens not present in normal individuals but, to date, none has succeeded. Persons with MS do have increased immune responses to a variety of myelin antigens, including myelin basic protein, proteolipid protein, and myelin/oligodendrocyte glycoprotein,[15-21] and increased numbers of activated T cells responsive to these antigens.[15,22] In addition, many of the myelin antigens recognized by MS (and normal) T cells are potent autoantigens capable of inducing experimental autoimmune encephalomyelitis (EAE), an animal model for MS.[23,24] The presence of increased numbers of myelin-reactive cells in persons with MS clearly indicates sensitization to such proteins. However, it is not clear whether the heightened immune responses to these antigens are primary or secondary to the disease process, nor is it known what role these responses play either in disease initiation or perpetuation.

There is a well-documented association between MS disease activity and antecedent infections[25,26] (personal observations). The study by Sibley and associates showed a clear association between infections, usually viral, and attacks or worsening of disease. Although preexistent symptoms of MS will worsen during the acute phase of an infection, especially if there is an associated fever, true disease exacerbations occur days to weeks after recovery.

Several mechanisms could explain the association between infection and the worsening of an organ-restricted, inflammatory, possibly autoimmune, disease:

1. Infections result in increased concentrations of circulating cytokines. Some of these, such as tumor necrosis factor or interferon-γ, in addition to having direct effects on oligodendrocytes, could alter the blood–brain barrier, allowing easier entry of myelin-specific immunocompetent cells and/or antibodies. Cytokines could also nonspecifically activate anti-myelin T cells resident within the CNS of patients with MS.
2. Infections result in immune responses to the infectious organism's hsp. These immune responses could cross-react with phylogenetically conserved hsp expressed by oligodendrocytes in areas of inflammation.[27]
3. Immune responses to an infectious agent's hsp could cross-react with myelin antigens, resulting in myelin destruction.
4. A combination of the above effects may be important.

A variety of approaches have been used to determine whether hsp, or immune responses to hsp, are involved in the pathogenesis of MS. These included studies on (1) the expression of hsp in the brains of persons with MS; (2) immune responses to hsp in MS patients; and (3) cross-reactivity between hsp and CNS myelin.

In addition, several laboratories studied the distribution of γ/δ T cells in MS brains and spinal fluids.[28-31] Although most T cells that respond to hsp express the α/β receptor complex, a high proportion ($\geq 50\%$) of T cells expressing γ/δ receptors respond to hsp. Results of these studies revealed that there were increased numbers of γ/δ T cells around areas of demyelination as well as in the spinal fluids during acute exacerbations, and that, in cerebrospinal fluid (CSF), greater numbers of γ/δ cells were found in individuals with shorter duration of disease.[30] These data provide circumstantial support for the hypothesis that immune responses to hsp may play a role in the pathogenesis of MS.

Expression of hsp in MS Central Nervous System

Several laboratories studied expression of hsp in areas of MS demyelination. Selmaj and his associates[31,32] demonstrated expression of HSP 65 in immature oligodendrocytes at the edges of MS plaques. There also was constitutive expression of HSP 72 in MS and non-MS brain, especially in astrocytes. Wucherpfenning *et al.*[28] demonstrated expression of HSP 60 in foamy macrophages at the edges of acute plaques and expression of HSP 90 in reactive astrocytes. In our studies we used a panel of 20 monoclonal and polyvalent antibodies to human and mycobacterial hsp to immunocytochemically stain fixed, frozen sections of normal and MS brain.[33] Patterns of staining varied with different antibodies. Some antibodies stained cell bodies of neurons and astrocytes. Others stained neurofilaments. A small number of antibodies (discussed below) stained normal myelin. In sections of spinal cord, staining of both central and peripheral myelin was observed. We could not detect increased staining at the edges of either acute or chronic plaques, and demyelinated areas did not stain at all. Thus, there are epitopes on normal myelin that are recognized by monoclonal antibodies to mycobacterial hsp.

Using a different approach, a number of laboratories studied the expression of hsp by glial cells *in vitro*. Again results varied with the techniques and antibodies used for the assays. Selmaj *et al.*,[32] Freedman *et al.*,[34] and Satoh *et al.*[35] identified oligodendrocytes as cells expressing hsp. Selmaj *et al.* detected constitutive HSP 65 expression in oligodendrocytes but not astrocytes, yet noted some HSP 70/72 expression in astrocytes. Satoh *et al.* detected constitutive expression of HSP 60 in cultured murine oligodendrocytes and "marginally detectable" levels in most astrocytes. Expression of HSP 60 was increased in oligodendrocytes following heat stress. Freedman *et al.* detected constitutive expression of HSP 60 and HSP 70/72 expression in oligodendrocytes with increased expression of HSP 70/72 following heat stress. No astrocytes expressed HSP 70/72 and only a small percentage of astrocytes expressed HSP 60 proteins. In contrast, Marini and co-workers,[36] using tissue cultures of rat astrocytes and neurons, demonstrated heat-inducible expression of HSP 70 predominantly in astrocytes, but oligodendrocytes may have been absent from these cultures. Using purified cultures of rat astrocytes, Dwyer *et al.*[37] demonstrated that such cells synthesized hsp of 30–34, 68, 70, 89, and 97 kDa and that exposure to heat readily induced expression of HSP 65.

Because MS is an inflammatory disease, concentrations of cytokines are increased in MS brain.[38,39] De Souza *et al.*[27] studied the effects of cytokines on the expression of hsp in mixed cultures of human glial cells.[33,34] A mixture of cytokines induced expression of HSP 72, predominantly in oligodendrocytes. The specific cytokines involved in this induction were IL-1, interferon-γ, and tumor necrosis factor-α. Birnbaum *et al.* (unpublished observations) prepared cultures of purified murine astrocytes and exposed them to heat shock with or without exposure to a mixture of cytokines. Cytokines alone induced small amounts of HSP 70/72. However the combination of heat shock and cytokine exposure augmented expression of HSP 70/72 2–11-fold. The particular cytokines involved in this phenomenon were interferon-γ and tumor necrosis factor-α.

It is apparent from the above data that results can vary widely, depending on the specificities of the antibodies used and the particular methods. Nevertheless, good evidence exists that some antibodies to hsp bind to normal myelin while others bind to oligodendrocytes, or astrocytes. In addition, the inflammatory milieu within MS brains increases the expression of hsp within glia, increasing the possibility that immune responses to hsp of infectious agents could cross-react with their human homologues or with cross-reactive myelin epitopes.

Immune Responses to hsp in MS Patients and Controls

Work in this area can be divided into studies involving cellular immune responses and those involving humoral responses.

Two groups described cellular immune responses to heat shock proteins in persons with MS and other neurologic diseases (OND), Salvetti et al.[40] and our laboratory.[41] Salvetti et al. studied peripheral blood T cell proliferative responses to recombinant HSP 65 and HSP 70 from *M. bovis* in 31 persons with MS, 19 individuals with OND, and 19 normal controls. Proliferative responses to HSP 70 were significantly more frequent in persons with MS compared to OND and healthy controls. Responses to HSP 65 were equivalent in the three groups. Lines of T cells were established from 10 patients with MS and 12 healthy controls, using PPD as the antigen. Again, HSP 70 reactive lines were significantly more common in MS patients than in healthy controls. Interestingly, cytofluorometric analyses of PPD responsive lines revealed that only a minority of responding cells expressed γ/δ T cell receptors. Our laboratory studied T cell proliferative responses to *M. tuberculosis,* tetanus toxoid, and recombinant HSP 65 from *M. leprae.* T cells were concurrently collected from the peripheral bloods and spinal fluids of 20 persons with MS and 9 persons with inflammatory neurologic diseases other than MS. Cells were cultured *in vitro* and stimulated with the above antigens. Significantly increased spinal fluid lymphocyte proliferative responses to mycobacterial sonicate, relative to responses from paired peripheral blood lymphocytes, were present in 14 of the 20 specimens from patients with MS compared to 2 of 9 specimens from patients with OND ($p < 0.025$). Spinal fluid lymphocytes also responded to tetanus toxoid, but differences between blood and spinal fluid were not statistically significant. Lymphocytes from one patient with MS responded only to recombinant HSP 65. When MS patients were classified according to duration of disease, 9 of 10 patients with duration less than two years had spinal fluid T cells responding to *M. tuberculosis* compared to 5 of 10 with disease longer than two years ($p < 0.012$). These data supplement the observations of Shimonkevitz et al.[30] that described increased numbers of activated γ/δ cells predominantly in spinal fluids from persons with recent onset MS.

Additional data in support of the hypothesis that immune responses to hsp play a role in autoimmune demyelination are the observations of Mor and Cohen.[42] These investigators prepared T cells from the spinal cords, blood, spleen, and lymph nodes of rats during the acute phase of EAE or during recovery from EAE. Using limiting dilution analyses, they determined the frequency of T cell responses to the myelin protein, myelin basic protein (MBP), and to recombinant HSP 65 and HSP 70. As expected, responses to MBP were enriched in the spinal cords of rats during and after acute EAE. However, there was also enrichment of T cells responsive to HSP 65. T cell lines established from spinal cord lymphocytes responded to MBP,

HSP 65, and HSP 70. When EAE was induced with an anti-MBP responsive T cell line, similar patterns of enrichment for MBP and HSP 65 reactive T cells were noted, indicating that responses to hsp occurred in the absence of exposure to adjuvant mycobacteria.

Studies of humoral immune responses to hsp in MS are mainly the work in our laboratory[43,44] and that of Freedman and his associates.[45] We used immunoblots to detect antibodies to native and recombinant mycobacterial and bacterial hsp in paired spinal fluids and sera from persons with MS and OND. Antibodies to many hsp, including those of the 60 kDa and 70 kDa families, were present in CSF and sera from all patient groups. Patterns of antibodies varied between CSF and sera, and between patients, but no disease-distinctive patterns were seen. When anti-hsp antibodies were analyzed for isotypes, patients with MS had higher concentrations of anti-hsp IgA antibodies than did OND patients. This suggested an *in situ* synthesis of such antibodies within the CNS in persons with MS. Prabhakar *et al.* studied antibody concentrations to recombinant HSP 60 using an ELISA. Titers of antibodies in MS spinal fluids were significantly higher than those seen in persons with OND and the higher titers correlated with the presence of oligoclonal bands in MS CSF, but not OND CSF. In another recent study Gao *et al.*[46] demonstrated the presence of antibodies to mycobacterial HSP 65 and human HSP 60 in spinal fluids of persons MS as well as those with other neurologic illnesses. In this study, immune responses to hsp were not disease specific.

The presence of immune responses to hsp in spinal fluids of persons with a variety of chronic inflammatory CNS diseases is not unexpected because exposure to cytokines and inflammatory cells increases expression of these proteins and could result in an accumulation of anti-hsp T cells and antibodies in this anatomic compartment. However, since all of the above studies used large protein molecules as antigens, immune responses to particular hsp epitopes could not be detected nor were differences in cytokine secretion studied. Patterns of immune responses to particular hsp peptides vary among individuals, depending on differences in their major histocompatibility complex (MHC) genes and their different illnesses.[47] Such differences in patterns of immune response, especially those related to individual MHC genotypes, may be important in determining susceptibility to autoimmune diseases such as MS.

Modulation of Experimental Autoimmune Encephalomyelitis by Immunization with hsp

Although studies with MS patient materials have suggested that immune responses to hsp may play a role in pathogenesis, the best evidence for such a phenomenon comes from studies of an animal model of MS, EAE.

As noted above, we found that certain anti-hsp antibodies stain normal myelin. We extended these observations by performing immunoblots with normal human myelin as antigen.[33] A panel of 20 anti-stress protein antibodies was assayed for the ability to bind to normal human myelin proteins separated on SDS-PAGE. Three monoclonal antibodies, specific for either mycobacterial or human hsp, stained bands of normal myelin proteins. One murine monoclonal to *M. leprae* HSP 65, IIH9, stained a 44–46 kDa doublet. This doublet was the same size as the myelin protein 2′,3′, cyclic 3′ nucleotide phosphodiesterase (CNP). To study this observation further, purified CNP was used in immunoblots. IIH9 bound to CNP in a pattern identical to that seen with whole myelin. A nonapeptide region of sequence homology was identified between the epitope of HSP 65 recognized by IIH9 and CNP. This peptide (hsp-CNP peptide) was synthesized and used in immunblots. IIH9 strongly bound to this peptide, proving that this region of sequence homology was responsible for the observed cross-reactivity.

To determine whether immune responses to this peptide had biologic consequences, we immunized rats with hsp-CNP peptide, using either complete or incomplete Freund's adjuvant, the only difference between the two adjuvants being the presence of heat-killed *M. tuberculosis* in the complete Freund's adjuvant (CFA). No clinical disease or histologic changes in the CNS were observed. Four weeks later, animals were challenged with guinea-pig spinal cord in CFA. Those animals that originally received peptide in CFA developed accelerated and enhanced EAE. Those animals previously immunized with peptide in incomplete Freund's adjuvant (IFA) either remained healthy (40%) or developed very mild EAE. Differences between the two groups were statistically significant. Thus, an immune response to an hsp peptide having sequence homology with a myelin protein modulated the course of EAE.

In an attempt to determine the mechanisms involved in the protection offered by peptide immunization we measured spleen cell proliferative responses of rats immunized with hsp-CNP peptide upon stimulation with either recombinant, mycobacterial HSP 65, hsp-CNP peptide, or no antigen. Cells were collected at two time points, 12 and 31 days after peptide immunization. As expected, strong proliferative responses were seen at both time points with cells from animals given peptide in CFA, that is, adjuvant containing mycobacteria. In contrast, day 12 spleen cells from rats given hsp-CNP peptide in IFA did not respond to HSP 65. This too was expected because IFA contains no mycobacteria. However, by day 31 there was a dramatic change. Spleen cells from rats given peptide in IFA proliferated to HSP 65 stimulation as strongly as cells from rats given peptide in CFA. No proliferative responses were seen in spleen cells from any group when stimulated by hsp-CNP peptide alone. This latter observation is not unexpected since hsp-CNP peptide is a B-cell determinant. We interpret these observations to indicate that epitope spreading may have occurred following immunization with hsp-CNP peptide in IFA. In other words, even though there were no proliferative responses to peptide alone, sufficient T-cell stimulation was induced to allow diversification of the response to other epitopes of HSP 65. By 31 days after immunization, numbers of these HSP 65 responsive cells could be detected in our proliferative assays. The phenomenon of epitope spreading or diversification of immune responses initiated by restricted peptide epitopes is an important one that has significant implications in terms of determining patterns of immune response in any chronic inflammatory process, including MS.[48,49]

We next measured antibodies to HSP 65 and hsp-CNP peptide in sera from rats immunized 12 and 31 days previously with hsp-CNP peptide in either CFA or IFA. Antibodies to peptide were present in all animal groups. Only one of three rats immunized with peptide in CFA had antibodies to HSP 65 at 12 or 31 days after immunization. In contrast, antibodies to HSP 65 were seen in rats given peptide in IFA, both 12 days previously (1 of 3 rats) and 31 days previously (4 of 4 rats). These results support our hypothesis that, as a result of immunization with hsp-CNP peptide, epitope spreading occurred such that antibodies to other determinants of HSP 65 were evoked.

Immune responses can be categorized by the patterns of cytokines secreted by activated T cells. Th1 responses are those in which T cells secrete IL-2 and interferon-γ. Th2 responses are those in which T cells secrete IL-4 and IL-5.[50,51] Th1 responses have been implicated in the pathogenesis of cell-mediated diseases such as MS and EAE.[52] We wished to determine the patterns of immune responses to hsp-CNP peptide in terms of Th1 versus Th2. To do this we determined the isotypes of the IgG anti-peptide antibodies. IgG2a antibodies require secretion of interferon-γ. Thus, their presence indicates a Th1 pattern of response.[53] IgG1 antibodies arise in the presence of IL-4 and are an indicator of a Th2 pattern of T-cell response.[53] Anti-peptide antibodies from peptide-CFA immunized rats were a mixture of IgG1 and IgG2a isotypes on day 12 after immunization. By day 31, anti-peptide antibodies were almost exclusively IgG2a, indicating the presence of a strong Th1 response. In contrast, anti-peptide antibodies in the IFA immunized group were mainly IgG1 at both time points, though some IgG2a isotypes were detected on day 31. Thus, protection against EAE was associated with a Th2 pattern of response. These data are in agreement with other observations showing that Th1 responses are responsible for the development of EAE[52,54,55] and that Th2 cytokines, such as TGF-β, protect against EAE.[56]

Lewis rats are susceptible to acute EAE but rarely go on to have relapses. To study a model of EAE more closely resembling MS, we induced EAE in the SJL mouse by immunization with an encephalitogenic peptide of proteolipid protein, PLP139-151, emulsified in CFA. This results in a chronic relapsing form of EAE that has many similarities to MS. Following immunization with peptide, animals develop an acute illness from which almost all recover completely over a period of 10–14 days. One to three weeks after recovery mice begin to have spontaneous relapses of disease. Recovery from these attacks is often incomplete, and some animals develop chronic progressive disability. To study the role of hsp in this model mice were injected intravenously with HSP 60. Controls received either bovine serum albumin (BSA) or PLP139-151. One week later animals were immunized with PLP139-151 in CFA to induce EAE. All animals became ill with EAE, though as expected lesser numbers of mice receiving intravenous PLP139-151 developed EAE and those that did had very mild disease. Mice were then carefully followed over the ensuing three months. Mice given i.v. BSA recovered from their acute illness and went on to have mild to moderate relapses with good recovery between attacks. The few mice that became ill in the i.v. PLP139-151 group recovered completely and never experienced relapses. Mice pretreated with HSP 60 had disease as severe as BSA pretreated mice indicating that their acute EAE was not modified by exposure to HSP 60. However, over the ensuing three months HSP 60-treated animals experienced a significant increase in the severity and frequency of their relapses as well as sustaining incomplete recovery between attacks. Although the reasons for this effect remain to be elucidated, it is clear in this model that immune responses to hsp play an important role, not in the acute phase of EAE induced by peptide, but in the relapses that occur subsequent to recovery. An understanding of the mechanisms involved in this phenomenon may shed light on the causes of relapses in persons with MS.

One way to explain the above observations is to postulate that there is cross-reactivity between hsp and myelin. Data from several laboratories other than our own suggest that such cross-reactivity occurs. In 1975 Wisniewski and Bloom[57] noted primary demyelination in the brains of guinea pig sensitized to tuberculin who were then subsequently challenged with PPD intracranially. The investigators interpreted these data to indicate that demyelination was the result of a passive bystander effect, induced by the localized delayed hypersensitivity response. In retrospect, an alternative explanation is that demyelination occurred because of a specific cross-reactivity between myelin and PPD. Additional observations that support this alternative conclusion come from several different laboratories,[58–61] all of them demonstrating that exposure of EAE-susceptible animals to either *B. pertussis* or *M. tuberculosis* rendered them highly resistant to subsequent development of EAE.

Yet in the experiments described in the previous paragraph we successfully induced EAE in animals exposed to *M. tuberculosis* in CFA. These disparities in results may be due to the differences in the time intervals between initial exposure to *M. tuberculosis* and rechallenge.

SUMMARY

Stress or heat shock proteins are constitutively expressed in normal CNS tissues, in a variety of cell types (oligodendrocytes, astrocytes, and neurons). Their presence may protect cells from various stresses, such as hypoxia, anoxia, and excessive excitatory stimulation. Increased amounts of hsp are expressed in various cells of the CNS during acute toxic-metabolic states and in chronic degenerative and inflammatory diseases. Increased expression of hsp may lead to immune responses to these proteins.

Antibodies to mycobacterial hsp bind to normal human myelin and to oligodendrocytes in regions of MS demyelination. Cellular immune responses to hsp occur with increased frequency and magnitude in persons with MS, especially those with recent onset of disease. In addition, there are populations of T cells expressing γ/δ antigen receptors in the brains and spinal fluids of persons with MS, suggesting an *in situ* immune response to hsp. Humoral immune responses to hsp are found in CSF, but no disease specificity has been documented. Some myelin proteins have sequence homology with particular hsp. One instance is the homology between a peptide of mycobacterial HSP 65 and the myelin protein CNP. Our data in EAE suggest that immune responses to either cross-reactive epitopes or whole hsp can modify the course of both acute and chronic relapsing EAE.

These data support the hypothesis that an immune response to an infectious agent's hsp could result in a cross-reactive immune response to CNS myelin, or to responses to endogenous, CNS-expressed hsp, resulting in demyelination. This may be an important mechanism in the pathogenesis of MS.

REFERENCES

1. HARTL, F. U. 1996. Molecular chaperones in cellular protein folding. Nature **381:** 571–579.
2. MÖLLER, G. 1991. Heat-shock proteins and the immune system. Immunol. Rev. **121:** 5–220.
3. MORIMOTO, R. I., A. TISSIÈRES & C. GEORGOPOULOS. 1990. Stress Proteins in Biology and Medicine. Cold Spring Harbor Laboratory. Cold Spring Harbor, NY.
4. MORIMOTO, R. I., A. TISSIÈRES & C. GEORGOPOULOS. 1994. The Biology of Heat Shock Proteins and Molecular Chaperones. Cold Spring Harbor Monogr. Ser. Cold Spring Harbor, NY.
5. VAN EDEN, W. & D. B. YOUNG. 1996. Stress Proteins in Medicine. Marcel Dekker. New York.
6. JONES, D. B., A. F. COULSON & G. W. DUFF. 1993. Sequence homologies between hsp60 and autoantigens. Immunol. Today **14:** 115–118.
7. LAMB, J. R., V. BAL, P. MENDEZ-SAMPERIO, A. MEHLERT, *et al.* 1989. Stress proteins may provide a link between the immune response to infection and autoimmunity. Int. Immunol. **1:** 191–196.
8. QUAYLE, A. J., K. B. WILSON, S. G. LI, K. J. KJELDSEN, *et al.* 1992. Peptide recognition, T cell receptor usage and HLA restriction elements of human heat-shock protein (hsp) 60 and mycobacterial 65-kDa hsp-reactive T cell clones from rheumatoid synovial fluid. Eur. J. Immunol. **22:** 1315–1322.

9. STEINHOFF, U., B. SCHOEL & S. H. KAUFMANN. 1990. Lysis of interferon-gamma activated Schwann cell by cross-reactive CD8+ alpha/beta T cells with specificity for the mycobacterial 65 kd heat shock protein. Int. Immunol. **2:** 279–284.

10. KAUFMANN, S. H. E. 1990. Heat shock proteins and the immune response. Immunol. Today **11:** 129–136.

11. RES, P. C. M., D. TELGT, J. M. VAN LAAR, M. O. POOL, *et al.* 1990. High antigen reactivity in mononuclear cells from sites of chronic inflammation. Lancet **336:** 1406–1408.

12. KANTENGWA, S., Y. R. DONATI, M. CLERGET, P. I. MARIDONNEAU, *et al.* 1991. Heat shock proteins: An autoprotective mechanism for inflammatory cells? Semin. Immunol. **3:** 49–56.

13. ELIAS, D. & I. R. COHEN. 1994. Peptide therapy for diabetes in NOD mice. Lancet **343:** 704–706.

14. OTTENHOFF, T. H., P. TORRES, J. T. DE LAS AGUAS, R. FERNANDEZ, *et al.* 1986. Evidence for an HLA-DR4-associated immune-response gene for *Mycobacterium tuberculosis.* A clue to the pathogenesis of rheumatoid arthritis? Lancet **2:** 310–313.

15. ALLEGRETTA, M., J. A. NICKLAS, S. SRIRAM & R. J. ALBERTINI. 1990. T cells responsive to myelin basic protein in patients with multiple sclerosis. Science **247:** 718–721.

16. BAXEVANIS, C. N., G. J. RECLOS, C. SERVIS, E. ANASTASOPOULOS, *et al.* 1989. Peptides of myelin basic protein stimulate T lymphocytes from patients with multiple sclerosis. J. Neuroimmunol. **22:** 23–30.

17. HAFLER, D. A., D. S. BENJAMIN, J. BURKS & H. L. WEINER. 1987. Myelin basic protein and proteolipid protein reactivity of brain- and cerebrospinal fluid-derived T cell clones in multiple sclerosis and postinfectious encephalomyelitis. J. Immunol. **139:** 68–72.

18. JOHNSON, D., D. A. HAFLER, R. J. FALLIS, M. B. LEES, *et al.* 1986. Cell-mediated immunity to myelin-associated glycoprotein, proteolipid protein, and myelin basic protein in multiple sclerosis. J. Neuroimmunol. **13:** 99–108.

19. LIBLAU, R., L. E. TOURNIER, J. MACIAZEK, G. DUMAS, *et al.* 1991. T cell response to myelin basic protein epitopes in multiple sclerosis patients and healthy subjects. Eur. J. Immunol. **21:** 1391–1395.

20. LISAK, R. P. & B. ZWEIMAN. 1977. In vitro cell-mediated immunity of cerebrospinal-fluid lymphocytes to myelin basic protein in primary demyelinating diseases. N. Engl. J. Med. **297:** 850–853.

21. PETTE, M., K. FUJITA, B. KITZE, J. N. WHITAKER, *et al.* 1990. Myelin basic protein-specific T lymphocyte lines from MS patients and healthy individuals. Neurology **40:** 1770–1776.

22. ZHANG, J., S. MARKOVIC-PLESE, B. LACET, J. RAUS, *et al.* 1994. Increased frequency of interleukin 2-responsive T cells specific for myelin basic protein and proteolipid protein in peripheral blood and cerebrospinal fluid of patients with multiple sclerosis. J. Exp. Med. **179:** 973–984.

23. FRITZ, R. B., C. H. CHOU & D. E. McFARLIN. 1983. Relapsing murine experimental allergic encephalomyelitis induced by myelin basic protein. J. Immunol. **130:** 1024–1026.

24. TUOHY, V. K., R. A. SOBEL & M. B. LEES. 1988. Myelin proteolipid protein-induced experimental allergic encephalomyelitis. Variations of disease expression in different strains of mice. J. Immunol. **140:** 1868–1873.

25. SIBLEY, W. A., C. R. BAMFORD & K. CLARK. 1985. Clinical viral infections and multiple sclerosis. Lancet **1:** 1313–1315.

26. PANITCH, H. S. 1994. Influence of infection on exacerbations of multiple sclerosis. Ann. Neurol. **36:** S25–S28.

27. DE SOUZA, S. D., J. P. ANTEL & M. S. FREEDMAN. 1994. Cytokine induction of heat shock protein expression in human oligodendrocytes: An interleukin-1-mediated mechanism. J. Neuroimmunol. **50:** 17–24.

28. WUCHERPFENNIG, K. W., J. NEWCOMBE, H. LI, C. KEDDY, *et al.* 1992. Gamma delta T-cell receptor repertoire in acute multiple sclerosis lesions. Proc. Natl. Acad. Sci. USA **89:** 4588–4592.

29. HVAS, J., J. R. OKSENBERG, R. FERNANDO, L. STEINMAN, *et al.* 1993. Gamma delta T cell receptor repertoire in brain lesions of patients with multiple sclerosis. J. Neuroimmunol. **46:** 225–234.

30. SHIMONKEVITZ, R., C. COLBURN, J. A. BURNHAM, R. S. MURRAY, *et al.* 1993. Clonal expansions of activated gamma/delta T cells in recent-onset multiple sclerosis. Proc. Natl. Acad. Sci. USA **90:** 923–927.

31. SELMAJ, K., C. F. BROSNAN & C. S. RAINE. 1991. Colocalization of lymphocytes bearing gamma delta T-cell receptor and heat shock protein hsp65+ oligodendrocytes in multiple sclerosis. Proc. Natl. Acad. Sci. USA **88:** 6452–6456.

32. SELMAJ, K., C. F. BROSNAN & C. S. RAINE. 1992. Expression of heat shock protein-65 by oligodendrocytes in vivo and in vitro: Implications for multiple sclerosis. Neurology **42:** 795–800.

33. BIRNBAUM, G., L. KOTILINEK, P. SCHLIEVERT, H. B. CLARK, *et al.* 1996. Heat shock proteins and experimental autoimmune encephalomyelitis. I. Immunization with a peptide of the myelin protein 2′,3′ cyclic nucleotide 3′ phosphodiesterase that is cross reactive with a heat shock protein alters the course of EAE. J. Neurosci. Res. **44:** 381–396.

34. FREEDMAN, M. S., N. N. BUU, T. C. RUIJS, K. WILLIAMS, *et al.* 1992. Differential expression of heat shock proteins by human glial cells. J. Neuroimmunol. **41:** 231–238.

35. SATOH, J., H. NOMAGUCHI & T. TABIRA. 1992. Constitutive expression of 65-kDa heat shock protein (HSP65)-like immunoreactivity in cultured mouse oligodendrocytes. Brain Res. **595:** 281–290.

36. MARINI, A. M., M. KOZUKA, R. H. LIPSKY & T. S. J. NOWAK. 1990. 70-Kilodalton heat shock protein induction in cerebellar astrocytes and cerebellar granule cells in vitro: Comparison with immunocytochemical localization after hyperthermia in vivo. J. Neurochem. **54:** 1509–1516.

37. DWYER, B. E., R. N. NISHIMURA, J. DE VELLIS & K. B. CLEGG. 1991. Regulation of heat shock protein synthesis in rat astrocytes. J. Neurosci. Res. **28:** 352–358.

38. SELMAJ, K., C. S. RAINE, B. CANNELLA & C. F. BROSNAN. 1991. Identification of lymphotoxin and tumor necrosis factor in multiple sclerosis lesions. J. Clin. Invest. **87:** 949–954.

39. HOFMAN, F. M., D. R. HINTON, K. JOHNSON & J. E. MERRILL. 1989. Tumor necrosis factor identified in multiple sclerosis brain. J. Exp. Med. **170:** 607–612.

40. SALVETTI, M., C. BUTTINELLI, G. RISTORI, M. CARBONARI, *et al.* 1992. T-lymphocyte reactivity to the recombinant mycobacterial 65- and 70-kDa heat shock proteins in multiple sclerosis. J. Autoimmunity **5:** 691–702.

41. BIRNBAUM, G., L. KOTILINEK & L. ALBRECHT. 1993. Spinal fluid lymphocytes from a subgroup of multiple sclerosis patients respond to mycobacterial antigens. Ann. Neurol. **34:** 18–24.

42. MOR, F. & I. R. COHEN. 1992. T cells in the lesion of experimental autoimmune encephalomyelitis. Enrichment for reactivities to myelin basic protein and to heat shock proteins. J. Clin. Invest. **90:** 2447–2455.

43. BIRNBAUM, G. & P. SCHLIEVERT. 1992. Antibodies to mycobacterial antigens in the spinal fluids and blood from patients with multiple sclerosis and other neurologic diseases. Neurology **42:** 247.

44. BIRNBAUM, G. & L. KOTILINEK. 1993. Antibodies to 70-kd heat shock protein are present in CSF and sera from patients with multiple sclerosis. 45th Annual Meeting of the American Academy of Neurology, New York, April.

45. PRABHAKAR, S., E. KURIEN, R. S. GUPTA, S. ZIELINSKI, *et al.* 1994. Heat shock protein immunoreactivity in CSF—Correlation with oligoclonal banding and demyelinating disease. Neurology **44:** 1644–1648.

46. GAO, Y. L., C. S. RAINE & C. F. BROSNAN. 1994. Humoral response to hsp 65 in multiple sclerosis and other neurologic conditions. Neurology **44:** 941–946.

47. MUTIS, T., Y. E. CORNELISS, G. DATEMA, P. J. VAN DEN ELSEN, *et al.* 1994. Definition of a human suppressor T-cell epitope. Proc. Natl. Acad. Sci. USA **91:** 9456–9460.

48. LEHMANN, P. V., E. E. SERCARZ, T. FORSTHUBER, C. M. DAYAN, *et al.* 1993. Determinant spreading and the dynamics of the autoimmune T-cell repertoire. Immunol. Today **14:** 203–208.

49. MCRAE, B. L., C. L. VANDERLUGT, M. C. DEL CANTO & S. D. MILLER. 1995. Functional evidence for epitope spreading in the relapsing pathology of experimental autoimmune encephalomyelitis. J. Exp. Med. **182:** 75–85.

50. MUTIS, T., Y. E. CORNELISSE & T. H. OTTENHOFF. 1993. Mycobacteria induce CD4+ T cells that are cytotoxic and display Th1-like cytokine secretion profile: Heterogeneity in cytotoxic activity and cytokine secretion levels. Eur. J. Immunol. **23:** 2189–2195.

51. MUTIS, T., E. M. KRAAKMAN, Y. E. CORNELISSE, J. B. HAANEN, *et al.* 1993. Analysis of cytokine production by mycobacterium-reactive T cells. Failure to explain mycobacterium leprae-specific nonresponsiveness of peripheral blood T cells from lepromatous leprosy patients. J. Immunol. **150:** 4641–4651.

52. VAN DER VEEN, R. C. & S. A. STOHLMAN. 1993. Encephalitogenic Th1 cells are inhibited by Th2 cells with related peptide specificity: Relative roles of interleukin (IL)-4 and IL-10. J. Neuroimmunol. **48:** 213–220.

53. LIN, M. S. & Y. W. CHEN. 1993. B cell differentiation. II. Isotype potential of a single B cell. Cell. Immunol. **150:** 343–352.

54. VAN DER VEEN, R. C., J. A. KAPP & J. L. TROTTER. 1993. Fine-specificity differences in the recognition of an encephalitogenic peptide by T helper 1 and 2 cells. J. Neuroimmunol. **48:** 221–226.

55. MUSTAFA, M., C. VINGSBO, T. OLSSON, A. LJUNGDAHL, *et al.* 1993. The major histocompatibility complex influences myelin basic protein 63-88-induced T cell cytokine profile and experimental autoimmune encephalomyelitis. Eur. J. Immunol. **23:** 3089–3095.

56. STEVENS, D. B., K. E. GOULD & R. H. SWANBORG. 1994. Transforming growth factor-beta 1 inhibits tumor necrosis factor-alpha/lymphotoxin production and adoptive transfer of disease by effector cells of autoimmune encephalomyelitis. J. Neuroimmunol. **51:** 77–83.

57. WISNIEWSKI, H. M. & B. R. BLOOM. 1975. Primary demyelination as a nonspecific consequence of a cell-mediated immune reaction. J. Exp. Med. **141:** 346–359.

58. VANDENBARK, A. A., D. R. BURGER & R. M. VETTO. 1975. Cell-mediated immunity in experimental allergic encephalomyelitis: Cross-reactivity between myelin basic protein and mycobacteria antigens. Proc. Soc. Exp. Biol. Med. **148:** 1223–1226.

59. MOSTARICA-STOJKOVIC, M., S. VUKMANOVIC, M. PETROVIC, Z. RAMIC, *et al.* 1988. Dissection of the adjuvant and suppressive effects of mycobacteria in experimental allergic encephalomyelitis production. Int. Arch. Allergy Appl. Immunol. **85:** 82–86.

60. HEMPEL, K., A. FREITAG, B. FREITAG, B. ENDRES, *et al.* 1985. Unresponsiveness to experimental allergic encephalomyelitis in Lewis rats pretreated with complete Freund's adjuvant. Int. Arch. Allergy Appl. Immunol. **76:** 193–199.

61. LEHMANN, D. & A. BEN NUN. 1992. Bacterial agents protect against autoimmune disease. I. Mice pre-exposed to Bordetella pertussis or Mycobacterium tuberculosis are highly refractory to induction of experimental autoimmune encephalomyelitis. J. Autoimmunity **5:** 675–690.

Central Neurogenic Neuroprotection: Central Neural Systems That Protect the Brain from Hypoxia and Ischemia

DONALD J. REIS,[a] EUGENE V. GOLANOV,
ELENA GALEA, AND DOUGLAS L. FEINSTEIN

Department of Neurology and Neuroscience
Cornell University Medical College
New York, New York

INTRODUCTION

The brain is highly dependent upon a continuous and abundant supply of oxygen and glucose for its metabolism. Thus, even modest reductions in regional cerebral blood flow (rCBF) impair neuronal function and, if briefly sustained, result in neuronal death. Yet there are naturalistic behaviors during which rCBF may fall below thresholds which normally would compromise neuronal function. These include the marked hypoxemia sustained during submersion in diving vertebrates and the reductions in rCBF associated with profound suppression of cerebral metabolism (measured as regional cerebral glucose utilization, rCGU) in hibernating mammals. The fact that the reductions in rCBF are associated with a stereotyped pattern of behavior implies the presence within brain of neuronal systems dedicated to its own protection.

Our laboratory has been investigating some of the mechanisms by which the brain may control its own survival in the face of hypoxia and/or ischemia. Here we discuss two ways by which the brain may confront these threats. The first, a *reflex central neurogenic vasodilation*, is a rapid reflex cerebrovascular vasodilation generated from excitation of oxygen-sensitive neurons in the rostral ventrolateral medulla oblongata (RVLM) which initiates adjustments of the systemic and cerebral circulations to divert blood to, and increase blood flow within, the brain. The second, *conditioned central neurogenic neuroprotection*, results from excitation of pathways, yet unknown, which are represented in the cerebellar fastigial nucleus (FN) to produce prolonged protection from cerebral ischemia.

REFLEX CENTRAL NEUROGENIC VASODILATION

Primary Vasodilation and Oxygen-conserving Responses

During submersion, diving vertebrates undergo a rapid set of reflex autonomic adjustments in which differentiated excitation of sympathetic neurons is critical. The response, the *diving reflex*,[1] is a specific example of a group of related responses

[a] Address correspondence to Donald J. Reis, M.D., Division of Neurobiology, 411 East 69th Street, New York, NY 10021. E-mail: djreis@mail.med.cornell.edu

generically defined by Wolf[2] as *oxygen-conserving reflexes*. Within seconds after submersion, there is a powerful and differentiated activation of sympathetic nerves to muscle, gut, and kidney, reducing organ flow to a minimum and redirecting blood to brain and heart. The elevation in rCBF initiated by hypoxemia (and presumably submersion) is not associated with elevations in rCGU[3,4] and hence represent a *primary cerebrovascular vasodilation.*[5]

Simulation of the Oxygen-conserving Reflex and Primary Vasodilation Evoked from Oxygen-sensitive Neurons of Rostral Ventrolateral Medulla

The sympathetically mediated vasomotor responses of the oxygen-conserving reflex can be replicated by electrical or chemical stimulation of a small population of neurons, mostly adrenergic, lying within a small subnucleus, the C1 area of the RVLM.[6] These tonically active reticulospinal sympathoexcitatory neurons play a critical role in circulatory control, maintaining resting (tonic) arterial pressure (AP), and mediating the vasomotor component of most cardiovascular reflexes, including those arising from arterial baro- and chemoreceptors, from pain afferents, and in association with emotional behaviors.[6]

Electrical and chemical stimulation of the RVLM not only activates the systemic circulation to elevate AP, but also elevates rCBF[7-9] (FIGS. 1 and 2). The elevations in rCBF elicited from RVLM are stimulus locked, widespread, and greatest in the cerebral cortex (FIG. 2).

Neurons of the RVLM also mediate much of the sympathetic and cerebrovascular responses to hypoxemia[10] (FIG. 3). Local microinjection of sodium cyanide (NaCN) into the RVLM dose-dependently and site-selectively increases sympathetic nerve activity, elevates AP, generates expiratory apnea (FIG. 3A) and also bradycardia [not shown].[10] It thereby replicates in full the oxygen-conserving/diving reflex.[1] The hypoxia sensitivity is restricted only to the sympathoexcitatory reticulospinal vasomotor neurons of the region: They are the only neurons in the region excited by microinjection or iontophoresis of NaCN (FIG. 3C) or by hypoxemia (FIG. 3E).[11] Exposure of slices of RVLM to hypoxia or NaCN results in excitation of pacemaker neurons (FIG. 3D) (corresponding to sympathoexcitatory neurons of RVLM). Hypoxic excitation is direct and not transneuronal because the response persists after synaptic transmission is blocked *in vivo*[12] and can be replicated *in vitro* after treatment with tetrodotoxin.[13]

Two lines of evidence indicate that these RVLM neurons are essential for the expression of the cerebrovascular vasodilation elicited by hypoxia. First, electrical stimulation of RVLM in intact or spinalized rats site-specifically and dose-dependently elevates rCBF, but not rCGU.[14] In this manner it replicates hypoxic vasodilation.[4,15] The response can only be attributed to stimulation of the reticulospinal sympathoexcitatory neurons since these are the only neurons in the region excited by the agents.[11] Second, bilateral lesions of RVLM, but not adjacent regions, reduce by over 50% the elevation of rCBF produced by hypoxemia (FIG. 4). The fact that such lesions do not affect the vasodilation elicited by hypercarbia indicates that the response is stimulus selective.[14,16] Thus much of the cerebrovascular vasodilation elicited in the cerebral cortex by hypoxemia is a reflex which results from excitation of oxygen-sensitive brainstem neurons, and not by a direct effect of hypoxia on blood vessels[17] nor by stimulation of arterial chemoreceptors whose activity, while regulating blood flow to most vascular beds, is without effect on the cerebral circulation.[18]

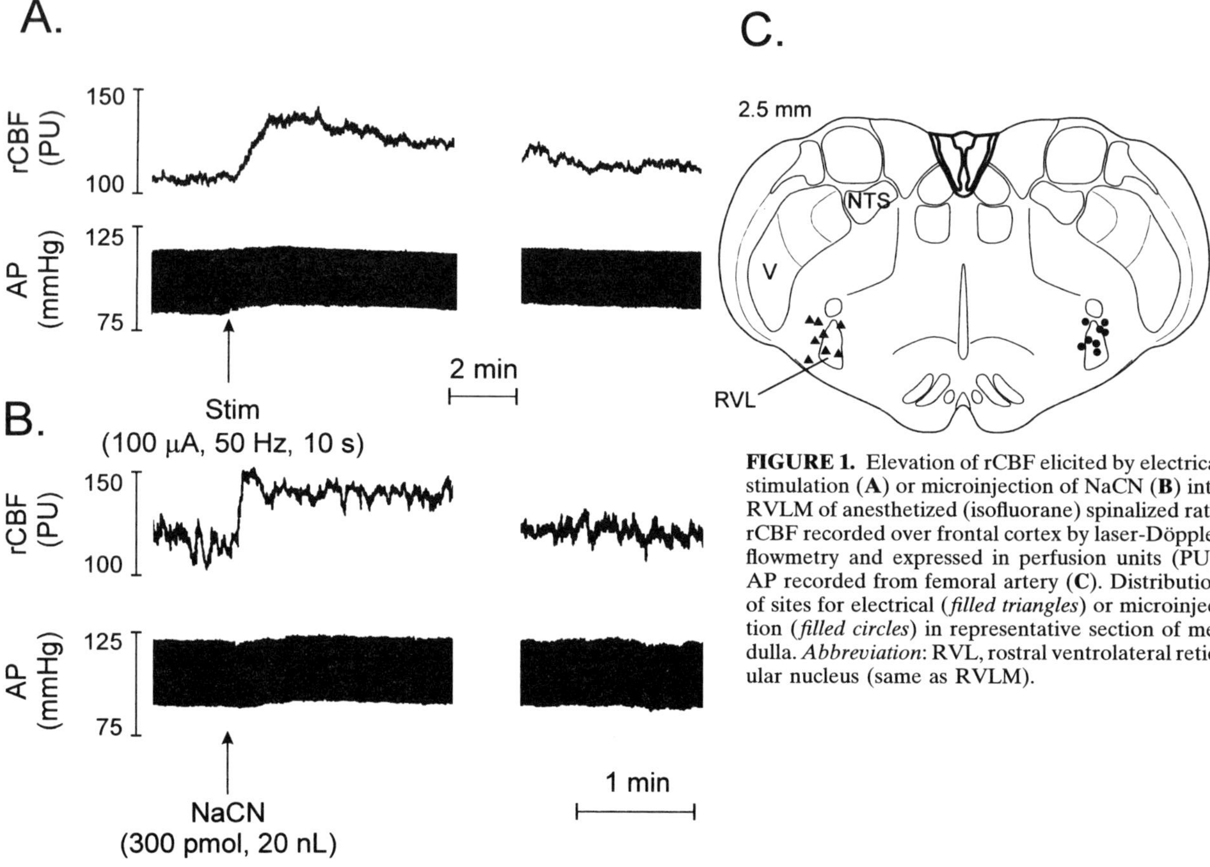

FIGURE 1. Elevation of rCBF elicited by electrical stimulation (**A**) or microinjection of NaCN (**B**) into RVLM of anesthetized (isofluorane) spinalized rats. rCBF recorded over frontal cortex by laser-Döppler flowmetry and expressed in perfusion units (PU). AP recorded from femoral artery (**C**). Distribution of sites for electrical (*filled triangles*) or microinjection (*filled circles*) in representative section of medulla. *Abbreviation*: RVL, rostral ventrolateral reticular nucleus (same as RVLM).

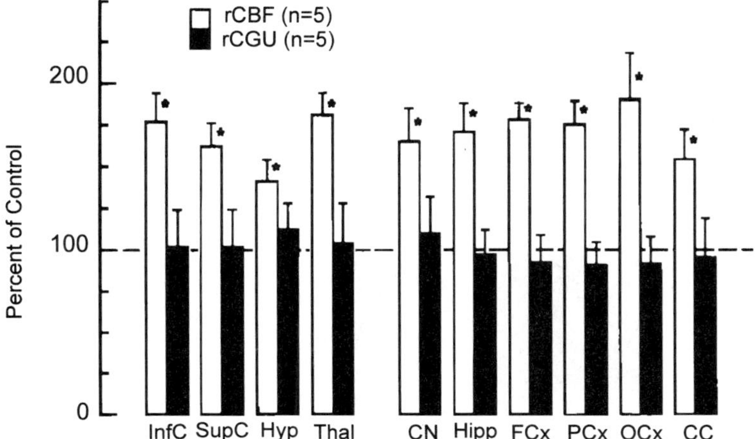

FIGURE 2. Effect of electrical stimulation of the rostral ventrolateral medulla (RVLM) on regional cerebral blood flow (rCBF) and regional cerebral glucose utilization (rCGU) in anesthetized rat. rCBF and rCGU were measured regionally in tissue homogenates by methods of Kety and Sokoloff,[69] respectively. Simulation of RVLM significantly (*$p < 0.05$) increased rCBF throughout the brain without altering rCGU. *Abbreviations*: CC, corpus callosum; CN, caudate nucleus; Fcx, frontal cortex; Hipp, hippocampus; Hyp, hypothalamus; InfC, inferior colliculus; Ocx, occipital cortex; Pcx, parietal cortex; SupC, superior colliculus; Thal, thalamus. (From Underwood *et al.*[9] Reprinted with permission from the *Journal of Cerebral Blood Flow and Metabolism*.)

Functional Considerations

Thus, reticulospinal sympathoexcitatory neurons of the RVLM rapidly and reflexly readjust the circulation to divert blood to brain. The effect is mediated in two ways. First, by initiating a primary vasodilation, rCBF is directly increased. The absence of any stimulus-initiated elevations of rCGU is relevant, because it means that the selective increase in rCBF provides more glucose and oxygen to the cortex than would be required if such stimulation also increased rCGU. The fact that the vasodilation is generalized suggests that rCBF is increased to protect brain regions from hypoxemia even if not metabolically active. Second, the same neurons of RVLM that increase rCBF also excite spinal preganglionic neurons.[8] This elicits widespread vasoconstriction and may increase AP. Since the cerebrovascular bed is dilated and cerebrovascular autoregulation attenuated, any elevation in AP will passively elevate rCBF.

This reflex central neurogenic vasodilation is initiated by stimuli primarily affecting neurons in RVLM. With the exception of selective brainstem ischemia (*the cerebral ischemic reflex*),[19] relevant stimuli will be those that affect the whole brain and would include hypoxemia and/or global ischemia. Activation of this system, however, is locked to the stimulus and is short-lived (longer periods of hypoxia or circulatory arrest are pathological). Moreover, it is only effective if the cerebral circulation is intact. Unlike conditioned central neurogenic protection (below) activation of neurons of the RVLM do not appear to be cytoprotective.[20]

The neuronal pathways through which excitation of oxygen-sensitive neurons

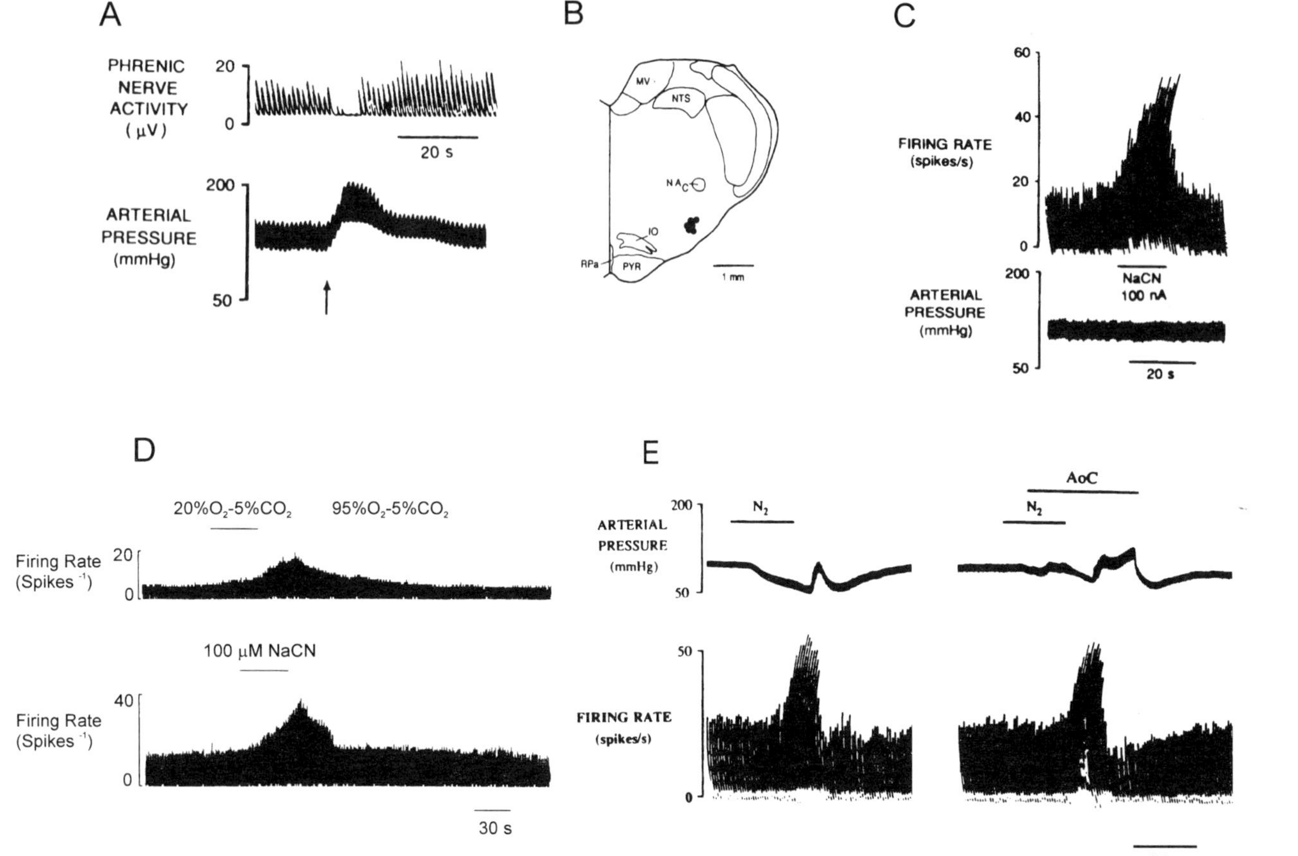

FIGURE 3. Neurons of RVLM are selectively excited by NaCN and hypoxia. (**A**) Microinjection of 300 pmol of NaCN (15 nL) into RVLM elevates AP (*lower trace*) and inhibits integrated phrenic nerve activity (*upper trace*). (**B**) Injection sites of **A** highly localized to RVLM. *Abbreviations*: MV, medial vestibular nucleus; Nac, nucleus ambiguus compactus; NTS, nucleus tractus solitarii; RIA, n. rapae pallidus; PYR, pyramid. (**C**) Iontophoretically applied NaCN excites sympathoexcitatory reticulospinal neurons of RVLM. (Since only one RVLM neuron was stimulated, AP did not rise). (**D**) Effect of hypoxia or NaCN on the activity of pacemaker neurons (corresponding to sympathoexcitory reticulospinal neurons) recorded in slice of RVLM. (**E**) Hypoxemia excites RVLM neuron. Hypoxemia was produced in anesthetized rat by substitution of N_2 (*bar*) for O_2 resulting, after 10 s, in a reduction of PaO_2 to 28 mmHg. In *left panel*, AP was not altered. In right, the fall of AP was blocked by transiently constricting the abdominal aorta (AoC). (Adapted from Reis *et al.*[6])

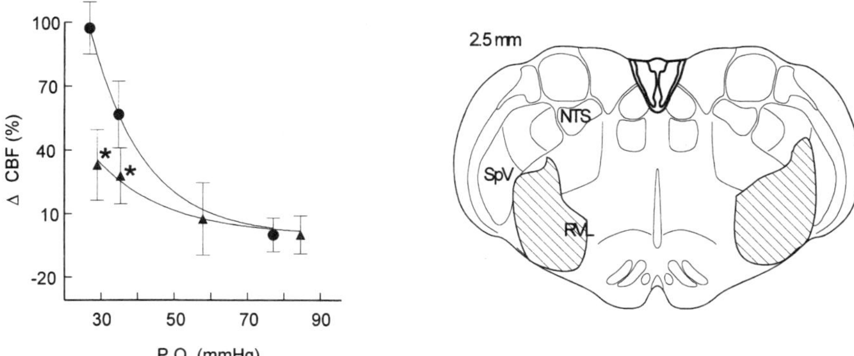

FIGURE 4. Hypoxic cerebrovascular vasodilation before and after bilateral lesions of RVLM in anesthetized spinalized rat. **Left panel:** Changes in rCBF, measured by laser-Döppler flowmetry before (*closed circles*) and after (*closed triangles*) placement of bilateral lesions of RVLM (average size in five animals). Note that lesions progressively attenuate the response to deepening levels of hypoxia to >50%.The same lesions failed to alter cerebrovascular vasodilation to hypercarbia. Control lesions in adjacent brainstem sites were without effect. *Abbreviations*: NT, nucleus tractus solitarii; RVL, rostral ventrolateral medulla; SpV, spinal trigeminal tract. (Modified from Golanov and Reis.[14])

in RVLM reflexively protects the cerebral cortex from hypoxia are indirect.[21] Rather, the projection is polysynaptic, reaching cortex through as-yet-undefined projections to upper brainstem and/or thalamus. The subcortical-cortical efferent vasodilator pathway does not directly regulate cerebral vessels. Rather, it appears to excite a small population of cortical neurons that seem to be dedicated to transducing a neuronal signal into vasodilation.[22,23] This system also appears to relay the central neurogenic vasodilation elicited from other brain regions, including the fastigial nucleus (FN)[22] and nucleus tractus solitarii (NTS).[24] By elevating rCBF independently of rCGU, it can also play the role of providing the brain with oxygen and metabolic substrates in anticipation of hypoxic need.

CENTRAL NEUROGENIC NEUROPROTECTION

The Fastigial Nucleus and Primary Vasodilation

Neurons of the RVLM are also the principal relay for the potent vasopressor and cerebrovascular vasodilator responses evoked by electrical stimulation of the cerebellar FN. This *fastigial pressor response* (FPR) consists of a marked elevation in AP and reductions in blood flow to skeletal muscle, kidney, and gut.[25] It also consists of a primary vasodilation, usually greater than that elicited from RVLM, and with rCBF in the cortex elevated over 200% without change in rCGU. Both the systemic and cerebrovascular components are abolished by bilateral lesions of the RVLM.[26,27] The neuronal elements within the FN mediating the FPR appear to be axons of brainstem neurons that project via collaterals to innervate cerebellum and also RVLM,[28] since microinjection of excitatory amino acids into the FN fails to replicate the FPR; however, after selective excitotoxic destruction of FN neurons,[27,29] combined with ablation of the cerebellar cortex, the FPR persists. On the other hand, stimulation of FN neurons with excitatory amino acids elicits a dose-dependent and site-selective *fall* of AP, rCBF, and rCGU; the *fastigial depressor reflex* (FDR)[27,29] is abolished when FN neurons are destroyed by excitotoxins. The FDR also appears to depend upon the integrity of the RVLM.[26]

Neuroprotection Evoked by Stimulation of the Fastigial Nucleus

That stimulation of the FN generated a potent elevation of rCBF not associated with change in metabolism also raised an intriguing question: Could stimulation of the FN protect the brain from ischemia? This rationale related to newer knowledge of the biology of focal ischemic infarctions. Specifically, they are not homogeneous but consist of two principal zones:[30,31] A central region in which rCBF and rCGU are deeply depressed and in which neurons undergo necrotic damage, the *ischemic core*;[32] and a region surrounding the core, the *ischemic penumbra*,[32] that is character-ized by a less robust reduction in rCBF, an elevation in rCGU,[32–34] and by electrical instability,[35,36] and in which neuronal death may be prolonged or delayed.[37,38] It is within the penumbra that the excessively released excitatory amino acids, notably L-glutamate, may promote excitotoxicity[39] by promoting the entry of Ca^{2+} through voltage-gated and NMDA receptor-coupled channels,[40] and that can be salvaged by treatments interfering with some of the processes, including blockade of NMDA receptors,[41] blockade of α-2-adrenergic and/or imidazoline receptors,[42] or blockade of Ca^{2+} channels.[43] Conceivably, elevating rCBF to this zone might reduce the neuronal damage associated with focal ischemia.

We therefore undertook a series of experiments in which we stimulated the FN for one hour in anesthetized rats and at the same time permanently occluded the middle cerebral artery (MCA). Changes in AP and/or blood gases were carefully controlled. At the end of stimulation, wounds were closed and the animals returned to their cages. Twenty-four hours later they were killed and the volume and distribu-tion of the cerebral infarction were examined. Controls were rats in which an electrode was inserted in the FN, but not stimulated (sham-stimulation), or animals in which the cerebellar dentate nucleus (DN), a region whose activation does not elevate rCBF[44] or other inert areas of cerebellar white matter, was stimulated.

As demonstrated in our initial study[45] and confirmed numerous times thereaf-ter,[20,46,47] one hour of FN stimulation reduced, by almost 50%, the volume of a focal cerebral infarction (FIG. 5).[45] Sham-stimulation or stimulation of the DN was without effect.[45] Topographically the area of salvage, the retrievable zone, corresponded to the ischemic penumbra, whereas the area unaffected by stimulation, the irretrievable zone, corresponded to the ischemic core. Our experiment therefore demonstrated, for the first time, that excitation of the CNS could protect the brain from isch-emic injury.

Central Neurogenic Neuroprotection Does Not Result from Changes in Cerebral Blood Flow or Metabolism

We initiated our first study to examine the possibility that a neurogenically initiated elevation of rCBF not coupled to any alteration in rCGU is neuroprotective. However, three subsequent studies have provided evidence that salvage is not related to changes in cerebral blood flow.

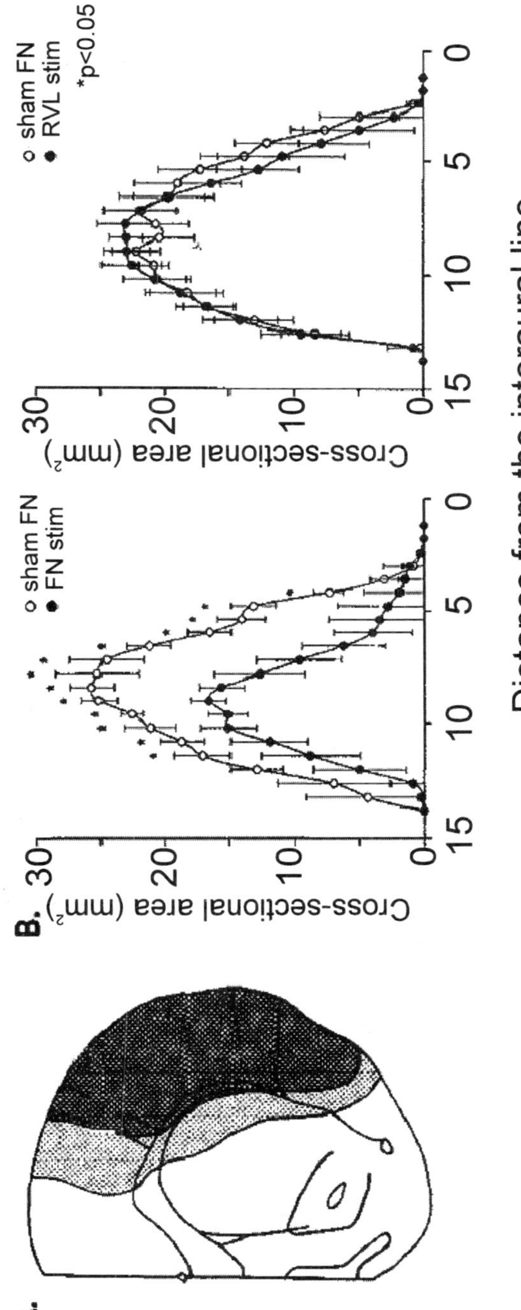

FIGURE 5. Stimulation of FN is neuroprotective whereas stimulation of RVLM is not. (**A**) Cross section of rat brain showing a composite of the extent of the average ischemic lesion in seven rats resulting from occlusion of the MCA 24 h earlier following 1 h of FN stimulation (*dark shading*) or sham-stimulation (*dark plus light shading*) just before occlusion. The dark shading corresponds to the ischemic core. Light shading corresponds to the ischemic penumbra. (**B**) Cross sectional areas of rat brains showing areas of lesions plotted along the rostral-caudal axis. Data are shown for groups of 5–7 rats with real (*closed circles*) or sham (*open circles*) stimulation of FN (*left panel*) or RVLM (*right panel*). Note that stimulation of FN, but not RVLM, reduces lesion volume in ischemic penumbra. (*$p < 0.01$; $n = 5$–7). (Adapted from Yamamoto *et al.*, 1993 [20].)

In the first study,[20] we continuously measured rCBF in anesthetized rats by laser-Döppler flowmetry. rCBF was measured simultaneously over the ischemic core (irretrievable zone), ischemic penumbra (retrievable zone), and nonaffected brain (FIG. 6). Measurements were made before, during, and after middle cerebral artery occlusion (MCAO) alone or during one hour of electrical stimulation of the FN. As a control, in other rats the RVLM was stimulated because this also elicits a primary vasodilation.[8,9] At the end of the stimulation epoch, rats were returned to their cages and 24 h later they were sacrificed and ischemic injury determined. Immediately after MCAO, as expected,[20] rCBF was reduced and did not recover over the course of the experiment. As shown in FIGURE 6, the reduction in rCBF was greatest in the core, least in the penumbra, and unchanged in unaffected areas of brain. In the absence of MCAO, stimulation of FN or RVLM increased rCBF in all three areas (not shown). After MCAO, stimulation of FN or RVLM failed to increase rCBF in ischemic areas (FIG. 6). However, it significantly reduced lesion volumes by salvaging brain in areas in the penumbra where rCBF remained significantly reduced.[20] Although stimulation of RVLM had comparable effects on rCBF in unaffected brain, it did not reduce lesion size.

The study indicated, therefore, that FN stimulation can salvage ischemic brain in the absence of an elevation of rCBF. Moreover, although stimulation of the RVLM evoked elevations in rCBF in unaffected areas comparable to those elicited from cerebellum, the fact that it failed to affect the lesion demonstrates that not all areas from which rCBF can be elevated when stimulated are equally neuroprotective. Thus the central neural pathways governing vasodilation and neuroprotection must differ. Finally, since the magnitude of ischemia was comparable in salvaged and unsalvaged brains, neurogenic neuroprotection cannot be attributed to differences in the ischemic stimulus itself.

A second study confirmed and extended these observations.[46] Changes in rCBF and rCGU were measured autoradiographically by the Kety (rCBF) and Sokoloff methods (rCGU), respectively, just after an hour of FN- or sham-stimulation in rats subjected to MCAO. Stimulation did not elevate rCBF or reduce an elevated rCGU in the area destined to be salvaged. Thus, it did not rectify the disproportion between enhanced rCGU and reduced rCBF (i.e., "misery perfusion"[48]) in the penumbra.

Central Neurogenic Neuroprotection Can be Preconditioned

The most convincing evidence that salvage cannot be attributed to enhanced perfusion was provided in our third study in which we examined the duration of protection provided by one hour of cerebellar stimulation.[49] In this investigation we stimulated rats to one hour of real or sham-stimulation of the FN. The MCA was occluded various times thereafter. We discovered that one hour of cerebellar simulation was capable of protecting the brain from focal ischemia, even when the MCA was occluded 10 days later. Protection, however, was not present when MCAO was performed 30 days later, indicating the effects of stimulation, although long-lasting, are not permanent (FIG. 7). The prolonged and "conditioned" neuroprotection cannot be attributed to changes in rCBF, because, while rCBF recovers within a few minutes after the stimulus is terminated,[20] protection persists for weeks. We have termed this form of neuroprotection *central neurogenic neuroprotection.*

What Mechanisms Can Account for Central Neurogenic Neuroprotection?

Central neurogenic neuroprotection, therefore, cannot be attributed to increasing rCBF, nor reducing rCGU. We are presently investigating two other mechanisms

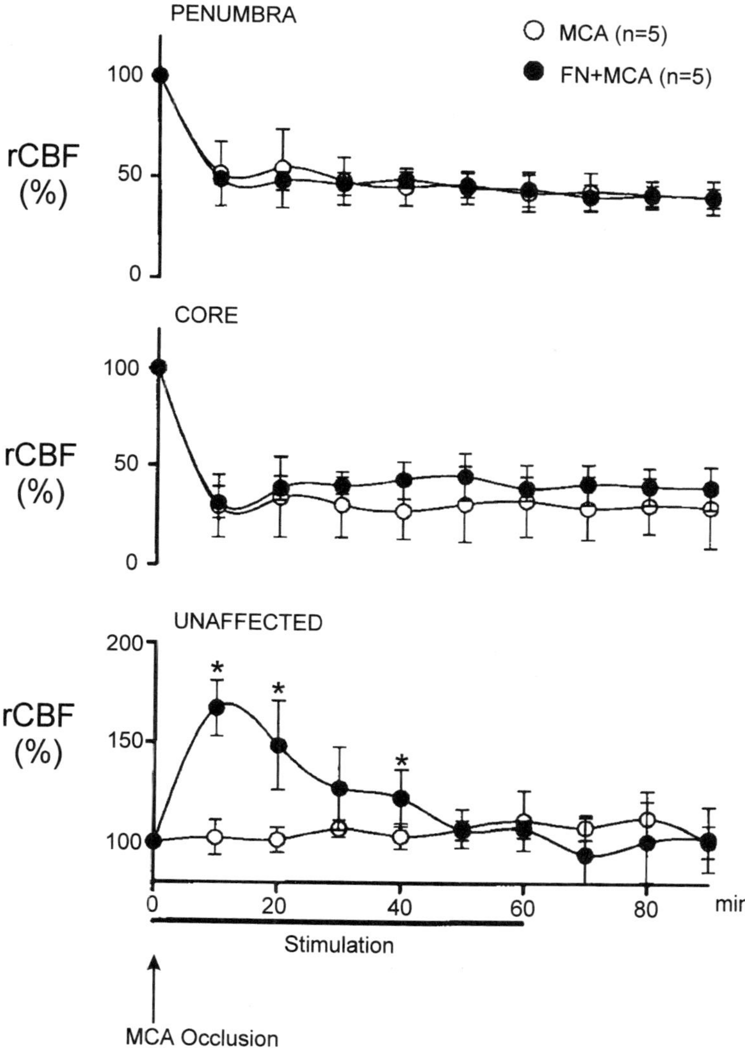

FIGURE 6. Stimulation of FN does not increase rCBF in areas of salvage. Changes in rCBF were measured by laser-Döppler flowmetry over the area corresponding to ischemic penumbra (*upper trace*), ischemic core (*middle trace*), and unaffected contralateral hemisphere (*lower trace*) following MCA occlusion. In one group only the MCA was occluded (*open circles*). In the other the FN was stimulated for 1 h following MCA occlusion (*closed circles*). Note that reduction in rCBF in core and penumbra is not affected by FN stimulation despite the fact that penumbra was subsequently shown to be salvaged in the same animals. See text for details. (Modified from Yamamoto *et al.*[20])

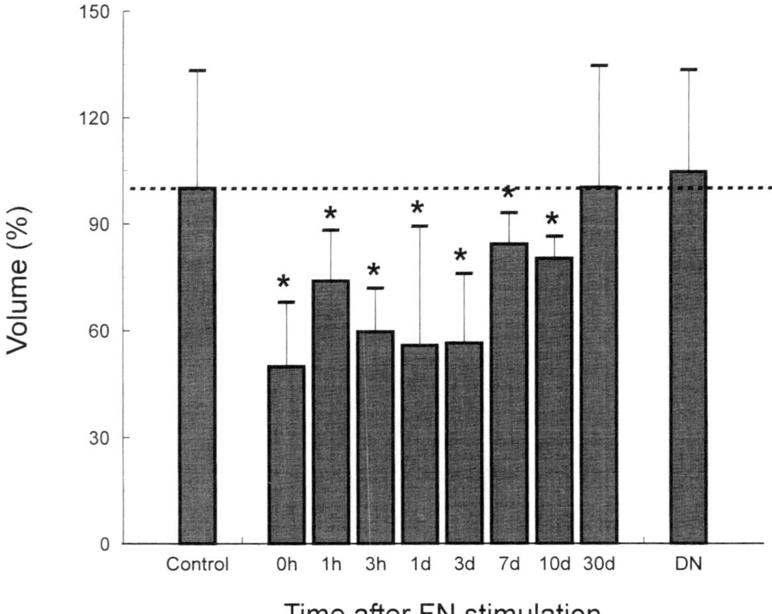

FIGURE 7. Stimulation of FN reversibly protects the brain for 10 days. In rats and matched controls the FN was stimulated or sham stimulated for 1 h. The MCA was occluded at various times thereafter as shown on y-axis. Twenty-four hours thereafter rats were killed and infarction volumes computed. Dotted line indicates 100% infarction volume in the sham-stimulated animals (*$p < 0.05$, $n = 5$ for each group at each time point). The DN was stimulated 72 h before in a single group. Note prolonged and reversible protection. (From Reis *et al.*[49])

that may account for at least some of the salvage: (1) a decrease in electrical excitability and (2) a down-regulation in the immune-reactivity of cerebral microvessels.

Changes in Electrical Excitability

Focal ischemia is associated with the immediate appearance of electrical instability in the ischemic penumbra characterized by recurrent waves of depolarization.[35,36] These periinfarction depolarizing waves (PIDs)[50] have been likened to cortical spreading depression (SD), the slowly moving surface negative DC shift initiated by locally depolarizing the cerebral cortex with KCl or an electrical pulse.[51,52] It has been proposed that the expression of PIDs contributes to infarction volumes, because the frequency of PIDs directly correlates with lesion size[35] and suppression of their expression results in neuroprotection.[53] The deleterious effects of PIDs have been attributed to the fact that each depolarizing event requires substantial energy to repolarize membranes. It has been argued[50] that depleted ATP and the inability of rCBF to rise in the penumbra to provide substrate accelerate the collapse of local metabolic machinery and promote cell death.

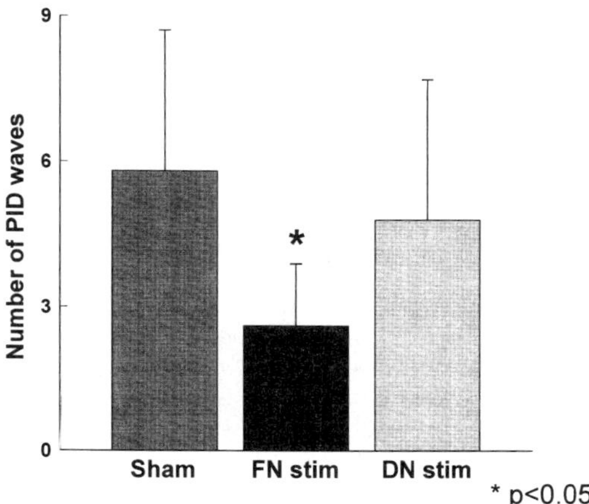

FIGURE 8. FN stimulation reduces total number of post-infarction depolarizing waves (PIDs) expressed in ischemic penumbra immediately following MCA occlusion. In anesthetized rats, the FN or DN were stimulated or FN sham-stimulated for 1 h before occluding the MCA and recording of electrical activity over the ischemic penumbra for 3 h and number of events assessed. Note that FN, but not sham or DN, stimulation significantly ($p < 0.05$) reduced PID numbers ($n = 5$/group). (From Golanov and Reis.[49])

If the hypothesis is correct, a reduction in neuronal excitability might suppress expression of PIDs and, secondarily, protect ischemic brain. Reduced excitability might be mediated by alterations in ion channels, particularly by mechanisms which open K-channels to hyperpolarize the membranes. That cerebellar stimulation might reduce the excitability of the cortex has been suggested by several studies demonstrating that electrical stimulation of the cerebellum decreases electrical excitability and elevates seizure thresholds in the cerebral cortex.[54,55]

We tested the hypothesis in several ways. First we examined whether FN stimulation would alter the expression of PIDs as reflected by alteration in the onset latency and number of events appearing over three hours after MCAO, when performed immediately and 72 hours after MCAO. Stimulation of FN for one hour significantly delayed the appearance of PIDs and reduced their numbers by over 50% when the MCAO was occluded at the same time[56] (FIG. 8). When the MCA was occluded 72 h after FN stimulation, the expression of PIDs was completely suppressed. Stimulation of the DN, as control, had no effect. Second, we investigated whether stimulation of the FN would elevate the threshold for evoking cortical SD (measured coulomb of stimulus current). The threshold for eliciting a SD in a hemisphere was determined in anesthetized rats subjected to one hour of FN or DN stimulation immediately prior to the test stimulus. We observed that stimulating the FN, but not DN, significantly elevated the threshold for inducing SDs by ~75% (from 1.6 ± 0.6 [mean $\pm$ SD] to 2.1 [$p < 0.05$, $n = 5$]).

To assess the contribution of K^+-channels to protection, 1 μmol of the K^+_{ATP} channel blocker glibenclimide (in 5 mL saline) was injected intracerebroventricularly (i.c.v.) ($n = 5$) 15 min before stimulating FN (1 h) followed by MCAO. Controls ($n = 5$) received i.c.v. saline and had lesions which were $146 + 19$ mm^3 in volume. Saline had no effect on lesion reduction (89 ± 13 mm^3) compared to FN stimulation alone. Glibenclimide abolished the neuroprotection (142 ± 25 mm^3, n.s. from control). In rats in which the FN was stimulated 72 h earlier, glibenclimide administered 15 min before MCAO also blocked the neuroprotection (95 $\pm$ 23 mm^3 FN stimulation vs. 139 $\pm$ 11 mm^3 FN stimulation + glibenclimide; $p < 0.05$). These findings are consistent with the possibility that FN stimulation may elicit prolonged opening of K-channels, possibly of the K_{ATP} subclass, leading to hyperpolarization of neurons and diminished excitability. Consistent with the hypothesis Heurtaux *et al.* have demonstrated[57] that ischemic preconditioned neuroprotection against global ischemic degeneration of neurons of the CA1 subzone can be blocked by treatment by blockade of the K_{ATP}-channel.

These results are consistent with an interpretation that conditional stimulation of FN may reduce the excitability of the cerebral cortex by opening K-channels, possibly of the K_{ATP} subclass. The molecular mechanism accounting for the prolonged changes in electrical excitability by this mechanism remains to be determined. Does it result from post-translational modification of potassium channel functions? To modification in subunit composition? Is it neuronal or glial?

Down-regulation of Immunoreactivity in Microvessels

A second mechanism that we have discovered which may contribute to conditioned neuroprotection is modification of immunoreactivity of brain in response to ischemic injury. Focal and global ischemia triggers in brain a cascade of inflammatory reactions that serve, as in most tissues, to isolate and destroy the damaged area and to begin the reparative processes. Two classes of cells are central to the development of post-ischemic inflammation in brain: vascular endothelium and microglia. In response to tissue injury, the microvascular endothelium almost immediately expresses a group of molecules, including intercellular cell adhesion molecule (ICAM-1) and the vascular cell adhesion molecule (VCAM-1),[58,59] that promote adherence and subsequent migration of leukocytes and monocytes/macrophages into brain.[59,60] These infiltrating cells can release cytokines, nitric oxide (NO), and free-oxygen radicals contributing to cell death and enhancement of the inflammatory responses. In addition, vascular cells express the inducible isoform of nitric oxide synthase (iNOS) to generate NO that may promote vasodilation and cellular necrosis. The inflammatory cascade may exacerbate ischemic damage. Blockade of such proinflammatory cytokines as IL-1β, inhibition of the migration of circulating leukocytes or monocytes into ischemic brain, or inhibition of iNOS activity, can decrease—up to 50%—the size of focal ischemic infarctions.[61–63] Thus, suppression of immunoreactivity by stimulation of the FN might underlie, in part, neuronal salvage. That this might be the case is supported by several findings.

In our first study we investigated whether conditional stimulation of the FN might suppress the expression of iNOS in ischemic brain. We characterized the time course and magnitude of the induction of iNOS mRNA within the ischemic core, penumbra, and cerebral cortex contralateral to the focal ischemic infarction in rat. We observed that MCAO induced iNOS mRNA in the ischemic core and penumbra, but not unaffected brain. The onset occurred within six hours, and peaked at 14–24 h to recover 48 h later.[64] Immunoreactive iNOS was localized in microvessels, invading macrophages and microglia within core and penumbra. When the FN was stimulated 14 h prior to MCAO, the amount of iNOS mRNA, measured 24 h later, was reduced by >90% in the ischemic penumbra, the area salvaged, but not in the core (FIG. 9). Reduction was manifested by an absence of iNOS immunoreactivity in microvessels in the penumbra and a reduced number of infiltrating monocytes. These observations, however, raised the questions: Does the

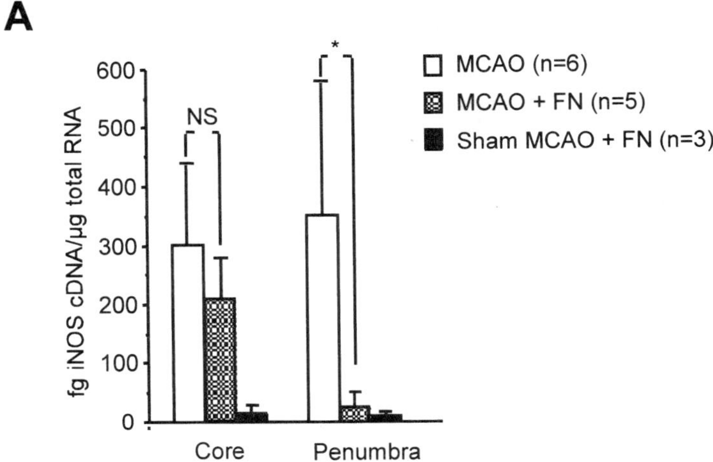

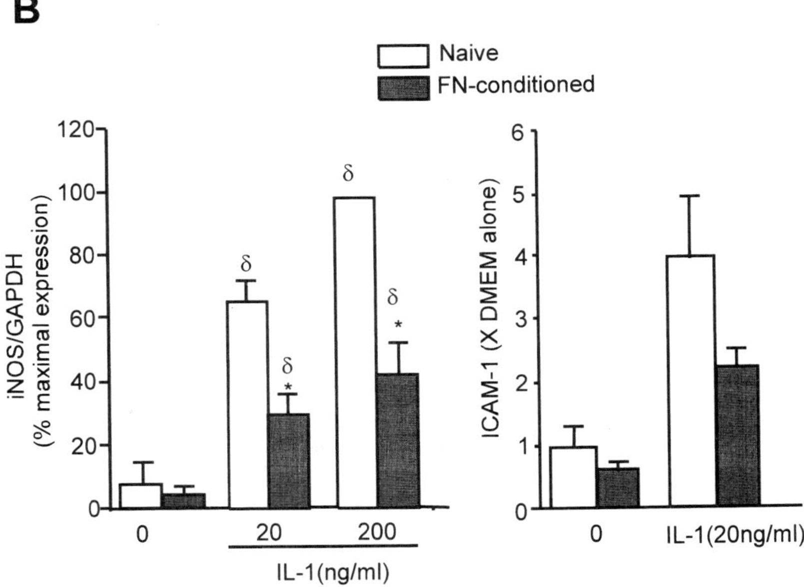

FIGURE 9. Stimulation of FN down-regulates expression of iNOS and ICAM-1 mRNA. (**A**) iNOS mRNA (assessed by RT-PCR) is increased in ischemic core and penumbra 15 h following MCA occlusion alone. FN stimulation, 72 h earlier, almost abolishes the increase in iNOS in the penumbra (salvaged zone), but not in the ischemic core. (**B**) Changes in up-regulation by IL-1β of iNOS (*left*) and ICAM-1 (*right*) mRNA in isolated microvessels of rat brain evoked by FN stimulation. Microvessels were isolated and incubated with IL-1β for 5 h and mRNAs measured by RT-PCR. In naive rats, treatment increases both mRNAs. Stimulation of FN for 1 h 72 h prior to sacrifice reduces by ~50% the stimulated increase in both mRNAs. iNOS mRNA expressed as ratio of iNOS to GAPDH mRNA. ICAM-1 expressed as multiple of control value (incubation in DMEM). (Data from ref. 64.)

conditioned stimulus itself inhibit expression of the proinflammatory molecules? Alternatively, is the blunted response secondary to the reduced necrosis in the zone?

To address these issues, we have studied the immune reactivity of cerebral microvessels analyzed *ex vivo*. We first demonstrated that incubation of microvessels isolated from the brains of otherwise untreated rats with IL-1β (20 ng/mL) induces the expression of the mRNAs for iNOS and ICAM-1. However, comparable treatment of rats 48–72 h after stimulating the FN for one hour reduces expression of both mRNAs by ~50% at all doses of the cytokine.

Stimulation of the DN has no effect (FIG. 9). The results suggest that FN stimulation may reduce immunoreactivity of cerebral microvessels. The molecular mechanism responsible for the effect may be related to inhibition of the transcription factor NFkβ, whose expression will initiate transcription of an array of proinflammatory molecules.

IS CENTRAL NEUROGENIC NEUROPROTECTION RESTRICTED TO FOCAL ISCHEMIA?

Will central neurogenic neuroprotection elicited from FN only salvage neurons from focal ischemia? To answer the question we recently investigated the effects of cerebellar stimulation on the delayed death of hippocampal neurons of the CA1 group evoked by transient global ischemia produced by reversible four-vessel occlusion[65] and the loss of striatal neurons generated by microinjection of the excitotoxin ibotenic acid.[66] We observed that the loss of CA1 neurons elicited by 10 min of ischemia is reduced by 57% (from 33 ± 11 cells/mm to 141 ± 6 cells/mm), while the volume of the necrotic lesion elicited by microinjection of 360 nL 23 nM ibotenate is reduced by 80% by stimulation of the FN for one hour 72 h earlier. Thus, the neuroprotection afforded by conditional stimulation of the FN may affect a variety of forms of neuronal injury, not all of which are ischemic.

SUMMARY

The brain can protect itself from ischemia and/or hypoxia by two distinct mechanisms which probably involve two separate systems of neurons in the CNS. One, which mediates a *reflexive neurogenic neuroprotection*, emanates from oxygen-sensitive sympathoexcitatory reticulospinal neurons of the RVLM. These cells, excited within seconds by reduction in blood flow or oxygen, initiate the systemic vascular components of the oxygen conserving (diving) reflex. They profoundly increase rCBF without changing rCGU and, hence, rapidly and efficiently provide the brain with oxygen. Upon cessation of the stimulus the systemic and cerebrovascular adjustments return to normal. The system mediating reflex protection projects via as-yet-undefined projections from RVLM to upper brainstem and/or thalamus to engage a small population of neurons in the cortex which appear to be dedicated to transducing a neuronal signal into vasodilation. It also appears to relay the central neurogenic vasodilation elicited from other brain regions, including excitation of axons innervating the FN. This mode of protection would be initiated under conditions of global ischemia and/or hypoxemia because the signal is detected by medullary neurons.

The second neuroprotective system is represented in intrinsic neurons of the cerebellar FN and mediates a *conditioned central neurogenic neuroprotection*. The response can be initiated by excitation of intrinsic neurons of the FN and does not appear dependent upon RVLM. The pathways and transmitters that mediate the effect are unknown. The neuroprotection afforded by this network is long-lasting, persisting for almost two weeks, and is associated with reduced excitability of cortical neurons and reduced immunoreactivity of cerebral microvessels. This mode of neuroprotection, moreover, is not restricted to focal ischemia, as we have demonstrated that it also protects the brain against global ischemia and excitotoxic cell death. That the brain may have neuronal systems dedicated to protecting itself from injury, at first appearing to be a novel concept, is, upon reflection, not surprising since the brain is not injured in naturalistic behaviors characterized by very low levels of rCBF, diving[1] and hibernation.[67] An understanding of the pathways, transmitters, and molecules engaged in such protection may provide new insights into novel therapies for a range of disorders characterized by neuronal death.

REFERENCES

1. BLIX, A. S. & B. FOLKOW. 1983. Cardiovascular adjustments to diving in mammals and birds. *In* Sect. 2, The Cardiovascular System. E. M. Renkin & C. C. Michel, Eds: 917–945. American Physiological Society. Bethesda, MD.
2. WOLF, S. 1966. Sudden death and the oxygen-conserving reflex. Am. Heart J. **71:** 840–841.
3. PULSINELLI, W. A. & T. E. DUFFY. 1979. Local cerebral glucose metabolism during controlled hypoxemia in rats. Science **204:** 626–629.
4. EDVINSSON, L., E. T. MACKENZIE & J. MCCULLOCH. 1993. Cerebral blood flow and metabolism. Raven Press. New York.
5. REIS, D. J. & C. IADECOLA. 1989. Central neurogenic regulation of cerebral blood flow. *In* Neurotransmissiom and Cerebrovascular Function. J. Seylaz & R. Sercombe, Eds: 369–390. Elsevier. Amsterdam.
6. REIS, D. J., E. V. GOLANOV, D. A. RUGGIERO & M.-K. SUN. 1994. Sympatho-excitatory neurons of the rostral ventrolateral medulla are oxygen sensors and essential elements in the tonic and reflex control of the systemic and cerebral circulations. J. Hypertens. **12:** S159–S180.
7. SAEKI, Y., A. SATO, Y. SATO & A. TRZEBSKI. 1989. Stimulation of rostral ventrolateral medullary neurons increases cortical cerebral blood flow via activation of the intracerebral neural pathway. Neurosci. Lett. **107:** 26–32.
8. GOLANOV, E. V. & D. J. REIS. 1994. Nitric oxide and prostanoids participate in cerebral vasodilation elicited by electrical stimulation of the rostral ventrolateral medulla. J. Cereb. Blood Flow Metab. **14:** 492–502.
9. UNDERWOOD, M. D., C. IADECOLA, A. F. SVED & D. J. REIS. 1992. Stimulation of C1 area neurons globally increases regional cerebral blood flow but not metabolism. J. Cereb. Blood Flow Metab. **12:** 844–855.
10. SUN, M.-K., I. T. JESKE & D. J. REIS. 1992. Cyanide excites medullary sympathoexcitatory neurons in rats. Am. J. Physiol. **262:** R182–R189.
11. SUN, M.-K. & D. J. REIS. 1993. Differential responses of barosensitive neurons of rostral ventrolateral medulla to hypoxia in rats. Brain Res. **609:** 333–337.
12. SUN, M.-K. & D. J. REIS. 1993. Hypoxic excitation of medullary vasomotor neurons in rats are not mediated by glutamate or nitric oxide. Neurosci. Lett. **157:** 219–222.
13. SUN, M.-K. & D. J. REIS. 1994. Hypoxia-activated Ca^{2+} currents in pacemaker neurones of rat rostral ventrolateral medulla in vitro. J. Physiol. (Lond.) **476:** 101–116.
14. GOLANOV, E. V. & D. J. REIS. 1996. Contribution of oxygen-sensitive neurons of the rostral ventrolateral medulla to hypoxic cerebral vasodilatation in the rat. J. Physiol. (Lond.) **495:** 201–216.
15. HAMER, J., S. HOYER, E. ALBERTI & F. WEINHARDT. 1976. Cerebral blood flow and oxidative brain metabolism during and after moderate and profound arterial hypoxaemia. Acta Neurochir. **33:** 141–150.

16. UNDERWOOD, M. D., C. IADECOLA & D. J. REIS. 1994. Lesions of the rostral ventrolateral medulla reduce the cerebrovascular response to hypoxia. Brain Res. **635:** 217–223.

17. KONTOS, H. A. 1987. Regulation of the cerebral microcirculation in hypoxia and ischemia. *In* Oxygen Transport and Utilization. C. W. Bryan-Brown & S. M. Ayres, Eds: 311–317. Society of Critical Care Medicine. Fullerton, CA.

18. HEISTAD, D. D. & H. A. KONTOS. 1983. Cerebral circulation. *In* Handbook of Physiology. Circulation. Vol. III. Peripheral circulation and organ blood flow. J. T. Shepherd and F. M. Abboud, Eds.: 137–182. American Physiological Society. Bethesda, MD.

19. KUMADA, M., R. A. DAMPNEY & D. J. REIS. 1979. Profound hypotension and abolition of the vasomotor component of the cerebral ischemic response produced by restricted lesions of medulla oblongata in rabbit: Relationship to the so-called tonic vasomotor center. Circ. Res. **45:** 63–70.

20. YAMAMOTO, S., E. V. GOLANOV & D. J. REIS. 1993. Reductions in focal ischemic infarctions elicited from cerebellar fastigial nucleus do not result from elevations in cerebral blood flow. J. Cereb. Blood Flow Metab. **13:** 1020–1024.

21. RUGGIERO, D. A. & D. J. REIS. 1988. Neurons containing phenylethanolamine-N-methyltransferase: A component of the baroreceptor reflex? *In* Epinephrine in the Central Nervous System. J. M. Stolk, D. C. U'Prichard & K. Fuxe, Eds: 291–307. Oxford University Press. New York.

22. GOLANOV, E. V. & D. J. REIS. 1996. Cerebral cortical neurons with activity linked to central neurogenic spontaneous and evoked elevations in cerebral blood flow. Neurosci. Lett. **209:** 101–104.

23. IADECOLA, C., S. P. ARNERIC, H. D. BAKER, L. W. TUCKER & D. J. REIS. 1987. Role of local neurons in cerebrocortical vasodilation elicited from cerebellum. Am. J. Physiol. **252:** R1082–R1091.

24. GOLANOV, E. V. & D. J. REIS. 1995. Synchronization of EEG activity in cerebral cortex by stimulation of nucleus tractus solitarii (NTS) in rat: Coupling to cerebral blood flow and mediation by rostral ventrolateral medulla (RVL). Soc. Neurosci. **21:** 1669.

25. DOBA, N. & D. J. REIS. 1972. Changes in regional blood flow and cardiodynamics evoked by electrical stimulation of the fastigial nucleus in the cat and their similarity to orthostatic reflexes. J. Physiol. (Lond.) **227:** 729–747.

26. CHIDA, K., M. D. UNDERWOOD, M. MIYAGAWA, H. KAWAMURA, C. IADECOLA, T. TAKASU & D. J. REIS. 1990. Participation of the rostral ventrolateral medulla in the cerebral blood flow of rats: Effects of stimulation and lesions on systemic and cerebral circulations. Ther. Res. **11:** 77–85.

27. CHIDA, K., C. IADECOLA & D. J. REIS. 1990. Lesions of rostral ventrolateral medulla abolish some cardio- and cerebrovascular components of the cerebellar fastigial pressor and depressor responses. Brain Res. **508:** 93–104.

28. RUGGIERO, D. A., M. ANWAR, E. V. GOLANOV & D. J. REIS. 1997. The pedunculopontine tegmental nucleus issues collaterals to the fastigial nucleus and rostral ventrolateral reticular nucleus in the rat. Brain Res. **760:** 272–276.

29. CHIDA, K., C. IADECOLA, M. D. UNDERWOOD & D. J. REIS. 1986. A novel vasodepressor response elicited from the rat cerebellar fastigial nucleus: The fastigial depressor response. Brain Res. **370:** 378–382.

30. ASTRUP, J., B. K. SIESJÖ & L. SYMON. 1977. Thresholds in cerebral ischemia—the ischemic penumbra. Stroke **8:** 51–57.

31. HOSSMANN, K. A. 1994. Viability thresholds and the penumbra of focal ischemia. Ann. Neurol. **36:** 557–565.

32. NEDERGAARD, M., A. GJEDDE & N. H. DIEMER. 1986. Focal ischemia of the rat brain: Autoradiographic determination of cerebral glucose utilization, glucose content and blood flow. J. Cereb. Blood Flow Metab. **6:** 414–424.

33. PASCHEN, W., G. MIES & K. A. HOSSMANN. 1992. Threshold relationship between cerebral blood flow, glucose utilization, and energy metabolites during development of stroke in gerbils. Exp. Neurol. **117:** 325–333.

34. PEEK, K. E., A. H. LOCKWOOD, M. IZUMIYAMA, E. W. YAP & J. LABOVE. 1989. Glucose metabolism and acidosis in the metabolic penumbra of rat brain. Metab. Brain Dis. **4:** 261–272.

35. MIES, G., T. IIJIMA & K. A. HOSSMANN. 1993. Correlation between peri-infarct DC shifts and ischaemic neuronal damage in rat. Neuroreport **4:** 709–711.

36. NEDERGAARD, M. & J. ASTRUP. 1986. Infarct rim: Effect of hyperglycemia on direct current potential and [14c]2-deoxyglucose phosphorylation. J. Cereb. Blood Flow Metab. **6:** 607–615.

37. CHEN, J., K. L. JIN, M. Z. CHEN, W. PEI, K. KAWAGUCHI, D. A. GREENBERG & R. P. SIMON. 1997. Early detection of DNA strand breaks in the brain after transient focal ischemia—Implications for the role of DNA damage in apoptosis and neuronal cell death. J. Neurochem. **69:** 232–245.

38. LINNIK, M. D., J. A. MILLER, J. SPRINKLECAVALLO, P. J. MASON, F. Y. THOMPSON, L. R. MONTGOMERY & K. K. SCHROEDER. 1995. Apoptotic DNA fragmentation in the rat cerebral cortex induced by permanent middle cerebral artery occlusion. Mol. Brain Res. **32:** 116–124.

39. CHOI, D. W. 1992. Excitotoxic cell death. J. Neurobiol. **23:** 1261–1276.

40. AHERN, K. V., H. S. LUSTIG, J. CHAN & D. A. GREENBERG. 1993. Calcium indicators and excitotoxicity in cultured cortical neurons. Neurosci. Lett. **162:** 169–172.

41. WAHLESTEDT, C., E. V. GOLANOV, S. YAMAMOTO, F. YEE, H. ERICSON, H. YOO, C. E. INTURRISI & D. J. REIS. 1993. Antisense oligodeoxynucleotides to NMDA-r1 receptor channel protect cortical neurons from excitotoxicity and reduce focal ischaemic infarctions. Nature **363:** 260–263.

42. MAIESE, K., L. PEK, S. B. BERGER & D. J. REIS. 1992. Reduction in focal cerebral ischemia by agents acting at imidazole receptors. J. Cereb. Blood Flow Metab. **12:** 53–63.

43. BOWERSOX, S. S., T. SINGH & R. R. LUTHER. 1997. Selective blockade of N-type voltage-sensitive calcium channels protects against brain injury after transient focal cerebral ischemia in rats. Brain Res. **747:** 343–347.

44. GOLANOV, E. V. & D. J. REIS. 1995. Vasodilation evoked from medulla and cerebellum is coupled to bursts of cortical EEG activity in rats. Am. J. Physiol. **268:** R454–R467.

45. REIS, D. J., M. D. UNDERWOOD, S. B. BERGER, M. KHAYATA & N. I. ZAIENS. 1989. Fastigial nucleus stimulation reduces the volume of cerebral infarction produced by occlusion of the middle cerebral artery in rat. *In* Neurotransmission and Cerbrovascular Function I. J. Seylaz and E. T. MacKenzie, Eds.: 401–404. Elsevier Science Publishers B. V. Amsterdam.

46. GOLANOV, E. V., S. YAMAMOTO & D. J. REIS. 1996. Electrical stimulation of cerebellar fastigial nucleus fails to rematch blood flow and metabolism in focal ischemic infarctions. Neurosci. Lett. **210:** 181–184.

47. ZHANG, F. G. & C. IADECOLA. 1992. Stimulation of the fastigial nucleus enhances EEG recovery and reduces tissue damage after focal cerebral ischemia. J. Cereb. Blood Flow Metab. **12:** 962–970.

48. BARON, J. C., M. G. BOUSSER, A. REY, A. GUILLARD, D. COMAR & P. CASTAIGNE. 1981. Reversal of focal "misery-perfusion syndrome" by extra-intracranial arterial bypass in hemodynamic cerebral ischemia. A case study with 15O positron emission tomography. Stroke **12:** 454–459.

49. REIS, D. J., E. V. GOLANOV, K. KOBYLARZ & S. YAMAMOTO. 1997. Conditioned neuroprotection from ischemic infarction elicited by electrical stimulation of the cerebellar fastigial nucleus (fn) in rat. Brain Res. In press.

50. HOSSMANN, K. A. 1996. Periinfarct depolarizations. Cerebrovasc. Brain Metab. Rev. **8:** 195–208.

51. OCHS, S. 1962. The nature of spreading depression in neural networks. Int. Rev. Neurobiol. **4:** 1–69.

52. CHOPP, M. 1996. Spreading depression. Cephalalgia **16:** 77–87.

53. MIES, G., K. KOHNO & K. A. HOSSMANN. 1994. Prevention of periinfarct direct current shifts with glutamate antagonist NBQX following occlusion of the middle cerebral artery in the rat. J. Cereb. Blood Flow Metab. **14:** 802–807.

54. HABLITZ, J. J. & G. REA. 1976. Cerebellar nuclear stimulation in generalized penicillin epilepsy. Brain Res. Bull. **1:** 599–601.

55. MANZONI, T., S. SAPIENZA & A. URBANO. 1968. EEG and behavioural sleep-like effects

induced by fastigial nucleus in unrestrained, unanaesthetized cat. Arch. Ital. Biol. **106:** 61–72.

56. GOLANOV, E. V. & D. J. REIS. 1997. Neuroprotective electrical stimulation of the cerebellar fastigial nucleus suppresses peri-infarction depolarizing waves. J. Cereb. Blood Flow Metab. **17:** S456.

57. HEURTEAUX, C., I. LAURITZEN, C. WIDMANN & M. LAZDUNSKI. 1995. Essential role of adenosine, adenosine A1 receptors, and ATP-sensitive K^+ channels in cerebral ischemic preconditioning. Proc. Natl. Acad. Sci. USA **92:** 4666–4670.

58. WANG, X. A., A. L. SIREN Y. LIU & G. Z. FEURSTEIN. 1994. Upregulation of intercellular adhesion molecule ICAM-1 on brain microvascular endothelial cells in rat ischemic cortex. Brain Res. Mol. Brain Res. **26:** 61–68.

59. SCHROETER, M. S., A. L. JANDER, O. W. WITTE & G. STOLL. 1994. Local immune responses in the rat cerebral cortex after middle cerebral artery occlusion. J. Neuroimmunol. **55:** 195–203.

60. MEERSCHAERT, J. & M. B. FURIE. 1995. The adhesion molecules used by monocytes for migration across endothelium include cd11a/cd18, cd11b/cd18 and vla-4 on monocytes and Icam-1, vcam-1 and other ligands on endothelium. J. Immunol. **154:** 4099–4112.

61. RELTON, J. K. & N. J. ROTHWELL. 1992. Interleukin-1 receptor antagonist inhibits ischaemic and excitotoxic neuronal damage in the rat. Brain Res. Bull. **29:** 243–246.

62. ZHANG, F. & C. IADECOLA. 1994. Reduction of focal cerebral ischemic damage by delayed treatment with nitric oxide donors. J. Cereb. Blood Flow Metab. **14:** 574–580.

63. IADECOLA, C., F. Y. ZHANG & X. H. XU. 1995. Inhibition of inducible nitric oxide synthase ameliorates cerebral ischemic damage. Am. J. Physiol. **37:** R286–R292.

64. GALEA, E., D. L. FEINSTEIN, E. V. GOLANOV, S. GLICKSTEIN & D. J. REIS. 1997. Reduction of inflammatory reactivity of brain microvessels by stimulation of the cerebellar fastigial nucleus: Role of MAD-3 (NFkB inhibitor). J. Cereb. Blood Flow Metab. **17(Suppl. 1):** S567.

65. GLICKSTEIN, S., B. A. TURNER, E. V. GOLANOV, S. REGUNATHAN & D. J. REIS. 1997. Electrical stimulation of cerebellar fastigial nucleus protects against excitotoxic degeneration of striatal neurons. J. Cereb. Blood Flow Metab. **17:** S457.

66. LIU, F., E. V. GOLANOV & D. J. REIS. 1996. Electrical stimulation of the cerebellar fastigial nucleus reduces the delayed neuronal death produced by global cerebral ischemia. Soc. Neurosci. **22:** 71

67. FRERICHS, K. U., C. KENNEDY, L. SOKOLOFF & J. M. HALLENBECK. 1994. Local cerebral blood flow during hibernation, a model of natural tolerance to cerebral ischemia. J. Cereb. Blood Flow Metab. **14:** 193–205.

68. SAKURADA, O., C. KENNEDY, J. JEHLE, J. D. BROWN, G. L. CARBIN & L. SOKOLOFF. 1978. Measurement of local cerebral blood flow with iodo[^{14}C]antipyrine. Am. J. Physiol. **234:** H59–H66.

69. SOKOLOFF, L., M. REIVICH, C. KENNEDY, M. H. DES ROSIERS, C. S. PATLAK, K. D. PETTIGREW, O. SAKURADA & M. SHINOHARA. 1977. The [^{14}C]deoxyglucose method for the measurement of local cerebral glucose utilisation: Theory, procedure, and normal values in the conscious and anesthetized albino rat. J. Neurochem. **28:** 897–916.

Ischemic Brain Injury and the Therapeutic Window

W. A. PULSINELLI,[a] M. JACEWICZ,[a] D. E. LEVY,[b]
C. K. PETITO,[c] AND F. PLUM[d]

[a]Department of Neurology
University of Tennessee College of Medicine
Memphis, Tennessee 38163

[b]Knoll Pharmaceutical
30 North Jefferson Road
Whippany, New Jersey 07981

[c]Department of Pathology
University of Miami School of Medicine
Miami, Florida 33136

[d]Department of Neurology and Neuroscience
Cornell University Medical College
New York, New York 10021

THE THERAPEUTIC WINDOW IN BRAIN ISCHEMIA

Following the onset of brain ischemia, an interval exists during which treatment may lessen the degree and extent of brain damage, accelerate functional recovery, and improve long-term neurologic outcome. This time period has been termed the *therapeutic window.*

Whether brain ischemia arises from cardiac arrest or from focal ischemic stroke, several present options for treating stroke were not even considered possible only a decade ago. Now, pharmacologic, surgical, radiologic-interventional, and other methods are becoming increasingly available, thereby forcing physicians to revise outdated, previously nihilistic, attitudes toward stroke. For the newer therapies to be effective, however, it has become clear that treatment must begin early and fall within the therapeutic window. Although this concept appears straightforward, the pathophysiology of brain ischemia is far from fully understood, and we cannot attach specific time limits which can describe the therapeutic window for all individuals with ischemic brain injury. In fact, for each stroke victim, the therapeutic window will vary with distinct limits determined by ischemia severity, brain temperature, amount of cerebral edema and other metabolic conditions, and by whether the cause of ischemia is focal (stroke) or global (cardiac arrest). In fact, different regions of focally ischemic brain in the same individual probably exhibit distinct therapeutic windows: intensely ischemic areas will require treatment within minutes of ischemia onset to avoid infarction, while surrounding marginally perfused areas may still benefit from treatment delivered many hours after ischemia onset. These considerations often make it difficult to predict the therapeutic window for the ischemically threatened brain.

TIME LIMITS FOR THE THERAPEUTIC WINDOW

Although the therapeutic window may be difficult to ascertain in any given patient, specific time limits have been defined in well controlled animal models of brain ischemia as discussed below.[1-7] However, several caveats should be kept in mind. These time limits reflect our past inability, clinically and experimentally, to reverse the pathologic process of cell death. As future research clarifies the fundamental mechanisms of ischemic brain injury, cellular changes previously considered irreversible may yield to newer therapies and become reversible, thereby expanding the therapeutic window. Furthermore, we can now hope that early treatment (e.g., immediate administration of a pharmacologic cocktail by emergency medical staff) may alter the course of ischemia pathophysiology and widen the therapeutic window for additional intervention (e.g., thrombolysis). If we consider that additional or delayed neurologic deterioration in humans not infrequently occurs many hours after the initial insult, this delayed injury may be amenable to therapy well outside the time constraints defined by animal studies.[8] Currently, the time limits for the therapeutic window have been based on animal experiments in which a histopathologically defined end point was correlated with the duration of transient ischemia. Future studies may identify a more accurate and/or earlier measure of irreversible ischemic injury and thereby lead to a more precise time point for the transition between reversible injury and irreversible damage. Thus, it seems likely that new discoveries will replace current definitions of the therapeutic window within which ischemic damage can be reduced.

THE REPERFUSION AND CYTOPROTECTIVE WINDOWS

Every brain cell, including those exquisitely sensitive to even brief ischemia (e.g., CA1 pyramidal neurons), can withstand a certain limited duration of ischemia without being destroyed.[9] The *reperfusion window* refers to the longest period of time that brain cells can withstand ischemia and recover fully once blood flow is restored.[10] The reperfusion window for global ischemia (cardiac arrest) differs markedly from that for focal ischemic stroke, as discussed below.

It is now clear for both global and focal cerebral ischemia that cellular and biochemical events promoting injury continue even after cerebral recirculation is fully achieved.[9,11,12] This late developing injury has been termed *maturation* or *delayed injury,* and can be partially reversed with pharmacologic and other cytoprotective manipulations.[3,9,11-14] The time period during which cytoprotective agents may reduce brain damage has been termed the *cytoprotective window.* This window may encompass part or all of the reperfusion window and may extend minutes to hours into the recirculation period. Together, the reperfusion and the cytoprotective windows comprise the therapeutic window.

TEMPORAL PROFILE OF HISTOPATHOLOGIC DAMAGE

Global Cerebral Ischemia

Global cerebral ischemia produces a discrete regional loss of neurons, the extent and topography of which depend largely on the duration and degree of oxygen deprivation. A complete or nearly complete loss of cerebral blood flow, as occurs in cardiac arrest, must be reversed within minutes if the normothermic patient is to recover without clinically significant cognitive loss. Transient, severe ischemia will damage neurons that are highly sensitive to oxygen deprivation. These include the pyramidal neurons in the CA1 zone of the hippocampus, Purkinje cells of the cerebellum, pyramidal neurons of cortical layers 3, 5, and 6, and the medium-sized neurons of the striatum.[3] Brief global ischemia (5–10 min) causes most CA1 neurons to die, while sparing most medium-sized neurons of the striatum. The latter are damaged if ischemia lasts for 15–30 min. Thus, different neuronal populations have distinct reperfusion windows depending on the hierarchy of sensitivity to ischemia: 5 min for CA1 neurons and 15 min for the medium-sized striatal neurons.

The time for an ischemically stressed neuronal population to reach irreversible injury (currently defined by the earliest detection of histologic necrosis) is termed the maturation time of ischemic damage. Surprisingly, the rank order of neuronal sensitivity to ischemia does not correlate with the length of the maturation time. Thus, after 15–30 min of global ischemia, medium-sized striatal neurons undergo rapid breakdown with histopathologic damage detectable within 3–12 h. In contrast, CA1 neurons fatally injured by 5–10 min of global ischemia do not undergo a histologic stage of damage for up to 24–72 h.[3] Accordingly, not only are there distinct reperfusion windows for discrete neuronal populations, but the cytoprotective windows for the threatened neurons can vary from a few hours to several days.

Focal Cerebral Ischemia

As with global cerebral ischemia, the degree and duration of focal cerebral ischemia determine the extent of histologic damage. Unlike the diffuse, severe drop in cerebral blood flow produced by cardiac arrest, the pattern of ischemia following focal occlusion of a brain artery (e.g., by embolism) is more complex and less predictable. Focal cerebral ischemia is typically incomplete, and the ischemic topography varies depending on the availability of blood flow through vascular collaterals. The latter is governed by autosomal recessive hereditary factors that dictate the caliber of collateral connections between the anterior cerebral and middle cerebral artery (MCA) territories.[15-17] Accordingly, the occlusion of the middle cerebral artery in one patient with small caliber collaterals results in a rapid, catastrophic infarction of the entire MCA territory whereas in another patient with large caliber collaterals, similar occlusion produces only minor blood flow reductions and little or no adverse clinical effect. More typically, however, the cerebral blood flow (CBF) reductions in the MCA territory feature a region of severe ischemia (area furthest from the collateral blood supply) and a region of intermediate ischemia (area closest to the collateral blood supply). The former region, called the *ischemic core*, lies in the central area of the ischemic vascular territory and the latter region, called the *ischemic penumbra* or the *penumbral zone*, surrounds the ischemic core and occupies the periphery of the involved vascular territory.

The ischemic penumbra was originally defined as electrically (synaptically) quiescent brain tissue capable of recovery with recirculation.[18] This concept has more recently been expanded to describe a physiologically unstable region in which ion membrane gradients and energy metabolites fluctuate,[19,20] in conjunction with dynamic alterations in protein synthesis,[21,22] gene expression,[21,23] and a host of other cellular functions, most or all of which can recover with the timely restoration of CBF.

Vulnerable neurons in the ischemic core are irreversibly injured during the first hour of ischemia, but glia and other brain cells succumb (infarction) only if ischemia persists beyond the first hour.[4,24] Brain infarction appears first in the ischemic core and then, with the persistence of ischemia, extends outward into the penumbral zone. In rodents, the penumbral zone is progressively lost during the first 2–3 h of ischemia,[4–7,24] whereas in primates this zone is lost over approximately 4 h.[1,2] Thus, for the typical focally ischemic region, separate reperfusion windows exist for central regions of severe ischemia and for the more peripheral regions of intermediate and milder degrees of ischemia. To salvage the ischemic core (which may involve a small or a large portion of the arterial territory at risk depending on collateral CBF), cerebral reperfusion must occur rapidly, as soon as possible within the first hour of ischemia onset. In contrast, reperfusion as late as 3–4 h after ischemia onset may rescue the penumbral zone, depending at least in part on the relative intensity of the preceding ischemia (moderate versus mild).

The cytoprotective window for the ischemic core differs markedly from that for the ischemic penumbra. Although cytotoxic effects in the ischemic core can be delayed with cerebral hypothermia, under ordinary clinical conditions salvage of the ischemic core requires prompt recirculation. Pharmacologic intervention alone cannot save the ischemic core. By contrast, in regions of intermediate or mild ischemia, drugs can reach the injured tissue in sufficient concentration and in a timely fashion. In the ischemic penumbra, drugs can selectively block one or more cellular processes that may be instrumental in achieving injury (e.g., NMDA and AMPA glutamate receptor antagonists hinder pathologic calcium ion fluxes). Other drugs may reversibly shut down less essential cell functions in order to spare limited energy supplies for other more critical purposes (i.e., restoring homeostasis). Finally, as the first wave of neurons die, the oxygen requirement of the surviving tissue falls so that remaining neurons may survive indefinitely at the lowered blood flow level or die off at a less rapid rate. Thus, cytoprotective agents have the potential for increasing neuronal salvage in the ischemic penumbra without the necessity for improved circulation. Clearly, early reperfusion and early treatment with cytoprotective agents offer the best prospects for neurologic recovery in focal ischemic stroke.

THERAPEUTIC WINDOW: CLINICAL ASPECTS

It has not been possible to perform systematic studies of selective neuronal damage in survivors of cardiac arrest. Nevertheless, the available data show that the temporal and spatial characteristics of global ischemic brain injury in humans is much the same as that for experimental animals.[25] This suggests that the shortest maturation times for ischemic damage measure 3–13 h after cardiac arrest (medium-sized striatal neurons), whereas the longest maturation times may take as much as 24–72 h (hippocampal CA1 neurons). The latter offers a relatively long period for potential cytoprotective intervention, and importantly involves neurons whose integrity is essential for memory functions, especially in the ability to acquire new information. Preliminary evidence now exists that certain drugs (e.g., AMPA receptor antagonists) can attenuate the destruction of CA1 neurons when administered hours after global ischemia.

In focal ischemic stroke, the therapeutic window is difficult to determine in any individual patient because of uncertainties regarding the severity and duration of ischemia. In the least complicated example—that of permanent occlusion of a cerebral artery—infarction evolves in the threatened territory over a time course resembling that for primates, in which the reperfusion window is approximately

4 h. Adding a few hours of maturation time to the reperfusion window results in a therapeutic window of about 6 h, but possibly as long as 12 h. If the ischemic insult is unstable, with recurrent waves of ischemia and reperfusion, the therapeutic window may well be accordingly prolonged. In any event, it should be apparent from this type of analysis that the earlier therapy is started, the greater the prospects for successful cytoprotection, recirculation, and neurologic outcome.

REFERENCES

1. JONES, T. H., M. B. MORAWETZ, R. M. CROWELL, F. W. MARCOUX, S. J. FITZGIBBON, U. DEGIROLAMI & R. G. OJEMANN. 1981. Thresholds of focal cerebral ischemia in awake monkey. J. Neurosurg. **54:** 773–782.
2. CROWELL, R. M., F. W. MARCOUX & U. DEGIROLAMI. 1981. Variability and reversibility of focal cerebral ischemia in unanesthetized monkeys. Neurology **31:** 1295–1302.
3. PULSINELLI, W., J. BRIERLEY & F. PLUM. 1982. Temporal profile of neuronal damage in a model of transient forebrain ischemia. Ann. Neurol. **11:** 491–498.
4. KAPLAN, B., S. BRINT, J. TANABE, X. WANG & W. PULSINELLI. 1991. Temporal thresholds for neocortical infarction in rats subjected to reversible focal cerebral ischemia. Stroke **22:** 1032–1039.
5. YIP, P. K., Y. Y. HE, C. Y. HSU, N. GARG, P. MARANGOS & E. L. HOGAN. 1991. Effect of plasma glucose on infarct size in focal cerebral ischemia-reperfusion. Neurology **41:** 899–905.
6. XUE, D., Z. G. HUANG, K. E. SMITH & A. M. BUCHAN. 1992. Immediate or delayed hypothermia prevents focal cerebral infarction. Brain Res. **587:** 66–72.
7. LI, Y., M. CHOPP, J. H. GARCIA, Y. YOSHIDA, A. G. ZHANG & S. R. LEVINE. 1992. Distribution of the 72-kd heat-shock protein as a function of transient focal cerebral ischemia in rats. Stroke **23:** 1292–1298.
8. FISHER, M. & J. H. GARCIA. 1996. Evolving stroke and the ischemic penumbra. Neurology **47:** 884–888.
9. PULSINELLI, W. 1992. Pathophysiology of acute ischemia stroke. Lancet **339:** 533–536.
10. PULSINELLI, W. 1995. The ischemic penumbra in stroke. Sci. Am. Sci. Med. Jan/Feb: 16–25.
11. GINSBERG, M. D. 1993. Emerging strategies for the treatment of ischemic brain injury *In* Molecular and Cellular Approaches to the Treatment of Ischemic Brain Disease. S. G. Waxman, Ed. Vol. 71: 207–237. Raven Press. New York.
12. CHOI, D. W. 1990. Methods for antagonizing glutamate neurotoxicity. Cerebrovasc. Brain Metab. Rev. **2:** 105–147.
13. KIRINO, T. 1982. Delayed neuronal death in the gerbil hippocampus following ischemia. Brain Res. **237:** 57–69.
14. ITO, U., M. SPATZ, J. T. WALKER & I. KLATZO. 1975. Experimental cerebral ischemia in Mongolian gerbils. Acta Neuropathol. **32:** 209–223.
15. COYLE, P., D. J. ODENHEIMER & C. F. SING. 1984. Cerebral infarction after middle cerebral artery occlusion in progenies of spontaneously stroke-prone and normal rats. Stroke **15:** 711–716.
16. COYLE, P. 1986. Different susceptibilities to cerebral infarction in spontaneously hypertensive (SHR) and normotensive Sprague-Dawley rats. Stroke **17:** 520–525.
17. JACEWICZ, M. 1992. Hypertension in SHR and predisposition to cerebral infarction (editorial). Hypertension **19:** 47–48.
18. ASTRUP, J., L. SYMON & B. K. SIESJO. 1981. Thresholds in cerebral ischemia: The ischemic penumbra. Stroke **12:** 723–725.
19. TAKEDA, Y., M. JACEWICZ, T. S. NOWAK & W. A. PULSINELLI. 1993. DC-potential and energy metabolites in focal ischemia. J. Cereb. Blood Flow Metab. **13:** S450.
20. GINSBERG, M. D. & W. A. PULSINELLI. 1994. The ischemic penumbra, injury thresholds and the therapeutic window for acute stroke. Ann. Neurol. **36:** 553–554.
21. JACEWICZ, M., M. KIESSLING & W. A. PULSINELLI. 1986. Selective gene expression in focal cerebral ischemia. J. Cereb. Blood Flow Metab. **6:** 263–272.

22. HOSSMANN, K. A. 1994. Viability thresholds and the penumbra of focal ischemia. Ann. Neurol. **36:** 557–565.
23. NOWAK, T. S. & M. JACEWICZ. 1994. The heat shock/stress response in focal cerebral ischemia. Brain Pathol. **4:** 67–76.
24. JACEWICZ, M., J. TANABE & W. A. PULSINELLI. 1992. The CBF threshold and dynamics for focal cerebral infarction in spontaneously hypertensive rats. J. Cereb. Blood Flow Metab. **12:** 359–370.
25. PETITO, C., E. FELDMANN, W. A. PULSINELLI & F. PLUM. 1987. Delayed hippocampal damage in humans following cardiorespiratory arrest. Neurology **37:** 1281–1286.

APPENDIX

Cornell Medical College
Cerebrovascular Disease Research Center
(1960–1994)

Fred Plum, M.D.
Chairman and Director

D. Barbut	S. Goldman	W. Pulsinelli
S. Brint	B. Hingfeldt	D. Rawlinson
A. Buchan	M. Horwich	D. Reis
J. Caronna	D. Howse	N. Renvoir
M. Cavazutti	C. Iadecola	J. Sage
R. Collins	M. Jacewicz	L. Salford
A. Cooper	B. Kaplan	J. Schaefer
N. Cruz	R. Kraig	B. Sigsbee
G. Dienel	M. Kiessling	A. Slivka
U. Dirnagl	J. Lai	W. Talman
J. Dougherty	D. Levy	J. Tanabe
T. Duffy	A. Lockwood	B. Troy
M. Erlich	K. Maiese	R. Van Uitert
A. Francis	S. Mora	B. Volpe
G. Gibson	M. Nedergaard	T. Voorhies
A. Gjedde	C. Petito	C. Wasterlain

The Cornell Cerebrovascular Disease Research Center was one of the first two large disease-related Program Projects established by the National Institutes of Health (NIH). Irving Wright initiated the program in 1960 and Fletcher McDowell carried it forward at the Cornell Division of Bellevue Hospital in 1962. When Bellevue became totally the responsibility of New York University in 1968, the Center was moved to new laboratories at Cornell Medical College constructed for Don Reis, Jerome Posner, and Fred Plum.

The wonderful productivity of the people who joined the Center at one time or another fulfilled the wise early farsightedness of NIH in construction of disease-related centers of excellence. Among the 50 or more faculty and fellows listed above as members of the Center during Fred Plum's management, all but six have continued in academic, clinical or laboratory neuroscience. Thirty-two remained active investigators for many years either within the Center or at other institutions in the United States or other countries. Indeed, several once-members of the Center have gone on to direct their own high-quality stroke-related research laboratories and clinical programs elsewhere. Twelve have become departmental or division chairmen in the U.S. or abroad and have continued to attack problems in cerebral vascular disease and metabolism. All, in a variety of ways, have made important contributions to understanding the field and the advances it has brought to patients.

Included among the hundreds of contributions which emanated from the Center over the years are the following:

- The concept that increased neurophysiologic activity in the brain increased regional lactate concentrations and cerebral blood flow disproportionately to the rate of oxygen consumption; this finding of nonhypoxic lactacidosis led directly to current techniques developed by others to identify changes in focal brain metabolism by positron emission tomography or functional magnetic resonance imaging in response to regional cerebral metabolic activity
- The finding that acute global brain ischemia leads to delayed neuronal necrosis in rodents and humans after days-long intervals
- Observations that hyperammonemia leads indirectly rather than directly to brain metabolic dysfunctions and, by inference, that the process must reflect indirect rather than direct mechanisms causing neurologic abnormalities in hepatic coma
- The discovery that severe hypoxia can damage brain neurons and astrocytes both *in vivo* and *in vitro* by inducing severe intracellular acidosis
- The finding that increased cerebral blood flow accompanying CO_2 inhalation or functional hypertension can temporarily open the blood–brain barrier to large proteins; if the hyperemia is brief, the alien proteins are pumped out again.

Finally, the Stroke Center early demonstrated that the treatment of stroke improves the outcome from stroke. Outcome studies by the Center's investigators produced reliable indicants of signs and symptoms early in the course of the disease that accurately predicted future function of individual patients. The ultimate value of the data eventually became embodied in treatment protocols that shortened patient stay and accelerated recovery.

Whole-Body Hyperthermia and ADPRT Inhibition in Experimental Treatment of Brain Tumors[a]

L. G. SALFORD,[b,g] A. BRUN,[c] E. KJELLÉN,[d] R. W. PERO,[e] AND R. B. R. PERSSON[f]

[b]Division of Experimental Neurooncology
Department of Neurosurgery
[c]Division of Neuropathology, Department of Pathology
[d]Department of Oncology
[e]Department of Molecular Ecogenetics
[f]Department of Medical Radiation Physics
Lund University Hospital and Lund University
Lund, Sweden

INTRODUCTION

Patients with astrocytomas are still beyond cure despite extensive surgery, improved radiotherapy, and combination chemotherapy. Median survival time after first operation for an astrocytoma grade III–IV[1] is at best only about 14 months, and only exceptional cases survive more than 10 years.[2] It must be concluded that the therapies in clinical use are inefficient and that every effort should be made to find alternatives that selectively eradicate the tumor cells.

An astrocytoma grade III–IV has a tendency to grow like an octopus, with a central core and several extensions into the surrounding normal brain. In many cases, the actively proliferating part of the tumor—the front part—which appears like "raw fish-meat" to the neurosurgeon, is well delineated toward the normal brain.[3] This might lead us to believe that if the entire front of the tumor and the central necrotic areas could be removed during an operation, a cure might be achieved. However, even hemispherectomies fail to radically remove the tumor.[4,5] We can conclude that malignant cells are spread diffusely in the brain, having migrated from the tumor even into portions of the brain distant from the tumor itself. These migrating "guerrilla cells" may be very difficult to reveal both by histopathological and other methods, but their existence is proven by clinical experience,[5] morphological studies,[6,7] and by our own studies in the seemingly normal tissue surrounding malignant gliomas.[8–12]

The migrating cells hide from antineoplastic agents behind an intact blood–brain barrier and are impossible to reach surgically. Attempts to cure astrocytomas by local treatment seem to be doomed to fail. However, whole-body hyperthermia (WBH), alone or as an adjuvant, may be an attractive therapeutic alternative

[a]This work was supported by the Swedish Cancer Society, The Medical Faculty, Lund University, The Lund University Hospital, Einar Björkelunds Foundation, John and Augusta Perssons Foundation, Berta Kamprads Foundation, and the Crafoord Foundation, Lund.

[g]Address correspondence to Leif G. Salford, M.D., Ph.D., Division of Experimental Neurooncology, Department of Neurosurgery, Lund University Hospital, S-221 85 Lund, Sweden.

because it is cytotoxic, has shown radiosensitizing properties,[13] and reaches every malignant cell in the brain. Hyperthermia has also been shown to enhance the effects of chemotherapy and immunotherapy.[14–17]

The problems with treatment of WBH in rodents have been discussed.[14,18] We have demonstrated that WBH is feasible in a rat glioma model and have studied the effect of WBH, alone or combined with nicotinamide (NAM) and with variations in tumor burden, reporting only animals surviving at least 19 days after inoculation of the glioma cells.

NAM was chosen because it has been shown to be an effective radiosensitizer in animal tumor models.[19,20] NAM was also chosen because it acts as an inhibitor of ADPRT (poly adenosine diphosphate ribosyl transferase), a chromatin-bound enzyme activated by DNA strand breaks and suggested to be important in the DNA repair system.[17,21]

MATERIAL AND METHODS

Animal model

The Fischer-344 rat strain used in our laboratory was originally provided by the Department of Immunology, Karolinska Institute, Stockholm. Fischer rats of both sexes, weighing 200–300 g, were used in the experiments. The animals had free access to water and pellets (SAN-bolagcn, Malmö, Sweden).

By stereotactic technique, 5 μL nutrient solution with either 1,000 or 5,000 rat glioma cells (RG2 cell line) were injected with a Hamilton syringe into the head of the right caudate nucleus in 120 Fischer-344 rats out of which 60 served as controls. One group of animals ($n = 102$) received 1,000 cells and another group ($n = 18$) received 5,000.

The rat glioma cell line RG2, originally an ethyl nitrosourea-induced glioma rat tumor, has proven to grow very well in infinite cell culture cycles for two decades.[22] When at least 1,000 cells of the RG2 cell line are inoculated in the brain of our rats, well-delineated tumors develop in 100% of the animals.[23] The tumors cause neurological symptoms after about three weeks, and the untreated tumors by then have reached a diameter of 3–6 mm. At inoculation, every animal to be treated was matched to a control animal that was inoculated with the same amount of identical tumor cells immediately before or after the animal to be treated. Animals ($n = 8$–12) were inoculated at each instance.

Hyperthermia Treatment

WBH was induced by a radiant heat device (Enthermics Inc., Menomonee Falls, WI) in 40 animals at 42 °C. All animals were under general anesthesia during the treatment. Chloral hydrate, 5%, 6 mL/kg body weight, was given i.p. initially. One femoral vein was cannulated and during the treatment, additional chloral hydrate could be given i.v. to keep the animals under deep anesthesia. Isotonic NaCl (5 mL) was given s.c. as substitution before the treatment. In the preparation for this study, we had problems in repeatedly treating animals at 42.0 °C. This was solved with saline substitution before the hyperthermia sessions.

Rectal temperature was measured with a thermistor probe (ATS, Lund Science, Lund, Sweden). The temperature was elevated during about 20 min and could be kept at exactly 42.0 °C during the following 30 min. Following hyperthermia treatment the animals were allowed to return to normal temperature and to wake up from anesthesia. WBH was given from day 7 after transplantation and twice a week thereafter.

Animals that died before the completion of four hyperthermia treatments or before day 19 after inoculation were not evaluated for response. This limit was chosen to restrict the variation in tumor size and also to get a substantial amount of treatment to separate treated and untreated groups of animals.

Nicotinamide Treatment

Nicotinamide (NAM) has been shown to be an effective radiosensitizer in animal tumor models at a dose of 200 mg/kg body weight given in close connection with radiotherapy.[19,20] In the present study, NAM (200 mg/kg b.w.) was given intraperitoneally 45 min before hyperthermia treatment to 47 of the WBH-treated animals.

Treatment Protocols

Four different treatment protocols were used:

1. WBH at 42.0 °C, 1,000 RG2 cells, 13 treated animals plus 13 controls.
2. NAM only, 1,000 RG2 cells, 20 treated animals plus 20 controls.
3. WBH at 42.0 °C plus NAM, 1,000 RG2 cells, 18 treated animals plus 18 controls.
4. WBH at 42.0 °C plus NAM, 5,000 RG2 cells, 9 treated animals plus 9 controls.

Evaluation of Response

Whenever a treated animal or its matched control within a simultaneously inoculated group of 8–12 animals started to develop neurological signs of tumor growth, all animals within the group were sacrificed by perfusion-fixation of the brains under chloral hydrate anesthesia. This technique was initiated in our laboratories in 1971 by Professor Fred Plum during his sabbatical in Lund, Sweden.[24] All brains were examined histopathologically by one of the authors (A.B.) who was uninformed about the previous treatment of the animals. After paraffin embedding, five coronal slices from each animal were studied microscopically in Cresyl violet staining. In this way, the whole telencephalon was covered except for the frontal and occipital poles. The slice with the largest tumor portion was chosen for a simplified calculation of tumor size: the largest diameter was multiplied with its perpendicular diameter resulting in the surface of a square. No attempts were made to adjust for the exact form of the tumor as the values of interest are correlations between tumors of treated animals and their controls.

Statistics

Student's *t* test for paired samples was used for the statistical evaluation.

TABLE 1. Effect of WBH and/or NAM upon the Growth of 1,000 or 5,000 RG2 Rat Glioma Cells Inoculated in the Brain of Fischer-344 Rats

	n	Tumor Size (mm^2)	Significance
Group 1: WBH at 42 °C, 1,000 RG2 cells; 13 treated animals plus 13 controls			
Treated animals	13	10.8 ± 6.9	n.s. ($p = 0.316$)
Controls	13	8.4 ± 5.6	
Group 2: NAM only, 1,000 RG2 cells; 20 treated animals plus 20 controls			
Treated animals	20	12.2 ± 8.2	n.s.
Controls	20	12.0 ± 7.3	
Group 3: WBH at 42.0 °C plus NAM, 1,000 RG2 cells; 18 treated animals plus 18 controls			
Treated animals	18	4.0 ± 4.8	$p = 0.031$
Controls	18	8.7 ± 7.8	
Group 4: WBH at 42.0 °C plus NAM, 5,000 RG2 cells; 9 treated animals plus 9 controls			
Treated animals	9	23.1 ± 7.7	n.s.
Controls	9	24.0 ± 9.7	

WBH, whole-body hyperthermia; NAM, nicotinamide.

RESULTS

All animals, treated as well as controls, developed tumors. These were rounded, polycyclic with well-defined boundaries. On histopathological examination, the tumors were usually solid with minor necrotic areas without correlation to treatment, tumor size or time from inoculation to death. No signs of brain damage were found outside the tumor areas—neither necrosis, gliosis nor inflammatory changes—that could be ascribed to the treatment.

The majority of the animals were sacrificed on day 20 or day 21 after inoculation. A few animals were sacrificed on day 19 (group 1) and on days 22 and 23 (group 4).

The effect of hyperthermia and/or NAM treatment is shown in TABLE 1. WBH 42 °C as single treatment had no inhibitory effect upon the growth of 1,000 inoculated tumor cells (group 1); neither had NAM as single treatment (group 2). WBH 42 °C in combination with NAM had no inhibitory effect upon the growth of 5,000 inoculated tumor cells (group 4). However, when only 1,000 cells had been inoculated (group 3) did the combined treatment with WBH 42 °C and NAM have a significant inhibitory effect ($p < 0.05$).

DISCUSSION

WBH has the advantage of reaching every cell in the body. It should be ideal at least as an adjuvant therapy against malignant brain tumors with their migrating cells spreading into the normal brain tissue, protected from therapeutic drugs behind an intact blood–brain barrier.

As stated previously, we had problems in repeatedly treating animals at 42.0 °C. With saline infusion s.c. before the hyperthermia sessions, we had only about 5% mortality during the treatment. Animals that died before the completion of four hyperthermia treatments, or before day 19 after inoculation, were not evaluated for response.

We chose to inoculate only 1,000 glioma cells in the majority of animals in order to allow even minor effects of the treatment to be demonstrated. Our results indicate that a rectal temperature of 42 °C during 4–5 WBH treatments has no impact on the tumor growth in our model. We did not measure the intracerebral temperature during these experiments, but assumed that the technique used with radiant heat provided a uniform temperature in the body. It should be noted, however, that brain temperature in neurosurgical patients has been shown to exceed the rectal temperature in 90% of all measurements, with the largest measured gradient 2.3 °C and with a mean value of 0.33 °C.[25] Thus, we cannot exclude the possibility that our treatment has reached temperatures above 42 °C in the brain, but no pathology beyond that caused by the tumors was observed at histological examination of the brains, and the animals did not show signs of brain damage during the WBH treatment.

Hosotani *et al.*[26] have recently pointed out that WBH in cats with implanted intracerebral tumors that reached the temperature 41.8 ± 15 °C (mean ± SD) for two hours, also led to increased peritumoral brain edema and significant increase of intracranial pressure. Our animals were not sacrificed in connection with the WBH sessions, but histopathological examination did not reveal increased peritumoral edema in the treatment animals as compared to the untreated. Neither did we see clinical signs of increased intracranial pressure in the WBH-treated animals during the hours after treatment.

Ibuchi *et al.*[27] have reported that a clear difference in heat sensitivity exists *in vitro* between normal rat brain cells and rat glioma cells induced by Rous sarcoma virus, when temperatures between 43 and 44 °C are reached. At 42 °C the proliferation of both normal and glioma cells was only slightly inhibited. This finding supports our negative results for WBH as single treatment.

Because WBH at 42 °C had no effect at all, we decided to combine this maximal possible temperature, with an appropriate ADPRT inhibitor in order to enhance any DNA damage possibly produced by the hyperthermia. ADPRT inhibitors have been shown not only to enhance cytotoxicity, but also to reduce the thermotolerance in V79 cells.[28] We chose NAM which is identical to vitamin B3, because members of our group have worked with this compound in conjunction with experimental studies on radiosensitizing effects of hyperthermia.

NAM given as single treatment in group 2 was found to have no effect upon tumor growth when 1,000 cells were given. The addition of WBH 42.0 °C as in group 3, however, proved to have a significant effect at the $p < 0.05$ level. The low number of tumor cells inoculated possibly provides a laboratory counterpart to the clinical situation where a patient, who has recently undergone an extensive resection of his glioma, has only relatively few tumor cells left behind in the brain. When 5,000 glioma cells were inoculated (group 4) and identical treatment as in group 3 given, no effect could be demonstrated. This supports the suggestion that the treatment may be of value when a discrete tumor burden is at hand.

The mean values for tumor size show large standard deviations. This is an expression for the large spread of tumor size from animal to animal. We ascribe this to possible small variations in exact number of cells that are sucked into the Hamilton syringe and which then reach the target point in the caudate nucleus during the stereotactic inoculation. The condition of the cells may differ from day to day and also depend upon when in their division cycle they are harvested. Even if the Fischer-344 rats that we used have been inbred for several years, minor differences in their response to inoculated tumor cells may exist. This underlines the utmost importance of matching every treated animal with its control before simultaneous inoculation of identical cells in identical amounts.

The controls in groups 1 and 3 developed similar tumor sizes, about 8 mm², whereas the controls in group 2 were about 12 mm². An explanation is that the experiments in group 2 were performed several months later than the others. It should also be stressed that the difference between the mean values for the control groups is not significant ($p = 0.140$, Student's t test, independent samples).

The number of cells inoculated has a clear effect upon the tumor growth. We had earlier shown that 500 cells develop identifiable tumors within four weeks only in 1 of 10 animals. When 5,000 cells were inoculated, the controls developed tumors twice the size of those after inoculation of 1,000 cells.

It has been shown that malignant gliomas have a relative alkalinity intracellularly, both in rat models including RG2[29] and in the human situation, as shown with PET scan[30] and with magnetic resonance spectroscopy.[31,32] The relative alkalinity intracellularly may be a prerequisite for proliferation of the cancer cells as it is in embryonal cells.[33,34] Hossman *et al.*[29] suggest that tumor blood perfusion is more critical for clearance of acid equivalents than for glucose supply. It has been proposed that the glycolytic rate of tumors should be increased by hyperthermia to provoke intracellular acidosis and resulting necrosis.[35]

Hyperthermia may have another possible mechanism important for the impairment of clearance of acid equivalents, because it has been shown that the morphologically immature tumor vessels are more vulnerable to heat than the normal tissue blood vessels.[36] Already at a temperature level of 42 °C, the tumor blood flow often decreases during or after heating due to damage to the tumor vasculature.[37] It has been shown that tumor pH significantly drops following hyperthermia.[38]

Gliomas have a higher glycolytic rate compared to oxygen uptake.[39] Reduction of aerobic glycolysis by inhibition of mitochondrial hexokinase, which is increased in malignant gliomas, can be achieved with lonidamine, which also inhibits glycolysis. We plan to combine WBH with this drug in coming experiments. Another possibility is to combine WBH with inhibition of the pentose phosphate shunt (which is the major alternative pathway to glycolysis) with 6-amino nicotinamide.[40,41] This compound inhibits glucose 6-phosphate dehydrogenase, which has activity 3–10 times higher in neuroectodermal tumors than in adjacent normal brain.[42]

Malignant brain tumors such as astrocytomas and glioblastomas are not localized tumors because they send migrating cells into the surrounding normal brain. Local treatment, including interstitial hyperthermia[43] may prolong survival but does not seem to have potential for cure. In contrast, WBH is a logical way to reach all tumor cells. It seems that WBH on its own is not effective, but our present results give some hope that WBH in combination with other therapies influencing cell metabolism will improve future therapies against malignant brain tumors.

SUMMARY

Malignant primary brain tumors have hitherto been incurable. One reason for this may be the migrating tumor cells that spread into the surrounding normal brain, creating the basis for the inevitable recurrences. Therefore, local therapy may have a temporary effect, but for a cure, the treatment must reach all the tumor cells. Whole-body hyperthermia (WBH) is such a general treatment, which we have studied in a rat glioma model. Cells of the RG2 rat glioma cell line were inoculated in the right caudate nucleus of Fischer-344 rats, which were then either controls or treated with WBH, induced by a radiant heat device for 4–5 sessions of 30 min at body temperature 42 °C (rectal), and/or nicotinamide (NAM), an effective radiosensitizer in animal tumor models and an inhibitor of ADPRT (poly adenosine diphosphate ribosyl transferase), a chromatin-bound enzyme suggested to be important in the DNA repair system. We have shown that WBH 42 °C alone, or in combination with NAM, has no effect upon tumor growth if a larger number of RG2 cells (5,000) are inoculated. If only 1,000 cells are inoculated, a significant inhibitory effect ($p < 0.05$) is observed on tumor growth as compared to the untreated control animals. Thus, WBH is feasible, and in some circumstances effective, in a rat glioma model. WBH in combination with other therapies influencing cell metabolism may be of value in future postoperative treatment of human malignant brain tumors.

ACKNOWLEDGMENTS

The authors are grateful to Dr. Anders Hugander, Department of Surgery, Jönköping Hospital, for help with the radiant heat device; and to Susanne Strömblad, Catarina Blennow, Kerstin Sturesson, and Juan Riosecco for excellent technical assistance.

REFERENCES

1. KERNOHAN, J. W., R. F. MABON, H. J. SVIEN & A. W. ADSON. 1949. A simplified classification of the gliomas. Mayo Clin. Proc. **24:** 71–75.
2. SALFORD, L. G., A. BRUN & S. NIRFALK. 1988. Ten year survival among patients with supratentorial astrocytoma grade III and IV. J. Neurosurg. **69:** 506–509.
3. BRUN, A., H. KRISTENSEN & L. G. SALFORD. Natural growth and spread of highly malignant cerebral astrocytomas. Submitted.
4. DANDY W. E. 1933. Physiological studies following of the right cerebral hemisphere in man. Johns Hopkins Hospital Bull. **53:** 31–51.
5. BELL, E., JR. & L. J. KARNOSH. 1949. Cerebral hemispherectomy. J. Neurosurg. **6:** 285–293.
6. BURGER, P. C., E. R. HEINZ, T. SHIBATA & P. KLEIHUES. 1988. Topographic anatomy and CT correlations in the untreated glioblastoma-multiforme. J. Neurosurg. **68:** 698–704.
7. DAUMAS-DUPORT, C., V. MONSAIGNEON, S. BLOND, C. MUNARI, A. MUSOLINA, J. P. CHODKIEWICZ & O. MISSIR. 1987. Serial stereotactic biopsies and CT scan in gliomas: Correlative study in 100 astrocytomas, oligo-astrocytomas and oligodendrocytomas. J. Neuro-Oncol. **4:** 317–328.
8. SALFORD, L. G., B. BALDETORP, A. BRUN, G. HALLENCREUTZ & B. STENSTAM. 1988. DNA content in human astrocytomas and surrounding brain tissue. Acta Neurochir. **91:** 162–163.
9. SALFORD, L. G., R. W. PERO, A. T. AAS & A. BRUN. 1992. Metoclopramide as a sensitizer of 1,3-BIS(2-chloroethyl)-1-nitrosourea (BCNU) treatment of brain tumors in the rat. Anti-Cancer Drugs **3:** 267–272.
10. SALFORD, L. G., R. B. R. PERSSON, A. BRUN, C. CEBERG, P. C. KONGSTAD & L. MIR. 1993. A new brain tumour therapy combining bleomycin with in vivo electropermeabilization. Biochem. Biophys. Res. Commun. **194(2):** 938–943.
11. SALFORD, L. G., C. P. CEBERG, A. BRUN, A. PERSSON & R. B. R. PERSSON. 1996. Foundations for boron neutron capture therapy of high-grade astrocytomas. *In* Neutron Capture Therapy for Cancer. Plenum Press. New York.
12. SJÖHOLM, H., K. LJUNGGREN, R. ADELI, A. BRUN, R. B. R. PERSSON, S. E. STRAND & L. G. SALFORD. 1995. Necrosis of malignant gliomas after intratumoral injection of thallium-201 in vivo in the rat. Anti-Cancer Drugs **6:** 109–114.
13. BEN-HUR, E., M. M. ELKIND & B. V. BRONK. 1974. Thermally enhanced radioresponse of cultured Chinese hamster cells: Inhibition of repair of subethal damage and enhancement of lethal damage. Radiat. Res. **58:** 38–51.
14. HAHN, G. M. 1982. Hyperthermia and Cancer. Plenum Press. New York.

15. OLESON, J. R. & M. W. DEWHIRST. 1983. Hyperthermia: An overview of current progress and problems. Curr. Probl. in Cancer **1:** 1–62.

16. ROBINS, H. I. 1984. Role of whole-body hyperthermia in the treatment of neoplastic disease: Its current status and future prospects. Cancer Res. **44:** 4878–4883.

17. ROBINS, H. I., G. G. JONSSON, E. L. JACOBSON, C. L. SCHMITT, J. D. COHEN & M. K. JACOBSON. 1991. Effect of hyperthermia in vitro and in vivo on adenine and pyridine nucleotide pools in human peripheral lymphocytes. Cancer **67:** 2096–2102.

18. ROBINS, H. I., R. A. STEEVES, L. M. SHECTERLE, P. A. MARIN, A. MILLER, B. PALIVAL, A. J. NEVILLE & W. H. DENNIS. 1984. Whole body hyperthermia (41–42°C): A simple technique for unanesthetized mice. Med. Phys. **11(6):** 833–839.

19. HORSMAN, M. R., D. M. BROWN, M. J. LEMMON, J. M. BROWN & W. W. LEE. 1986. Preferential tumour radiosensitization by analogs of nicotinamide and benzamid. Int. J. Radiat. Oncol. Biol. Phys. **12:** 1307–1310.

20. HORSMAN, M. R., D. J. CHAPLIN & J. M. BROWN. 1987. Radiosensitization by nicotinamide in vivo: A greater enhancement of tumour damage compared to that of normal tissues. Radiat. Res. **109:** 479–489.

21. PERO, R. W., L. G. SALFORD, L.-G. STRÖMBLAD & C. ANDERSSON. 1992. Mononuclear leukocyte ADP-ribosylation as an indicator of immune function in malignant-glioma patients treated with bethamethasone for cerebral edema. J. Neurosurg. **77:** 601–606.

22. WECHSLER, W., P. KLEIHUES, S. MATSUMOTO, K. J. ZÜLCH, S. IVANKOVIC, T. PREUSS-MAN & H. DRUCKREY. 1969. Pathology of experimental neurogenic tumors chemically induced during prenatal and postnatal life. Ann. N. Y. Acad. Sci. **159:** 360–408.

23. AAS, A. T., C. BLENNOW, A. BRUN, S. STRÖMBLAD & L. G. SALFORD. 1995. The RG2 rat glioma model in actual experimental neuro-oncology. J. Neuro-Oncol. **23:** 175–183.

24. SALFORD, L. G., F. PLUM & J. B. BRIERLEY. 1973. Graded Hypoxia oligemia in rat brain. II. Neuropathological alterations and their implications. Arch. Neurol. **29:** 234–238.

25. MELLERGÅRD, P. & C.-H. NORDSTRÖM. 1991. Intracerebral temperature in neurosurgical patients. Neurosurgery **28:** 709–713.

26. HOSOTANI, K., K. KATSUMURA, M. KABUTO, Y. HANDA, T. KUBOTA & M. HAYASHJI. 1993. Effect of whole-body hyperthermia on the development of peritumoral brain edema. Acta Neuropathol. (Berl.) **69:** 139–147.

27. IBUCHI, Y., R. TANAKA, Y. YAMADA & H. HONDO. 1988. Selective heat-sensitivity of glioma cells (Abstr.). 5th International Symposium on Hyperthermic Oncology. Kyoto, Japan. P2–C2.

28. MIYAKOSHI, J., W. ODA & C. INAGAKI. 1985. Effects of m-aminobenzamide on the response of Chinese hamster cells to hyperthermia and/or radiation. Radiat. Res. **102:** 359–366.

29. HOSSMAN, K. A., G. MIES, W. PASCHEN, L. SZABO, E. DOLAN & W. WECHSLER. 1986. Regional metabolism of experimental brain tumours. Acta Neuropathol. (Berl.) **69:** 139–147.

30. ROTTENBERG, D. A., J. Z. GINOS, K. J. KEARFOTT, L. JUNCK & D. D. BIGNER. 1984. In vivo measurement of regional brain tissue pH using positron emission tomography. Ann. Neurol. **15(Suppl.):** S98–S102.

31. OBERHAENSLI, R. D., D. HILTON-JONES, P. J. BORE, L. J. HANDS, R. P. RAMPLING & G. K. RADDA. 1986. Biochemical investigation of human tumours in vivo with phosphorous-31 magnetic resonance spectroscopy. Lancet **2:** 8.

32. CADOUX-HUDSON, T. A. D., M. J. BLACKLEDGE, R. RAJAGOPALAN, D. J. TAYLOR & G. K. RADDA. 1989. Human primary brain tumour metabolism in vivo: A phosphorus magnetic resonance spectroscopy study. Br. J. Cancer **60:** 430–436.

33. OBER, S. S. & A. B. PARDEE. 1987a. Intracellular pH is increased after transformation of Chinese hamster embryo fibroblasts. Proc. Natl. Acad. Sci. USA **88:** 2766–2770.

34. OBER, S. S. & A. B. PARDEE. 1987b. Both protein kinase C and calcium mediate activation of the Na+/H+ antiporter in Chinese hamster embryo fibroblasts. J. Cell Physiol. **132(2):** 311–317.

35. OVERGAARD, J. 1976. Influence of extracellular pH on the viability and morphology of tumour cells exposed to hyperthermia. J. Natl. Cancer Inst. **56:** 1243–1250.

36. SONG, C. W. 1988. Physiological and environmental factors in thermal injury of tissues (Abstr.). International Symposium on Hyperthermic Oncology L-9: p 12.

37. REINHOLD, H. S. & A. V. D. BERG-BLOK. 1980. Features and limitations of the "in vitro" valuation of tumour response by optical means. *In* Proceedings of the Ninth L.H. Gray Memorial Conference, Cambridge, England. Br. J. Cancer.

38. BICHER, H. I., F. W. HETZEL, T. S. SANDHU, S. FRINAK, P. VAUPEL, M. D. O'HARA & T. O'BRIEN. 1980. Effects of hyperthermia on normal and tumour microenvironment. Radiology **137**: 523–530.

39. VICTOR, J. V. & A. WOLF. 1937. Metabolism of brain tumours. Research publications. Assoc. Res. Nerv. Ment. Dis. **16**: 44–58.

40. POLITIS, M. J. 1989. 6-AN selectively causes necrosis in reactive anstroglia cells in vivo. J. Neurol. Sci. **41**: 994–1010.

41. LEVANTE, S., L. A. ZOTTER, D. ENG, J. GAVALCHIN & J. A. WINFIELD. 1990. In-vitro and in-vivo tumoricidal effects of 6-aminonicotinamide on human glial tumors (Abstr). *In* Cancer in the Nervous System. M.D. Anderson Cancer Center, Nov. 3–6.

42. PAXTON, H. D. 1959. Quantitative histochemistry of brain tumours and analogous normal tissue. Neurology **9**: 367–370.

43. STEA, B., J. KITTELSON, J. R. CASSADY, A. HAMILTON, N. GUTHKELCH, B. LULU, E. OBBENS, K. ROSSMAN, W. SHAPIRO, A. SHETTER & T. CETAS. 1992. Treatment of malignant gliomas with interstitial irradiation and hyperthermia. Int. J. Radiat. Oncol. Biol. Phys. **24**: 657–667.

Molecular Pathology of Cerebral Ischemia: Delayed Gene Expression and Strategies for Neuroprotection[a]

COSTANTINO IADECOLA[b] AND M. ELIZABETH ROSS

Laboratory of Cerebrovascular Biology and Stroke
Department of Neurology
University of Minnesota Medical School
Minneapolis, Minnesota 55455

INTRODUCTION

Early concepts on the pathogenesis and treatment of ischemic stroke were based on the assumption that energy failure is the sole determinant of ischemic brain damage. Consequently, cerebral ischemia was thought to result in immediate and irretrievable brain injury. Evidence accumulated during the last two decades, however, has challenged this postulate. Studies in animal models have demonstrated that the rapidity and severity of the brain damage depend on the intensity of the ischemic insult. Thus, in the center of the ischemic territory, wherein the reduction in flow is most severe ($<20\%$ of the preischemic value), rapid energy failure results in loss of ionic gradients and cell death.[1] At the outskirts of the area of ischemia, where collateral flow from adjacent arterial territories prevents severe ischemia, the brain damage develops at a slower pace (FIG. 1). This peripheral region corresponds to the so-called ischemic penumbra, an area in which neurons are functionally compromised but still viable.[2,3]

In the early phase of cerebral ischemia, factors threatening neuronal survival in the penumbra include mainly glutamate excitotoxicity, free radical damage, and energy failure resulting from recurrent depolarization waves.[4,5] However, at later times other mechanisms come into play. The initial ischemic event activates a variety of genetic programs that unfold over the course of hours and days. Recent evidence indicates that some of the gene products deriving from these molecular events are deleterious to the ischemic brain and contribute to the late stages of tissue damage. These new developments suggest novel strategies for stroke therapies targeted at the late stages of ischemic brain damage. In this paper some of these molecular events will be reviewed with focus on two genes expressed in the post-ischemic period: inducible nitric oxide synthase (iNOS) and cyclooxygenase (COX-2).

[a] This work was supported by grants from the National Institutes of Health (NS31318, NS34179 and NS35806), the American Heart Association (Grant-in-aid, Established Investigator Award), and the Searle-Monsanto Company.

[b] Address correspondence to C. Iadecola, M.D., Laboratory of Cerebrovascular Biology and Stroke, Department of Neurology, University of Minnesota Medical School, Box 295 UMHC, 420 Delaware Street S.E., Minneapolis, MN 55455. E-mail: iadec001@maroon.tc.umn.edu

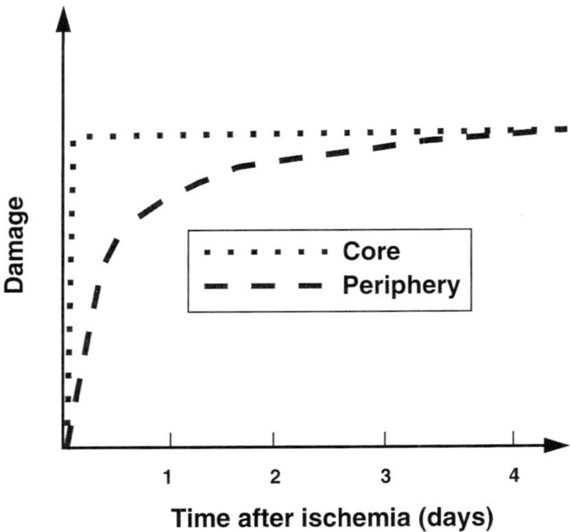

FIGURE 1. Illustration of the time course of development of brain damage following cerebral ischemia. Evidence reviewed in the text suggests that the damage develops rapidly in the center of the ischemic region and more slowly at the periphery.

PROGRESSION OF CEREBRAL ISCHEMIC DAMAGE AND THE "THERAPEUTIC WINDOW"

Several lines of evidence suggest that cerebral ischemic damage develops at a pace slower than previously believed (TABLE 1). Careful analysis of hematoxylin and eosin stained sections at different times after occlusion of the rat middle cerebral artery (MCA) indicates that brain damage develops over hours to days depending on the brain region.[6] Neuronal death progresses rapidly in regions where the ischemia is most severe. However, in areas surrounding the ischemic core, potentially viable cells are still observed more than 12 h after MCA occlusion.[6,7] In addition, studies by positron emission tomography indicate that viable tissue, defined by hemodynamic and metabolic criteria, is still present many hours after stroke in human or in monkey.[8–10] More recently, magnetic resonance based techniques have been employed to define the temporal profile of the brain damage. These studies have also shown that the development of irretrievable tissue damage is relatively slow, progressing over the course of several days in some cases.[11,12] These observations, collectively, suggest that the brain can potentially be "rescued" from infarction many hours after onset of ischemia and challenge the widespread notion of a "therapeutic window" of 3–6 h.[13] This realization is of critical importance for stroke therapy because most patients reach medical attention at a time when current therapeutic strategies are no longer effective.[14,15] Therefore, it would be highly desirable to develop therapeutic interventions that can be instituted many hours after the onset of ischemia.

Interventions targeted at the delayed evolution of the damage require an understanding of the mechanisms responsible for such a progression. Most studies to date have focused on events, such as excitotoxicity, calcium overload, and free radical production, that occur in the acute stages of cerebral ischemia.[1,4,5] Although these pathogenic processes are critical for the initiation of cerebral ischemic damage, they occur in the early stages of the ischemic cascade and, consequently, are unlikely to be responsible for the progression of the damage that occurs several hours to

TABLE 1. Evidence for Delayed Progression of Cerebral Ischemic Damage in the Post-ischemic Period

Evidence	Species/Model	Technique	Refs.
Histological			
•Maturation of irreversible damage between 4 and 46 h after focal ischemia	Wistar rat, transient or permanent MCAO	H&E	7, 29
•Delayed neuronal injury (red neurons) observed at >12 h after ischemia		H&E	7, 29
•Reversal of neuronal damage at 72 h in penumbral regions	Fisher rat, permanent MCAO	H&E	6
Flow-metabolism			
•Expansion of hypometabolic area up to 24 h or more	Baboon, MCAO	PET	10
•Potentially viable tissue (CMRO2 >1.4 mL/100 mL/min) up to 17 h after stroke	Human, MCA stroke	PET	9
•Potentially viable tissue (increased OEF/reduced flow) up to 48 h after stroke	Human, MCA stroke	PET	8
Magnetic resonance			
•Signal characteristics suggestive of irreversible brain damage develop over days	Human, MCA stroke	DWI, PWI, T_2	11, 12
	Fisher rat, permanent MCAO	DWI, PWI	63

Abbreviations: CMRO2, cerebral metabolic rate for oxygen; DWI, diffusion-weighted imaging; H&E, hematoxylin and eosin; MCAO, middle cerebral artery occlusion; OEF, oxygen extraction fraction; PET, positron emission tomography; PWI, perfusion-weighted imaging; T2: T_2-weighted imaging.

days after induction of ischemia. In recent years molecular biological investigations have revealed that a wide variety of genes are expressed both in the early and late stages of cerebral ischemia. Evidence is accumulating that the products of some of these genes have an important impact on the cellular events occurring in the ischemic brain and, ultimately, on the progression of the damage.

EVENTS ASSOCIATED WITH FOCAL CEREBRAL ISCHEMIA

Focal cerebral ischemia triggers a complex array of cellular and molecular changes. A brief description of some of the molecular and cellular events occurring in the first 4–5 days after stroke is presented below.

Molecular Events

Cerebral ischemia activates a number of molecular programs that result in the *de novo* expression or up-regulation of a wide variety of genes (FIG. 2). Within 30 min after occlusion of the rat MCA there is expression of immediate early genes, for example, c-fos, c-jun, in neurons (FIG. 2). The duration of the early gene expression is regionally diverse. In the center of the ischemic region, the expression

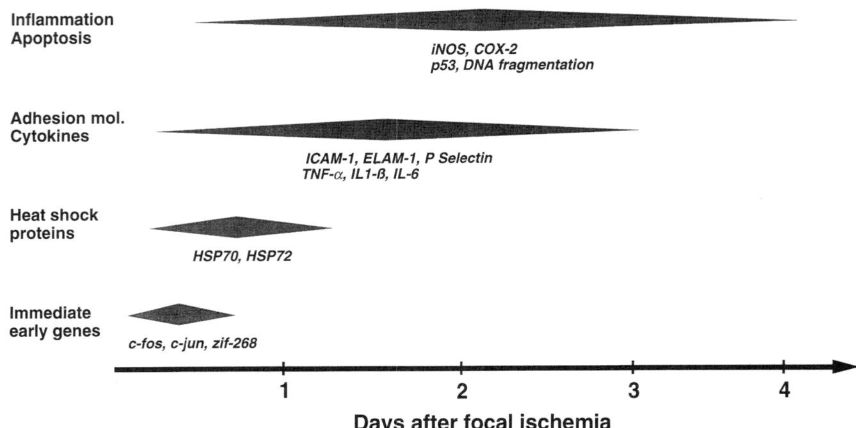

FIGURE 2. Time course of expression of selected genes following focal cerebral ischemia. Immediate early genes are turned on first, followed by genes encoding for heat shock proteins, adhesion molecules, cytokines, and inflammation-related proteins. In the late stages of cerebral ischemia, gene products related to apoptosis are expressed, for example, p53, and DNA fragmentation is observed. *Abbreviations*: COX-2, cyclooxygenase 2; HSP, heat shock protein; IL, interleukin; iNOS, inducible nitric oxide synthase; ICAM-1, intercellular adhesion molecule 1; ELAM-1, endothelial-leukocyte adhesion molecule 1; TNF-α, tumor necrosis factor α.

peaks at 3–4 h and returns to baseline within 24–48 h (see ref. 16 for a review). However, in the peripheral area, the expression continues to increase up to 4 days.[17] The induction of early genes is thought to be related to calcium-mediated activation of second messenger systems, which, in turn, act on the promoter of early genes to initiate transcription.[16] The role of early gene expression in the pathogenesis of cerebral ischemia remains to be defined. Early gene proteins activate transcription of a wide variety of genes through interaction with a number of promoter elements, such as activator protein 1 (AP-1) or cAMP/calcium response elements (CRE).[18] Therefore, early gene expression leads to activation of other genes whose products are involved in cerebral ischemic damage.

A second wave of gene expression involves heat shock proteins (hsp) (see ref. 19 for a review; FIG. 2). Hsp gene expression is limited to regions in which cerebral blood flow decreases below 50% of normal and is thought to occur only in injured cells that remain viable after ischemia. Accordingly, in areas of severe ischemia, hsp are observed predominantly in vascular cells, which are more resistant to ischemic cell death than neurons.[20] In regions of less severe ischemia, that is, the penumbra, hsp induction is observed in neurons (e.g., ref. 21). Hsp, therefore, seem to be induced in cells that are destined to survive and may have a protective role.

A third wave of gene expression includes genes encoding inflammatory cytokines (TNFα, IL1β, IL6, MCP-1) and adhesion molecules (ICAM-1, ELAM-1, P-selectin)[22–24] (FIG. 2). Cytokines are thought to induce expression of adhesion molecules on the cerebral vasculature which, in turn, leads to transendothelial migration of blood-borne inflammatory cells into the ischemic brain. In addition, cytokines may contribute to the initiation of a fourth wave of gene expression involving the inflammation-related genes iNOS and COX-2 (FIG. 2). During the late phase of the damage, there is also evidence of internucleosomal DNA fragmentation and expression of gene products involved in programmed cell death such as p53.[25–27] These findings raise the possibility that apoptosis plays a role in the delayed cell death that occurs at the infarct border.

Cellular Events

Neurons are more sensitive to ischemia than are glial cells, which, in turn, are more susceptible than endothelial cells.[20] Within 30 min after ischemia neurons in the core region appear shrunken and scalloped.[7] Neurons then become swollen and exhibit vacuolation in dendrites.[7] A few hours after induction of ischemia neutrophils adhere to the cerebral endothelium and invade the ischemic brain (see ref. 28 for a review). This process is part of the inflammatory reaction that involves the ischemic brain and is thought to be initiated by expression of cytokines and adhesion molecules (see ref. 24 for a review). The neutrophilic infiltration peaks at 24–48 h and then begins to subside. At this time, macrophages start to accumulate in the ischemic brain and become the predominant cell in the late stages of infarction. Substantial evidence exists that post-ischemic inflammation contributes to cerebral ischemic damage. For example, neutrophil depletion prior to induction of ischemia or administration of antibodies against cytokine receptors or adhesion molecules reduces the inflammatory reaction and ameliorates the damage produced by MCA occlusion (see refs. 22 and 23 for reviews).

Astrocytes and microglia also participate in the cellular reaction that follows focal cerebral ischemia. Shortly after MCA occlusion, astrocytes become swollen[7] and within the next several hours they become activated, overexpressing glial fibrillary acidic protein.[29] The bulk of the astrocytic reaction occurs at the periphery of the infarct and results in the formation of the glial scar.[30] Microglial cells become reactive and proliferate.[31] Microvessels also proliferate starting 5–7 days after MCA occlusion.[30]

These data suggest that important cellular and molecular events are initiated by the ischemic insults and continue to evolve for several days after induction of ischemia. Although the pathogenic significance of post-ischemic gene expression is not entirely clear, recent evidence from our laboratory suggests that some of these genes play an important role in the delayed progression of the damage.

INDUCIBLE NITRIC OXIDE SYNTHASE GENE EXPRESSION

Nitric oxide (NO) is a free radical that in brain can act either as a molecular messenger or a neurotoxin (FIG. 3). As a molecular messenger, NO is thought to be involved in synaptic plasticity, morphogenesis, transmitter release, neuroendocrine function, and regulation of the cerebral circulation.[32–34] As a toxin, NO has been implicated in the mechanisms of the neurotoxicity associated with central nervous system infections, inflammation, MPTP, AIDS, dementia, and cerebral ischemia.[35–43] In cerebral ischemia, NO derived from neuronal NOS is involved in glutamate-mediated neurotoxicity and contributes to the early stages of ischemic brain damage.[37,42,44] However, recent studies from our laboratory indicate that NO produced by iNOS participates also in the tissue damage that occurs in the late stages of cerebral ischemia.

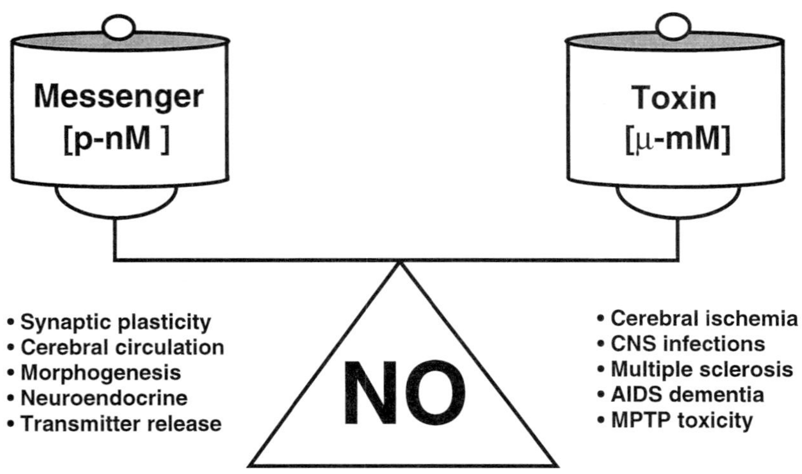

FIGURE 3. Selected effects of nitric oxide (NO) in the central nervous system. At low concentrations, NO acts as a molecular messenger and, as such, is thought to be involved in a wide variety of regulatory processes. At high concentrations, NO is cytotoxic and may mediate neurotoxicity in several neurological disorders.

NO Synthesis and NO Synthases

NO is synthesized from the oxidation of L-arginine, a process catalyzed by the enzyme NOS. Products of the reaction are NO, L-citrulline, and water. Three isoforms of NOS have been characterized (TABLE 2). Neuronal NOS (nNOS; NOS I) is expressed constitutively in selected neuronal populations and is activated by

TABLE 2. Isoforms of Nitric Oxide Synthase

Characteristics	NOS I	NOS II	NOS III
Other name	bNOS, nNOS	iNOS	eNOS
Human chromosome	12	17, 14 (?)	7
Molecular mass	≈160 kDa	≈133 kDa	≈130 kDa
Quaternary structure	Dimer	Dimer	Unknown
Typical cell	Neuron	Macrophage	Endothelium
Intracellular localization	Cytosolic and membrane bound	Cytosolic	Mainly membrane bound
Expression	Constitutive, inducible (?)	Inducible	Constitutive
Regulation	Ca-CaM	Transcription	Ca-CaM
NO output	Pulse (pmol)	Continuous (μmol)	Pulse (pmol)

Abbreviations: Ca-CaM, calcium-calmodulin; NOS, nitric oxide synthase.

calcium-induced binding of calmodulin to the enzyme. Endothelial NOS (eNOS; NOS III) is constitutively expressed in endothelial cells and is also activated by Ca^{2+}-calmodulin. Thus, eNOS and nNOS produce NO intermittently, only when the intracellular calcium concentration increases. The inducible (immunological) isoform of NOS (iNOS; NOS II) is usually not present in cells but its expression is transcriptionally induced by certain stimuli, typically endotoxins and cytokines.[45] iNOS catalytic activity is not calcium-dependent and, consequently, the enzyme is continuously active and produces large amounts of NO. NO produced by iNOS is thought to mediate the antimicrobial and antineoplastic effects of macrophages.[45] Mechanisms of NO cytotoxicity include DNA damage, energy failure, and oxidative damage (see ref. 46 for a review).

iNOS and Cerebral Ischemia

As reviewed above, cerebral ischemia is associated with an inflammatory reaction that contributes to the development and progression of the tissue damage. However, the mechanisms by which inflammation exerts this effect are not completely understood. Although microvascular plugging by intravascular leukocytes may worsen the severity of ischemia in the acute phase, toxic products released by infiltrating inflammatory cells may also play a role.[28] Because iNOS is induced during inflammation in many tissues, it is conceivable that iNOS is expressed after cerebral ischemia and contributes to the damage. We, therefore, undertook a series of studies to determine whether iNOS is induced in the post-ischemic brain and, if so, to define its role in the mechanisms of the damage. In these studies we used a rat model of focal cerebral ischemia produced by transient or permanent occlusion of the MCA. iNOS mRNA and protein in the post-ischemic brain were determined by the reverse-transcription polymerase chain reaction (RT-PCR) and immunocytochemistry, respectively (FIG. 4). iNOS enzymatic activity was determined by the citrulline conversion assay of Bredt and Snyder modified for detection of calcium-independent NOS activity.[47] We found that iNOS mRNA is expressed after focal cerebral ischemia.[40,48] However, the temporal pattern of expression and the predominant cellular localization are different depending on whether the ischemia is permanent or transient. In transient ischemia, iNOS and mRNA expression peaks at 12 h and returns to baseline at 4 days.[40,48] iNOS immunoreactivity is observed both in cerebral vessels (endothelial cells and smooth muscle cells) and in inflammatory cells throughout the injured brain.[40,48] In permanent ischemia, iNOS mRNA is first observed at 12 h, peaks at 48 h, and disappears by 7 days.[48] iNOS immunoreactivity is observed in neutrophils invading the infarct border.[48] Both in permanent and transient ischemia, iNOS enzymatic activity is increased in the post-ischemic brain, suggesting that iNOS is catalytically active.[40,48,49]

Role of iNOS Expression in Ischemic Brain Damage

The data reviewed above demonstrate that iNOS is expressed following cerebral ischemia. In subsequent studies we investigated whether NO produced by iNOS is deleterious to the ischemic brain. For this purpose we used aminoguanidine, a relatively selective inhibitor of iNOS. We found that aminoguanidine (100 mg/kg; i.p.; b.i.d.), administered starting 24 h after permanent MCA occlusion, reduces post-ischemic iNOS activity and decreases infarct size by 33%.[39] Aminoguanidine did not affect resting cerebral blood flow, arterial pressure, rectal temperature,

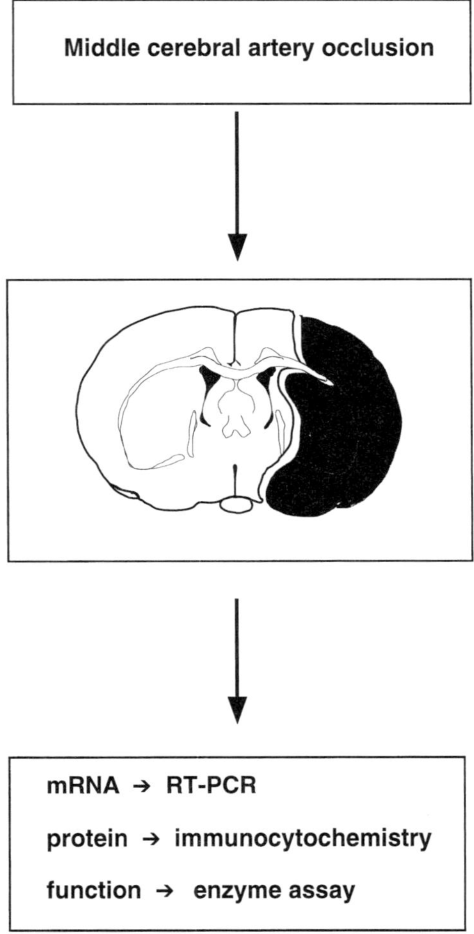

FIGURE 4. Strategy for studying iNOS and COX-2 expression following focal cerebral ischemia. Rats were sacrificed at different time points after MCA occlusion. mRNA was determined in tissue samples from the ischemic brain by the reverse transcription polymerase chain reaction (RT-PCR). The cellular localization of the protein was determined immunocytochemically in paraffin-embedded brain sections using antibodies directed against the iNOS or COX-2 protein. iNOS or COX-2 function was tested by measuring enzymatic activity in brain homogenates from the ischemic brain.

plasma glucose or arterial hematocrit.[39] The reduction in infarct size was abolished if the NO precursor L-arginine was co-administered with aminoguanidine.[39] In contrast, we found that co-administration of D-arginine does not abrogate the effect of aminoguanidine. These findings are consistent with the hypothesis that the protective effect of aminoguanidine is related to inhibition of the L-arginine-NO biosynthetic pathway. Similar reductions in stroke size were obtained if aminoguanidine was administered after transient MCA occlusion.[40]

We then studied the effect of the NO precursor L-arginine on cerebral ischemic damage. Because iNOS is continuously active, NO production is limited by the availability of substrates and cofactors. Consequently, administration of L-arginine in the post-ischemic period would be expected to enhance NO production and worsen ischemic damage. Consistent with this prediction, we found that L-arginine, but not the inactive isomer D-arginine, enlarges the size of the infarct produced by MCA occlusion.[50] L- or D-arginine were administered 24 h after MCA occlusion.[50]

The aminoguanidine data suggest that NO produced by iNOS is deleterious to the brain and that it contributes to the progression of cerebral ischemic damage. However, aminoguanidine has also pharmacological effects unrelated to iNOS inhibition that could confound the interpretation of the results (see ref. 39). To provide nonpharmacological evidence that iNOS is involved in ischemic brain damage, we also used knockout mice with a null mutation of the iNOS gene.[51] After MCA occlusion, iNOS knockouts failed to express iNOS mRNA, a finding that confirms the lack of iNOS expression in these animals. The infarct produced by MCA was 30–40% smaller in iNOS knockouts than in wild-type controls (B6 or SV129 mice).[52] The experiments on the iNOS knockouts, therefore, support the conclusion that iNOS expression is deleterious to the post-ischemic brain.

Factors Responsible for Post-Ischemic iNOS Expression

The mechanisms of post-ischemic iNOS induction remain to be determined. Ischemia is followed by expression of cytokines in the injured brain (see previous sections). Therefore, iNOS expression could be triggered by cytokines probably through the transcription factors interferon regulatory 1 (IRF-1) and nuclear factor κb. These transcription factors are known to bind to the iNOS promoter region and to activate iNOS transcription (see ref. 46 for a review). Indeed, preliminary results from our laboratory suggest that IRF-1 is an important pathway for post-ischemic iNOS expression because knockout mice lacking the IRF-1 have reduced iNOS expression.[53] The iNOS promoter also contains consensus sequences for the hypoxia regulatory factor 1 (HIF-1).[54] It is therefore conceivable that hypoxia may activate iNOS expression through up-regulation of HIF-1. However, presently no experimental evidence exists to support this possibility.

CYCLOOXYGENASE GENE EXPRESSION

COX, or prostaglandin H2 synthase, is a rate-limiting enzyme for prostanoid synthesis present in two isoforms. COX-1 is constitutively expressed and participates in normal cellular functions.[55] COX-2 is not expressed in most normal tissues but is induced during inflammation.[56] COX-2 is thought to be responsible for the cytotoxicity associated with inflammation, an effect mediated by at least two mechanisms. First, COX-2 activity is associated with production of free radicals that are toxic to cells.[57,58] Second, COX-2 produces toxic prostanoids.[56] Because COX-2 is expressed during inflammation, we sought to determine whether COX-2 is also expressed in brain after cerebral ischemia, a condition associated with an inflammatory reaction.

COX-2 Expression and Cerebral Ischemia

Cerebral ischemia produced by transient occlusion of the rat MCA up-regulates COX-2 mRNA in the post-ischemic brain. The expression was first detected 6 h

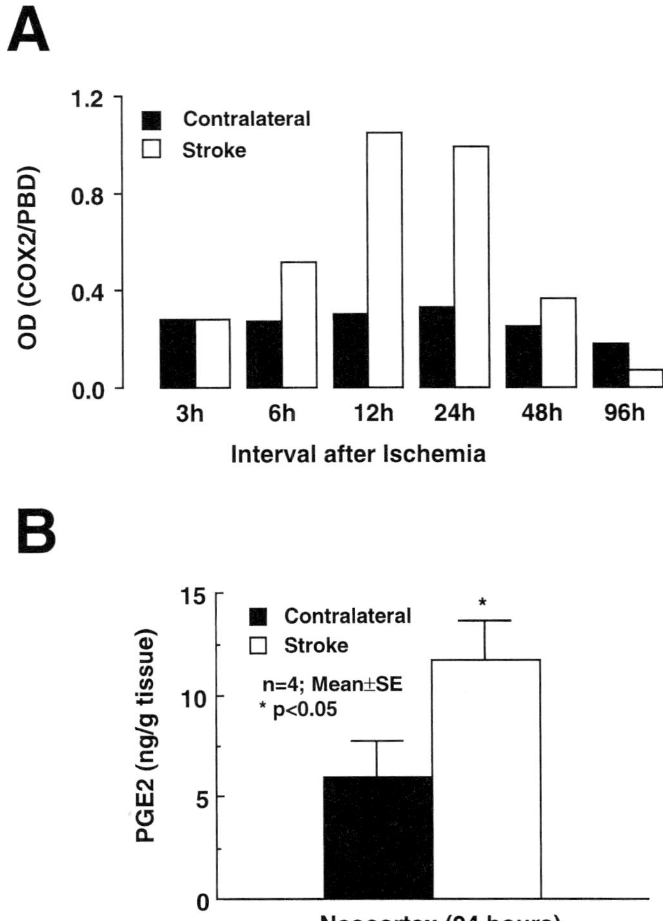

FIGURE 5. (**A**) Up-regulation of COX-2 mRNA in the rat brain following MCA occlusion. Total RNA was extracted from the ischemic brain (stroke) and contralaterally (contralateral), reverse transcribed into DNA and amplified by PCR. Products were run on a gel and the density of the COX-2 band was normalized by that of a housekeeping gene porphobilinogen deaminase (PBD). COX-2 expression is present at 6 h and peaks at 12 h. COX-2 mRNA does not increase in the brain contralateral to the stroke. (**B**) Effect of MCA occlusion on the brain concentration of PGE_2, one of the COX-2 reaction products. PGE_2 increases in the post-ischemic brain but not contralaterally. The PGE_2 accumulation indicated that COX-2 enzymatic activity is increased in the post-ischemic brain.

after ischemia and peaked at 12 h[59] (FIG. 5A). Competitive RT-PCR revealed a fivefold up-regulation of COX-2 mRNA. We then used immunocytochemistry to determine whether COX-2 mRNA up-regulation is associated with an increase in the COX-2 protein. In the brain of sham-operated rats, few immunoreactive cells were observed in the cerebral cortex, piriform cortex, hippocampus and amygdala, as previously described.[60] After cerebral ischemia, a marked induction of COX-2 immunoreactivity was found in neurons in the ischemic hemisphere. Immunoreactive neurons were located at the medial border of the ischemic lesion.[59] Some positive neurons were found in the transitional region between the normal and infarcted brain, a locus that corresponds to the anatomical location of the ischemic penumbra. These neurons had shrunken cytoplasm and nucleus, consistent with the morphological characteristics of ischemic neurons. Other neurons had a normal morphology and were located in the cingulate cortex adjacent to the infarct.

To determine whether the COX-2 up-regulation results in increased synthesis of prostaglandins, we measured PGE_2, one of the products of the COX-2 pathway, in the post-ischemic brain. In sham-operated rats, low levels of PGE_2 were found in the cerebral cortex. However, 24 h after MCA occlusion, PGE_2 was markedly increased only in the ischemic brain (FIG. 5B).[59] Thus, the up-regulation in COX-2 message and protein is associated with increased catalytic activity, supporting the contention that COX-2 is functional.

Role of COX-2 Expression in Cerebral Ischemia

To study the role of COX-2 in cerebral ischemic damage, we used the relatively selective COX-2 inhibitor NS-398. This agent inhibits COX-2 1,000 times more potently than COX-1.[61,62] NS-398 (20 mg/kg; i.p.) was administered starting 6 h after permanent occlusion of the rat MCA. NS-398 attenuates the increase in PGE_2 produced by cerebral ischemia, suggesting that this drug is effective in blocking COX-2 activity.[59] NS-398 reduced the size of the stroke produced by permanent MCA occlusion by approximately 30% (FIG. 6A). The area "rescued" from infarction involved mainly the medial border of the lesion, a site corresponding to the region in which the COX-2 positive neurons are located (FIG. 6B). NS-398 did not affect arterial pressure, rectal temperature, plasma glucose, arterial blood gases or arterial hematocrit.[59] These data suggest that the up-regulation of COX-2 in neurons is deleterious to the ischemic brain.

SUMMARY AND CONCLUSIONS

The evidence reviewed in this paper suggests that molecular and cellular events occurring in the late stages of cerebral ischemia (>6 h) play an important role in the evolution of ischemic brain damage. We focused our inquiry on two inflammation-related genes iNOS and COX-2. iNOS is expressed in inflammatory and vascular cells in the post-ischemic brain. Pharmacological inhibition of iNOS activity ameliorates ischemic damage, whereas knockout mice lacking the iNOS gene are relatively protected from the consequences of cerebral ischemia. COX-2 is expressed in neurons at the infarct border and inhibition of COX-2 activity improves ischemic brain damage. These results indicate that expression of iNOS and COX-2 contributes to the late stages of ischemic brain damage. Consequently, inhibition of iNOS and COX-2 could be a valuable addition to treatment strategies for ischemic stroke. Most efforts to date have targeted the acute phase of cerebral ischemia. Inhibition of iNOS or COX-2 offers the prospect of treatments directed to the late stages of the damage. However, additional preclinical studies would be necessary before these new treatment strategies can be tested in human stroke.

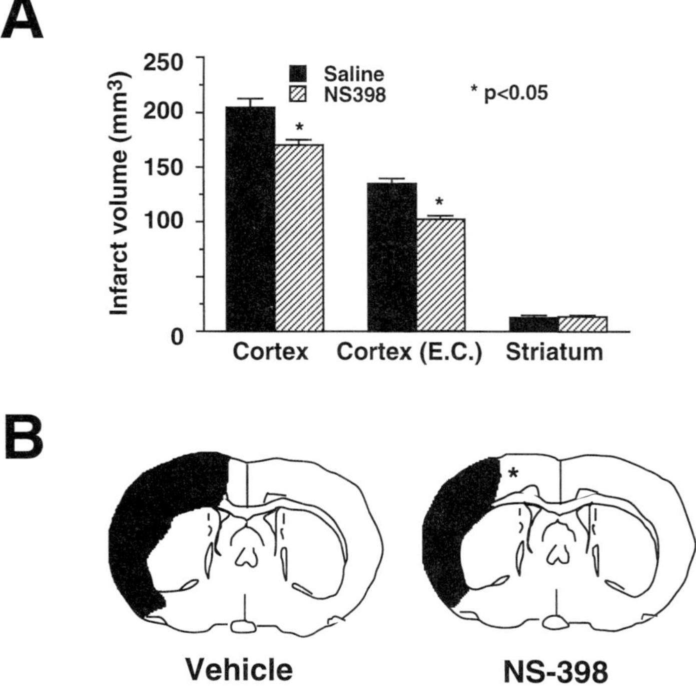

FIGURE 6. Effect of the relatively selective inhibitor of COX-2 NS398 on focal cerebral ischemic damage. NS398 was administered i.p. starting 6 h after permanent MCA occlusion in spontaneously hypertensive rats. (**A**) NS398 reduces the size of the infarct in the cerebral cortex but not in the striatum. The reduction in stroke size persists after correction for swelling (cortex E.C.). (**B**) Representative brain section illustrating the location of the tissue spared from infarction by NS398. The salvaged area is located at the medial border of the infarct. This region (*asterisk*) corresponds to the area in which COX-2 immunoreactive neurons are located following cerebral ischemia. The data support the hypothesis that NS398 blocks COX-2 activity in these neurons and prevents them from dying.

ACKNOWLEDGMENTS

This contribution is dedicated to Dr. F. Plum who taught us the importance of clinically relevant basic research. We thank Dr. D. J. Reis for his guidance and continued support and Dr. R. W. Price for providing the inspiration and encouragement for these studies. Drs. S. Nogawa and F. Zhang participated in the work described here. Ms. Karen MacEwan provided editorial assistance.

REFERENCES

1. HOSSMANN, K.-A. 1994. Viability thresholds and the penumbra of focal ischemia. Ann. Neurol. **36:** 557–565.

2. ASTRUP, J., L. SYMON, N. M. BRANSTON & N. A. LASSEN. 1977. Cortical evoked potential and extracellular K+ and H+ at critical levels of brain ischemia. Stroke **8:** 51–57.

3. ASTRUP, J., B. K. SIESJÖ & L. SYMON. 1981. Thresholds in cerebral ischemia—The ischemic penumbra. Stroke **6:** 723–725.

4. CHOI, D. W. 1990. Cerebral hypoxia: Some new approaches and unanswered questions. J. Neurosci. **10:** 2493–2501.

5. CHAN, P. H. 1996. Role of oxidants in ischemic brain damage. Stroke **27:** 1124–1129.

6. DERESKI, M. O., M. CHOPP, R. A. KNIGHT, L. C. RODOLOSI & J. H. GARCIA. 1993. The heterogeneous temporal evolution of focal ischemic neuronal damage in the rat. Acta Neuropathol. **85:** 327–333.

7. GARCIA, J. H., Y. YOSHIDA, H. CHEN, Y. LI, Z. G. ZHANG, J. LIAN, S. CHEN & M. CHOPP. 1993. Progression from ischemic injury to infarct following middle cerebral artery occlusion in the rat. Am. J. Pathol. **142:** 623–635.

8. HEISS, W.-D., M. HUBER, G. R. FINK, K. HERLOZ, U. PIETRZYK, R. WAGNER & K. WEINHARD. 1992. Progressive derangement of periinfarct viable tissue in ischemic stroke. J. Cereb. Blood Flow Metab. **12:** 193–203.

9. MARCHAL, G., V. BEAUDOUIN, P. RIOUX, V. DE LA SAYETTE, F. LE DOZE, F. VIADER, J.-M. DERLON & J.-C. BARON. 1996. Prolonged persistence of substantial volumes of potentially viable brain tissue after stroke. Stroke **27:** 599–606.

10. TOUZANI, O., A. R. YOUNG, J. M. DERLON, V. BEADOUIN, G. MARCHAL, P. RIOUX, F. MEZENGE, J. C. BARON & E. T. MACKENZIE. 1995. Sequential studies of severely hypometabolic tissue volumes after permanent middle cerebral occlusion: A positron emission tomographic investigation in anesthetized baboons. Stroke **26:** 2112–2119.

11. WARACH, S., J. GAA, B. SIEWERT, P. WIELOPOLSKI & R. R. EDELMAN. 1995. Acute human stroke studied by whole brain echo planar diffusion-weighted magnetic resonance imaging. Ann. Neurol. **37:** 231–241.

12. WELCH, K. M. A., J. WINDHAM, R. A. KNIGHT, V. NAGESH, J. W. HUGG, M. JACOBS, D. PECK, P. BOOKER, M. O. DERESKY & S. R. LEVINE. 1995. A model to predict the histopathology of human stroke using diffusion and T2-weighted magnetic resonance imaging. Stroke **26:** 1983–1989.

13. BARON, J.-C., R. VON KUMMER & G. J. DEL ZOPPO. 1995. Treatment of acute ischemic stroke. Challenging the concept of a rigid and universal time window. Stroke **26:** 2219–2221.

14. BILLER, J., J. T. PATRICK, A. SHEPARD & H. P. ADAMS. 1993. Delay time between onset of ischemic stroke and hospital arrival. J. Stroke Cerebrovasc. Dis. **3:** 228–230.

15. MARSHALL, R. S. & J. P. MOHR. 1993. Current management of ischaemic stroke. J. Neurol. Neurosurg. Psychiatry **56:** 6–16.

16. KIESSLING, M. & K.-A. HOSSMAN. 1994. Focal cerebral ischemia: Molecular mechanisms and new therapeutic strategies. Brain Pathol. **4:** 21–95.

17. UEMURA, Y., N. W. KOWALL & M. A. MOSKOWITZ. 1991. Focal ischemia in rats causes time-dependent expression of c-fos protein immunoreactivity in widespread regions of ipsilateral cortex. Brain Res. **552:** 99–105.

18. AN, G., T. N. LIN, J. S. LIU, J. J. XUE, Y. Y. HE & C. Y. HSU. 1993. Expression of c-fos and c-jun family genes after focal cerebral ischemia. Ann. Neurol. **33:** 457–464.

19. NOWAK, T. S. & M. JACEWICZ. 1994. The heat shock/stress response in focal cerebral ischemia. Brain Pathol. **4:** 67–76.

20. PLUM, F. 1983. What causes infarction in ischemic brain?: The Robert Wartenberg lecture. Neurology **33:** 222–233.

21. KINOUCHI, H., F. R. SHARP, M. P. HILL, J. KOISTINAHO, S. M. SAGAR & P. H. CHAN. 1993. Induction of 70-kDa heat shock protein and hsp70 mRNA following transient focal cerebral ischemia in the rat. J. Cereb. Blood Flow Metab. **13:** 105–115.

22. FEUERSTEIN, G. Z., T. LIU & F. C. BARONE. 1994. Cytokines, inflammation, and brain injury: Role of tumor necrosis factor-alpha. Cerebrovasc. Brain Metab. Rev. **6:** 341–360.

23. ROTHWELL, N. J. & P. J. STRIJBOS. 1995. Cytokines in neurodegeneration and repair. Int. J. Dev. Neurosci. **13:** 179–185.

24. FEUERSTEIN, G. Z., X. WANGE & F. C. BARONE. Inflammatory mediators and brain

injury: The role of cytokines and chemokines in stroke and CNS diseases. *In* Cerebrovascular Diseases. M. D. Ginsberg & J. Bogousslavsky, Eds. Blackwell Science. Cambridge, MA. In press.

25. MacManus, J. P., I. E. Hill, E. Preston, I. Rasquinha, T. Walker & A. M. Buchan. 1995. Differences in DNA fragmentation following transient ischemia or decapitation ischemia in rats. J. Cereb. Blood Flow Metab. **15:** 728–737.

26. Li, Y., M. Chopp, Z. G. Zhang, C. Zaloga, L. Niewenhuis & S. Gautam. 1994. p53-immunoreactive protein and p53 mRNA expression after transient middle cerebral artery occlusion in rats. Stroke **25:** 849–855.

27. Charriaut-Marlangue, C., I. Margaill, M. Plotkine & Y. Ben-Ari. 1995. Early endonuclease activation following reversible focal ischemia in the rat brain. J. Cereb. Blood Flow Metab. **15:** 385–388.

28. Kochanek, P. M. & J. M. Hallenbeck. 1992. Polymorphonuclear leukocytes and monocyte/macrophages in the pathogenesis of cerebral ischemia and stroke. Stroke **23:** 1367–1379.

29. Chen, H., M. Chopp, L. Schultz, G. Bodzin & J. H. Garcia. 1993. Sequential neuronal and astrocytic changes after transient middle cerebral artery occlusion in the rat. J. Neurol. Sci. **118:** 109–116.

30. Clark, R. K., E. V. Lee, C. J. Fish, R. F. White, W. J. Price, Z. L. Jonak & G. Z. Feuerstein. 1993. Development of tissue damage, inflammation and resolution following stroke: An immunohistochemical and quantitative planimetric study. Brain Res. Bull. **31:** 565–572.

31. Morioka, T., A. N. Kalehua & W. J. Streit. 1993. Characterization of microglial reaction after middle cerebral artery occlusion in the rat brain. J. Comp. Neurol. **327:** 123–132.

32. Garthwaite, J. & C. L. Boulton. 1995. Nitric oxide signaling in the central nervous system. Annu. Rev. Physiol. **57:** 683–706.

33. Iadecola, C. 1993. Regulation of the cerebral microcirculation during neural activity: Is nitric oxide the missing link? Trends Neurosci. **16:** 206–214.

34. Zhang, J. & S. H. Snyder 1995. Nitric oxide in the nervous system. Annu. Rev. Pharmacol. Toxicol. **35:** 213–233.

35. Bo, L., T. M. Dawson, S. Wesselingh, S. Mork, S. Choi, P. A. Kong, D. Hanley & B. D. Trapp. 1994. Induction of nitric oxide synthase in demyelinating regions of multiple sclerosis brains. Ann. Neurol. **36:** 778–786.

36. Cross, A. H., T. P. Misko, R. F. Lin, W. F. Hickey, J. L. Trotter & R. G. Tilton. 1994. Aminoguanidine, an inhibitor of inducible nitric oxide synthase, ameliorates experimental autoimmune encephalomyelitis in SJL mice. J. Clin. Invest. **93:** 2684–2690.

37. Dawson, V. L., T. M. Dawson, E. D. London, D. S. Bredt & S. H. Snyder. 1991. Nitric oxide mediates glutamate neurotoxicity in primary cortical cultures. Proc. Natl. Acad. Sci. USA **88:** 6368–6371.

38. Hewett, S. J., C. A. Csernansky & D. W. Choi. 1994. Selective potentiation of NMDA-induced neuronal injury following induction of astrocytic iNOS. Neuron **13:** 487–494.

39. Iadecola, C., F. Zhang & X. Xu. 1995. Inhibition of inducible nitric oxide synthase ameliorates cerebral ischemic damage. Am. J. Physiol. **268:** R286–R292.

40. Iadecola, C., F. Zhang, R. Casey, H. B. Clark & M. E. Ross. 1996. Inducible nitric oxide synthase gene expression in vascular cells following transient focal cerebral ischemia. Stroke **27:** 1373–1380.

41. Koprowski, H., Y. M. Zheng, K. E. Heber, N. Fraser, L. Rorke, Z. F. Fu, C. Hanlon & B. Dietzschold. 1993. In vivo expression of inducible nitric oxide synthase in experimentally induced neurologic diseases. Proc. Natl. Acad. Sci. USA **90:** 3024–3027.

42. Nowicki, J. P., D. Duval, H. Poignet & B. Scatton. 1991. Nitric oxide mediates neuronal death after focal cerebral ischemia in the mouse. Eur. J. Pharmacol. **204:** 339–340.

43. Hantraye, P., E. Brouillet, R. Ferrante, S. Palfi, R. Dolan, R. T. Matthews & M. F. Beal. 1996. Inhibition of neuronal nitric oxide synthase prevents MPTP-induced parkinsonism in baboons. Nature Med. **2:** 1017–1021.

44. HUANG, A., P. L. HUANG, N. PANAHIAN, T. DALKARA, M. C. FISHMAN & M. A. MOSKOWITZ. 1994. Effects of cerebral ischemia in mice deficient in neuronal nitric oxide synthase. Science **265:** 1883–1885.
45. NATHAN, C. 1995. Inducible nitric oxide synthase: Regulation subserves function. Curr. Top. Microbiol. Immunol. **196:** 1–4.
46. IADECOLA, C. 1997. Bright and dark sides of nitric oxide in ischemic brain damage. Trends Neurosci. **20:** 132–138.
47. ROSS, M. E. & C. IADECOLA. 1996. Nitric oxide synthase expression in cerebral ischemia: Neurochemical, immunocytochemical and molecular approaches. *In* Methods in Enzymology. L. Packer, Ed.: 408–426. Academic Press. Orlando, FL.
48. IADECOLA, C., F. ZHANG, X. XU, R. CASEY & M. E. ROSS. 1995. Inducible nitric oxide synthase gene expression in brain following focal cerebral ischemia. J. Cereb. Blood Flow Metab. **15:** 378–384.
49. IADECOLA, C., X. XU, F. ZHANG, E. E. EL-FAKAHANY & M. E. ROSS. 1995. Marked induction of calcium-independent nitric oxide synthase activity after focal cerebral ischemia. J. Cereb. Blood Flow Metab. **14:** 52–59.
50. ZHANG, F., R. CASEY, M. E. ROSS & C. IADECOLA. 1996. Aminoguanidine ameliorates and L-arginine worsens brain damage from intraluminal middle cerebral artery occlusion. Stroke **27:** 317–323.
51. MACMICKING, J. D., C. NATHAN, G. HOM, N. CHARTRAIN, D. S. FLETCHER, M. TRUMBAUER, K. STEVENS, Q. W. XIE, K. SOKOL, N. HUTCHINSON, H. CHEN & J. S. MUDGETT. 1995. Altered responses to bacterial infection and endotoxic shock in mice lacking inducible nitric oxide synthase. Cell **81:** 641–650.
52. IADECOLA, C., F. ZHANG, R. CASEY & M. E. ROSS. 1996. Knockout mice lacking the inducible nitric oxide synthase gene are resistant to cerebral ischemia. Soc. Neurosci. Abstr. **22:** 1693 (Abstr.).
53. IADECOLA, C., F. ZHANG, X. XU & T. MAK. 1996. Knockout mice lacking IRF1 transcription factor do not express inducible nitric oxide synthase and have smaller infarcts after middle cerebral artery occlusion. Stroke **27:** 27A (Abstr).
54. MELILLO, G., T. MUSSO, A. SICA, L. S. TAYLOR, G. W. COX & L. VARESIO. 1995. A hypoxia-responsive element mediates a novel pathway of activation of the inducible nitric oxide synthase promoter. J. Exp. Med. **182:** 1683–1693.
55. SMITH, W. L. & D. L. DEWITT. 1995. Biochemistry of prostaglandin endoperoxide H synthase-1 and synthase-2 and their differential susceptibility to nonsteroidal anti-inflammatory drugs. Semin. Nephrol. **15:** 179–194.
56. SEIBERT, K., J. MASFERRER, Y. ZHANG, S. GREGORY, G. OLSON, S. HAUSER, K. LEAHY, W. PERKINS & P. ISAKSON. 1995. Mediation of inflammation by cyclooxygenase-2. Agents Actions Suppl. **46:** 41–50.
57. KONTOS, H. A., E. P. WEI, J. T. POVLISHOCK, W. D. DIETRICH, C. J. MAGIERA & E. F. ELLIS. 1980. Cerebral arteriolar damage by arachidonic acid and prostaglandin G2. Science **209:** 1242–1245.
58. CHAN, P. H. & R. A. FISHMAN. 1980. Transient formation of superoxide radicals in polyunsaturated fatty acid-induced brain swelling. J. Neurochem. **35:** 1004–1007.
59. NOGAWA, S., F. ZHANG, E. ROSS & C. IADECOLA. 1997. Cyclooxygenase-2 gene expression in neurons contributes to ischemic brain damage. J. Neurosci. **17:** 27–46.
60. BREDER, C. D., D. DEWITT & R. P. KRAIG. 1995. Characterization of inducible cyclooxygenase in rat brain. J. Comp. Neurol. **355:** 296–315.
61. REITZ, D. B., J. J. LI, M. B. NORTON, E. J. REINHARD, J. T. COLLINS, G. D. ANDERSON, S. A. GREGORY, C. M. KOBOLDT, W. E. PERKINS, K. SEIBERT, *et al.* 1994. Selective cyclooxygenase inhibitors: Novel 1,2-diarylcyclopentenes are potent and orally active COX-2 inhibitors. J. Med. Chem. **37:** 3878–3881.
62. MASFERRER, J. L., B. S. ZWEIFEL, P. T. MANNING, S. D. HAUSER, K. M. LEAHY, W. G. SMITH, P. C. ISAKSON & K. SEIBERT. 1994. Selective inhibition of inducible cyclooxygenase 2 in vivo is antiinflammatory and nonulcerogenic. Proc. Natl. Acad. Sci. USA **91:** 3228–3232.
63. KNIGHT, R. A., M. O. DERESKI, J. A. HELPERN, R. J. ORDIDGE & M. CHOPP. 1994. Magnetic resonance imaging assessment of evolving focal cerebral ischemia. Comparison with histopathology in rats. Stroke **25:** 1252–1261.

Ketogenic Diet and the Brain

SAMI I. HARIK,[a,e] ALI S. AL-MUDALLAL,[b]
JOSEPH C. LaMANNA,[b] W. DAVID LUST,[c]
AND BARRY E. LEVIN[d]

[a]Department of Neurology
University of Arkansas College of Medicine
Little Rock, Arkansas

Departments of Neurology[b] and Neurosurgery[c]
Case Western Reserve University School of Medicine
Cleveland, Ohio

[d]Department of Neurosciences
New Jersey School of Medicine and Dentistry
Newark, New Jersey

INTRODUCTION

Clinical and basic neuroscientists have had an interest in ketogenic diets since the beginning of this century. The clinical interest in this subject was kindled by the observations of Wilder that ketosis induced by starvation or by ketogenic diet had a beneficial effect on seizures.[1] Later, clinical evidence confirmed this observation, and experiments in mice and rats demonstrated that diet-induced ketosis increased the threshold for electroshock convulsions.[2,3] Although the anticonvulsant effects of the ketogenic diet withstood the test of time, its use has declined with the introduction of effective antiepileptic medications. However, despite the plethora of such medications, there has been a recent resurgence of interest in the ketogenic diet for intractable seizure disorders particularly in infants and children.[4,5]

The mechanisms that underlie the anticonvulsant properties of ketogenic diets remain unknown. Chief among the hypotheses was brain acidosis, first proposed by Lennox in 1928.[6] Against this hypothesis were the findings of DeVivo *et al.* who reported similar creatine phosphokinase mass action ratios in the brains of rats receiving ketogenic diet and control rats, suggesting that the brain pH was not altered in diet-induced ketosis.[7] There is a paucity of direct measurements of brain intracellular pH in experimental animals or in human subjects taking ketogenic diets.

From the basic neuroscience standpoint, controversy exists as to whether the mammalian brain uses ketone bodies as substrates for a considerable portion of its oxidative metabolism. Under normal conditions, the mammalian brain relies almost entirely on glucose for its metabolism[8] although it has all the enzymes needed to metabolize ketone bodies (β-hydroxybutyrate and acetoacetate) as alternate sources of energy.[9] The landmark study by Owen *et al.* suggested, based on arteriovenous differences, that the adult human brain uses ketone bodies as the principal energy substrates during starvation, resulting in a remarkable decrease in brain

[e] Address correspondence to Sami I. Harik, M.D., University of Arkansas for Medical Sciences, Department of Neurology, 4301 W. Markham, Slot 500, Little Rock, AR 72205. E-mail: sharik@neurology.uams.edu

glucose consumption.[10] Despite this evidence for a glucose-sparing effect of ketonemia in starving humans, the cerebral metabolic rate for glucose (measured by the 2-deoxyglucose method) in awake rats was not significantly decreased when blood ketone bodies were elevated by short-term starvation and β-hydroxybutyrate infusions.[11]

Our objective in this paper is to review recent work from our laboratories that was aimed at resolving controversies that pertain to long-term diet-induced ketosis. Adult rats were maintained on a novel ketogenic diet that is avidly consumed by rats and which induced moderate elevations in blood β-hydroxybutyrate and acetoacetate levels for about six weeks. Two groups of control rats were used in all our experiments. The first group consumed regular laboratory chow, and the second group consumed a diet rich in carbohydrates (instead of fats) and had the same protein content as the ketogenic diet. At the end of the experiment, we measured intracellular brain pH, cerebral cortical metabolites, and regional cerebral metabolic rate for glucose in rats maintained on the ketogenic diet and in the control groups. The work reviewed here was recently published.[12,13]

METHODS

Adult male Wistar rats weighing about 325 g and housed in individual cages were divided into three groups. The first group received regular laboratory chow *ad libitum*. The second group received a ketogenic diet deriving about 90% of its caloric value from fat and 10% from protein (TABLE 1). To avoid excessive weight gain in these rats, we restricted their intake to 10 g of this diet per rat per day. To control for the lower protein content of the ketogenic diet, we employed a third group of rats that received a high-carbohydrate diet deriving about 10% of its caloric value from proteins and 78% from carbohydrates. The rats in groups 1 and 3 had unlimited access to their diets. Rats in all groups added weight to a comparable extent. At weekly intervals, the rats were weighed and samples of tail venous blood were obtained for measurement of β-hydroxybutyrate and acetoacetate. The rats were maintained on the different diets for about six weeks.

At the end of the experiment, some of the rats were used to determine the regional cerebral metabolic rate for glucose by the 2-deoxyglucose autoradiographic

TABLE 1. Caloric Composition of the Diets

	Regular Lab Chow[a]	Ketogenic[b]	High-CHO[c]
Protein	27%	10.4% (17.6%)	10.4% (10.2%)
Carbohydrate	56%	0%	78.1% (76.2%)
Fat	17%	89.6% (67.3%)	11.5% (5.0%)
Kcal/g of diet	3.50	6.76	3.90

Diet contents by weight are in parentheses.

[a] Values were estimated from the information supplied by the vendor.

[b] The ketogenic diet contained 100 g casein (80 mesh), 1.5 g DL-methionine, 50 g cellulose (BW200), 50 g corn oil, 338.5 g Crisco, 35 g salt mix S10001, 0.25 g vitamin mix V11501, and 2 g choline bitartrate.

[c] The high-carbohydrate diet contained 100 g casein (80 mesh), 1.5 g DL-methionine, 751.5 g dextrose, 50 g cellulose, 50 g corn oil, 35 g salt mix S10001, 10 g vitamin mix V10001 (which includes about 10 g of sucrose), and 2 g choline bitartrate.

(Table is from ref. 12.)

method.[14] In other rats, we measured cerebral metabolites by freeze trapping.[15] The frozen brains were removed in a cold box and samples of the parietal cortex were extracted and analyzed for glucose, glucose-6 phosphate, glycogen, lactate, citrate, β-hydroxybutyrate, acetoacetate, ATP, creatine phosphate, and γ-aminobutyric acid (GABA). Intracellular brain pH was measured in other rats by the neutral red technique.[16]

RESULTS

Rats in all groups gained weight to a comparable extent during the six weeks of the experiment. From preliminary observations, we knew that rats consuming the ketogenic diet had to be restricted to about 10 g of the high-fat diet per rat per day to prevent excessive weight gain relative to the other groups of rats that were given unlimited access to their diets. Because the weight gain was similar in all groups of rats, we assumed that the caloric consumption was likewise similar.

As expected, rats consuming the high-fat diet had significantly higher blood β-hydroxybutyrate and acetoacetate levels than rats in the other two groups. The higher blood concentrations of ketone bodies were evident at one week after starting the ketogenic diet, and the hyperketonemia stabilized after four weeks with blood β-hydroxybutyrate levels of about 0.5 mM and blood acetoacetate levels of about 0.2 mM, which were about 10-fold higher than those in the other groups of rats.[13] Except for the higher blood ketone bodies in rats maintained on the ketogenic diet, no differences were found in the physiologic variables, including plasma glucose levels and arterial pH, among the three groups of rats.[12,13]

No significant differences were found among the three groups of rats in their intracellular cerebral cortical pH (Fig. 1). Intracellular pH was measured at

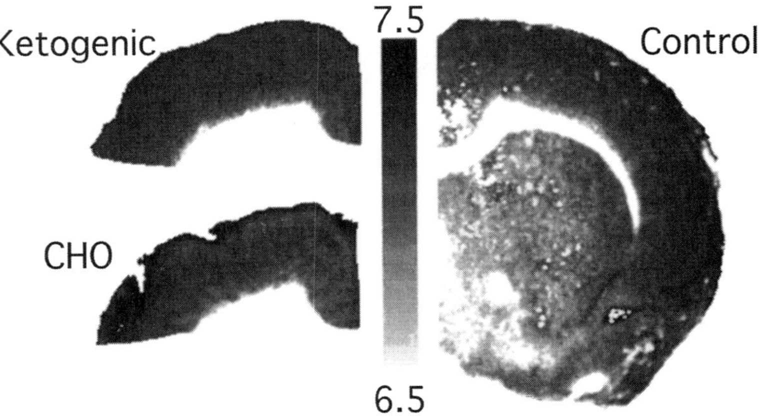

FIGURE 1. Right-hand portion of this figure shows half of a coronal brain section from a rat on regular lab chow. This is a digitalized optical density ratio image where the gray scale was calibrated to pH. Left-hand side of the figure depicts examples of the cerebral cortex from rats on the ketogenic diet (*top*) and the high-carbohydrate diet (*bottom*). A gray-scale calibration stripe from pH 6.5 to pH 7.5 is provided in the center. Darker areas represent more alkaline pH conditions. The pH of the cerebral cortex was similar in the three groups.

TABLE 2. Regional CMRglc Results[a]

Region	Regular Lab Chow	Ketogenic	High-CHO
Cerebral Cortex			
Sensorimotor	87.1 ± 10.5	76.2 ± 12.7	65.9 ± 2.1
Somatosensory	90.5 ± 10.1	73.2 ± 6.0	69.8 ± 4.8
Auditory	98.6 ± 7.7	96.5 ± 12.0	85.5 ± 7.7
Visual	86.8 ± 5.9	76.0 ± 5.7	57.0 ± 3.6[b]
Hippocampus	65.9 ± 8.8	56.9 ± 3.9	49.9 ± 5.5
Caudate-putamen	81.6 ± 5.8	63.6 ± 6.9	57.8 ± 3.1[b]
Medial geniculate	84.3 ± 5.2	78.7 ± 6.9	59.6 ± 2.7[b]
Superior colliculus	79.7 ± 6.0	71.7 ± 7.5	49.9 ± 3.5[b]

[a] Data are mean ± SEM values for regional glucose utilization (μmol · 100 gm^{-1} · min^{-1}) in five rats in each group. (Table is from ref. 12.)

[b] Denotes that the values for rats fed a high-carbohydrate diet were significantly different ($p < 0.05$) from the group fed regular lab chow by ANOVA and post hoc Scheffe test. No significant differences were found between the results of the ketogenic group and either of the two other groups.

7.01 ± 0.04 (mean ± SEM) in rats taking regular laboratory chow, 7.02 ± 0.05 in rats on the ketogenic diet, and 7.05 ± 0.03 in rats on the high-carbohydrate diet.[13] Also, there were no significant differences in cerebral levels of ATP, phosphocreatine or GABA among the three groups of rats (results not shown). Thus, diet-induced ketosis did not produce cerebral acidosis.

The regional cerebral metabolic rates for glucose in rats receiving regular laboratory chow were similar to those obtained in other studies in awake rats. We found no significant differences in regional cerebral metabolic rates for glucose between rats that were fed the ketogenic diet and rats maintained on regular laboratory chow. Thus, the ketogenic diet had no significant cerebral glucose-sparing effects in these rats. However, rats maintained on the high-carbohydrate diet had significantly lower regional cerebral metabolic rates for glucose in the visual cortex, caudate-putamen, medial geniculate, and superior colliculus than in the other groups of rats (TABLE 2). The trend in all other regions was for a lower metabolic rate for glucose in the brains of rats maintained on the high-carbohydrate diet.[12]

There were no significant differences in the cerebral levels of glucose, glycogen, lactate, and citrate among the three groups of rats (TABLE 3). However, cerebral

TABLE 3. Cerebral Cortical Metabolites[a]

	Regular Lab Chow	Ketogenic	High-CHO
Glucose	21.03 ± 1.01	22.73 ± 1.13	19.58 ± 2.24
Glycogen	29.40 ± 5.47	21.73 ± 7.22	21.78 ± 3.39
Glucose 6-phosphate	1.86 ± 0.64	1.70 ± 0.88	5.91 ± 1.64[b]
Lactate	14.50 ± 1.21	17.04 ± 1.26	19.36 ± 1.29
Citrate	3.57 ± 0.03	3.74 ± 0.32	3.45 ± 0.06
β-hydroxybutyrate	0.07 ± 0.03	0.75 ± 0.18[b]	0.19 ± 0.02

[a] Data represent means ± SEM in nmol of metabolite/mg cerebral cortex protein for three rats maintained on the regular lab chow and four rats maintained on each of the other two diets. (Table is from ref. 12.)

[b] Denotes significant differences ($p < 0.05$) from the other two groups using the Kruskal-Wallis nonparametric ANOVA followed by the Mann-Whitney test.

glucose 6-phosphate was two- to threefold higher in rats taking the high-carbohydrate diet (TABLE 3). As expected, brain hydroxybutyrate was severalfold higher in rats taking the ketogenic diet, indicating that the higher blood concentrations of β-hydroxybutyrate in these rats resulted in an abundance of this energy substrate in their brains.[12]

DISCUSSION

These experiments addressed several issues related to ketogenic and other unbalanced diets. The first was methodological; we describe a diet that induces moderate ketosis and that is avidly consumed by rats. Many previously used rat models of diet-induced ketosis entailed gastric gavage several times per day, a tedious and difficult procedure. In most models of diet-induced ketosis in rats and mice, the animals did not gain as much weight as controls. The ketogenic diet that we used was so avidly taken by the rats that we had to restrict access to it to prevent excessive weight gain. The ketogenic diet that we used induced only moderate ketonemia of about 0.75 mM although it contained a marginal amount of protein and no carbohydrates. In contrast, children consuming a ketogenic diet achieve ketonemia of 2–3 mM.[4] Thus, we believe that adult male Wistar rats do not achieve the robust ketonemia that is observed in children. A considerable amount of preliminary work was performed before we arrived at the final ketogenic diet described in TABLE 1. The protein content of the diet had to be decreased considerably to prevent gluconeogenesis. Increasing the fat content of the ketogenic diet to more than 90% would have produced a more robust ketosis but at the expense of further decreasing the protein content of the diet. It is important to note that the moderate ketosis that we obtained was not associated with hypoglycemia or with other abnormalities of measured physiological variables over the 6-week duration of the experiment.[12,13]

Another question was whether intracellular cerebral acidosis occurred in ketotic rats. Direct measurements of cerebral pH by the neutral red method demonstrated no evidence of cerebral acidosis (FIG. 1). The neutral red method was previously found to yield the same results as those obtained by [31P]nuclear magnetic resonance spectroscopy.[17] The lack of cerebral acidosis in ketotic rats is consistent with the findings of DeVivo et al. who calculated cerebral pH from creatine phosphokinase mass action ratios.[7] Davidian et al. also reported lack of cerebral acidosis in mice that were given a ketogenic diet for four weeks, which was supplemented twice daily with medium chain triglycerides given by stomach tube.[18] We did not find altered cerebral GABA levels in rats receiving the ketogenic diet. Thus, we believe that the antiseizure effects of the ketogenic diet are unlikely to be mediated by either cerebral acidosis or by increased cerebral GABA concentrations.

The third objective of our studies was to determine if the long-term provision of ketone bodies to the brain would result in their considerable use as substrates for cerebral metabolism, thereby decreasing the reliance of the brain on glucose as the major metabolic fuel. We conducted the study over several weeks to ensure facilitation of the blood-to-brain transport of ketone bodies and to allow the putative induction, if any, of brain enzymes that metabolize ketone bodies. Given that brain oxygen consumption is not altered by ketogenic diet[19,20] if ketone bodies were metabolized to a considerable extent by the brain of adult rats maintained on ketogenic diet, we would expect that these rats would decrease their cerebral metabolic rate for glucose. Despite the severalfold increase in the concentration of cerebral β-hydroxybutyrate in rats that were maintained on the ketogenic diet

(TABLE 3), no significant decreases were found in regional cerebral metabolic rates for glucose in these rats (TABLE 2). These findings suggest that ketone bodies, despite their availability, are not metabolized to a significant extent by the brain when glucose is available. It is possible that when glucose availability is limited, such as in the recently described clinical entity where glucose transport at the blood–brain barrier is defective,[21] then the brain would use ketone bodies. Another possible explanation for our findings is that ketone body metabolism by the brain does not affect glucose phosphorylation but may inhibit pyruvate metabolism and increase brain-to-blood pyruvate or lactate release. Against this latter possibility is the absence of increased cerebral lactate in rats consuming the ketogenic diet.

The unexpected finding from our study was the diminished regional cerebral metabolic rates for glucose in rats that were maintained on the high-carbohydrate diet (TABLE 2). This group of rats was intended as another control group for rats taking the ketogenic diet. The considerable reduction of about 25% in the overall brain glucose phosphorylation in rats maintained on the high-carbohydrate diet suggests cerebral metabolic dysfunction. The increased cerebral glucose 6-phosphate in these rats suggests inhibition of enzymes downstream from hexokinase and provides a good explanation for the decreased cerebral hexokinase activity which is measured by the 2-deoxyglucose method.

The decreased brain glucose utilization in rats receiving the high-carbohydrate diet occurred despite similar plasma glucose levels and comparable cerebral glucose and lactate levels in all three groups of rats. Thus, the decreased brain glucose utilization in rats maintained on the high-carbohydrate diet cannot be attributed to alterations in the "lump constant"[14] nor to changes in brain:plasma glucose ratios. It should be noted that all diets contained mineral and vitamin supplements, including a minimum of 0.1 mg of thiamine per rat per day (TABLE 1), so our results cannot be explained by simple vitamin deficiencies.

The mechanisms underlying the decreased regional cerebral metabolic rate for glucose in rats receiving the high-carbohydrate diet remain to be elucidated. Nonetheless, our results call attention to the similarities between the low cerebral metabolic rate for glucose in rats receiving the high-carbohydrate diet on the one hand and the encephalopathies that occurred in some World War II prisoners of war,[22,23] and in victims of the recent epidemic of neurologic disorders that afflicted some Cubans (adults and children)[24] on the other hand. Both clinical situations may have been caused by a diet that is marginal in its protein content and high in its carbohydrate content. The high-carbohydrate diet that we describe here may be a useful animal model for the study of the effects of poorly balanced diets on the growing and adult mammalian brain. Poor diets and other causes of malnutrition are a major worldwide health problem, particularly in less developed countries.

REFERENCES

1. WILDER, R. M. 1921. Effects of ketonuria on the course of epilepsy. Mayo Clin. Bull. **2:** 307–308.
2. UHLEMANN, E. R. & A. H. NEIMS. 1972. Anticonvulsant properties of the ketogenic diet in mice. J. Pharmacol. Exp. Ther. **180:** 231–238.
3. APPLETON, D. B. & D. C. DEVIVO. 1974. An animal model for the ketogenic diet. Epilepsia **15:** 211–227.
4. NORDLI, D. R., JR., D. KOENIGSBERGER, J. SCHROEDER & D. C. DEVIVO. 1992. Ketogenic diets. *In* The Medical Treatment of Epilepsy. S. R. Resor, Jr., Ed.: 455–471. Marcel Dekker. New York.

5. KINSMAN, S. L., E. P. G. VINING, S. A. QUASKEY, D. MELLITS & J. M. FREEMAN. 1992. Efficacy of the ketogenic diet for intractable seizure disorders: Review of 58 cases. Epilepsia **33(6):** 1132–1136.

6. LENNOX, W. G. 1928. Ketogenic diet in the treatment of epilepsy. N. Engl. J. Med. **199:** 74–75.

7. DEVIVO, D. C., M. P. LECKIE, J. S. FERRENDELLI & D. B. McDOUGAL, JR. 1978. Chronic ketosis and cerebral metabolism. Ann. Neurol. **3:** 331–337.

8. SIESJO, B. K. 1978. Brain Energy Metabolism.: 101–125. John Wiley & Sons. New York.

9. SOKOLOFF, L. 1973. Metabolism of ketone bodies by the brain. Annu. Rev. Med. **24:** 271–280.

10. OWEN, O. E., A. P. MORGAN, H. G. KEMP, J. M. SULLIVAN, M. G. HERRERA & G. J. CAHILL, JR. 1967. Brain metabolism during fasting. J. Clin. Invest. **46:** 1589–1595.

11. CORDDRY, D. H., S. I. RAPOPORT & E. D. LONDON 1982. No effect of hyperketonemia on local cerebral glucose utilization in conscious rats. J. Neurochem. **38:** 1637–1641.

12. AL-MUDALLAL, A. S., B. E. LEVIN, W. D. LUST & S. I. HARIK. 1995. Effects of unbalanced diets on cerebral glucose metabolism in the adult rat. Neurology **45:** 2261–2265.

13. AL-MUDALLAL, A. S., J. C. LAMANNA, W. D. LUST & S. I. HARIK. 1996. Diet-induced ketosis does not cause cerebral acidosis. Epilepsia **37:** 258–261.

14. SOKOLOFF, L., M. REIVICH, C. KENNEDY, *et al.* 1977. The [^{14}C]deoxyglucose method for the measurement of local cerebral glucose utilization: Theory, procedure, and normal values in conscious and anesthetized albino rats. J. Neurochem. **28:** 897–916.

15. LUST, W. D., A. J. RICCI, W. R. SELMAN & R. A. RATCHESON. 1989. Methods of fixation of nervous tissue for use in the study of cerebral energy metabolism. *In* Neuromethods, Vol. 11, Carbohydrates and Energy Metabolism. A. A. Boulton, G. B. Baker & R. F. Butterworth, Eds.: 1–41. Humana Press. Clifton, NJ.

16. LAMANNA, J. C., J. K. GRIFFITH, B. R. CORDISCO, C.-W. LIN & W. D. LUST. 1992. Intracellular pH in rat brain in vivo and in brain slices. Can. J. Physiol. Pharmacol. **70:** S269–S277.

17. GRIFFITH, J. K., B. R. CORDISCO, C.-W. LIN & J. C. LAMANNA. 1992. Distribution of intracellular pH in the rat brain cortex after global ischemia as measured by color film histophotometry of neutral red. Brain Res. **573:** 1–7.

18. DAVIDIAN, N. M., T. C. BUTLER & D. T. POOLE. 1978. The effect of ketosis induced by medium chain triglycerides on intracellular pH of mouse brain. Epilepsia **19:** 369–378.

19. HAWKINS, R. A., D. H. WILLIAMSON & H. A. KREBS. 1971. Ketone-body utilization by adult and suckling rat brain in vivo. Biochem. J. **122:** 13–18.

20. RUDERMAN, R. B., P. S. ROSS, M. BERGER & M. N. GOODMAN. 1974. Regulation of glucose and ketone-body metabolism in brain of anaesthetized rats. Biochem. J. **138:** 1–10.

21. DEVIVO, D. C., R. R. TRIFILETTI, R. I. JACOBSON, G. M. RONEN, R. A. BEHMAND & S. I. HARIK. 1991. Defective glucose transport across the blood-brain barrier as a cause of persistent hypoglycorrhachia, seizures, and developmental delay. N. Engl. J. Med. **325:** 703–709.

22. DENNY-BROWN, D. E. 1946. Neurological conditions resulting from prolonged and severe dietary restriction (case reports in prisoners-of-war, and general review). Medicine **26:** 41–113.

23. SPILLANE, J. D. 1947. Nutritional Disorders of the Nervous System. Livingstone. Edinburgh, UK.

24. ROMAN, G. C. 1994. Epidemic neuropathy in Cuba: A plea to end the United States economic embargo on a humanitarian basis. Neurology **44:** 1784–1786.

Nitroxidergic Transmission in the Nucleus Tractus Solitarii[a]

W. T. TALMAN[b]

Neurology Service
Department of Veterans Affairs Medical Center
and
Departments of Neurology and Neuroscience
University of Iowa
Iowa City, Iowa 52246

INTRODUCTION

Over the past two decades many studies have led to a totally new concept of signal transduction. It is now appreciated that the radical nitric oxide (NO·), produced by constitutive nitric oxide synthase (NOS), may play an important role in endothelium-derived relaxation[1,2] and in inhibition of platelet aggregation.[3] More recently, investigations have suggested that NO· may also participate as an interneuronal messenger.[4] The idea that a soluble gas might act on target neurons after freely passing through their cell membranes was first met with considerable skepticism,[5,6] but now it has wide acceptance.[6] Although understanding of signal transduction mechanisms underlying such transmission is incomplete, activation of the cytoplasmic enzyme soluble guanylate cyclase (sGC) with formation of cyclic GMP (cGMP) is known to play a role.[7] Some have suggested that sGC, through which NO· may in part mediate its actions, may serve as a "receptor" for the molecule.[8] Classic receptor mechanisms of neurotransmission are thought to be unnecessary. Through this putative signal transduction mechanism, NO· has been thought to contribute to synaptic transmission both in the central and in the peripheral nervous system.[4,9]

A major contribution to the hypothesized role of NO· in neurotransmission came with studies suggesting that activation of the *N*-methyl-D-aspartate (NMDA) receptor leads to release of NO· from central neuronal processes.[10,11] Likewise, activation of NMDA receptors was found to be associated with activation of sGC and formation of cGMP.[12]

In earlier studies we showed that activation of NMDA receptors within the nucleus tractus solitarii (NTS), the primary site of termination of cardiovascular afferent nerves, leads to prominent changes in arterial blood pressure and heart rate and that NMDA receptors are integral to the baroreceptor reflex.[13] Studies from other laboratories also suggested that nitroxidergic mechanisms play a role

[a] This work was supported in part by a Department of Veterans Affairs Clinical Investigatorship and Merit Review and by grants from the National Institutes of Health, R01-HL32205 and PO1-HL14388.

[b] Address correspondence to William T. Talman, M.D., Department of Neurology, University of Iowa, Iowa City, IA 52242. E-mail: william-talman@uiowa.edu

in cardiovascular control through the NTS.[14-18] Therefore, we sought to test that hypothesis and to determine whether NO·, administered into the NTS, elicits cardiovascular responses.

EVIDENCE FOR NITROXIDERGIC NEURONAL ELEMENTS IN NUCLEUS TRACTUS SOLITARII

We recently extended work also done by others and showed that mechanisms for biosynthesis of NO· are present in the NTS.[19] We used three methods to demonstrate that NOS was present in NTS neurons and terminal fields. First, NADPH diaphorase was stained with nitroblue tetrazolium. This technique is felt to correlate *generally* with other methods for visualizing the location of NOS;[20-22] however, to confirm more directly the presence of the protein we also used immunohistochemical methods with an antibody (Transduction Labs, Lexington, KY) to rat neuronal NOS. Finally, to confirm that NOS may be produced in the NTS we also used techniques of *in situ* hybridization for NOS mRNA. The cDNA probe was provided by Dr. David Bredt. These studies provide evidence that NO· may be synthesized in NTS. The physiological relevance of nitroxidergic pathways in NTS has been suggested by others who have shown that NOS is reduced in the NTS after removal of a nodose ganglion.[15,18] Thus, vagal afferents, some of which may contribute to cardiovascular reflex transmission, may synthesize NO·. However, in addition to formation of the radical itself, NOS in the NTS could also lead to synthesis of other NO·-containing compounds. For example, S-nitrosothiols could be expected to rapidly form as a result of nitrosation of thiol groups by NO⁺, one of the redox products of NO· itself.[23,24] Indeed, one recent report provided direct evidence for synthesis of S-nitrosothiols by brain.[25]

ACTIONS OF NITRIC OXIDE DONORS IN THE NUCLEUS TRACTUS SOLITARII

Because NO· itself is extremely labile and because NO· could be found in brain as an S-nitrosothiol, we initially sought to evaluate effects elicited by the radical. We microinjected (25–50 nL) NO· donors unilaterally into the NTS of adult male Sprague-Dawley rats that were anesthetized with chloralose (60 mg/kg followed by 20 mg/kg/h). Microinjection of S-nitrosocysteine (SNC), an S-nitrosothiol known to release NO·, led to cardiovascular responses that were similar to those elicited when glutamate or NMDA was injected into the NTS.[13,26,27] Others have reported similar findings when injections were made into the NTS of conscious rats.[28,29] Although these results were consistent with a role for NO· in NTS, we extended the studies to the effects produced by microinjecting other NO· donors at homologous sites in NTS. In contrast to the responses produced by SNC, microinjection into NTS of S-nitrosoglutathione (GSNO), S-nitrosoacetylpenicillamine (SNAP), sodium nitroprusside (SNP) or glyceryltrinitrate (GTN) did not produce responses like those produced by S-nitrosocysteine (250 pmoles). The doses of these compounds ranged between 10 and 1000 pmoles. One of the compounds, glyceryltrinitrate, actually elicited small pressor responses and never produced depressor responses. Direct microinjection of a concentrated solution of NO· itself did not significantly alter either arterial pressure or heart rate. Because NO· is extremely labile, it was possible that the injectate might no longer have contained the gas in solution when the injection was made. Therefore, we made similar injections from the same injection system into a closed tube filled with nitrogen and measured NO· in the headspace by the chemiluminescence technique.[30] These studies confirmed that NO· persisted in the injectate in concentrations of approximately 2 mM, 200 μM, and 100 μM. The maximal concentration (2 mM) of NO· was limited by the gas-water partition coefficient.

A UNIQUE ROLE FOR S-NITROSOCYSTEINE IN THE NUCLEUS TRACTUS SOLITARII

Because SNC was the only S-nitrosothiol that elicted pronounced changes in arterial pressure and heart rate when injected into NTS, we sought to determine whether responses to the compound differed if the dextro- or levoisomer of the parent thiol cysteine were used in the synthesis of SNC. We found that L-SNC elicited dose-dependent (10 to 250 pmoles) depressor and bradycardic responses that were significantly greater than those elicited by injection of the dextroisomer (D-SNC) at the same site.[31] For example, L-SNC at a dose of 250 pmoles elicited a 300% greater decrease of arterial pressure than did D-SNC at the same dose (see FIG. 1).

The differing responses to the two isomers could have resulted if differing amounts of NO· were released when the compounds were introduced into the NTS. Two assays, one biological and one chemical, were used to address this issue. In the bioassay, dose-related responses of arterial pressure and heart rate were determined when L-SNC and D-SNC were injected intravenously in anesthetized rats. The vasodilatation produced under such circumstances is accepted as being the result of NO· release. In our studies the dose-related depressor responses were identical. In contrast to responses seen with injections into NTS, the depressor responses elicited by i.v. injection were associated with reflex tachycardia. In the chemical assay we again used chemiluminescence to analyze the amount of NO· in the headspace and found that L- and D-SNC released identical amounts of NO· when exposed to homogenates of whole-brain tissue. Thus, responses elicited by L- and D-SNC did not differ because of different amounts of NO· being released by the two isomers. In these experiments, as with all the S-nitrosothiol studies, the compounds were always freshly prepared by standard techniques[32] prior to each experiment. Synthesis was confirmed by spectrophotometry.

The foregoing data did not support our hypothesis that NO· was itself acting in NTS to produce cardiovascular responses. We sought to further test whether NO· released by L-SNC into the extracellular space mediated responses to the S-nitrosothiol. Reduced, or oxy- (Fe^{++}), hemoglobin was used to "scavenge" NO· that might have been released from L-SNC. L-SNC (250 pmoles) was injected both before and after microinjection of oxyhemoglobin at the same site. Neither a dose of 5 pmoles ($n = 5$) nor a dose of 40 pmoles ($n = 6$) had any effect on responses to L-SNC. In that a 40-pmole dose could have scavenged as much as 160 pmoles of NO·, this dose should have significantly reduced responses to L-SNC if those responses were the result of actions of NO·.

Cleavage of an S-nitrosothiol yields the disulfide cystine as well as nitrogen monoxide. Therefore, we sought to determine whether cystine was responsible for the actions of L-SNC. Microinjection of cystine (50–500 pmoles; $n = 4$) into the NTS had no significant effect on either arterial pressure or heart rate. However, microinjection of L-cysteine ($n = 6$) itself produced dose-dependent (threshold dose

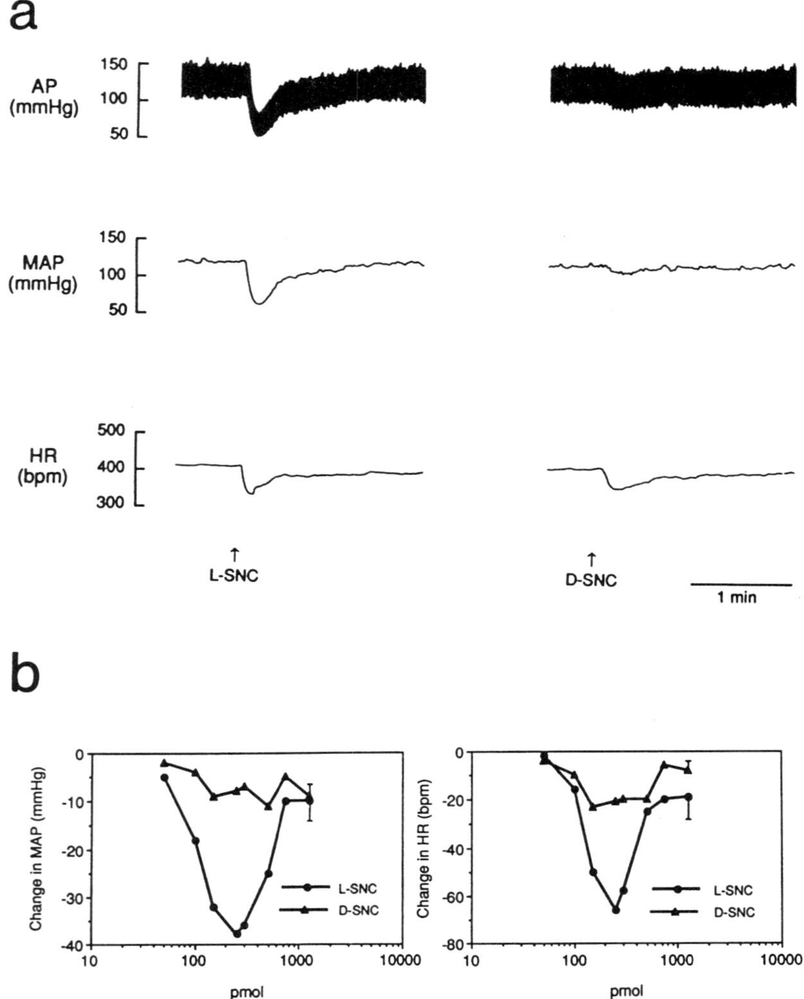

FIGURE 1. (a) Microinjection (50 nL) into the NTS of L-S-nitrosocysteine (L-SNC; 150 pmoles, *left*) elicits greater reductions of pulsatile arterial pressure (AP), mean arterial pressure (MAP), and heart rate (HR) than does microinjection of D-S-nitrosocysteine (D-SNC; 150 pmoles, *right*). Microinjections were made unilaterally into the NTS of rats that were anesthetized with chloralose. **(b)** Dose-related reductions of MAP (*left*) and HR (*right*) elicited by microinjection of L-SNC are significantly greater than those elicited by D-SNC. Doses of L-SNC from 100 to 500 pmoles elicited significant ($p < 0.05$) responses in six rats. (From Ohta et al.[31] Reprinted with permission of *Brain Research*.)

50 pmoles; maximally effective dose 500 pmoles) changes in both variables. If L-SNC were acting through its cysteine moiety, it might be expected to elicit its responses through activation of excitatory amino acid receptors that are found in abundance in NTS. However, although responses to L-cysteine (200 pmoles) were abolished by injection into NTS of the excitatory amino acid antagonist kynurenic acid, responses to L-SNC (250 pmoles) were not affected. The dose of kynurenic acid (1 nmole) would be expected to selectively affect responses to ionotropic excitatory amino acid agonists in the NTS.[13,27]

Although L-SNC did not seem to be acting through excitatory amino acid receptors, it might still have led to synthesis of NO$^{\cdot}$ and consequent activation of sGC in target cells.[11] Indeed, when the sGC inhibitor methylene blue (250 pmoles) was injected into NTS prior to L-SNC, responses to L-SNC were significantly reduced.[33] Microinjection of methylene blue bilaterally into NTS also attenuated the Bezold Jarisch reflex elicited by intravenous infusion of serotonin.[34] These data suggested that L-SNC, like NO$^{\cdot}$, may be acting through sGC. However, because methylene blue may also inhibit NOS,[35] we sought to determine whether blockade of NOS by injection of L-nitroarginine methyl ester (L-NAME; 1 μmole) into the NTS altered responses to L-SNC (250 pmoles) injected at the same site up to 60 min later. The inhibitor had no effect on responses to L-SNC (250 pmoles).

In sum, the data from our experiments suggested that SNC may be mediating cardiovascular responses through stereospecific actions in NTS and that those actions were independent of release of NO$^{\cdot}$ into the extracellular space. In support of SNC's acting as a more classic neurotransmitter, our recent work has demonstrated that synaptosomal fractions of whole-brain homogenates demonstrate saturable, specific binding of GSNO that is displaced by SNC.[36] Thus, SNC may act in brain through mechanisms that are similar to those mediating the actions of more classic neurotransmitters.

In further physiologic studies we have found that GSNO, which did not elicit cardiovascular responses when injected into the NTS but did compete with SNC for binding, may be an endogenous antagonist for S-nitrosothiol binding sites. Depressor and bradycardic responses elicited by SNC injected into the NTS were significantly reduced by microinjection of GSNO at the same site.

COMPARISONS WITH OTHER STUDIES OF NITROXIDERGIC MECHANISMS IN NUCLEUS TRACTUS SOLITARII

For the most part, studies of the physiologic relevance of nitroxidergic mechanisms in cardiovascular reflex control by the NTS have used indirect means. For example, one such study made efforts to increase the amount of NO$^{\cdot}$ produced in NTS by injecting the NO$^{\cdot}$ precursor L-arginine and showed the injection led to decreased arterial pressure and heart rate.[17] NOS does act on L-arginine to synthesize NO$^{\cdot}$; therefore the study was thought to support a role for NO$^{\cdot}$ in cardiovascular control by the NTS. Although increased NO$^{\cdot}$ may have resulted from the injections, the study does not conclusively show that the cardiovascular responses were due to NO$^{\cdot}$. Instead, the presumably augmented NO$^{\cdot}$ synthesis may have in turn led to increased production of S-nitrosothiols. Under these circumstances, an S-nitrosothiol, like SNC, could have been responsible for the responses seen. In support of such a chain of events, thiols are found in abundance in biological tissues where concentrations of cysteine and gluthathione may be among the highest.[37] Other studies suggest a role for NO$^{\cdot}$ in the NTS because of the cardiovascular effects of NOS inhibitors administered into the nucleus.[14,38] However, the difficulty measuring authentic NO˙ and SNC in biological samples[25] makes it imprudent to directly apply these findings to NO˙ as the end product of NOS.

Our studies suggest that NO˙ itself does not elicit cardiovascular and autonomic responses when released into NTS and that those responses reported with administration of NO˙ precursors or inhibitors may be the result of production of an S-nitrosothiol such as SNC. Actions produced by SNC may in turn follow binding of the compound to a site on target cell membranes. Thus, the actions of SNC would be directed toward cells that contain binding sites and would differ from NO˙ for which there are no recognized classic receptors. Indeed, it is unclear how specificity of action might occur with NO˙ signal transduction. The radical may diffuse up to 1000 μm from a point source[5,39,40] and, therefore, could affect two million or more synapses in the neighborhood of the cell from which it is released.[5] If sGC were the only second messenger through which NO˙ acts, specificity of action could occur if NO˙-generating, NOS-positive, nerve elements were adjacent to nerve elements that contain sGC and form cGMP.[8] However, although presynaptic terminals that contain one of the enzymes are often adjacent to postsynaptic membranes that contain the other,[8] exceptions have been described.[22,41]

In fact, there would be no necessity to have such close apposition of the source with the site of action if NO˙ diffused great distances from its site of release. On the other hand, a terminal adjacent to a target cell membrane would be consistent with release of a transmitter, perhaps an S-nitrosothiol, that acts at a more traditional receptor. In such a case the signal transduction mechanisms beyond the receptor may in some case be through sGC, whereas in other cases another mechanism would prevail. NO˙ then could play a role as a constituent of a more classic transmitter but could, under other circumstances and in other locations, act as a freely diffusible independent neuronal messenger.

NO˙, which has a half-life measured in seconds,[42] rapidly forms peroxynitrites, NO$^+$ and NO$^-$.[24,43] This extreme lability of the diffusible messenger would greatly limit the extent of the molecule's effects and contribute to its specificity of action, but another contribution might obtain as a result of the altered redox state of NO˙. One of the potential mechanisms of action of NO˙ relies upon a one electron transfer and formation of the nitrosonium NO$^+$ ion which, unlike NO˙, readily nitrosylates thiols to form S-nitrosothiols.[23,24] As suggested in this paper, formation of S-nitrosothiols may provide another avenue for specific actions of NO˙. Because thiols—particularly cysteine, glutathione, and protein thiols—are major components of biological systems where they are found in concentrations of 1–10 mM,[37] rapid formation of S-nitrosothiols could be expected upon synthesis of NO˙.[37] Once formed, these S-nitrosothiols could concentrate in the cell of origin, the extracellular fluid, or target cells where they could serve as a reservoir of NO˙[44] or even a stored form of transmitter. Recent studies have confirmed that brain synthesizes S-nitrosothiols when presented with native thiols.[25] Such S-nitrosothiol synthesis would naturally occur in regions like the NTS where NO˙ itself is synthesized through actions of NOS on L-arginine.[45]

Although these endogenous S-nitrosothiols could certainly release NO˙, they could also independently participate in cell-to-cell signaling.[46] Like NO˙ these compounds are also labile but, unlike NO˙, they may be stored and released in response to stimuli.[47] Even though the compounds may produce many of the same physiological responses as NO˙ and might be thought to manifest their physiological activity through release of NO˙, their actions have been shown to be unrelated to the speed with which they release NO˙.[46] Furthermore, although some S-nitrosothiols pass quickly through cell membranes[32] and, like NO˙, activate sGC,[32,47] membrane transport is not essential for their action.[32]

CONCLUSION

Our studies do not eliminate a role for NO˙ in transmission in NTS, but they do suggest that S-nitrosothiols may contribute to cell-to-cell signaling independent of their acting as NO˙ donors. We conjecture that S-nitrosothiols, acting at distinct binding sites, participate in transmission of cardiovascular reflex signals in the NTS of rats. It is unclear whether S-nitrosothiols contribute similarly to signal transduction at other central sites.

ACKNOWLEDGMENTS

The following colleagues have contributed to the scientific publications that are reviewed in this chapter: Drs. James Bates, Stephen Lewis, Li-Hsien Lin, Benedito Machado, Hisashi Ohta, Jun-ichi Taguchi, and Ming Yin.

REFERENCES

1. FURCHGOTT, R. F. & P. M. VANHOUTTE. 1989. Endothelium-derived relaxing and contracting factors. FASEB J. **3:** 2007–2018.
2. AMEZCUA, J. L., G. J. DUSTING, R. M. J. PALMER & S. MONCADA. 1988. Acetylcholine induces vasodilatation in the rabbit isolated heart through the release of nitric oxide, the endogenous nitrovasodilator. Br. J. Pharmacol. **95:** 830–834.
3. RADOMSKI, M. W., R. M. J. PALMER & S. MONCADA. 1987. The role of nitric oxide and cGMP in platelet adhesion to vascular endothelium. Br. J. Pharmacol. **92:** 181–187.
4. DAWSON, T. M., V. L. DAWSON & S. H. SNYDER. 1992. A novel neuronal messenger molecule in brain: The free radical, nitric oxide. Ann. Neurol. **32:** 297–311.
5. GARTHWAITE, J. 1995. Neural nitric oxide signalling. Trends Neurosci. **18:** 51–52.
6. NATHAN, C. & Q. XIE. 1994. Nitric oxide synthases: Roles, tolls, and controls. Cell **78:** 915–918.
7. KNOWLES, R. G., M. PALACIOS, R. M. J. PALMER & S. MONCADA. 1989. Formation of nitric oxide from L-arginine in the central nervous system: A transduction mechanism for stimulation of the soluble guanylate cyclase. Proc. Natl. Acad. Sci. USA **86:** 5159–5162.
8. SOUTHAM, E. & J. GARTHWAITE. 1993. The nitric oxide-cyclic GMP signalling pathway in rat brain. Neuropharmacol. **32:** 1267–1277.
9. DE MAN, J. G., P. A. PELCKMANS, G. E. BOECKXSTAENS, H. BULT, L. OOSTER-BOSCH, A. G. HERMAN & Y. M. VAN MAERCKE. 1991. The role of nitric oxide in inhibitory non-adrenergic non-cholinergic neurotransmission in the canine lower oesophageal sphincter. Br. J. Pharmacol. **103:** 1092–1096.
10. GARTHWAITE, J., G. GARTHWAITE, R. M. PALMER & S. MONCADA 1989. NMDA receptor activation induces nitric oxide synthesis from arginine in rat brain slices. Eur. J. Pharmacol. **172:** 413–416.
11. EAST, S. J. & J. GARTHWAITE. 1991. NMDA receptor activation in rat hippocampus induces cyclic GMP formation through the L-arginine-nitric oxide pathway. Neurosci. Lett. **123:** 17–19.
12. SOUTHAM, E., S. J. EAST & J. GARTHWAITE. 1991. Excitatory amino acid receptors coupled to the nitric oxide/cyclic GMP pathway in rat cerebellum during development. J. Neurochem. **56:** 2072–2081.
13. OHTA, H. & W. T. TALMAN. 1994. Both NMDA and non-NMDA receptors in the NTS participate in the baroreceptor reflex in rats. Am. J. Physiol. **267:** R1065–R1070.
14. HARADA, S., S. TOKUNAGA, M. MOMOHARA, H. MASAKI, T. TAGAWA, T. IMAIZUMI & A. TAKESHITA. 1993. Inhibition of nitric oxide formation in the nucleus tractus solitarius increases renal sympathetic nerve activity in rabbits. Circ. Res. **72:** 511–516.

15. LÜ, Y., Y.-Q. DING, B.-Z. QIN & J.-S. LI. 1994. The distribution and origin of axon terminals with NADPH diaphorase activity in the nucleus of the solitary tract of the rat. Neurosci. Lett. **171:** 70–72.

16. ZANZINGER, J., J. CZACHURSKI & H. SELLER. 1995. Effects of nitric oxide on sympathetic baroreflex transmission in the nucleus tractus solitarii and caudal ventrolateral medulla in cats. Neurosci. Lett. **197:** 199–202.

17. TSENG, C. J., H. Y. LIU, H. C. LIN, L. P. GER, C. S. TUNG & M. H. YEN. 1996. Cardiovascular effects of nitric oxide in the brain stem nuclei of rats. Hypertension **27:** 36–42.

18. RUGGIERO, D. A., E. P. MTUI, K. OTAKE & M. ANWAR. 1996. Central and primary visceral afferents to nucleus tractus solitarii may generate nitric oxide as a membrane-permeant neuronal messenger. J. Comp. Neurol. **364:** 51–67.

19. LIN, L.-H., S. BOUTELLE, A. SANDRA & W. T. TALMAN. 1995. Changes in expression of nitric oxide synthase in the dorsal vagal complex after nodose ganglionectomy or vagotomy in rat. Soc. Neurosci. Abstr. **21:** 625 (Abstr.).

20. HOPE, B. T., G. J. MICHAEL, K. M. KNIGGE & S. R. VINCENT. 1991. Neuronal NADPH diaphorase is a nitric oxide synthase. Proc. Natl. Acad. Sci. USA **88:** 2811–2814.

21. NAKOS, G. & R. GOSSRAU. 1994. When NADPH diaphorase (NADPHd) works in the presence of formaldehyde, the enzyme appears to visualize selectively cells with constitutive nitric oxide synthase (NOS). Acta Histochem. **96:** 335–343.

22. SCHMIDT, H. H. H. W., G. D. GAGNE, M. NAKANE, J. S. POLLOCK, M. F. MILLER & F. MURAD. 1992. Mapping of neural nitric oxide synthase in the rat suggests frequent co-localization with NADPH diaphorase but not with soluble guanylyl cyclase, and novel paraneural functions for nitrinergic signal transduction. J. Histochem. Cytochem. **40:** 1439–1456.

23. STAMLER, J. S. 1994. Redox signaling: Nitrosylation and related target interactions of nitric oxide. Cell **78:** 931–936.

24. STAMLER, J. S., D. J. SINGEL & J. LOSCALZO. 1992. Biochemistry of nitric oxide and its redox-activated forms. Science **258:** 1898–1902.

25. KLUGE, I., U. GUTTECK-AMSLER, M. CUÉNOD & K. Q. DO. 1995. S-nitrosoglutathione is endogenous in rat cerebellum. Soc. Neurosci. Abstr. **21:** 626 (Abstr.).

26. LEWIS, S. J., H. OHTA, B. H. MACHADO, J. N. BATES & W. T. TALMAN. 1991. Microinjection of S-nitrosocysteine into the nucleus tractus solitarii decreases arterial pressure and heart rate via activation of soluble guanylate cyclase. Eur. J. Pharmacol. **202:** 135–136.

27. TALMAN, W. T. 1989. Kynurenic acid microinjected into the nucleus tractus solitarius of rat blocks the arterial baroreflex but not responses to glutamate. Neurosci. Lett. **102:** 247–252.

28. MACHADO, B. H. & L. G. H. BONAGAMBA. 1992. Microinjection of S-nitrosocysteine into the nucleus tractus solitarii of conscious rats decreases arterial pressure but L-glutamate does not. Eur. J. Pharmacol. **221:** 179–182.

29. LEWIS, S. J., R. L. DAVISSON, J. N. BATES, A. K. JOHNSON, H. OHTA & W. T. TALMAN. 1992. Stereoselective actions of S-nitrosocysteine (SNC) suggests the presence of specific S-nitrosothiol receptors. FASEB J. **6:** A1165 (Abstr.).

30. MYERS, P. R., R. L. MINOR, JR., R. GUERRA, JR., J. N. BATES & D. G. HARRISON. 1990. Vasorelaxant properties of the endothelium-derived relaxing factor more closely resemble S-nitrosocysteine than nitric oxide. Nature **345:** 161–163.

31. OHTA, H., J. N. BATES, S. J. LEWIS & W. T. TALMAN. 1997. Actions of S-nitrosocysteine in the nucleus tractus solitarii are unrelated to release of nitric oxide. Brain Res. **746:** 98–104.

32. MATHEWS, W. R. & S. W. KERR. 1993. Biological activity of S-nitrosothiols: The role of nitric oxide. J. Pharmacol. Exp. Ther. **267:** 1529–1537.

33. MARTIN, W., G. M. VILLANI, D. JOTHIANADAN & R. F. FURCHGOTT. 1985. Selective blockade of endothelium-dependent and glyceryl trinitrate-induced relaxation by hemoglobin and by methylene blue in the rabbit aorta. J. Pharmacol. Exp. Ther. **232:** 708–716.

34. LEWIS, S. J., B. H. MACHADO, H. OHTA & W. T. TALMAN. 1991. Processing of cardiopulmonary afferent input within the nucleus tractus solitarii involves activation of soluble guanylate cyclase. Eur. J. Pharmacol. **203:** 327–328.

35. MAYER, B., F. BRUNNER & K. SCHMIDT. 1993. Inhibition of nitric oxide synthesis by methylene blue. Biochem. Pharmacol. **45:** 367–374.
36. TAGUCHI, J., H. OHTA & W. T. TALMAN. 1995. Identification and pharmacological characterization of an S-nitrosoglutathione binding site in rat brain. Soc. Neurosci. Abstr. **21:** 626 (Abstr.).
37. ARNELLE, D. R. & J. S. STAMLER. 1995. NO^+, NO^x, and NO^- donation by S-nitrosothiols: Implications for regulation of physiological functions by S-nitrosylation and acceleration of disulfide formation. Arch. Biochem. Biophys. **318:** 279–285.
38. MA, S., F. M. ABBOUD & R. B. FELDER. 1995. Effects of L-arginine-derived nitric oxide synthesis on neuronal activity in nucleus tractus solitarius. Am. J. Physiol. **268:** R487–R491.
39. GARTHWAITE, J. & C. L. BOULTON. 1995. Nitric oxide signaling in the central nervous system. Annu. Rev. Physiol. **57:** 683–706.
40. SCHUMAN, E. M. & D. V. MADISON. 1994. Nitric oxide and synaptic function. Annu. Rev. Neurosci. **17:** 153–183.
41. ZHANG, J. & S. H. SNYDER. 1995. Nitric oxide in the nervous system. Annu. Rev. Pharmacol. Toxicol. **35:** 213–233.
42. FEELISCH, M., M. TE POEL, R. ZAMORA, A. DEUSSEN & S. MONCADA. 1994. Understanding the controversy over the identity of EDRF. Nature **368:** 62–65.
43. PRYOR, W. A. & G. L. SQUADRITO. 1995. The chemistry of peroxynitrite: A product from the reaction of nitric oxide with superoxide. Am. J. Physiol. **268:** L699–L722.
44. STAMLER, J. S., O. JARAKI, J. OSBORNE, D. I. SIMON, J. KEANEY, J. VITA, D. SINGEL, C. R. VALERI & J. LOSCALZO. 1992. Nitric oxide circulates in mammalian plasma primarily as an S-nitroso adduct of serum albumin. Proc. Natl. Acad. Sci. USA **89:** 7674–7677.
45. MONCADA, S. 1992. The 1991 Ulf von Euler Lecture. The L-arginine : nitric oxide pathway. Acta Physiol. Scand. **145:** 201–227.
46. GASTON, B., J. M. DRAZEN, A. JANSEN, D. A. SUGARBAKER, J. LOSCALZO, W. RICHARDS & J. S. STAMLER. 1994. Relaxation of human bronchial smooth muscle by S-nitrosothiols *in vitro*. J. Pharmacol. Exp. Ther. **268:** 978–984.
47. IGNARRO, L. J. 1990. Nitric oxide: A novel signal transduction mechanism for transcellular communication. Hypertension **16:** 477–483.

A Model of Perinatal Hypoxic-Ischemic Brain Damage[a]

ROBERT C. VANNUCCI[b] AND SUSAN J. VANNUCCI[c]

Departments of Pediatrics (Pediatric Neurology)[b] and
Cellular and Molecular Physiology[c]
The Milton S. Hershey Medical Center
The Pennsylvania State University
Hershey, Pennsylvania 17033-0850

INTRODUCTION

The brain damage that results from perinatal cerebral hypoxia-ischemia is a major cause of acute mortality and chronic disability in infants and children. Statistics suggest an incidence of systemic asphyxia in 2–4 per 1,000 full-term infants and an incidence that approaches 60% in very low birthweight (premature) newborn infants. Between 20 and 50% of asphyxiated newborn infants who exhibit hypoxic-ischemic encephalopathy expire during the newborn period and, of the survivors, up to 25% exhibit permanent neuropsychologic handicaps in the form of cerebral palsy with or without associated mental retardation, learning disability or epilepsy (for review, see ref. 1). Given the magnitude of the problem, it is appropriate that researchers have developed models of fetal and neonatal hypoxic-ischemic brain damage in several animal species.

DEVELOPMENT AND PATHOLOGY OF THE MODEL

Over the past several years, we and our research colleagues have investigated a model of hypoxic-ischemic brain damage in the immature rat.[2] The 7-day postnatal rat was chosen for study because at this stage of development the animal's brain is histologically similar to that of a 32–34-week gestation human fetus or newborn infant, that is, cerebral cortical neuronal layering is complete, the germinal matrix is involuting, and white matter has undergone little myelination. The model has proved useful for numerous studies of perinatal hypoxic-ischemic brain damage and presently is used by numerous investigators throughout the United States and abroad.

The method to produce hypoxic-ischemic brain damage in the 7-day-old rat is based on the Levine preparation in the adult rat[3] and consists of unilateral common carotid artery ligation followed by systemic hypoxia produced by the inhalation of 8% oxygen–balance nitrogen. The rat pups are capable of surviving this severity of hypoxia for three or more hours before an appreciable mortality occurs. Measurements of systemic physiologic variables during the course of hypoxia reveal hypoxemia combined with hypocapnia produced by hyperventilation.[4] The hypocapnia

[a] This work is supported by National Institutes of Health Grants No. P01 HD30704 (to R.C.V.) and No. R29 HD31521 (to S.J.V.).

234

compensates for the metabolic acidosis caused by lactacidemia, such that systemic pH does not change from the control value. Mean systemic blood pressure during hypoxia decreases to a low of 23 mmHg (-23%) at 2 h.

Hypoxic-ischemic brain damage is a near universal finding in those immature rats surviving up to 3 h of systemic hypoxia. By 15–50 h of recovery, damage, largely restricted to the cerebral hemisphere ipsilateral to the common carotid artery occlusion, is observed in cerebral cortex, subcortical and periventricular white matter, striatum (basal ganglia), and hippocampus[2,5] (Fig. 1). Tissue injury takes the form of either selective neuronal necrosis (glia and blood vessels spared) or infarction (all elements destroyed). Neocortical damage is often laminar in distribution, with layers 3 and 5 + 6 bearing the brunt of injury as in the adult. However, cortical damage also appears as columns of dead neurons (ghosts) adjacent to columns of preserved neurons oriented at right angles to the pial surface. This pattern of damage has been described in premature human infants subjected to repeated bouts of hypoxia-acidosis with hypotension and is proposed to be the early pathologic lesion of ulegyria.[6] In the rat pups, there is also necrosis of subcortical and periventricular white matter, which originates in and spreads from so-called myelinogenic foci, areas which are presumed to be the sites of origin of the oligodendrocytes. The evolution of the ischemic cell change and the associated gliomesodermal reaction appear more rapid than that found in adults. Thus, at least in the immature rat, hypoxic-ischemic damage involving cerebral cortex, white matter, and deep gray matter structures (basal ganglia and thalamus) can coexist in the same animal and, of necessity, results from the same hypoxic-ischemic stress. What effect age and variations in the systemic hypoxic stress have on the severity and distribution of brain damage is presently under investigation.

The nature and time course of the edema which accompanies hypoxia-ischemia in the immature rat also has been elucidated.[7–9] During hypoxia-ischemia, water content of the cerebral hemisphere ipsilateral to the common carotid artery occlusion increases in near linear fashion to a maximum at 3 h. Tissue volume of the ipsilateral cerebral hemisphere was also determined at specific intervals during recovery from hypoxia-ischemia in immature rats recovering from either 1, 1.5, 2, or 3 h of hypoxia-ischemia. One hour of hypoxia-ischemia was associated with mild cerebral edema that peaked within 4 h of recovery and resolved entirely by 72 h. Hypoxia-ischemia of 1.5-h duration was associated with edema which peaked at 24 h of recovery but which was still present at 72 h. In contrast, 2 or 3 h of hypoxia-ischemia, which causes brain damage with infarction in the majority of animals, led to edema which increased progressively for up to three days of recovery and which was still prominent even at six days.

To investigate the integrity of the blood–brain barrier (BBB) during the recovery period following cerebral hypoxia-ischemia, horseradish peroxidase (HRP) was injected into 19 7-day-old postnatal rats from 0 to 24 h of recovery from 3 h of hypoxia-ischemia.[9] Extravasation of HRP from the vascular compartment into the brain parenchyma was seen in 17 of the 19 analyzed brains, an incidence of staining near identical to the 92% incidence of histologic alterations seen in the brains of immature rats exposed to the same duration of hypoxia-ischemia.[2] Tissue staining appeared as patchy areas of darkening surrounded by a pale background or as a diffuse darkening involving specific regions of the entire ipsilateral cerebral hemisphere. Focal areas of intense staining were apparent in cerebral cortex especially in the distribution of the middle cerebral artery, and in hippocampus, striatum, and thalamus. Staining was less well appreciated in subcortical and periventricular white matter. In cerebral cortex, staining was especially prominent in those areas known to be vulnerable to damage, specifically layers 3 and 5 + 6.[2] In addition, HRP

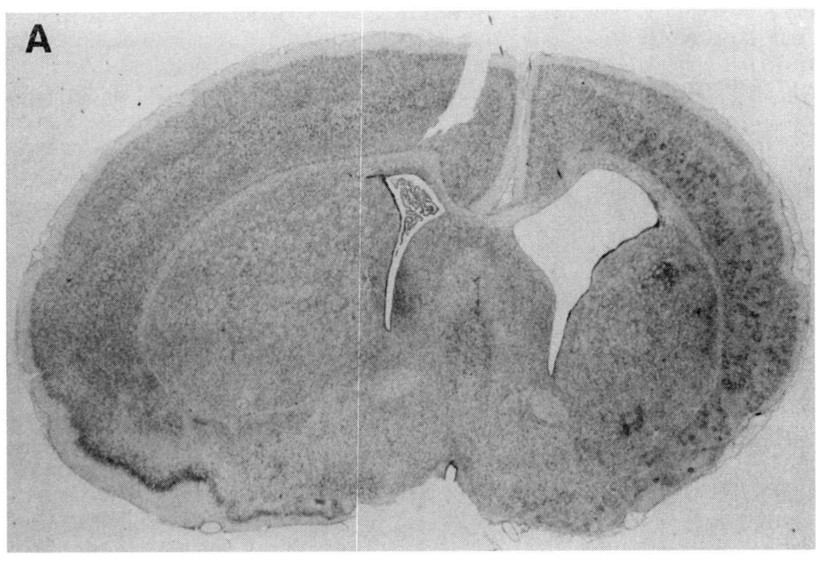

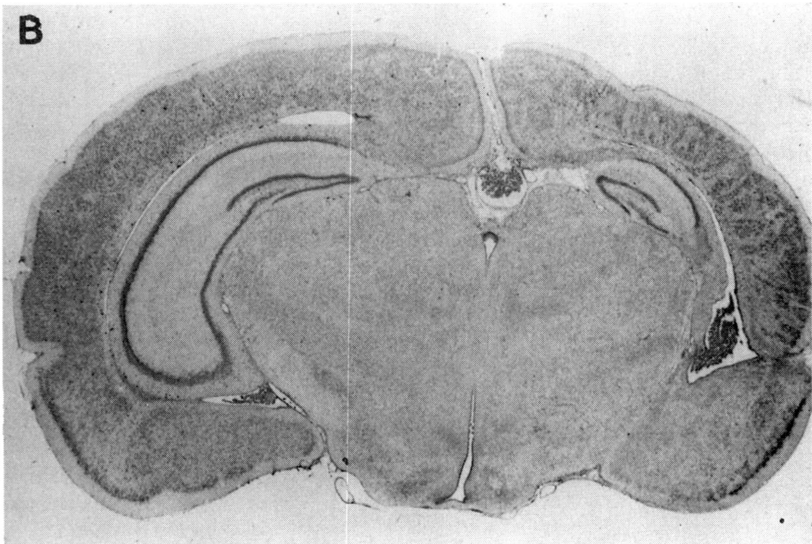

FIGURE 1. Brain damage in an immature rat model of cerebral hypoxia-ischemia. Shown are anterior (**A**) and posterior (**B**) coronal sections of brain from a rat that was subjected to unilateral cerebral hypoxia-ischemia at 7 days of postnatal age and sacrificed at 30 days. Note the damage involving the cerebral hemisphere ipsilateral to the common carotid artery occlusion (*right side*). A columnar pattern of ischemic neuronal necrosis is noted in cerebral cortex of both sections, in addition to injury involving the striatum, hippocampus, thalamus, and hypothalamus.

staining occasionally appeared as columns oriented at right angles to the pial surface alternating with columns of little or no staining, a finding previously observed on histologic examination.[2,5] HRP staining was never seen in the contralateral hemisphere. These findings indicate that cerebral edema is an early and inevitable accompaniment to the brain damage that results from perinatal cerebral hypoxia-ischemia. A vasogenic component of the edema is present and occurs in association with and reflects the severity of cerebral injury.

CEREBRAL BLOOD FLOW AND METABOLIC CORRELATES

Having established the pathologic characteristics of our rat model of perinatal hypoxic-ischemic brain damage, we initiated investigations to delineate those cerebral vascular and metabolic derangements that occur during the course of and following the insult. To ascertain the extent and distribution of the ischemic alterations that occur during hypoxia-ischemia, we modified the Sakurada technique[10] to measure regional cerebral blood flow (rCBF), using carbon-14 autoradiography with iodo-[14C]-antipyrine as the radioactive tracer.[11] Blood flows to individual structures of the ipsilateral cerebral hemisphere were not influenced by unilateral arterial occlusion alone. Hypoxia-ischemia was associated with decreases in rCBF of the ipsilateral cerebral hemisphere such that, by 2 h, flows to subcortical white matter, neocortex, striatum, and thalamus were 15, 17, 34, and 41% of control values, respectively. We found that the hierarchy of the blood flow reductions correlated closely with the distribution and extent of ischemic neuronal necrosis or infarction. More recently, we have used the radioactive tracer, isopropyl-[14C]-iodoamphetamine (IPIA) to measure rCBF during the course of hypoxia-ischemia.[12] This tracer provides greater spatial resolution of the brain structures visualized by autoradiography than does iodo-[14C]-antipyrine. By use of IPIA, a columnar distribution of preferential perfusion was seen within the cerebral cortex, which corresponds closely to the pathologic pattern of injury seen within this structure of the immature rat (FIG. 2). Similarly, perfusion deficits, especially of the dorsolateral striatum and ventrolateral thalamus, presumably account for the predilection of these regions to hypoxia-ischemia injury. However, the reduction in CBF was uniform throughout the pyramidal cell layer of the hippocampus which, accordingly, cannot account for the known vulnerability of selected regions of this structure to hypoxic-ischemic damage. In this instance, metabolic factors (intrinsic vulnerability) must play a dominant role (see below).

Having ascertained the cerebral vascular alterations that occur during the course of hypoxia-ischemia in the immature rat, we sought to determine those cerebral metabolic pertubations that characterize the model.[13] To assess regional cerebral glucose utilization (rCGU), we used a modification of the method of Sokoloff *et al.*,[14] using 2-deoxy-[14C]-glucose (2-DG) as the radioactive tracer. During the first 90 min of hypoxia-ischemia, the lumped constant increased from 0.55 (control) to 1.04, and 99% of 2-DG was converted to 2-DG-6-phosphate. Increases in cerebral glucose utilization (CGU) occurred in all of eight analyzed structures of the cerebral hemisphere ipsilateral to the carotid artery occlusion, ranging from 287% (frontal white matter) to 445% (striatum) of control values. Relatively comparable elevations in CGU (234–435% of controls) occurred in the contralateral cerebral hemisphere, which values were not significantly different from those of the ipsilateral hemisphere. The relatively proportionate increases in rCGU of the two cerebral hemispheres, only one of which sustains tissue injury, suggest interhemispheric differences in the

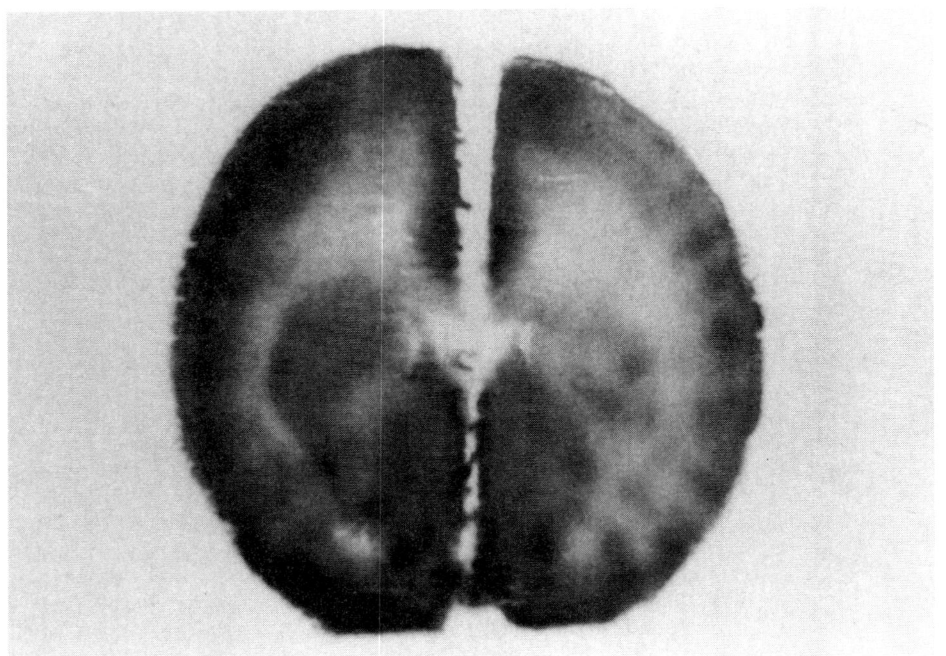

FIGURE 2. Cerebral blood flow (CBF) autoradiogram from an immature rat subjected to unilateral cerebral hypoxia-ischemia. Note the decrease in CBF to component structures of the cerebral hemisphere ipsilateral to the carotid artery occlusion (*right side*). A residual columnar perfusion deficit is apparent within the cerebral cortex; a perfusion deficit is also apparent within the dorsolateral striatum. (From Ringel *et al.*[12] Reprinted with permission from *Developmental Brain Research*.)

extent to which glucose is metabolized through anaerobic glycolysis to maintain cellular energy production. It is likely that in the ischemic hemisphere, most if not all of the available glucose is consumed anaerobically with little or no degradation via oxidative metabolism. Given the inefficiency of glycolysis to generate ATP, the high-energy phosphate reserves (ATP, ADP, phosphocreatine) would be rapidly depleted, as has been shown to occur in this animal model (see below). In contrast, glucose in the contralateral cerebral hemisphere is consumed at least to some extent by oxidative processes, thereby promoting optimal preservation of high-energy reserves.[4]

To ascertain regional alterations in glycolytic intermediates and high-energy phosphate reserves during perinatal hypoxia-ischemia, Welsh *et al.*[4] subjected 7-day-old postnatal rats to unilateral carotid artery ligation combined with 8% oxygen, during which their brains were rapidly frozen for later enzymatic, fluorometric analysis of selected cerebral metabolites. Phosphocreatine and ATP fell progressively to values <10% of control in the ipsilateral cerebral hemisphere during the course of hypoxia-ischemia of 3-h duration. AMP levels increased sharply in the ipsilateral hemisphere, with the total pool of adenylates (ATP + ADP + AMP) diminishing to 42% of controls by 3 h. Despite a slight increase in blood glucose

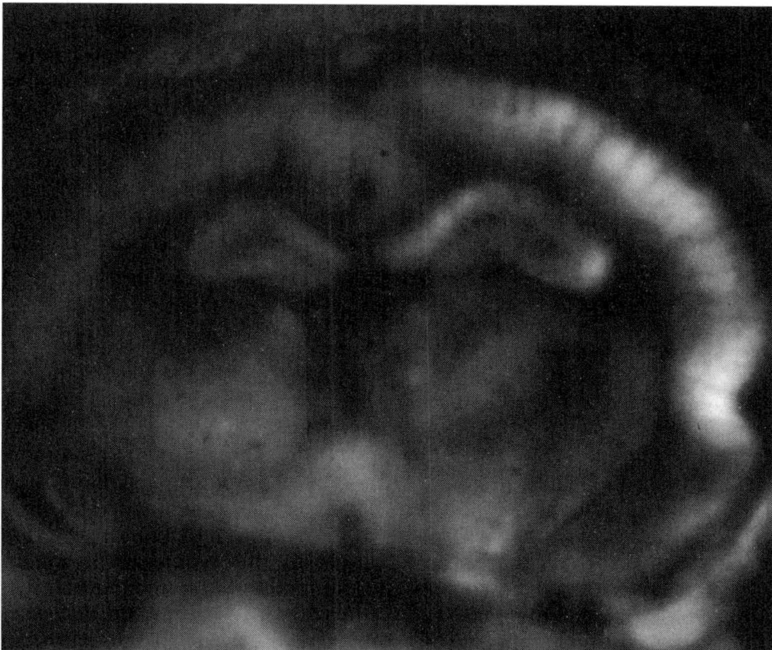

FIGURE 3. Columnar alterations of NADH tissue fluorescence during cerebral hypoxia-ischemia in the immature rat. A coronal brain specimen, frozen at 2 h of hypoxia-ischemia and fluoresced at low temperature with ultraviolet light, is shown. Columns of NADH fluorescence are apparent in the neocortex of the right cerebral hemisphere, ipsilateral to the carotid artery occlusion. (From Welsh *et al.*[4] Reprinted with permission from the *Journal of Cerebral Blood Flow and Metabolism.*)

at 20 min of hypoxia-ischemia, cerebral levels of glucose and glucose-6-phosphate were markedly reduced. Throughout the hypoxic insult, concentrations of all measured glycolytic intermediates, except lactate, were lower in the ipsilateral hemisphere compared to those of the contralateral hemisphere. The accumulation of brain lactate, which closely paralleled the increase in blood lactate, was minimally greater in the ipsilateral hemisphere, while the lactate/pyruvate ratio was three times that of the contralateral hemisphere.

Regional alterations in NADH fluorescence, as a reflection of the redox state of the tissue, appeared in the ipsilateral cerebral cortex and hippocampus after 1 h of hypoxia-ischemia.[4] A columnar pattern of NADH fluorescence occurred in neocortex, which closely mimics the pathologic distribution of brain damage seen in this model[2,5] (FIG. 3). Enhanced NADH fluorescence also occurred in the medial aspect of the CA1 and the entire CA2 and CA3 sectors of the ipsilateral hippocampus. At 2 and 3 h of hypoxia-ischemia, a prominent columnar depression of NADH fluorescence occurred, which persisted into and became more widespread during the recovery period following resuscitation of the animals. A correlation between depressed NADH fluorescence and depleted ATP and phosphocreatine, present as cortical columns during hypoxia and as larger regions during recovery, suggests that decreased formation of NADH may be limiting in the resynthesis of high-energy phosphate reserves (see below).

Yager *et al.*[15,16] measured selected glycolytic and tricarboxylic acid intermediates and high-energy phosphate reserves during hypoxia-ischemia in order to calculate intracellular pH (pHi), as well as the redox states of the cytoplasm and mitochondria at the terminus of the insult. At 3 h of hypoxia-ischemia, concentrations of glucose and pyruvate were depleted to 10 and 30% of controls, respectively, whereas lactate increased eightfold. Phosphocreatine, ATP, and total adenine nucleotides were decreased by 87, 72, and 50% of controls, respectively. Calculated pHi decreased from 7.0 (controls) to 6.6. The cytoplasmic NAD^+/NADH ratio decreased (increased reduction) to 10% of controls during hypoxia-ischemia; whereas paradoxically, mitochondrial NAD^+/NADH shifted toward oxidation. From the findings, Yager *et al.*[15,16] concluded that mitochondrial oxidation during hypoxia-ischemia resulted from a limitation of substrate supply, as reflected by near total depletions of intracellular glucose, pyruvate, and α-ketoglutarate, leading to a deficiency of reducing equivalents within mitochondria. The findings suggest that hypoxia-ischemia leads to an associated depletion of intracellular substrates, which, in turn, is ultimately responsible for or a major contributor to the brain damage that arises from perinatal hypoxia-ischemia. Furthermore, the near-identical increases in tissue lactate of the two cerebral hemispheres, only one of which exhibits intracellular acidosis, suggest that lactacidosis per se is not responsible for the brain damage, including infarction, resulting from perinatal cerebral hypoxia-ischemia.

In a recently completed study, Yager *et al.*[17] measured pHi as well as the redox state of mitochondria during the course of hypoxia-ischemia in the immature rat. Intracellular pH, calculated from the changes in high-energy phosphate reserves, of the cerebral hemisphere ipsilateral to the carotid artery occlusion decreased for the first 60 min of hypoxia-ischemia, plateauing at approximately 6.4. In the contralateral cerebral hemisphere, pHi remained within the normal range (7.04 ± 0.04 SEM). The mitochondrial redox state was calculated from the changes in pHi as well as from the changes in the substrate couple, acetoacetate : β-hydroxybutyrate. Based on the substrate couple, the calculated mitochondrial redox state was reduced initially and to a similar extent in both cerebral hemispheres. However, between 90 and 180 min of hypoxia-ischemia, mitochondrial NAD^+/NADH of the ipsilateral hemisphere became oxidized, compared to the control value, and especially to that of the contralateral cerebral hemisphere. The secondary oxidation of the ipsilateral hemisphere presumably reflected a partial depletion in accumulated reducing equivalents and coincided temporally with the duration of hypoxia-ischemia required to produce cerebral infarction. The findings suggest that perinatal cerebral hypoxia-ischemia is characterized more by a limitation of substrate rather than oxygen supply to brain, which might explain why glucose supplementation improves neuropathologic outcome, in contrast to that in adults (see below).

Because an excessive accumulation of calcium in neuronal and other tissues has been postulated to represent a "final common pathway" for cell death arising from hypoxia-ischemia, we believed it important to clarify the role of altered calcium flux into and distribution within the perinatal brain undergoing hypoxic-ischemic injury.[18] As in our previous studies, 7-day-old postnatal rats underwent unilateral common carotid artery ligation followed by 3 h of hypoxia with 8% oxygen. Either prior to or following hypoxia-ischemia, the animals received a s.c. injection of $[^{45}Ca]Cl_2$, and their brains were subjected to $[^{45}Ca]$-autoradiography at varying intervals thereafter. During hypoxia-ischemia, calcium flux into the ipsilateral cerebral hemisphere was prominent, especially in cerebral cortex, hippocampus, striatum, and thalamus. As in the NADH fluorescence study (see above), calcium

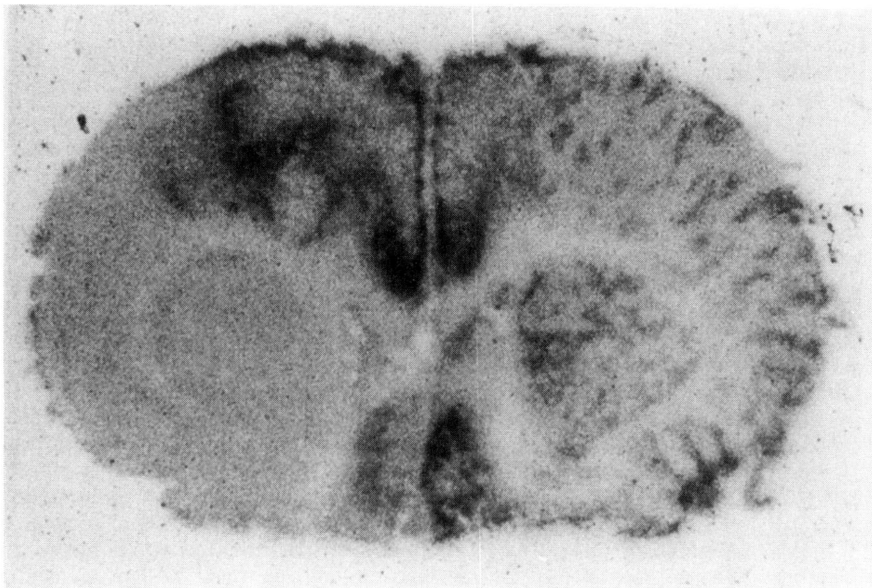

FIGURE 4. Distribution of $[^{45}C]Cl_2$ radioactivity in immature rat brain during hypoxia-ischemia. An autoradiogram of an anterior coronal section of brain is shown. A columnar pattern of radioactivity is prominent in the cerebral cortex. Contralateral radioactivity also is apparent which takes on a more laminar distribution, especially in the deeper layers of the cerebral cortex. (From Stein and Vannucci.[18] Reprinted with permission from the *Journal of Cerebral Blood Flow and Metabolism*.)

accumulation often occurred in a columnar distribution within cerebral cortex as well as in the medial aspect of the CA1 and in the CA2–3 sectors of the hippocampus (FIG. 4). Calcium accumulation was low at 1 h of recovery, with increasing intensities thereafter for up to 15 days. As during hypoxia-ischemia, the distribution of the radioactivity was most prominent in those structures that are known to be vulnerable to hypoxic-ischemic injury. We concluded that hypoxia-ischemia is associated with enhanced calcium uptake into the immature brain, which does not entirely dissipate, but rather progressively accumulates for up to 15 days of recovery. The findings implicate a disruption of intracellular calcium homeostasis as a major factor in the evolution of perinatal hypoxic-ischemic brain damage.

Studies also have been accomplished to characterize the cerebral vascular and metabolic alterations that persist well into the recovery period following resuscitation from hypoxia-ischemia in the immature rat.[8] Using our modification to measure rCBF in the small laboratory animals,[19] we have found that CBF is similar in both cerebral hemispheres at 30 min, 4 and 24 h of recovery from hypoxia-ischemia and not different from age-matched controls (50–65 mL/100 g/min). At 3 and 6 days of recovery, CBF in the ipsilateral cerebral hemisphere decreases to 30 and 26% of the contralateral hemisphere and 23 and 29% of control animals, respectively. Accordingly, an early hypoperfusion does not follow perinatal hypoxia-ischemia as occurs in adult animals.[20–22] A late hypoperfusion takes place that results from, rather than causes, tissue necrosis seen histologically at 15–50 h of recovery. Studies are now in progress to ascertain any intrahemispheric, regional alterations in CBF that occur during recovery from hypoxia-ischemia. Our preliminary results suggest that, like hemispheric CBF, there are no early perfusion deficits that might accentuate tissue injury.

To ascertain lingering alterations in glycolytic intermediates and high-energy phosphate reserves during recovery from hypoxia-ischemia, 7-day-old postnatal rats were subjected to unilateral common carotid artery ligation followed by 3 h of hypoxia with 8% oxygen.[4,15,16] As previously demonstrated, glucose in the cerebral hemisphere ipsilateral to the carotid artery occlusion was nearly completely exhausted during hypoxia-ischemia with a concurrent increase in lactate to 10 mmol/kg. During recovery, glucose promptly increased above control values, suggesting an inhibition of glycolytic flux, as documented by the measurement of cerebral hemispheric glucose utilization at 24 h of recovery. Tissue lactate declined rapidly during recovery but remained slightly elevated in the ipsilateral hemisphere for 12 h. Phosphocreatine and ATP in the ipsilateral hemisphere were 14 and 26% of controls at the end of hypoxia-ischemia; total adenine nucleotides also were partially depleted (-46%). During the first hour of recovery, mean phosphocreatine was replenished to within 90% of baseline, whereas mean ATP was incompletely restored to 68–81% of controls. Individual ATP and total adenine nucleotide values were >2 SD below control levels in 17 of 24 (71%) brains at all intervals of recovery. Both ATP and total adenine nucleotides were inversely correlated with tissue water content, reflecting the extent of cerebral edema, at 10 min and 42 h of recovery. Thus, following perinatal cerebral hypoxia-ischemia, ATP and total adenine nucleotides never recover completely in brains undergoing damage, but rather are permanently depleted to levels that appear to reflect the severity of tissue injury, at least as determined by the severity of cerebral edema. Recovery of phosphocreatine to near normal levels can occur despite evolving brain damage.

The rate of CGU as well as the rate of cerebral energy utilization (CEU) also has been assessed in immature rats during recovery from cerebral hypoxia-ischemia.[23] CGU was determined using a modification of the Sokoloff technique with 2-DG as the radioactive tracer. CEU was determined using the Lowry decapitation technique. Postnatal rats (7-day-old) previously subjected to hypoxia-ischemia, underwent those procedures necessary for the measurement of either CGU or CEU at 1, 4, or 24 h of recovery. At 1 h of recovery, CGU of the cerebral hemisphere ipsilateral to the carotid artery ligation was 97% of the control rate (8.7 μmol/100 g/min) but was only 48% of controls in the contralateral hemisphere. At 4 h of recovery, CGU was increased 49% above baseline in the ipsilateral hemisphere, decreasing thereafter to 84% of controls at 24 h. CGU of the contralateral hemisphere normalized by 4 h of recovery. An inverse correlation between endogenous concentrations of ATP or PCr and CGU in the ipsilateral hemisphere was apparent at 4 h of recovery. CEU of the ipsilateral cerebral hemisphere was 64 and 46% of controls (3.47 mmol ~P/kg/min) at 4 and 24 h, respectively ($p < 0.05$), and 77% of controls at 4 h of recovery. CEU of the contralateral hemisphere was unchanged from controls at all measured intervals. Correlation of the alterations in CGU with those in CEU at the same intervals indicated that substrate supply exceeds energy utilization during early recovery from hypoxia-ischemia. The discrepancy in substrate supply and energy utilization combined with a persistent disruption of the cerebral energy state implies the existence of an uncoupling of mitochondrial oxidative phosphorylation as one of the mechanisms for the occurrence of perinatal hypoxic-ischemic brain damage.

More recently, studies from our laboratory have investigated the effects of these alterations in energy demand on the proteins involved in substrate supply, the

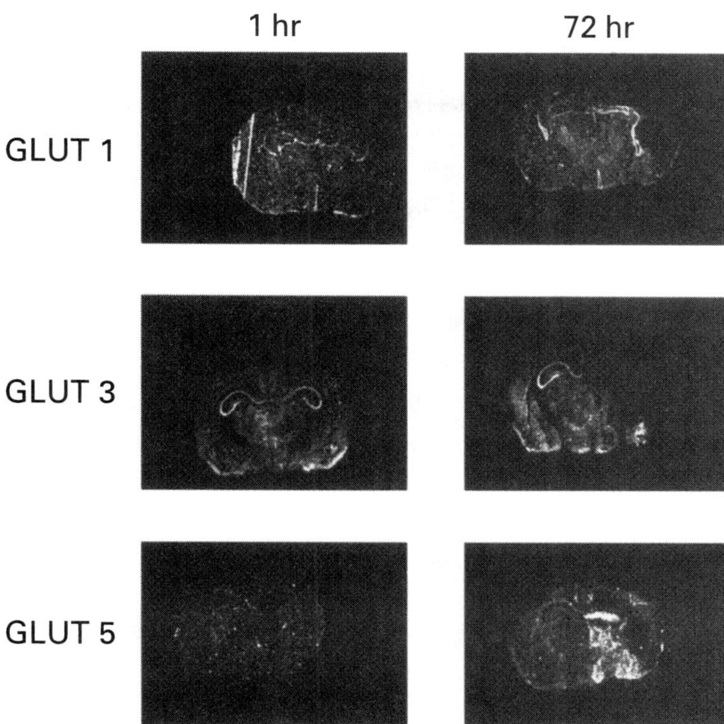

FIGURE 5. Glucose transporter expression following cerebral hypoxia-ischemia in the immature rat. Seven-day postnatal rats were subjected to unilateral cerebral hypoxia-ischemia for 2.5 h.[2] Dark-field illumination micrographs are shown of *in situ* hybridization analyses for GLUT1, 3, and 5 in adjacent sections from rat pups at 1 and 72 h of recovery. Hemisphere ipsilateral to the carotid artery ligation is on the right.

facilitative glucose transporter proteins. The transport of glucose into most mammalian cells is by means of facilitated diffusion, mediated by the glucose transporter proteins, or GLUTs. The facilitative glucose transporters now comprise a 7-gene, 6-protein family, and are named GLUT1–7, for the order in which they were cloned (for review, see ref. 24). The predominant glucose transporter isoforms in brain are GLUT1, which is detected at high concentrations as a highly glycosylated form (55 kDa GLUT1) in the BBB, and also as a less glycosylated form present throughout the parenchyma, predominantly in glia; GLUT3, which is the neuronal glucose transporter; and GLUT5 in microglia.[25] The levels of all of these proteins are quite low in immature rat brain, representing approximately 10% of their adult concentrations at 7 days, and might well be limiting to CGU at this age.[26] The effects of cerebral hypoxia-ischemia on the gene expression of GLUTs 1, 3, and 5 at 1 and 72 h of recovery are depicted in FIGURE 5. GLUT1 mRNA is elevated immediately following the insult, and this is most apparent in the microvessels of the contralateral (left) hemisphere. This is in agreement with studies of ischemia in adult rat or gerbil brain.[27–29] Hypoxia alone has been shown to increase GLUT1 protein in the BBB,[30] consistent with the present observations in the contralateral, nonligated hemisphere. Glucose deprivation of cerebral endothelial cells in culture has been shown to increase GLUT1 mRNA levels, probably by a posttranscriptional mechanism for mRNA stabilization.[31] Western blot analysis of ipsilateral and contralateral hemispheres in the immature rat has shown significant increases in 55 kDa GLUT1 at 4 h of recovery from hypoxia-ischemia.[32] By 72 h of recovery, although GLUT1 in the BBB has returned to normal levels, there is clearly increased expression in reactive astrocytes, which is especially apparent in the necrotic hippocampus. Increased GLUT1 mRNA in GFAP-positive astrocytes has been demonstrated in adult rat brain following focal ischemia,[28] and this might constitute part of the stress response of GLUT1 in these cells. A recent study demonstrated an increased expression in the glucose-regulated protein (GRP)-78 in astrocytes exposed to hypoxia/re-oxygenation *in vitro*,[33] and GLUT1 has been shown to be regulated in a coordinate fashion to GRP-78.[34]

An increase in neuronal GLUT3 is also part of the early hypoxic-ischemic response, especially in certain discrete areas, such as the pyriform cortex and hippocampus, in both the immature (FIG. 5) and adult rat brain.[28] This early increase is also seen in increased protein levels in the immature brain,[32] although it is quickly followed by striking decreases with impending neuronal death, underscoring the extreme vulnerability of neurons to hypoxia-ischemia. In addition to normal mechanisms in neighboring glial cells, which come into play in an attempt to protect the neurons, an increase in the neuronal glucose transport capacity *in vivo*, achieved

TABLE 1. Physiologic and Therapeutic Variables That Influence the Severity of Hypoxic-Ischemic Brain Damage in the Immature Rat

Variable	Influence on Outcome
Hyperglycemia	
Moderate (250–350 mg/dL)	No difference in pathologic outcome[53]
Extreme (500–600 mg/dL)	Protective[54]
Post-hypoxic-ischemic	Increases brain damage[55]
Hypoglycemia	
Insulin-induced	Increases mortality; no difference in pathologic outcome[56]
Fasting	Protective[56]
Hypothermia	
Mild and moderate	Highly protective[57–59]
Carbon dioxide	Hypocapnia, delirious; mild hypercapnia, protective[60]
Glucocorticosteroids	
Acute therapy	Increases mortality; no difference in pathologic outcome[61]
Chronic therapy	Decreases brain damage[62–64]
MK-801	Highly protective[65–67]
Calcium channel blockers	Protective[68,69]
Free radical inhibitors and scavengers (pre- and post-treatment)	Protective[70–72]
Nitric oxide inhibitors	Protective[73,74]
Nerve growth factor	Protective[75]

by overexpression of the GLUT1 gene with a herpes simplex viral vector, has recently been shown to protect adult rat striatal neurons from ischemia.[35]

GLUT5 expression is clearly a part of the later hypoxic-ischemic response in the immature rat and is consistent with the timing and localization of the microglial response to neuronal necrosis. A similar GLUT5 response has been seen in adult rat brain following focal ischemia although the insults are of less severity than those depicted in FIGURE 5, which do not involve significant necrosis, and also do not stimulate such an extensive microglial/GLUT5 response.[36,37]

OTHER INVESTIGATIONS

Using our model of hypoxic-ischemic brain damage in the immature rat, numerous investigators throughout the United States and abroad have studied mechanisms of brain damage, brain plasticity, and therapeutic interventions in relation to perinatal cerebral hypoxia-ischemia. These investigations have provided major insight into the manner in which hypoxia-ischemia damages the perinatal brain and why the distribution of injury differs from that of the adult. Studies have focused on neurotransmitter status and glutamate neurotoxicity during hypoxia-ischemia,[38–40] nitric oxide neurotoxicity during hypoxia-ischemia,[41,42] brain plasticity during development following cerebral hypoxia-ischemia,[43–48] immediate early gene induction by cerebral hypoxia-ischemia,[49–51] and the evolution of magnetic resonance imaging abnormalities following perinatal cerebral hypoxia-ischemia,[52] among others. We and others also have applied various physiologic and therapeutic manipulations to the immature rat model of perinatal hypoxic-ischemic brain damage. The results of these endeavors are summarized in TABLE 1.

SUMMARY

In conclusion, our immature rat model has gained wide acceptance as the animal model of choice to study basic physiologic, biochemical, and molecular mechanisms of perinatal hypoxic-ischemic brain damage. In addition, the model has been used extensively to study those physiologic and therapeutic variables which either are deleterious or beneficial to the perinatal brain undergoing hypoxia-ischemia. As therapeutic interventions are tested in the animal setting, the results will provide important information regarding the effect of these agents in the human setting.

REFERENCES

1. VANNUCCI, R. C. 1989. Pathophysiology of acute perinatal brain injury. I. Hypoxia-ischemia. *In* Management of Labor. W. R. Cohen, D. B. Acker & E. A. Friedman, Eds.: 183–244. Aspen Publishers. Rockville, MD.
2. RICE, J. E., R. C. VANNUCCI & J. B. BRIERLEY. 1981. The influence of immaturity on hypoxic-ischemic brain damage in the rat. Ann. Neurol. **9:** 131–141.
3. LEVINE, S. 1960. Anoxic-ischemic encephalopathy in rats. Am. J. Pathol. **36:** 1–17.
4. WELSH, F. A., R. C. VANNUCCI & J. B. BRIERLEY. 1982. Columnar alterations of NADH fluorescence during hypoxia-ischemia in immature rat brain. J. Cereb. Blood Flow Metab. **2:** 221–228.
5. TOWFIGHI, J., N. ZEC, J. YAGER, C. HOUSMAN & R. C. VANNUCCI. 1995. Temporal

evolution of neuropathologic changes in an immature rat model of cerebral hypoxia-ischemia. A light microscopic study. Acta Neuropathol. **90:** 375–386.

6. NORMAN, M. G. 1981. On the morphogenesis of ulegyria. Acta Neuropathol. **53:** 331–332.

7. VANNUCCI, R. C. 1985. Pathogenesis of perinatal hypoxic-ischemic brain damage. *In* Perinatal Neurology and Neurosurgery. R. A. Thompson, J. R. Green & S. D. Johnson, Eds.: 17–39. Spectrum Publications. New York.

8. MUJSCE, D. J., M. A. CHRISTENSEN & R. C. VANNUCCI. 1990. Cerebral blood flow and edema in perinatal hypoxic-ischemic brain damage. Pediatr. Res. **27:** 317–326.

9. VANNUCCI, R. C., M. A. CHRISTENSEN & J. Y. YAGER. 1993. Nature, time-course and extent of cerebral edema in perinatal hypoxic-ischemic brain damage. Pediatr. Neurol. **9:** 29–34.

10. SAKURADA, P., C. KENNEDY, J. JEHLE, J. D. BROWN, C. L. CARBIN & L. SOKOLOFF. 1978. Measurements of local cerebral blood flow with iodo-[14C]-antipyrine. Am. J. Physiol. **234:** H59–H66.

11. VANNUCCI, R. C., D. T. LYONS & F. VASTA. 1988. Regional cerebral blood flow during hypoxia-ischemia in immature rats. Stroke **19:** 245–250.

12. RINGEL, M., R. M. BRYAN & R. C. VANNUCCI. 1991. Regional cerebral blood flow during hypoxia-ischemia in the immature rat: Comparison of iodoantipyrine and iodoamphetamine as radioactive tracers. Dev. Brain Res. **59:** 231–235.

13. VANNUCCI, R. C., M. A. CHRISTENSEN & D. T. STEIN. 1989. Regional cerebral glucose utilization in the immature rat: Effect of hypoxia-ischemia. Pediatr. Res. **26:** 208–214.

14. SOKOLOFF, L., M. REIVICH, C. KENNEDY, M. H. DES ROSIERS, C. S. PATLAK, K. D. PETTIGREW, O. SAKURADA & M. SHINOHARA. 1977. The [14C] deoxyglucose method for the measurement of local cerebral glucose utilization: Theory, procedure and normal values in the conscious and anesthetized albino rat. J. Neurochem. **28:** 897–916.

15. YAGER, J. Y., R. M. BRUCKLACHER & R. C. VANNUCCI. 1991. Cerebral oxidative metabolism and redox state during hypoxia-ischemia and early recovery in the immature rat. Am. J. Physiol. **261:** H1102–H1108.

16. YAGER, J. Y., R. M. BRUCKLACHER & R. C. VANNUCCI. 1992. Cerebral energy metabolism during hypoxia-ischemia and early recovery in the immature rat. Am. J. Physiol. **262:** H672–H677.

17. YAGER, J. Y., R. M. BRUCKLACHER & R. C. VANNUCCI. 1996. Paradoxical mitochondrial oxidation in perinatal hypoxia-ischemic brain damage. Brain Res. **712:** 230–238.

18. STEIN, D. T. & R. C. VANNUCCI. 1988. Calcium accumulation during the evolution of hypoxic-ischemic brain damage in the immature rat. J. Cereb. Blood Flow Metab. **8:** 834–842.

19. LYONS, D. T., F. VASTA & R. C. VANNUCCI. 1987. Autoradiographic determination of regional cerebral blood flow in the immature rat. Pediatr. Res. **21:** 471–476.

20. LEVY, D. E., R. L. VAN UITERT & C. L. PIKE. 1979. Delayed postischemic hypoperfusion: A potential damaging consequence of stroke. Neurology **29:** 1245–1252.

21. CROCKARD, A., F. IANNOTTI, A. T. HUNSTOCK, R. D. SMITH, R. I. HARRIS & L. SYMON. 1980. Cerebral blood flow and edema following carotid occlusion in the gerbil. Stroke **11:** 494–498.

22. MILLER, C. L., D. C. LAMPARD, K. ALEXANDER & W. A. BRONIN. 1980. Local cerebral blood flow following transient cerebral ischemia. Stroke **11:** 534–541.

23. VANNUCCI, R. C., J. Y. YAGER & S. J. VANNUCCI. 1994. Cerebral glucose and energy utilization during the evolution of hypoxic-ischemic brain damage in the immature rat. J. Cereb. Blood Flow Metab. **14:** 279–288.

24. PESSIN, J. E. & G. I. BELL. 1992. Mammalian facilitative glucose transporter family: Structure and molecular regulation. Annu. Rev. Physiol. **54:** 911–930.

25. MAHER, F., S. J. VANNUCCI & I. A. SIMPSON. 1994. Glucose transporter proteins in brain. FASEB J. **8:** 1003–1011.

26. VANNUCCI, S. J. 1994. Developmental expression of GLUT1 and GLUT3 glucose transporters in brain. J. Neurochem. **62:** 240–246.

27. GERHART, D. Z., R. L. LEINO, W. E. TAYLOR, N. D. BORSON & L. R. DREWES. 1994. GLUT1 and GLUT3 gene expression in gerbil brain following brief ischemia: An *in situ* hybridization study. Mol. Brain Res. **25:** 313–322.

28. LEE, W. & C. A. BONDY. 1993. Ischemic injury induces brain glucose transporter gene expression. Endocrinology **133:** 2540–2544.

29. MCCALL, A. L., M. MOHOLT-SIEBERT, A. M. VAN BUEREN, N. J. CHERRY, N. LESSOV, N. TIFFANY, M. THOMPSON, H. DOWNES & W. R. WOODWARD. 1995. Progressive hippocampal loss of immunoreactive GLUT3, the neuron-specific glucose transporter, after global forebrain ischemia in the rat. Brain Res. **670:** 29–38.

30. HARIK, S. I., R. A. BEHMAND & J. C. LAMANNA. 1994. Hypoxia increases glucose transport at blood-brain barrier. J. Appl. Physiol. **77(2):** 896–901.

31. BOADO, R. J. & W. M. PARDRIDGE. 1993. Glucose deprivation causes posttranscriptional enhancement of brain capillary endothelial glucose transporter gene expression via GLUT1 mRNA stabilization. J. Neurochem. **60:** 2290–2296.

32. VANNUCCI, S. J., L. B. SEAMAN & R. C. VANNUCCI. 1996. Effects of hypoxia-ischemia on GLUT1 and GLUT3 glucose transporters in immature rat brain. J. Cereb. Blood Flow Metab. **16:** 77–81.

33. HORI, O., M. MATSUMOTO, K. KUWABARA, Y. MAEDA, H. UEDA, T. OHTSUKI, T. KINOSHITA, S. OGAWA, D. M. STERN & T. KAMADA. 1996. Exposure of astrocytes to hypoxia/reoxygenation enhances expression of glucose-regulated protein 78 facilitating astrocyte release of the neuroprotective cytokine interleukin 6. J. Neurochem. **66:** 973–979.

34. WERTHEIMER, E., S. SASSON, E. CERASI & Y. BEN-NERIAH. 1991. The ubiquitous glucose transporter GLUT1 belongs to the glucose-regulated protein family of stress-inducible proteins. Proc. Natl. Acad. Sci. USA **88:** 2525–2529.

35. LAWRENCE, M. S., G. H. SUN, D. M. KUNIS, T. C. SAYDAM, R. DASH, D. Y. HO, R. M. SAPOLSKY & G. K. STEINBERG. 1996. Overexpression of the glucose transporter gene with a herpes simplex viral vector protects striatal neurons against stroke. J. Cereb. Blood Flow Metab. **16:** 181–185.

36. LI, K., S. J. VANNUCCI, F. MAHER, F. C. BARONE, P. G. LYSKO & I. A. SIMPSON. 1996. GLUT5 microglial response in adult and immature rat brain following stroke. Soc. Neurosci. Abstr. **22:** 1423.

37. VANNUCCI, S. J., L. B. SEAMAN, R. M. BRUCKLACHER & R. C. VANNUCCI. 1996. Effect of increasing intervals of hypoxia-ischemia on GLUT1 and GLUT3 glucose transporters and infarction in perinatal rat brain. Soc. Neurosci. Abstr. **22:** 1425.

38. SILVERSTEIN, F. S., B. NAIK & J. SIMPSON. 1991. Hypoxia-ischemia stimulates hippocampal glutamate efflux in perinatal rat brain: An in vivo microdialysis study. Pediatr. Res. **30:** 587–590.

39. ANDINE, P., M. SANDBERG, R. BAGENHOLM, A. LEHMANN & H. HAGBERG. 1991. Intra- and extracellular changes of amino acids in the cerebral cortex of the neonatal rat during hypoxia-ischemia. Dev. Brain Res. **64:** 115–120.

40. GORDON, K. E., J. S. SIMPSON, D. STATMAN & F. S. SILVERSTEIN. 1991. Effects of perinatal stroke on striatal amino acid efflux in rats studied with in vivo microdialysis. Stroke **22:** 928–932.

41. FERRIERO, D. M., I. J. ARCAVI, S. M. SAGAR, T. K. MCINTOSH & R. P. SIMON. 1988. Selective sparing of NADPH-diaphorase neurons in neonatal hypoxia-ischemia. Ann. Neurol. **24:** 670–676.

42. FERRIERO, D. M., R. A. SHELDON, S. M. BLACK & J. CHUAI. 1995. Selective destruction of nitric oxide synthase neurons with quisqualate reduces damage after hypoxia-ischemia in the neonatal rat. Pediatr. Res. **38:** 912–918.

43. SILVERSTEIN, F. S. & M. V. JOHNSTON. 1984. Effects of hypoxia-ischemia on monoamine metabolism in the immature brain. Ann. Neurol. **15:** 342–347.

44. SILVERSTEIN, F. S., K. BUCHANAN & M. V. JOHNSTON. 1986. Hypoxia-ischemia disrupts striatal high affinity ^{3}H-glutamate uptake into synaptosomes. J. Neurochem. **47:** 1614–1619.

45. SILVERSTEIN, F. S., L. TORK, J. BARKS & M. V. JOHNSON. 1987. Hypoxia-ischemia produces focal disruption of glutamate receptors in developing brain. Dev. Brain Res. **34:** 33–39.

46. PRZEDBORSKI, S., V. KOSTIC, V. JACKSON-LEWIS, J. L. CADET & R. E. BURKE. 1991. Effect of unilateral perinatal hypoxic-ischemic brain injury in the rat on dopamine

D1 and D2 receptors and uptake cites: A quantitative autoradiographic study. J. Neurochem. **57:** 1951–1961.

47. BURKE, R. E., J. KENT, N. KENYON & A. KARANAS. 1991. Unilateral hypoxic-ischemic injury in neonatal rat results in a persistent increase in the density of striatal tyrosine hydroxylase immunoperoxidase staining. Dev. Brain Res. **58:** 171–179.

48. ROMIJN, H. J., A. W. J. W. HANSZEN, M. J. D. VAN VOORST, R. M. BUIJS, R. BALAZS & D. F. SWAAB. 1992. Perinatal hypoxic-ischemic encephalopathy aspects. The proportion of GABA-immunoreactive neurons in the cerebral cortex of the rat. Brain Res. **592:** 17–28.

49. FERRIERO, D. M., H. Q. SOBERANO, R. P. SIMON & F. R. SHARP. 1990. Hypoxia-ischemia induces heat shock protein-like (HSP 72) immunoreactivity in neonatal rat brain. Dev. Brain Res. **53:** 145–150.

50. BLUMENFELD, K. S., F. A. WELSH, V. A. HARRIS & A. PESENSON. 1992. Regional expression of c-fos and heat shock protein-70 MRNA following hypoxia-ischemia in immature rat brain. J. Cereb. Blood Flow Metab. **12:** 987–995.

51. GUBITS, R. M., R. E. BURKE, G. CASEY-MCINTOSH, A. BANDELE & F. MUNELL. 1993. Immediate early gene induction after neonatal hypoxia-ischemia. Mol. Brain Res. **18:** 228–238.

52. RUMPEL, H., R. BUCHLI, J. GEHRMANN, A. AGUZZI, O. ILLI & E. MARTIN. 1995. Magnetic resonance imaging of brain edema in the neonatal rat: A comparison of short and long term hypoxia-ischemia. Pediatr. Res. **38:** 113–118.

53. VOORHIES, T. M., D. RAWLINSON & R. C. VANNUCCI. 1986. Glucose and perinatal hypoxic-ischemic brain damage in the rat. Neurology **36:** 1115–1118.

54. VANNUCCI, R. C. & D. J. MUJSCE. 1992. Effect of glucose on perinatal hypoxic-ischemic brain damage. Biol. Neonate **62:** 215–224.

55. SHELDON, R. A., J. C. PARTRIDGE & D. M. FERRIERO. 1992. Postischemic hyperglycemia is not protective to the neonatal rat brain. Pediatr. Res. **32:** 489–493.

56. YAGER, J. Y., M. A. CHRISTENSEN & R. C. VANNUCCI. 1992. Effect of insulin induced and fasting hypoglycemia on perinatal hypoxic-ischemic brain damage. Pediatr. Res. **31:** 138–142.

57. YOUNG, R. S. K., T. P. OLENGINSKI, S. K. YAGEL & J. TOWFIGHI. 1983. The effect of graded hypothermia on hypoxic-ischemic brain damage: A neuropathologic study in the neonatal rat. Stroke **14:** 929–934.

58. YAGER, J. Y., J. TOWFIGHI & R. C. VANNUCCI. 1993. Influence of mild hypothermia on hypoxic-ischemic brain damage in the immature rat. Pediatr. Res. **34:** 525–529.

59. THORESEN, M., R. BAGENHOLM, E. M. LOBERG, F. APRICENA & I. KJELLMER. 1996. Posthypoxic cooling of neonatal rats provides protection against injury. Arch. Dis. Child. **74:** F3–F9.

60. VANNUCCI, R. C., J. TOWFIGHI, D. F. HEITJAN & R. M. BRUCKLACHER. 1995. Carbon dioxide protects the perinatal brain from hypoxic-ischemic damage: An experimental study in the immature rat. Pediatrics **95:** 868–874.

61. ALTMAN, D. I., R. S. K. YOUNG & S. K. YAGEL. 1984. Effects of dexamethasone in hypoxic-ischemic brain injury in the neonatal rat. Biol. Neonate **46:** 149–156.

62. BARKS, J. D. E., M. POST & U. I. TUOR. 1991. Dexamethasone prevents hypoxic-ischemic brain damage in the neonatal rat. Pediatr. Res. **29:** 558–563.

63. KALAYCI, O., S. CATALTEPE & O. CATALTEPE. 1992. The effect of bolus methylprednisolone and prevention of brain edema in hypoxic-ischemic brain injury: An experimental study in 7-day old rat pups. Brain Res. **569:** 112–116.

64. TUOR, U. I., C. S. SIMONE, R. ARELLANO, K. TANSWELL & M. POST. 1993. Glucocorticoid prevention of neonatal hypoxic-ischemic damage: Role of hyperglycemia and anti-oxidant enzymes. Brain Res. **604:** 165–172.

65. MCDONALD, J. W., F. S. SILVERSTEIN & M. V. JOHNSTON. 1987. MK-801 protects the neonatal brain from hypoxic-ischemic damage. Eur. J. Pharmacol. **140:** 359–361.

66. HATTORI, H., A. M. MORIN, P. H. SCHWARTZ, D. G. FUJIKAWA & C. C. WASTERLAIN. 1989. Post-hypoxic treatment with MK-801 reduces hypoxic-ischemic damage in the neonatal rat. Neurology **39:** 713–718.

67. FORD, L. M., P. R. SANBERG, A. B. NORMAN & M. H. FOGELSON. 1989. MK-801 prevents

hippocampal neurodegeneration in neonatal hypoxic-ischemic rats. Arch. Neurol. **46:** 1090–1096.

68. SILVERSTEIN, F. S., K. BUCHANAN, C. HUDSON & M. V. JOHNSTON. 1986. Flunarizine limits hypoxia-ischemia induced morphologic injury in immature rat brain. Stroke **17:** 477–482.

69. GUNN, A. J., T. MYDLAR, L. BENNET, *et al.* 1989. The neuroprotective actions of a calcium channel antagonist, flunarizine, in the infant rat. Pediatr. Res. **25:** 573–576.

70. PALMER, C., R. C. VANNUCCI & J. TOWFIGHI. 1990. Reduction of perinatal hypoxic-ischemic brain damage with allopurinol. Pediatr. Res. **27:** 332–336.

71. PALMER, C., J. TOWFIGHI, R. L. ROBERTS & D. F. HEITJAN. 1993. Allopurinol administered after inducing hypoxia-ischemia reduces brain injury in 7-day old rats. Pediatr. Res. **33(4):** 405–411.

72. THORDSTEIN, M., R. BAGENHOLM, K. THIRINGER & I. KJELLMER. 1993. Scavengers of free oxygen radicals in combination with magnesium ameliorate perinatal hypoxic-ischemic brain damage in the rat. Pediatr. Res. **34:** 23–26.

73. TRIFILETTI, R. R. 1992. Neuroprotective effects of NG-nitro-L-arginine in focal stroke in the 7-day old rat. Eur. J. Pharmacol. **218:** 197–198.

74. HAMADA, Y., T. HAYAKAWA, H. HATTORI & H. MIKAWA. 1994. Inhibitor of nitric oxide synthesis reduces hypoxia-ischemia brain damage in the neonatal rat. Stroke. **35:** 10–14.

75. HOLTZMAN, R. A. SHELDON, W. JAFFE, Y. CHENG & D. M. FERRIERO. 1996. Nerve growth factor protects the neonatal brain against hypoxic-ischemic injury. Ann. Neurol. **39:** 114–122.

Red and White Brain

ROBERT C. COLLINS

Department of Neurology
UCLA School of Medicine
Reed Neurological Research Center
710 Westwood Plaza
Los Angeles, California 90095

RED AND WHITE MUSCLE

Muscles of animals are composed of different fiber types for the support of posture and movement. These fibers vary physiologically and metabolically from slow-twitch oxidative fibers (type I) to fast-twitch glycolytic ones (type IIa), with intermediate fiber types in between (IIb, fast-twitch oxidative-glycolytic). During long periods of tonic stimulation oxidative fibers are able to sustain continuous activity, whereas the glycolytic fibers become fatigued. The oxidative muscle fibers appear dark, or red, in the fresh state because of their high content of myoglobin and mitochondrial cytochrome enzymes (e.g., cytochrome oxidase). These fibers oxidize lipids to derive energy for muscle contraction and are surrounded by a high density of capillaries. The glycolytic fibers appear white because of their relative lack of cytochromes. They contain high levels of glycogen for fuel, and their capillary density is relatively low.

Type I fibers primarily support continuous tonic muscle activity, whereas type IIa fibers become active during short periods of phasic activity. For example, the red oxidative fibers in fish run in parallel along the long axis.[1] Continuous undulating contractions propel the fish slowly through the water. White fibers are anatomically organized at oblique angles where brief, fast contractions are used to generate maximal force for sharp turns and jumps. In birds, red muscle fibers are primarily found in leg muscles in support of antigravity postures and walking. Pectoral muscle used for flight muscles are predominantly white.

Experiments in mammals have revealed that the muscle fiber types are determined by the motor neurons that innervate them. The enzyme profile of the fibers of a motor unit innervated by a single motor neuron are identical.[2] Whole muscles in mammals are a mixture of fiber types. Denervating a muscle will cause its red fibers to change their metabolic profile towards white. However, this can be prevented by electrical stimulation of the denervated muscle.[3] By contrast, exercise and conditioning will increase the proportion of red fibers in a muscle. Also, electrical stimulation of motor nerves will increase the level of oxidative enzymes within type IIa fibers.[4] If the nerves to red and white muscles are cut and then crossed by reanastomosis, the muscle fiber types change over.[5] These studies indicate that motor neurons control the physiological and enzymatic profile of the muscle fibers they innervate.

METABOLIC ANATOMY OF BRAIN

In contrast to muscle that oxidizes glucose and fat for energy, the brain derives essentially all of its fuel from glucose alone, 95% by complete oxidation. Studies with

Sokoloff's [^{14}C]2-deoxyglucose autoradiographic technique for measuring discrete anatomical differences in glucose utilization have found up to an eightfold variation among regions for the metabolism of glucose.[6] A tight correlation exists between metabolism and blood flow in brain. Histochemical stains for brain capillaries have found a strong correlation among 23 anatomical sites measuring the intensity of glucose utilization and capillary density ($r = .88$, $p < 0.001$).[7] This would seem to suggest a simple relationship between glucose metabolism, blood supply, and physiological function. However, regional analysis of oxidative and glycolytic enzyme levels in brain has revealed a much more complicated pattern than found in muscle. Among a series of 18 different gray matter regions in rat brain, no correlation was found between the level of cytochrome oxidase and capillary density. Interestingly, a negative correlation was found between the level of the glycolytic enzyme lactic dehydrogenase and capillaries among these same structures ($r = -.54$, $p < 0.025$).[7]

Most brain regions are a heterogeneous mix of neurons and glia dispersed among afferent and efferent fibers. The highest rates of glucose utilization and the greatest concentration of cytochrome oxidase are found in the neuropil, not in cell bodies. This reflects the use of energy to support membrane cation pumps in axon terminals and dendrites in response to continuously fluctuating synaptic potentials. The highest rates of energy metabolism in the brain are found in the neuropil of sensory systems that are continuously responding to external or internal stimuli, such as the auditory and vestibular systems.

Studies of laminated structures in the brain have found histological patterns of oxidative and glycolytic metabolism that reflect organizational principles similar to red and white muscle. In the hippocampus, for example, the highest levels of glucose metabolism and capillary density are found among the tips of the dendrites of the pyramidal neurons in stratum lacunosum moleculare and the outer two-thirds of the dentate gyrus molecular layer.[7] These layers also contain the highest levels of the oxidative enzymes cytochrome oxidase, malate dehydrogenase, and citrate synthetase.[8] Glycolytic enzymes are relatively low here. By contrast, the glycolytic enzymes lactic dehydrogenase and phosphofructokinase are relatively high in stratum radiatum, stratum oriens, and the inner third of the dentate gyrus molecular layer, zones that are low in rates of glucose utilization, oxidative enzymes, and capillaries. Thus, there is a reciprocal pattern or mirror image of the distribution of oxidative and glycolytic metabolic systems in the hippocampus. This type of pattern is also found in other laminated structures such as the olfactory bulb and olfactory cortex.[7]

The special feature of laminated structures that allows this type of analysis is the segregation of afferent and efferent pathways in relation to specific cell layers. This pattern is simple in palaeocortex and archaecortex, but much more complex in six layered neocortex. In hippocampus the highest level of oxidative metabolism is localized to the terminal field of the perforant pathway from the entorhinal cortex. The zone with the highest level of glycolytic metabolism that lies along the inner third of the molecular layer of the dentate gurus is within the terminal zone of the hippocampal commissural association systems. These findings suggest that the pattern of metabolism in histological zones in brain is heavily influenced by the type of innervation.

PLASTICITY OF FUNCTIONAL METABOLISM

Experiments have found that the level of functional activity within afferent pathways in brain influences the enzyme profile for energy metabolism within the terminal field of innervation. Wong-Riley has found that decreasing the afferent activity in the auditory, visual, and somatosensory systems causes a decrease in the level of cytochrome oxidase in the relay nuclei of these pathways.[9] The enzymatic change can be reversed in the auditory system when quiescent nerves are reactivated by electrical stimulation. Similarly, injecting the sodium channel blocker tetrodotoxin into the eye of monkeys reversibly blocks vision and reversibly depresses cytochrome oxidase in visual structures: laminae in the lateral geniculate nucleus and ocular dominance columns in visual cortex.[10]

In the hippocampus, cutting the perforant pathway into the dentate gyrus causes an immediate and permanent reduction of 20% in cytochrome oxidase in the terminal field of the pathway in the outer two-thirds of the dentate gyrus molecular layer.[11] By contrast, the lactic dehydrogenase rich zone in the inner one-third progressively widens up to 75% over 90 days. The expansion of this zone reflects the sprouting of the commissural association system into the adjacent deafferented terminal field of the perforant pathway. If the perforant pathway is anesthetized rather than cut, then the depression of metabolic enzymes in the dentate gyrus occurs to the same magnitude but is reversible.[12] Similar to muscle, a decrease in the physiological activity of afferent neurons in brain per se will cause a decrease in the level of oxidative enzymes.

An increase in physiological activity within a pathway will cause changes in energy metabolizing enzymes in synaptic relays in brain.[13] For example, extensive treadmill exercise in rats will result in an increase in mitochondrial density in the forelimb zones of the cerebellum.[14] Interestingly, motor learning in rats causes an increase in new synapses in these zones but no increase in mitochondrial density. These studies indicate that prolonged repetitive use of existing synapses increases their capacity for energy metabolism whereas learning new behaviors results in new synapses with an expansion of the standard profile in metabolizing enzymes. Studies in hippocampus have found a correlation between cell firing and the level of cytochrome oxidase.[15] Studies in muscle have found that neuronal activity controls the genes that code for energy metabolizing enzymes.[16]

ACTIVATION OF FUNCTIONAL ZONES

Brief changes in neurological activity cause brief changes in metabolism and blood flow in brain regions subserving that activity. This has been appreciated since 1890 when Roy and Sherrington observed an increase in a cranial bruit in a patient with an occipital arteriovenous malformation when he opened his eyes to visual stimulation.[17] Stimulation of a brain area increases synaptic activity and cation pumping across membranes. This stimulates turnover of ATP, an increase in glucose and oxygen consumption, as well as lactate and CO_2 production. The magnitude of change in glucose utilization is proportional to the intensity[18] and frequency[19] of the stimulus as well as the receptive field properties of stimulated neurons. Simultaneously, nitric oxide is released into the surrounding tissue which is thought to be the main stimulus for local vasodilation.[20] Regional blood flow increases maximally within a second or two after stimulation, but then plateaus and becomes relatively refractory to further stimulation.[21] Measurements of changes in blood flow, metabolism, and local oxyhemoglobin concentration are now used to study maps of functional brain organization in humans with PET, SPECT, and functional MRI scans.

Physiological stimulation of brain causes an increase in glycolytic metabolism, but only a relatively slight increase in oxidative metabolism in experimental animals[22] as well as in humans.[23] Tissue lactate increases in a zone of activation[24] despite an increase in the availability of oxygen that occurs with local vasodilation and an increase in blood flow. This burst in glycolysis is similar to muscle metabolism where periodic phasic activity uses white glycolytic fibers.

In primary visual cortex of primates, zones or blobs of high cytochrome oxidase activity are interspersed in fields of relatively low levels of this oxidative enzyme.[25] 2-Deoxyglucose experiments have found that these oxidative zones can be preferentially activated by visual stimulation with color[26] or sharply contrasted grids of relatively low periodicity.[27] This has been interpreted to indicate that these zones are continuously active as an animal passively scans an environment filled with colored objects at a low spatial frequency. When a novel object is brought into scrutiny by visual attention and foveation, a shift occurs to analysis of high spatial frequency and fine-grained resolution of details. The visual cortical areas with relatively low oxidative capacity become activated. In this situation an increase in lactate would be expected.

RED AND WHITE BRAIN

Studies of the metabolic architecture of brain have revealed many parallels with the organization of metabolism in "red and white" muscle. First, the oxidative and glycolytic enzyme profile of a particular brain area is heavily influenced by the type of synaptic input. Second, oxidative enzymes are highest in areas that are tonically stimulated by ongoing physiological activity. Third, brief phasic activity stimulates glycolytic metabolism more than oxidative metabolism. Fourth, the relative balance of oxidative and glycolytic enzymes in any one area is a reflection of the history of the use of that area. Functional zones are continuously remodeling their metabolic architecture in response to changing needs.

REFERENCES

1. ROME, L. C., R. P. FUNKE, R. M. ALEXANDER, G. LUTZ, H. ALDRIDGE, F. SCOTT & M. FREADMAN. 1988. Why animals have different muscle fiber types. Nature **335:** 824–827.
2. NEMETH, P. M., L. SOLANI, D. A. GORDON, T. M. HAMM, R. M. REINKING & D. G. STUART. 1986. Uniformity of metabolic enzymes within individual motor units. J. Neurosci. **6:** 892–898.
3. NEMETH, P. M. 1982. Electrical stimulation of denervated muscle prevents decreases in oxidative enzymes. Muscle Nerve **5:** 134–139.
4. CHI, M. M.-Y., C. S. HINYZ, J. HENDRICKSON, S. SALMONS, R. P. HELLENDAHL, J. L. PARK, P. M. NEMETH & O. H. LOWRY. 1986. Chronic stimulation of mammalian muscle: Enzyme changes in individual fibers. Am. J. Physiol. **251** (Cell Physiol. 20): C633–642.
5. ROMANUL, F. C. A. & C. J. VAN DER MEULEN. 1966. Reversal of the enzyme profiles of muscle fibers in fast and slow muscles by cross-innervation. Nature **212:** 1369–1379.
6. SOKOLOFF, L., M. REIVICH, C. KENNEDY, M. H. L. DES ROSIERS, C. S. PATLAK, K. D. PETTIGREW, O. SAKURADA & M. SHINOHARA. 1977. The [14C]deoxyglucose method for the measurement of local cerebral glucose utilization: Theory, procedure and normal values in conscious and anesthetized albino rat. J. Neurochem. **28:** 897–916.
7. BOROWSKY, I. W. & R. C. COLLINS. 1989. Metabolic anatomy of brain: A comparison of regional capillary density, glucose metabolism, and enzyme activities. J. Comp. Neurol. **288:** 401–413.

8. WAGMAN, I. L. & R. C. COLLINS. 1988. Red and white metabolism in hippocampus. Neurology **38(Suppl. 1):** 181.
9. WONG-RILEY, M. T. T. 1989. Cytochrome oxidase: An endogenous marker for neuronal activity. Trends Neurosci. **12:** 1721–1778.
10. WONG-RILEY, M. & E. W. CARROLL. 1984. Effect of impulse blockade on cytochrome oxidase activity in monkey visual system. Nature **307:** 262–264.
11. BOROWSKY, I. W. & R. C. COLLINS. 1989. Histochemical changes in enzymes of energy metabolism in the dentate gyrus accompany deafferentation and synaptic reorganization. Neuroscience **33:** 253–262.
12. COLLINS, R. C. & I. W. BOROWSKY. 1991. Metabolic architecture of brain: Oxidative and glycolytic systems. *In* Brain Work and Mental Activity. Alfred Benzon Symposium 31. N. A. Lassen, D. H. Ingvar, M. E. Raichle & L. Friberg, Eds.: 111–122. Munksgaard. Copenhagen.
13. DIETRICH, W. D., D. DURHAM, O. H. LOWRY & T. A. WOOLSEY. 1982. "Increased" sensory stimulation leads to changes in energy-related enzymes in the brain. J. Neurosci. **2:** 1608–1613.
14. BLACK, J. E., K. R. ISAACS, B. J. ANDERSON, A. A. ALCANTARA & W. T. GREENOUGH. 1990. Learning causes synaptogenesis, whereas motor activity causes angiogenesis, in cerebellar cortex of adult rats. Proc. Natl. Acad. Sci. USA **87:** 5568–5572.
15. KAGEYAMA, G. H. & M. WONG-RILEY. 1982. Histochemical localization of cytochrome oxidase in the hippocampus: Correlation with specific neuronal types and afferent pathways. Neuroscience **7:** 2337–2361.
16. SEEDORF, U., E. LEBERER, B. J. KIRSCHBAUM & D. PETTE. 1986. Neural control of gene expression in skeletal muscle. Biochem. J. **239:** 115–120.
17. ROY, C. S. & C. S. SHERRINGTON. 1890. On the regulation of blood supply to the brain. J. Physiol. **11:** 85–108.
18. MIYAOKA, M., M. SHINOHARA, M. BATIPPS, P. D. PETTIGREW, C. KENNEDY & L. SOKOLOFF. 1979. The relationship between the intensity of the stimulus and the metabolic response in the visual system of the rat. Soc. Neurosci. Abstr. **5:** 411.
19. TOGA, A. W. & R. C. COLLINS. 1981. Metabolic response of optic centers to visual stimulation in albino rat: Anatomical and physiological considerations. J. Comp. Neurol. **199:** 443–464.
20. MONCADA, S., M. W. RADOMSK & M. J. PALMER. 1988. Endothelium-derived relaxing factor. Biochem. Pharmacol. **37:** 2495–2501.
21. CANNESTRA, A. F. & A. W. TOGA. 1996. Evidence for vascular refractory periods measured with optical intrinsic signals. In press.
22. COLLINS, R. C., D. W. MCCANDLESS & I. W. WAGMAN. 1987. Cerebral glucose utilization: Comparison of [^{14}C]deoxyglucose and [6-^{14}C]glucose quantitative autoradiography. J. Neurochem. **49:** 1564–1570.
23. FOX, P. T., M. E. RAICHLE, M. A. MINTUN & C. DENCE. 1988. Nonoxidative glucose consumption during focal physiologic neural activity. Science **241:** 462–464.
24. PRICHARD, J. W., D. L. ROTHMAN & E. J. NOVOTMY. 1989. Photic stimulation raises lactate in human visual cortex (Abstr.). Magn. Reson. Med. **8:** 1071.
25. LIVINGSTONE, M. & D. HUBEL. 1988. Segregation of form, color, movement, and depth: Anatomy, physiology, and perception. Science **240:** 740–749.
26. TOOTEL, R. B. H., M. S. SILVERMAN, S. L. HAMILTON, R. L. DE VALOIS & E. SWITKES. 1988. Functional anatomy of macaque striate visual cortex. III. Color. J. Neurosci. **8:** 1569–1593.
27. TOOTEL, R. B. H., M. S. SILVERMAN, S. L. HAMILTON, R. L. DE VALOIS & E. SWITKES. 1988. Functional anatomy of macaque striate visual cortex. V. Spatial frequency. J. Neurosci. **8:** 1610–1624.

Neuronal Survival: Cellular and Molecular Pathways of Protection[a]

KENNETH MAIESE[b]

Laboratory of Cellular and Molecular Cerebral Ischemia
Department of Neurology
Center for Molecular Medicine and Genetics
Wayne State University School of Medicine
Detroit, Michigan 48201

CENTRAL NERVOUS SYSTEM INJURY

Central nervous system (CNS) injury, with its resultant disability, is one of the most catastrophic and devastating medical conditions. Until recently, neuronal degeneration associated with CNS disorders, such as Alzheimer's disease, Parkinson's disease, Huntington's chorea, and cerebrovascular disease, was believed to be irreversible. Collectively, these disorders affect a large segment of the population with both physical and mental disability. For example, at least half of all nursing home residents are afflicted with Alzheimer's disease.[1] In addition, cerebrovascular disease is a significant cause of death and disability around the world with the occurrence of approximately 500,000 new strokes per year in the United States alone.[2] Hypoxic-ischemic insults remain a major cause of acute adult and perinatal brain injury that leads to neurologic dysfunction.

SIGNAL TRANSDUCTION PATHWAYS IN NEURONAL INJURY

It is now clear that modulation of particular signal transduction pathways in the CNS can profoundly influence the extent of neuronal injury. For example, the therapeutic window for the treatment of cerebral ischemia is narrow, less than 10 h, and requires rapid reversal of the toxic cellular events. Although the core of an ischemic insult suffers from loss of cerebral blood flow and metabolism, the penumbral zone, that is, the region surrounding the ischemic core, is characterized by decreased blood flow and patchy areas of hypermetabolism. Pharmacological manipulation with agents such as glutamate receptor antagonists[3] and imidazole receptor binding agents[4] has been shown to reduce the extent of ischemia within the penumbral zone. In addition, muscarinic agonists have been demonstrated to possibly influence neuronal plasticity.[5]

[a] This work was supported by an Alzheimer's Association Investigator-Initiated Grant, a Johnson and Johnson Focused Giving Award, and grants from the American Heart Association (National), NIH National Institute of Neurological Disorders and Stroke, and the United Cerebral Palsy Research Foundation.

[b] Address correspondence to Kenneth Maiese, M.D., Department of Neurology, 6E-19 UHC, Wayne State University School of Medicine, 4201 St. Antoine, Detroit, Michigan 48201. E-mail: kmaiese@med.wayne.edu

Protection during neuronal injury also is thought to be a result of preserving calcium homeostasis. Several studies implicate the importance of glutamate toxicity and preventing elevations in intracellular calcium.[6,7] We have demonstrated that during anoxia, calcium, either from external or internal calcium stores, appears to be one of the initial mediators of neurotoxicity in the ischemic cascade.[8] Yet, subsequent neuronal degeneration appears to be ultimately dependent on the nitric oxide (NO) pathway. Generation of NO, by a mechanism that may require intracellular cellular calcium release, can lead to the death of neurons.

Other work has focused on the modulation of several signal transduction pathways, which include protein kinase C (PKC)[9-11] and protein kinase A (PKA).[10,12] During ischemic neuronal injury, agents that decrease PKC activity may prevent neuronal damage.[13] Inhibition of PKC activity also has been shown to protect neurons during periods of glutamate and kainate toxicity.[11] In addition, we have demonstrated that modulation of PKC activity and PKA activity is protective against both anoxia and NO exposure in primary hippocampal neuronal cultures.[9,10,14]

NO production also has been linked to the neuronal death that occurs with cerebral injury. NO, a free radical, has been shown to decrease neuronal survival. NO is generated from several isoforms of the enzyme nitric oxide synthase (NOS) and has a half-life of approximately 30 s. Each isoenzyme of NOS, such as neuronal NOS (NOS-I), endothelial NOS (NOS-III), and inducible NOS (NOS-II), may differentially modulate neuronal survival. For example, mutant mice deficient in NOS-I experience reduced infarct volumes[15] but, in contrast, mice deficient in NOS-III suffer from increased infarct size.[16] During periods of ischemia, excessive N-methyl-D-aspartate (NMDA) receptor activation leads to both calcium influx into cells and the production of NO and cGMP.[17] NO is believed to be toxic to neurons under these conditions. In support of this, studies have documented reduction in glutamate neurotoxicity in neurons by the addition of inhibitors of NO production.[18] We have shown that NO contributes to anoxic neuronal death and that peptide growth factors are protective against NO toxicity.[19] In addition, NO toxicity is at least partially mediated through the modulation of PKC and PKA.[9,10]

Our laboratory has been interested in identifying the signal transduction pathways that modulate neuronal cell survival during ischemic disease. These include the cellular pathways of NO, PKC, peptide growth factors, and metabotropic glutamate receptors. We have been interested in the protective role of peptide growth factors because they control many facets of cell survival, some of which are complementary to the cell and others which are detrimental to the cell. The laboratory has also begun to focus on the neuroprotective role of the metabotropic glutamate receptors. Metabotropic glutamate receptors differ from ionotropic receptors, such as NMDA receptors, in that they offer neuronal protection through the regulation of specific signal transduction pathways. Our intentions are to identify the cellular and molecular mechanisms that modulate neuronal survival in order to define therapeutic modalities for the treatment of neuronal injury.

ROLE OF NITRIC OXIDE IN NEURONAL INJURY

In Vivo *Models*

In rat models, we have demonstrated that neurons in the CA1 regional normally express the enzyme NOS as evidenced by NADPH diaphorase staining and mRNA probes for constitutive NOS (cNOS), but astrocytes do not express the cNOS enzyme.[20,21] If these animals are subjected to transient global ischemia in a four-vessel occlusion model, the expression and distribution of NOS are altered. Over a course of one to 30 days postischemic insult, a population of reactive astrocytes in the CA1 region of the hippocampus express the inducible form of NOS.[22] These studies suggest that the hippocampus is capable of expressing both the constituent form of NOS in the neurons of CA1 and the inducible form of NOS in the surrounding astrocytic layer. These studies also suggest, but are not conclusive, that this induction of NOS in the astrocytes may be detrimental to the neurons in the CA1 layer during an ischemic insult.

In Vitro *Models*

We employ primary hippocampal neuronal cultures for our studies which are directly applicable to the neurodegenerative processes that occur in the CNS. Hippocampal neurons were selected because these neurons, especially CA1 pyramidal cells, are exceedingly sensitive to *in vivo* hypoxic insults.[23] Hippocampal neurons retain their sensitivity to excitatory amino acids and hypoxia *in vitro*.[24,25] Like cortical neurons, hippocampal neurons are sensitive to NO toxicity in culture[19] and are responsive to the growth factors bFGF and EGF *in vivo* and *in vitro*.[19]

In our experimental paradigms, the primary hippocampal neurons are generated from 1-day-old fetal rats. The neurons are allowed to flourish for approximately two weeks and develop synaptic connections during this period. Cultures are deprived of oxygen by placing them in an anoxic environment at 37 °C with 95% N_2 and 5% CO_2 for a 2-h period. To evaluate the effects of NO, we expose the cells to a NO generator, such as sodium nitroprusside (SNP) or 3-morpholino-sydnonimine (SIN-1). Neuronal cell survival is assessed 24 h following exposure to anoxia or a NO generator with the tryptan blue dye exclusion method.

Our *in vivo* work has linked the production of NO with anoxic neuronal cell death. To determine whether NO mediates hippocampal neuronal cell death during anoxia *in vitro*, we inhibited the production of NO in an oxygen-free environment with the NOS inhibitor, N^{ω}-methyl-L-arginine (NMA). Under conditions when anoxia was toxic to approximately 75% of the neurons, treatment with NMA (10, 50, 100, 300, and 1000 μM) increased hippocampal neuronal cell survival in a dose-dependent manner and resulted in a maximum neuronal survival of 70%. Application of L-arginine (1 mM), the natural substrate for NO production, during anoxia completely reversed the effect of NMA, suggesting that NMA protects against neuronal death by inhibiting NOS.[19]

Because inhibition of NO production is neuroprotective during anoxia, it is also important to establish whether NO is directly toxic to hippocampal neurons in culture. Hippocampal neurons were exposed to the NO generator SNP for 5, 30 or 60 min. In each case, increasing doses of SNP (1, 10, 25, 50, 100, 300, and 1000 μM) resulted in progressive neuronal degeneration with approximately 50% of neuronal cell death occurring at 50 μM. We also examined the effects of NO through the application of the agent SIN-1, which also spontaneously releases NO. A 5-minute exposure of SIN-1 (1, 10, 25, 50, 100, 300, and 1000 μM) elicited hippocampal neuronal cell death in a dose-dependent fashion illustrating that NO is the toxic agent. Thus, NO is directly toxic to hippocampal neurons in culture.[19]

In these experimental applications, it is important to employ the use of different agents with similar pharmacological properties, such as SNP and SIN-1, to achieve the same result. For example, there has been some concern that the toxicity of SNP may be a result of the release of cyanide rather than the generation of NO.[26] Yet, in our neuronal culture system, we have demonstrated that potassium cyanide cannot kill at the same rate or dose as either SNP or SIN-1. SNP releases nitric oxide, which has a very short half-life of approximately 30 s. A 5-min exposure of SNP or SIN-1 elicits the hippocampal neuronal cell death in a dose-dependent fashion. In contrast, the administration of potassium cyanide, another by-product of SNP, in similar concentrations to SNP requires several hours to decrease the survival of the hippocampal neurons.[19]

PKC: A "DOWN-STREAM" MEDIATOR OF ANOXIA AND NITRIC OXIDE TOXICITY

As previously noted, several signal transduction pathways can influence neuronal survival. For example, PKC can alter the toxic effects of both anoxia and NO. During cerebral ischemia, increased levels of PKC are present in the hippocampal CA1 region[27,28] and PKC activity can regulate the release of glutamate,[29] suggesting that PKC activation may lead to ischemic neuronal damage. During periods of global ischemia, agents that decrease PKC activity may prevent neuronal damage. *In vitro* experiments have linked PKC with both excitatory amino acid and NO toxicity. Inhibition of PKC activity has been shown to reduce neuronal death during periods of glutamate and kainate toxicity.[11] We have shown that inhibition of PKC activity is protective against both anoxia and NO exposure in primary hippocampal neuronal cultures.[9,10,14] In addition, NO can directly modulate the activity of PKC.[30]

Neuroprotection during Anoxia

Because inhibition of PKC activity reduces glutamate toxicity, it was predicted that down-regulation of PKC activity or inhibition of PKC activity might attenuate the toxic effects of anoxia. We therefore examined whether inhibition of PKC activity was protective during anoxia. In our culture system, we observe approximately 90% survival during normoxic conditions and approximately 30% survival during anoxia. We can alter the activity of PKC by several methods. We initially chose to work with phorbol esters. In rat primary neuronal cultures, a 10–20 h pretreatment with PMA (1 μM) down-regulates PKC activity.[31] Down-regulation of PKC by 24-h preincubation with phorbol-12-myristate-13-acetate (PMA) (1 μM) increased survival from 30% in untreated anoxic cultures to almost 80%. Administration of the inactive phorbol ester 4-phorbol-12,13-didecanoate (PDD) (1 μM), which is structurally similar to PMA but does not alter PKC, did not affect hippocampal survival. This suggests that the effect of PMA was due to the down-regulation of PKC. Another method to decrease the activity of PKC is to inhibit the enzyme directly with the agent H-7. If we inhibit activity of PKC with the administration of H-7, we increase survival from almost 30% to almost 82% in this set of cells.[10]

We also examined the role of acute PKC activation on neuronal survival during anoxia. A 1-h application of PMA (100 nM) is sufficient to activate PKC.[32] It has been previously shown that PMA doses of 100 nM are toxic and can inhibit neurite outgrowth.[33] During normoxia, acute treatment with PMA (100 nM) decreased neuronal survival from 91 to 31%. Activation of PKC by 1-h treatment with PMA (100 nM) prior to anoxia also was not protective.[9,10]

Neuroprotection during Nitric Oxide Toxicity

Since inhibition of PKC activity is protective during anoxia, we next studied whether down-regulation of this kinase was protective during NO toxicity. We exposed hippocampal neurons to the NO generator SNP 300 μM for 5 min. At this dose, approximately 80% of the neurons are killed by a mechanism that involves NO generation.[19] To determine whether PKC contributed to NO toxicity, we pretreated cultures with PMA (1 μM) 24 h prior to SNP administration to chronically down-regulate PKC activity. Survival increased from 22% in cultures treated only with NO to approximately 88% in cultures in which PKC had been down-regulated. Pretreatment (24 h) with PDD (1 μM), the inactive phorbol ester derivative, did not provide any protection, suggesting that down-regulation of PKC is responsible for the resistance of these cells to NO.[10]

We have previously shown that peptide growth factors protect against NO toxicity,[19] and both of these growth factors are known to activate PKC.[34,35] We therefore determined whether acute activation of PKC during exposure to NO could alter neuronal survival. We activated PKC by pretreating the cultures with PMA (100 nM) one hour prior to SNP administration. Without the administration of SNP, PMA (100 nM) was toxic to hippocampal neurons and decreased neuronal survival from approximately 90 to 30%. Acute activation of PKC also did not offer protection during NO exposure.

As with any pharmacological analysis, one must explore different means to obtain the same effect since any pharmacological agent may modulate several biological functions. Therefore, we assessed whether other pharmacological agents that directly inhibit PKC activity could prevent neurodegeneration during NO exposure. The agents H-7 and H-8 each can inhibit the activity of PKC. Following a 1-h pretreatment with either H-7 or H-8, neuronal survival increased from 20% with NO exposure only to approximately 70%. We also examined the agent, D-sphingosine, which inhibits PKC activity by competing the diacylglycerol for PKC activation. Administration of D-sphingosine (10 μM) increased neuronal survival and was protective during NO exposure[10] (FIG. 1).

The results generated from these pharmacological studies are consistent with the hypothesis that the inhibition of PKC activation can decrease NO toxicity. Both chronic down-regulation of PKC with phorbol esters and inhibition of PKC activity by H-7, H-8, and D-sphingosine were neuroprotective during NO administration, suggesting that NO may mediate neurodegeneration through PKC activation.

PEPTIDE GROWTH FACTORS AND NEURONAL INJURY

Growth factors have gained increasing prominence as agents necessary for the prevention of neuronal injury. During development of the nervous system, growth factors function to regulate cell division, neurite outgrowth, and cell survival.[36] Recent application of trophic factors has focused on the CNS. Clinical trials involving the administration of trophic factors are currently under development for the treatment of several disorders, such as cerebrovascular disease. The capacity of trophic agents to direct survival of neurons during development as well as injury argue for their potentially essential role in disorders of neuronal degeneration.

Of the growth factors, basic fibroblast growth factor (bFGF) and epidermal growth factor (EGF) are present throughout the brain and react with several cell types. Both growth factors have trophic effects on CNS neurons but may support cell survival through independent mechanisms.[37] In addition, bFGF also may modulate the neuroprotective ability of EGF.[38]

Basic FGF is found in high concentration in mammalian brain and binds strongly to heparin.[39] Recent interest in the ability of bFGF to promote neurite outgrowth

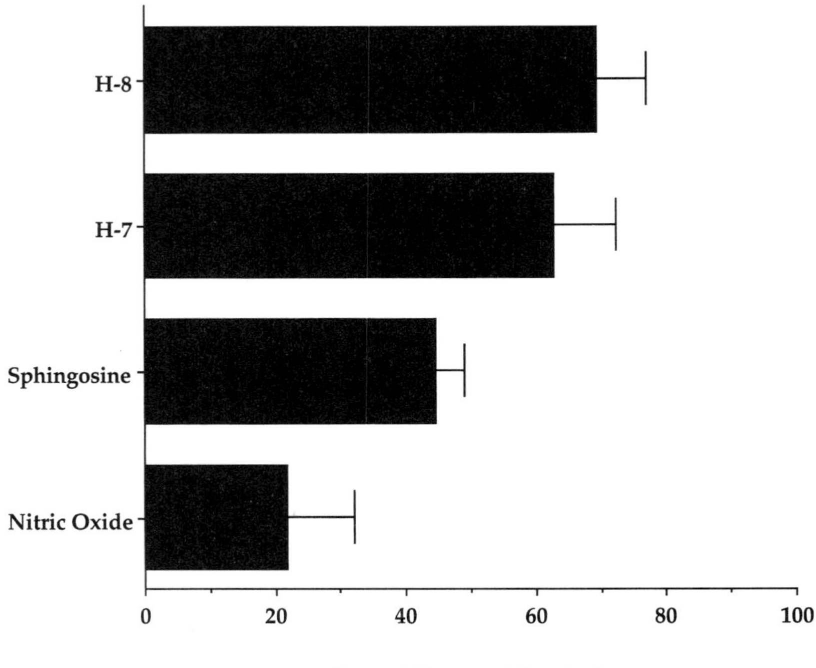

Percent Neuronal Survival

FIGURE 1. Inhibition of PKC activity is neuroprotective during NO exposure. Hippocampal cultures were pretreated with H-7 (10 μM), H-8 (10 μM), or sphingosine (10 μM) one hour prior to a 5-min SNP (300 μM) or a 5-min SIN-1 (300 μM) exposure. NO cultures received only SNP (300 μM) or SIN-1 (300 μM) administration. Neuronal survival was based on the percentage of the total number of neurons (viable + nonviable) and determined by trypan blue exclusion 24 h following exposure to NO. Each data point represents the mean and SD of $n = 10$ determinations (culture plates) from six separate experimental preparations.

and survival has directed the application of this trophic factor to the treatment of neuronal injury and degeneration. Basic FGF has been shown to stimulate neurite outgrowth in cells from the cortex, hippocampus, striatum, cerebellum, spinal cord, and parasympathetic ganglia.[36,40] During periods of neuronal injury, such as cerebral ischemia, the expression of bFGF is significantly increased.[41] Basic FGF can prevent the death of septal cholinergic neurons following their transection and promote regeneration in severed optic nerves.[42] Fibroblast growth factor is protective against focal cortical infarction,[43] global cerebral ischemia,[44] and NMDA toxicity.[45]

EGF promotes neuronal survival and neurite outgrowth in striatal, cortical, and cerebellar neurons in culture.[46] Similar to bFGF, EGF enhances survival of mesencephalic derived dopaminergic and GABAergic neurons.[47] EGF is neuroprotective during periods of anoxia and glutamate toxicity. Human recombinant EGF can increase cortical neuron survival *in vitro* during a 4-h period of anoxia when compared to control.[48] EGF attenuates neurotoxicity in neuronal cultures following exposure to potassium cyanide or NMDA toxicity.[24]

In addition to bFGF and EGF, it is also possible that a number of other peptide growth factors might be protective against cerebral injury. For example, transforming growth factor-β1 prevents glutamate neurotoxicity in rat neocortical cultures, protects mouse neocortex from ischemic injury *in vivo*,[49] and reduces focal infarct size.[50] Likewise, intraventricular injection of insulin-like growth factor 1 (IGF-1) reduces neuronal loss during transient cerebral ischemia.[51]

Neuroprotection during Anoxia

Basic FGF has been shown to prevent neuronal degeneration in hippocampal neurons during glutamate toxicity,[25] and EGF can increase hippocampal neuronal survival during both glutamate and potassium cyanide toxicity.[24] To examine the neuroprotective role of bFGF and EGF during anoxia, hippocampal neurons were pretreated with bFGF (10 ng/mL) or EGF (10 ng/mL) for 24 h and were subjected to anoxia for 8 h. In the absence of growth factors, approximately 35% of hippocampal neurons survived after the oxygen deprivation period. In contrast, bFGF increased hippocampal neuronal cell survival to 64%, and EGF increased neuronal survival to 63%. Thus, pretreatment with both bFGF and EGF protected hippocampal neurons from anoxia[19] and represents a significant degree of protection where one compares it with *in vivo* models of neuroprotection.[4]

Neuroprotection during Nitric Oxide Toxicity

It is conceivable that growth factors may protect against anoxia either by reducing the generation of NO or by eliminating the toxic by-products of NO downstream from its generation. To determine whether peptide growth factors could prevent NO toxicity, hippocampal cultures were pretreated with either bFGF or EGF 24 h prior to NO generation with SNP or SIN-1. Application of SNP or SIN-1 decreases neuronal survival from 90% to approximately 30%. Pretreatment with bFGF (10 ng/mL) or EGF (10 ng/mL) significantly decreased NO-induced neuronal degeneration. For example, compared to SNP or SIN-1 administration alone, hippocampal survival following bFGF administration increased from approximately 30 to 70%. In a similar fashion, EGF improved neuronal survival from approximately 30 to 75%. Combined administration of bFGF and EGF did not significantly improve neuronal survival. These results suggest that the protective mechanisms of peptide growth factors act downstream in the ischemic cascade, at or below the generation of NO, rather than upstream in the ischemic cascade at the level of anoxia[19] (FIG. 2).

Of interest in these experiments is our method of treatment. We are pretreating the hippocampal neurons with the trophic factors 24 h prior to an insult, either prior to anoxia or prior to NO. In addition, the growth factors are continuously replaced in the cell cultures during media changes. It is important to note that the effects of the growth factors are protective, but this type of pretreatment regimen is not clinically relevant. Unfortunately, one cannot predict when to begin treatment prior to the onset of cerebral injury. In addition, it is believed that reversible ischemic neuronal cell death may be obtainable only within a 4–6-h period following the initial insult.

Trophic factors may prevent neuronal degeneration following exposure to NO by altering cellular function such as calcium flux or gene regulation that render the cell resistant to the toxic effects of NO. Alternatively, the growth factors may protect neurons by reversing a previously sustained insult induced by exposure to NO. Thus, we examined whether trophic factors were protective with posttreatment

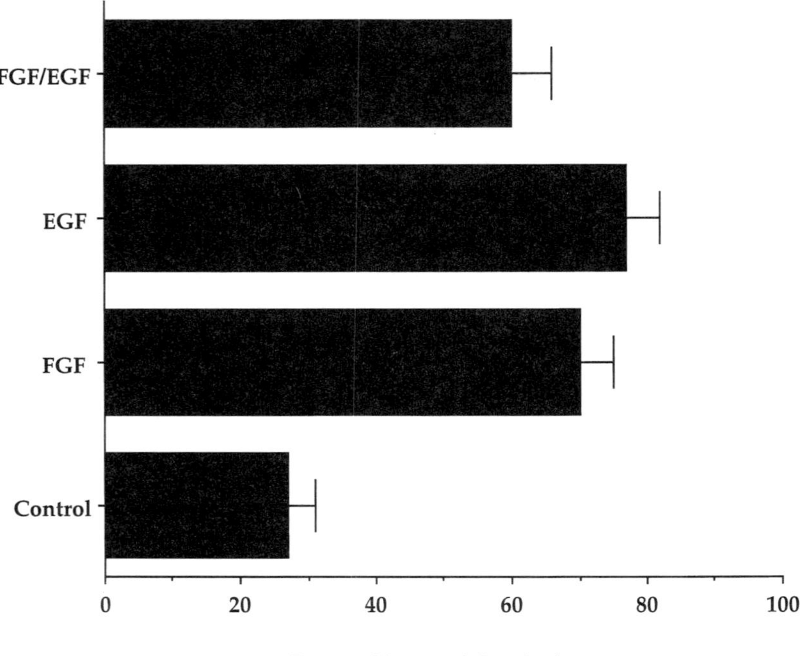

FIGURE 2. Peptide growth factors are neuroprotective during NO toxicity. Hippocampal cultures were pretreated with either bFGF (10 ng/mL), EGF (10 ng/mL), or combined bFGF (10 ng/mL) and EGF (10 ng/mL) treatment during a 5-min exposure to SNP (300 μM) or SIN-1 (300 μM). Neuronal survival was based on the percentage of the total number of neurons (viable + nonviable) and determined by trypan blue exclusion 24 h following exposure to NO. Each data point represents the mean and SD of $n = 10$ determinations (culture plates) from six separate experimental preparations. Control cultures received no growth factors and were exposed to SNP (300 μM) or SIN-1 (300 μM).

regimens and during "one-time" application posttreatment regimens. We administered bFGF (10 ng/mL), EGF (10 ng/mL), and combined bFGF (10 ng/mL) and EGF (10 ng/mL) either 24, 12, or 6 h prior to, at the time of, or 6 h following the onset of SNP (300 μM) administration. All cultures except the 6-h group received *continuous* treatment with bFGF and EGF. Pretreatment with either bFGF or EGF or the combination of bFGF and EGF at 24, 12, and 6 h protected hippocampal neurons from NO toxicity and increased neuronal survival from approximately 40 to 75%. In contrast, addition of growth factor at the time of SNP application (time = 0 h) provided only modest protection, and treatment with the growth factors 6 h after exposure to NO provided no significant protection from NO toxicity.[19]

To determine whether continued exposure to bFGF or EGF during application of NO was required for neuroprotection, hippocampal cultures were exposed to bFGF or EGF as described above, but cultures *did not* receive a continuous application of bFGF or EGF. Pretreatment with bFGF and EGF at 24, 12, and 6 h protected hippocampal neurons from NO toxicity to the same degree afforded by continuous trophic factor application. This suggests that continuous treatment with the trophic factors is not essential for protection from NO toxicity. For the posttreatment protocols, growth factor treatment at the time of SNP application or 6-h post SNP administration did not protect the hippocampal neurons.[19]

It is interesting to note that only a single application of the growth factors is needed to protect against NO toxicity. This suggests that bFGF and EGF are capable of altering a cell's physiology following a single exposure and allow that cell to be more tolerant or resistant to injury. This work may also suggest that NO, with an exceedingly short half-life of 30 s, results in an acute cellular stress that the growth factors are preventing or reversing. With either continuous application or one time application of the growth factors, our data also demonstrate that combined bFGF and EGF treatment does not significantly decrease neuronal degeneration following NO exposure when compared to individual application of the growth factors. As shown in nonneuronal cells,[38] it is possible that bFGF inhibits the protective effects of EGF.

Peptide Growth Factors and PKC

Basic FGF and EGF are protective during anoxia and NO toxicity,[19] and one of the mechanisms for their effect may involve modulation of PKC activity. We therefore examined whether the protective effect of the trophic factors was dependent on the regulation of PKC. We examined the effects of NO on hippocampal neuronal survival during chronic down-regulation of PKC and administration of the peptide growth factors (FIG. 3). To chronically down-regulate PKC activity, we pretreated cultures with PMA (1 μM) 24 h prior to NO. In combination, down-regulation of PKC and application of the trophic factors during NO decreased hippocampal neuronal survival. For example, neuronal survival was 68% with bFGF and 79% with EGF during NO, but decreased to 49% (bFGF) and 44% (EGF) with PKC down-regulation. Treatment with PDD (1 μM), an inactive phorbol ester derivative, did not alter the protective effects of the trophic factors, supporting the hypothesis that the effect of PMA (1 μM) was due to the down-regulation of PKC activity. In addition to down-regulation of PKC, inhibition of PKC activity with the agent H-7 and the addition of the growth factors also decreased neuronal survival during NO (FIG. 3).

Basic FGF and EGF are known to activate PKC.[34,35] We have shown previously that activation of PKC with PMA (100 nM) is toxic to hippocampal neurons during normoxic conditions.[9,10] We therefore determined whether acute activation of PKC during NO exposure could alter the protective effects of growth factors (FIG. 4). We activated PKC by pretreating the cultures with PMA (100 nM) one hour prior to NO. During NO exposure and the activation of PKC, the protective effects of the growth factors were decreased to a *greater degree* than during trials with inhibition of PKC activity. Addition of PMA (100 nM) with the application of the peptide growth factors decreased hippocampal neuronal survival for bFGF to 23% and for EGF to 31%. Because the combination of the growth factors and inhibition of PKC activity was toxic to hippocampal neurons during NO, this may suggest that bFGF and EGF require a minimum "threshold level" of PKC activity to be neuroprotective during an ischemic insult. Yet, if this threshold level of PKC activity is exceeded, such as during acute PKC activation with a PMA concentration of 100 nM, then neuroprotection by the growth factors during NO is lost and cerebral injury results.

Both the protective ability of peptide growth factors and the neuronal degeneration following exposure to NO are dependent upon the active modulation of

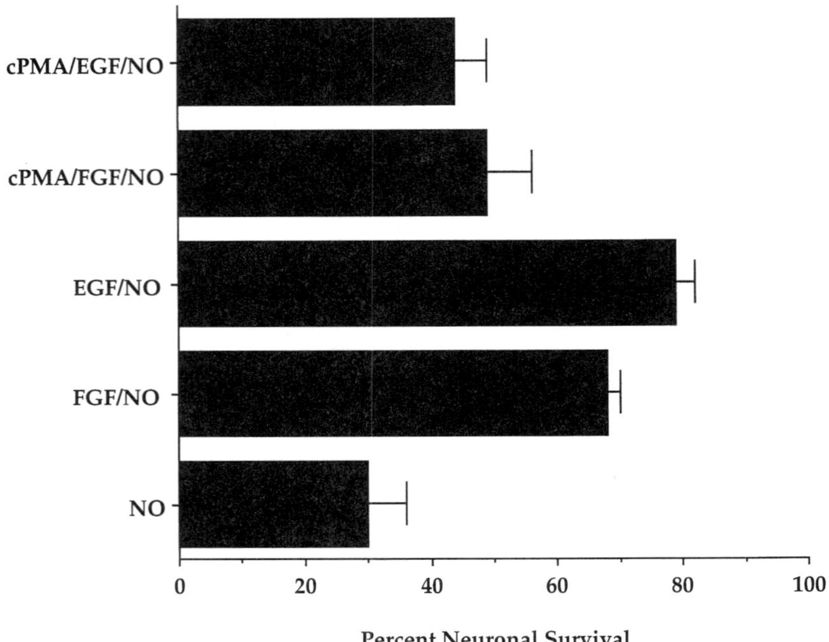

FIGURE 3. Down-regulation of PKC activity reduces the protective capacity of the peptide growth factors. Hippocampal neuronal cultures received bFGF (10 ng/mL), EGF (10 ng/mL), or a *chronic* 24-h pretreatment with PMA (1 μM, cPMA) with bFGF (10 ng/mL) or EGF (10 ng/mL) during NO exposure (SNP, 300 μM or SIN-1, 300 μM). Neuronal survival was based on the percentage of the total number of neurons (viable + nonviable) and determined by trypan blue exclusion 24 h following exposure to NO. Each data point represents the mean and SD of n = 8 determinations (culture plates) from four separate experimental preparations.

PKC.[9,10,14,30] In primary hippocampal neurons, we further characterized the ability of NO and bFGF and EGF to regulate *directly* the cellular activity of PKC. PKC activity was measured by a commercial P^{32} enzyme assay, and results were expressed as a percent change from baseline. Initially, neuronal cultures were exposed to the NO generators sodium nitroprusside (300 μM) and SIN-1 (300 μM) for 5 min, and PKC activity was assessed at 2, 6, and 24 h post NO exposure. PKC activity rapidly increased over baseline within 2 h (31 ± 8%) and gradually returned to baseline at 6 h (19 ± 8%) and 24 h (4 ± 5%) following NO administration. Treatment with PMA at a neuroprotective concentration of 1 μM down-regulated PKC activity by 88 ± 5% in normoxic cultures and actively reversed the NO-induced increase in PKC activity by 79 ± 6%. When administered alone, the trophic factors bFGF and EGF increased PKC activity over baseline by 26 ± 5% and 54 ± 11%, respectively. In contrast, bFGF and EGF individually *reduced* PKC activity in the presence of NO by approximately 45%. Our results illustrate that NO directly increases PKC activity and that the peptide growth factors actively down-regulate PKC activity during NO toxicity. These results suggest that NO toxicity and neuroprotection by bFGF and EGF are directly linked, in part, to the active modulation of the signal transduction pathways of PKC.[30]

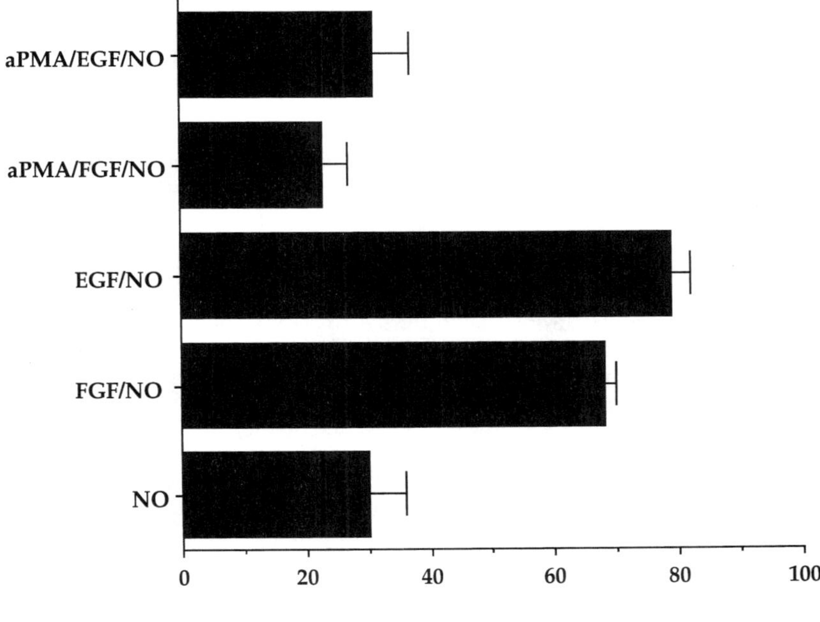

FIGURE 4. Activation of PKC during growth factor administration is toxic during NO exposure. Hippocampal neuronal cultures received bFGF (10 ng/mL), EGF (10 ng/mL), or an *acute* 1-h pretreatment with PMA (100 nM, aPMA) with bFGF (10 ng/mL) or EGF (10 ng/mL) during NO exposure (SNP, 300 μM or SIN-1, 300 μM). Neuronal survival was based on the percentage of the total number of neurons (viable + nonviable) and determined by trypan blue exclusion 24 h following exposure to NO. Each data point represents the mean and SD of n = 8 determinations (culture plates) from four separate experimental preparations.

METABOTROPIC GLUTAMATE RECEPTORS AND NEURONAL INJURY

Modulation of various neuronal cell receptors, such as glutaminergic, imidazole, and muscarinic,[4,5] can ultimately influence neuronal plasticity and survival during cerebral ischemia. Recently, the several cloned metabotropic receptor subtypes (mGluR1α, mGluR1β, and mGluR1c, mGluR2, mGluR3, mGluR4, mGluR5, mGluR6, mGluR7, and mGluR8) have been linked to the modulation of neuronal survival. They function through several signal transduction pathways such as cAMP, PKC, inositol phosphate, ion channel flux, and phospholipase D. Activation of the metabotropic receptors can reduce NMDA toxicity in retinal cells,[52] lessen epileptiform activity in the rat cortex,[53] and protect synaptic transmission during periods of hypoxia.[54,55]

The mechanisms that mediate neuroprotection by this group of receptors are not clear. During cerebral ischemia, glutamate receptor activation can lead to both calcium influx into neurons and the production of NO.[17] NOS is known to be induced in hippocampal astrocytes during this period[22] with the subsequent generation of

NO in the cerebral cortex.[56] In addition, glutamate receptors have been reported to stimulate directly NO production in neurons.[57] Inhibition of NO production during anoxia [14,19] is protective against neuronal cell death. Thus, changes in metabotropic glutamate receptor activity may represent one of the pathways that influences anoxic neuronal cell death and NO toxicity during cerebral ischemia.

Neuroprotection via the metabotropic glutamate receptors also may be mediated through specific signal transduction pathways. Metabotropic glutamate receptor function may require the activation of second messengers such as PKC.[58] PKC also can function as a feedback mechanism on metabotropic glutamate activity and can reduce the inhibitory effects of this receptor on excitatory transmission at corticostriatal synapses.[59] As previously described, PKC activation independently has been linked to ischemic neurodegeneration. Antagonism of PKC activity has been shown to reduce neuronal death during toxicity associated with glutamate, kainate, anoxia, and NO.[10,11,14]

Therefore, we examined whether metabotropic glutamate receptor activity modulated neuronal survival during anoxia and NO toxicity, and whether this modulation was dependent upon the PKC pathway. We focused on the ACPD and L-AP4 sensitive metabotropic glutamate receptors. These receptors have previously been linked to neuroprotection during cerebral ischemia[60] and NMDA toxicity[58] and have been associated with the inhibition of calcium currents[61] which could subsequently alter the production of NO.[8] We have demonstrated that *activation* of metabotropic glutamate receptors protects hippocampal neurons from anoxia and NO toxicity and that the mechanism of protection by these receptors may involve the modulation of PKC.

Neuroprotection through Activation of Metabotropic Glutamate Receptors

We evaluated the role of ACPD-sensitive metabotropic receptor subtypes, such as mGluR1α, mGluR2, and mGluR5, with the selective agonist 1S,3R-ACPD ((1S,3R)-1-aminocyclopentane-1,3-dicarboxylic acid)[62] during anoxia and NO toxicity. One hour prior to exposure to anoxia or SNP (300 μM), we administered increasing doses of 1S,3R-ACPD (10, 30, 100, 250, 500, 750, and 1000 μM). 1S,3R-ACPD was not toxic to the hippocampal neurons at concentrations up to 1000 μM (FIG. 5A). Increasing concentrations of 1S,3R-ACPD were neuroprotective against anoxia and NO toxicity, and the most significant effects occurred in the range of 250 to 1000 μM with neuronal survival increasing to approximately 75% (FIG. 5A). With this group of hippocampal cultures, survival increased from approximately 30% to a maximum of approximately 80% (FIG. 5A).

We next evaluated the neuronal metabotropic receptor mGluR4 in hippocampal neurons because this receptor can be pharmacologically isolated with the potent agonist L-AP4 (L(+)-2-amino-4-phosphonobutyric acid).[63] The ligand L-AP4 was administered one hour prior to the initiation of anoxia or exposure to SNP. L-AP4 was not toxic to the hippocampal neurons at any of the concentrations administered (10, 30, 100, 250, 500, 750, and 1000 μM) (FIG. 5B). Administration of L-AP4 increased hippocampal neuronal survival from approximately 45% to a maximum of 75% during anoxia and from approximately 30 to 60% during NO exposure. The most significant effects occurred in the range of 250 to 1000 μM (FIG. 5B).

Inhibition of Metabotropic Glutamate Receptor Activity
Does Not Confer Protection

The agent L-AP3 (L(+)-2-amino-3-phosphonopropionic acid) is a partial noncompetitive antagonist of ACPD-sensitive receptors.[64] Under conditions of mild

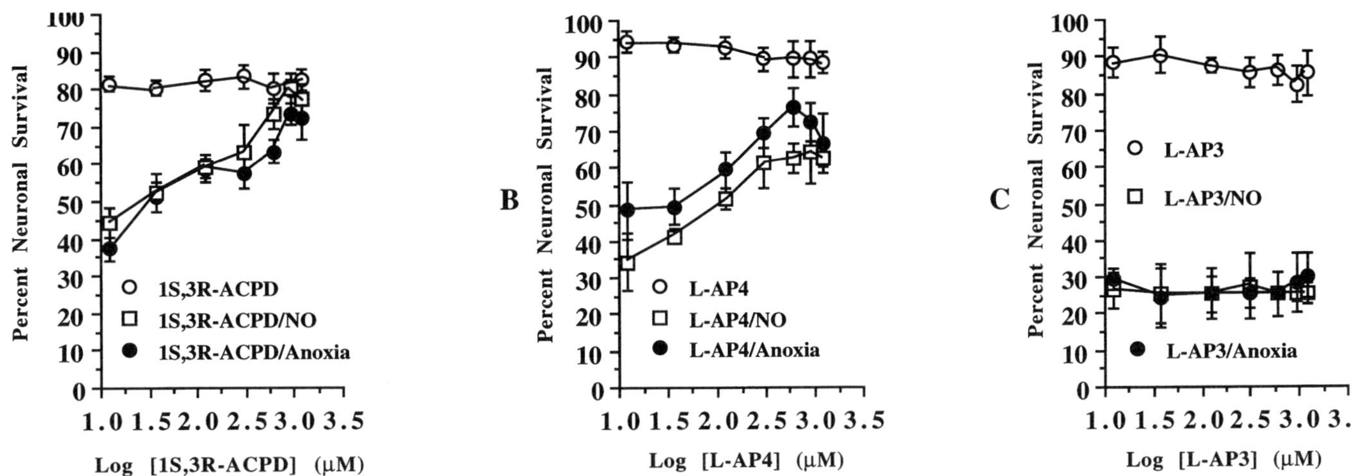

FIGURE 5. Metabotropic glutamate receptor activation is neuroprotective during anoxia and NO exposure. Hippocampal cultures were pretreated with increasing concentrations of (**A**) 1S,3R-ACPD, (**B**) L-AP4, and (**C**) L-AP3 one hour prior to an 8-h period of anoxia (*closed circles*), a 5-min exposure to SNP (300 μM) or SIN-1 (300 μM) (*open squares*), or in the absence of anoxia or NO (*open circles*). Neuronal survival was based on the percentage of the total number of neurons (viable + nonviable) and determined by trypan blue exclusion 24 h following exposure to anoxia or NO, or 25 h following exposure to the individual agents in the absence of anoxia or NO. Each data point represents the mean and SEM of $n = 10$ determinations (culture plates) from eight separate experimental preparations.

hypoxic injury, L-AP3 can protect synaptic transmission in rat CA1 neurons.[54] It appears that under specific environmental conditions, antagonism of the metabotropic receptor is necessary to modulate neuronal survival.

We therefore examined whether metabotropic receptor antagonism with L-AP3 during exposure to anoxia or NO could alter neuronal survival. L-AP3 was not toxic to hippocampal neurons, but modestly decreased survival from approximately 85 to 80% at dosese of 750–1000 μM (FIG. 5C). Administration of L-AP3 one hour prior to anoxia or SNP administration had no significant effect on neuronal survival (FIG. 5C). Neuronal survival ranged from 16 to 30% in cultures exposed only to anoxia or treated with only SNP. In cultures pretreated with L-AP3 (10–1000 μM) prior to anoxia or SNP administration, neuronal survival was not significantly altered and ranged from approximately 20 to 30%.

Metabotropic Glutamate Receptors and PKC

We next examined whether protection through metabotropic glutamate receptor activation during anoxia or NO exposure was dependent upon the PKC pathway. To determine whether PKC activity modulated the protective ability of metabotropic glutamate receptor activation during exposure to anoxia or SNP, we inhibited the activity of PKC with PMA (1 μM) or H-7 during the administration of the ligands 1S,3R-ACPD or L-AP4. Metabotropic receptor activation with 1S,3R-ACPD (750 μM) in conjunction with inhibition of PKC activity did not significantly alter neuronal survival during anoxia and NO exposure when compared to neuronal survival following treatment with 1S,3R-ACPD alone. The combined inhibition of PKC activity with PMA (1 μM) or H-7 and pretreatment with 1S,3R-ACPD (750 μM) increased neuronal survival to approximately 80% during anoxia, and to a maximum of 81% during NO exposure. This degree of protection is better than the neuronal survival observed with the individual inhibition of PKC activity (approximately 65%), but did not differ significantly from the neuronal survival observed with the individual treatment of 1S,3R-ACPD (750 μM) during NO administration (78%) and during anoxia (71%).

In contrast to the results observed with combined inhibition of PKC activity and treatment with 1S,3R-ACPD, combined inhibition of PKC activity and administration of L-AP4 (750 μM) significantly improved survival when compared to the individual treatment with PMA, H-7, or L-AP4. During anoxia, independent inhibition of PKC activity increased neuronal survival from 26 ± 3 to $63 \pm 4\%$ with PMA (1 μM) and to $62 \pm 3\%$ with H-7. Treatment with L-AP4 alone during anoxia increased neuronal survival to $70 \pm 5\%$. Neuronal survival was significantly improved to a maximum of 87% with combined inhibition of PKC activity and L-AP4 administration. This degree of improved survival with combined inhibition of PKC activity and metabotropic receptor activation by L-AP4 was paralleled during exposure to NO.

Our work suggests that the modulation of specific signal transduction pathways by metabotropic glutamate receptors may differ between normoxic and anoxic conditions. Although some metabotropic agonists can increase the activity of PKC in normoxic experimental systems,[65] our results illustrate that neuroprotection during anoxia and NO exposure by metabotropic glutamate receptor activation may require the active *inhibition* of PKC activity. This idea is supported by two observations. First, inhibition of PKC activity did not compromise neuronal protection by 1S,3R-ACPD or L-AP4 during anoxia or NO exposure. Second, protection by 1S,3R-ACPD during anoxia or NO exposure was not significantly enhanced by inhibition of PKC activity, suggesting that neuronal survival mediated by ACPD-sensitive metabotropic glutamate receptors may be, at least in part, dependent on the inhibition of PKC activity. Because combined treatment with L-AP4 and inhibition of PKC activity significantly improved neuronal survival over treatment with L-AP4 alone, these results suggest that L-AP4 metabotropic receptor subtypes, such as mGluR4, may increase neuronal survival during anoxia and NO toxicity by mechanisms that are both dependent and independent of PKC modulation. Our studies demonstrate that the mechanism of protection by metabotropic receptor agonists during both normoxia and anoxia or NO exposure differ, suggesting that *inhibition* rather than activation of PKC is the protective mechanism utilized by the metabotrophic receptor agonists.

NITRIC OXIDE, PKC, PEPTIDE GROWTH FACTORS, AND METABOTROPIC GLUTAMATE RECEPTORS IN NEURONAL INJURY

Generation of NO is one of the mediators of neuronal injury, and the detrimental effects of NO are, at least in part, modulated by the signal transduction pathways of PKC. Inhibition of PKC activity can protect hippocampal neurons during anoxia and NO exposure, but activation of PKC results in neuronal cell death.[9,10,14] In addition, NO can directly modulate the activity of PKC.[30]

The protective mechanisms of the peptide growth factors bFGF and EGF also appear to be linked to both the signal transduction pathways of NO and PKC.[14,19] The peptide growth factors are protective at or below the level of NO generation, but appear to require a minimum level of PKC activity. Yet, once a "threshold level" of PKC activation is exceeded during neuronal injury, the combination of the trophic factors and PKC activation becomes toxic to neurons. Our work further demonstrates that the peptide growth factors actively down-regulate PKC activity during NO exposure.[30]

CNS metabotropic glutamate receptors function differently at both the cellular and molecular level when compared to ionotropic glutamate receptors. Ionotropic receptors form ligand complexes that regulate neuronal ionic fluxes. In contrast, metabotropic glutamate receptors are coupled to second messenger systems and function through GTP-binding proteins. Active modulation of metabotropic glutamate receptor activity can prevent neuronal injury. Similar to the peptide growth factors, neuroprotection by metabotropic glutamate receptors occurs below the generation of NO.[66] The cellular mechanisms that mediate the protective effects of the metabotropic glutamate receptors are dependent, at least in part, on the pathway of PKC.[67] Further evaluation of the signal transduction pathways of NO, PKC, peptide growth factors, and metabotropic glutamate receptors may provide the foundation for the development of a therapeutic target against neuronal injury.

REFERENCES

1. KATZMAN, R. 1986. Alzheimer's disease. N. Engl. J. Med. **314(15):** 964–973.
2. AMERICAN HEART ASSOCIATION. 1991. Heart and Stroke Facts. Dallas, TX.
3. SIMON, R. P., J. H. SWAN, T. GRIFFITHS & B. S. MELDRUM. 1984. Blockade of *N*-methyl-D-aspartate receptors may protect against ischemic damage in the brain. Science **226:** 850–852.
4. MAIESE, K., L. PEK, S. B. BERGER & D. J. REIS. 1992. Reduction in focal cerebral ischemia by agents acting at imidazole receptors. J. Cereb. Blood Flow Metab. **12(1):** 53–63.

5. MAIESE, K., H. H. HOLLOWAY, D. M. LARSON & T. T. SONCRANT. 1994. Effect of acute and chronic arecoline treatment on cerebral metabolism and blood flow in the conscious rat. Brain Res. **641(1):** 65–75.

6. CHOI, D. W. 1988. Calcium-mediated neurotoxicity: Relationship of specific channel types and role in ischemic damage. Trends Neurosci. **11:** 465–469.

7. ROTHMAN, S. M. & J. W. OLNEY. 1986. Glutamate and the pathophysiology of hypoxic-ischemic brain damage. Ann. Neurol. **19:** 105–111.

8. MAIESE, K., J. WAGNER & L. BOCCONE. 1994. Nitric oxide: A downstream mediator of calcium toxicity in the ischemic cascade. Neurosci. Lett. **166(1):** 43–47.

9. MAIESE, K. 1994. Protein kinase C modulates the protective ability of peptide growth factors during anoxia. J. Auton. Nerv. Syst. **49:** S187–S193.

10. MAIESE, K., I. R. BONIECE, K. SKURAT & J. A. WAGNER. 1993. Protein kinases modulate the sensitivity of hippocampal neurons to nitric oxide toxicity and anoxia. J. Neurosci. Res. **36:** 77–87.

11. FAVARON, M., H. MANEV, H. ALHO, M. BERTOLINO, B. FERRET, A. GUIDOTTI & E. COSTA. 1988. Gangliosides prevent glutamate and kainate neurotoxicity in primary neuronal cultures of neonatal rat cerebellum and cortex. Proc. Natl. Acad. Sci. USA **85:** 7351–7355.

12. BREDT, D. S., C. D. FERRIS & S. H. SNYDER. 1992. Nitric oxide synthase regulatory sites. Phosphorylation by cyclic AMP dependent protein kinase, protein kinase C, and calcium/calmodulin protein kinase; identification of flavin and calmodulin binding sites. J. Biol. Chem. **267(16):** 10976–10981.

13. PHILLIS, J. W. & M. H. O'REGAN. 1996. Mechanisms of glutamate and aspartate release in the ischemic rat cerebral cortex. Brain Res. **730:** 150–164.

14. MAIESE, K. & L. BOCCONE. 1995. Neuroprotection by peptide growth factors against anoxia and nitric oxide toxicity requires modulation of protein kinase C. J. Cereb. Blood Flow Metab. **15:** 440–449.

15. PANAHIAN, N., T. YOSHIDA, P. L. HUANG, E. T. HEDLEY-WHYTE, T. DALKARA, M. C. FISHMAN & M. A. MOSKOWITZ. 1996. Attenuated hippocampal damage after global cerebral ischemia in mice mutant in neuronal nitric oxide synthase. Neuroscience **72(2):** 343–354.

16. HUANG, Z., P. L. HUANG, J. MA, W. MENG, C. AYATA, M. C. FISHMAN & M. A. MOSKOWITZ. 1996. Enlarged infarcts in endothelial nitric oxide synthase knockout mice are attenuated by nitro-L-arginine. J. Cereb. Blood Flow Metab. **16(5):** 981–987.

17. GARTHWAITE, J., G. GARTHWAITE, R. M. PALMER & S. MONCADA. 1989. NMDA receptor activation induces nitric oxide synthesis from arginine in rat brain slices. Eur. J. Pharmacol. **172:** 413–416.

18. IZUMI, Y., A. M. BENZ, D. B. CLIFFORD & C. F. ZORUMSKI. 1992. Nitric oxide inhibitors attenuate N-methyl-D-aspartate excitotoxicity in rat hippocampal slices [published erratum appears in Neurosci. Lett. **140(1):** 135]. Neurosci. Lett. **135(2):** 227–230.

19. MAIESE, K., I. BONIECE, D. DEMEO & J. A. WAGNER. 1993. Peptide growth factors protect against ischemia in culture by preventing nitric oxide toxicity. J. Neurosci. **13(7):** 3034–3040.

20. ENDOH, M., K. MAIESE, W. A. PULSINELLI & J. A. WAGNER. 1993. Reactive astrocytes express NADPH diaphorase in vivo after transient ischemia. Neurosci. Lett. **154(1–2):** 125–128.

21. ENDOH, M., K. MAIESE & J. WAGNER. 1994. Expression of the neural form of nitric oxide synthase by CA1 hippocampal neurons and other central nervous system neurons. Neuroscience **63:** 679–689.

22. ENDOH, M., K. MAIESE & J. WAGNER. 1994. Expression of the inducible form of nitric oxide synthase by reactive astrocytes after transient global ischemia. Brain Res. **651(1–2):** 92–100.

23. GINSBERG, M. D., D. I. GRAHAM & R. BUSTO. 1985. Regional glucose utilization and blood flow following graded forebrain ischemia in the rat: Correlation with neuropathology. Ann. Neurol. **18:** 470–481.

24. PAUWELS, P. J., H. P. VAN ASSOUW & J. E. LEYSEN. 1989. Attenuation of neurotoxicity

following anoxia or glutamate receptor activation in EGF- and hippocampal extract-treated neuronal cultures. Cell Signalling **1(1):** 45–54.

25. MATTSON, M. P., M. MURRAIN, P. B. GUTHRIE & S. B. KATER. 1989. Fibroblast growth factor and glutamate: Opposing roles in the generation and degeneration of hippocampal neuroarchitecture. J. Neurosci. **9(11):** 3728–3740.

26. BATES, J. N., M. T. BAKER, J. R. GUERRA & D. G. HARRISON. 1991. Nitric oxide generation from nitroprusside by vascular tissue. Evidence that reduction of the nitroprusside anion and cyanide loss are required. Biochem. Pharmacol. **42(Suppl):** S157–S165.

27. HARA, H., H. ONODERA & K. KOGURE. 1990. Protein kinase C activity in the gerbil hippocampus after transient forebrain ischemia: Morphological and autoradiographic analysis using [^{3}H]phorbol 12,13-dibutyrate. Neurosci. Lett. **120(1):** 120–123.

28. DOMANSKA-JANIK, K. & T. ZALEWSKA. 1992. Effect of brain ischemia on protein kinase C. J. Neurochem. **58(4):** 1432–1439.

29. LU, Y. M., B. F. LU, F. Q. ZHAO, Y. L. YAN & X. P. HO. 1993. Accumulation of glutamate is regulated by calcium and protein kinase C in rat hippocampal slices exposed to ischemic states. Hippocampus **3(2):** 221–227.

30. TENBROEKE, M., I. KUE, R. P. LISAK & K. MAIESE. 1996. Nitric oxide and peptide growth factors directly modulate protein kinase C activity. Soc. Neurosci. Abstr. **22:** 1460.

31. MATTHIES, H. J., H. C. PALFREY, L. D. HIRNING & R. J. MILLER. 1987. Down regulation of protein kinase C in neuronal cells: Effects on neurotransmitter release. J. Neurosci. **7:** 1198–1206.

32. LAI, W. S. & E. E. EL-FAKAHANY. 1988. Regulation of [^{3}H]phorbol-12,13-dibutyrate binding sites in mouse neuroblastoma cells: Simultaneous down-regulation by phorbol esters and desensitization of their inhibition of muscarinic receptor function. J. Pharmacol. Exp. Ther. **244:** 41–50.

33. MATTSON, M. P., P. DOU & S. B. KATER. 1988. Outgrowth-regulating actions of glutamate in isolated hippocampal pyramidal neurons. J. Neurosci. **8:** 2087–2100.

34. LI, M., P. MORLEY & B. K. TSANG. 1991. Epidermal growth factor elevates intracellular pH in chicken granulosa cells by activating protein kinase C. Endocrinology **129(6):** 2957–2964.

35. OURY, F., C. FAUCHER, I. RIVES, M. BENSAID, G. BOUCHE & J. M. DARBON. 1992. Regulation of cyclic adenosine 3′,5′-monophosphate-dependent protein kinase activity and regulatory subunit RII beta content by basic fibroblast growth factor (bFGF) during granulosa cell differentiation: Possible implication of protein kinase C in bFGF action. Biol. Reprod. **47(2):** 202–212.

36. WALICKE, P., M. W. COWAN, N. UENO, A. BAIRD & R. GUILLEMIN. 1986. Fibroblast growth factor promotes survival of dissociated hippocampal neurons and enhances neurite extension. Proc. Natl. Acad. Sci. USA **83:** 3012–3016.

37. KORNBLUM, H. I., H. K. RAYMON, R. S. MORRISON, K. P. CAVANAUGH, R. A. BRADSHAW & F. M. LESLIE. 1990. Epidermal growth factor and basic fibroblast growth factor: Effects on an overlapping population of neocortical neurons in vitro. Brain Res. **535:** 255–263.

38. HUFF, K. R. & W. SCHREIER. 1990. Fibroblast growth factor inhibits epidermal growth factor-induced responses in rat astrocytes. Glia **3(3):** 193–204.

39. SHING, Y., J. FOLKMAN, R. SULLIVAN, C. BUTTERFIELD, J. MURRAY & M. KLAGSBRUN. 1984. Heparin affinity: Purification of a tumor-derived capillary endothelial cell growth factor. Science **223:** 1296–1299.

40. WALICKE, P. A. 1988. Basic and acidic fibroblast growth factors have trophic effects on neurons from multiple CNS regions. J. Neurosci. **8:** 2618–2627.

41. TAKAMI, K., M. IWANE, Y. KIYOTA, M. MIYAMOTO, R. TSUKUDA & S. SHIOSAKA. 1992. Increase of basic fibroblast growth factor immunoreactivity and its mRNA level in rat brain following transient forebrain ischemia. Exp. Brain Res. **90(1):** 1–10.

42. SIEVERS, J., B. HAUSMANN, K. UNSICKER & M. BERRY. 1987. Fibroblast growth factors promote the survival of adult rat retinal ganglion cells after transection of the optic nerve. Neurosci. Lett. **76:** 157–162.

43. YAMADA, K., A. KINOSHITA, E. KOHMURA, T. SAKAGUCHI, J. TAGUCHI, K. KATAOKA &

T. HAYAKAWA. 1991. Basic fibroblast growth factor prevents thalamic degeneration after cortical infarction. J. Cereb. Blood Flow Metab. **11(3):** 472–478.

44. SASAKI, K., Y. OOMURA, K. SUZUKI, K. HANAI & H. YAGI. 1992. Acidic fibroblast growth factor prevents death of hippocampal CA1 pyramidal cells following ischemia. Neurochem. Int. **21(3):** 397–402.

45. FREESE, A., S. P. FINKLESTEIN & M. DI FIGLIA. 1992. Basic fibroblast growth factor protects striatal neurons in vitro from NMDA-receptor mediated excitotoxicity. Brain Res. **575:** 351–355.

46. MORRISON, R. S., R. F. KEATING & J. R. MOSKAL. 1988. Basic fibroblast growth factor and epidermal growth factor exert different trophic effects on CNS neurons. J. Neurosci. Res. **21:** 71–79.

47. FERRARI, G., G. TOFFANO & S. D. SKAPER. 1991. Epidermal growth factor exerts neuronotrophic effects on dopaminergic and GABAergic CNS neurons: Comparison with basic fibroblast growth factor. J. Neurosci. Res. **30:** 493–497.

48. KINOSHITA, A., K. YAMADA, T. HAYAKAWA, K. KATAOKA, T. MUSHIROI, E. KOHMURA & H. MOGAMI. 1990. Modification of anoxic neuronal injury by human recombinant epidermal growth factor and its possible mechanism. J. Neurosci. Res. **25:** 324–330.

49. PREHN, J. H., C. BACKHAUSS & J. KRIEGLSTEIN. 1993. Transforming growth factor-beta 1 prevents glutamate neurotoxicity in rat neocortical cultures and protects mouse neocortex from ischemic injury in vivo. J. Cereb. Blood Flow Metab. **13(3):** 521–525.

50. GROSS, C. E., M. M. BEDNAR, D. B. HOWARD & M. B. SPORN. 1993. Transforming growth factor-beta 1 reduces infarct size after experimental cerebral ischemia in a rabbit model. Stroke **24(4):** 558–562.

51. GUAN, J., C. WILLIAMS, M. GUNNING, C. MALLARD & P. GLUCKMAN. 1993. The effects of IGF-1 treatment after hypoxic-ischemic brain injury in adult rats. J. Cereb. Blood Flow Metab. **13:** 609–616.

52. SILIPRANDI, R., M. LIPARTITI, E. FADDA, J. SAUTTER & H. MANEV. 1992. Activation of the glutamate metabotropic receptor protects retina against N-methyl-D-aspartate toxicity. Eur. J. Pharmacol. **219(1):** 173–174.

53. SHEARDOWN, M. J. 1992. Metabotropic glutamate receptor agonists reduce epileptiform activity in the rat cortex. Neuroreport **3(10):** 916–918.

54. OPITZ, T. & K. G. REYMANN. 1991. Blockade of metabotropic glutamate receptors protects rat CA1 neurons from hypoxic injury. Neuroreport **2(8):** 455–457.

55. OPITZ, T. & K. G. REYMANN. 1993. (1S, 3R)-ACPD protects synaptic transmission from hypoxia in hippocampal slices. Neuropharmacology **32(1):** 103–104.

56. SATO, S., T. TOMINGA, T. OHNISHI & S. T. OHNISHI. 1993. EPR spin-trapping study of nitric oxide formation during bilateral carotid occlusion in the rat. Biochim. Biophys. Acta **1181:** 195–197.

57. MARIN, P., J. F. QUIGNARD, M. LAFON-CAZAL & J. BOCKAERT. 1993. Non-classical glutamate receptors, blocked by both NMDA and non-NMDA antagonists, stimulate nitric oxide production in neurons. Neuropharmacology **32(1):** 29–36.

58. KOH, J. Y., E. PALMER & C. W. COTMAN. 1991. Activation of the metabotropic glutamate receptor attenuates N-methyl-D-aspartate neurotoxicity in cortical cultures. Proc. Natl. Acad. Sci. USA **88(21):** 9431–9435.

59. SWARTZ, K. J., A. MERRITT, B. P. BEAN & D. M. LOVINGER. 1993. Protein kinase C modulates glutamate receptor inhibition of Ca^{2+} channels and synaptic transmission. Nature **361:** 165–168.

60. CHIAMULERA, C., P. ALBERTINI, E. VALERIO & A. REGGIANI. 1992. Activation of metabotropic receptors has a neuroprotective effect in a rodent model of focal ischaemia. Eur. J. Pharmacol. **216(2):** 335–336.

61. TROMBLEY, P. Q. & G. L. WESTBROOK. 1992. L-AP4 inhibits calcium currents and synaptic transmission via a G-protein-coupled glutamate receptor. J. Neurosci. **12(6):** 2043–2050.

62. SCHOEPP, D. D., B. G. JOHNSON, R. A. TRUE & J. A. MONN. 1991. Comparison of (1S,3R)-1-aminocyclopentane-1,3-dicarboxylic acid (1S,3R-ACPD)- and 1S,3R-ACPD-stimulated brain phosphoinositide hydrolysis. Eur. J. Pharmacol. **207(4):** 351–353.

63. SCHULTE, M. K., E. R. WHITTEMORE, J. F. KOERNER & R. L. JOHNSON. 1992. Structure-

function relationships for analogues of L-2-amino-4-phosphonobutanoic acid on the quisqualic acid-sensitive AP4 receptor of the rat hippocampus. Brain Res. **582(2):** 291–298.

64. ARAMORI, I. & S. NAKANISHI. 1992. Signal transduction and pharmacological characteristics of a metabotropic glutamate receptor, mGluR1, in transfected CHO cells. Neuron **8(4):** 757–765.

65. MANZONI, O. J., F. FINIELS-MARLIER, I. SASSETTI, J. BLOCKAERT, C. LE PEUCH & F. A. SLADECZEK. 1990. The glutamate receptor of the Qp-type activates protein kinase C and is regulated by protein kinase. C. Neurosci. Lett. **109(1–2):** 146–151.

66. MAIESE, K., R. GREENBERG, L. BOCCONE & M. SWIRIDUK. 1995. Activation of the metabotropic glutamate receptor is neuroprotective during nitric oxide toxicity in primary hippocampal neurons of rats. Neurosci. Lett. **194(3):** 173–176.

67. MAIESE, K., M. SWIRIDUK & M. TENBROEKE. 1996. Cellular mechanisms of protection by metabotropic glutamate receptors during anoxia and nitric oxide toxicity. J. Neurochem. **66:** 2419–2428.

On the Rate of Decarboxylation of Dopa to Dopamine in Living Mammalian Brain[a]

PAUL CUMMING,[b] PAUL DEEP,[b] OLIVIER ROUSSET,[b]
ALAN EVANS,[b] AND ALBERT GJEDDE[b–d]

[b]McConnell Brain Imaging Centre
Montreal Neurological Institute
3801 University Avenue
Montreal, PQ, Canada H3A 2B4

[c]PET Centre
Aarhus University Medical Institutions
44 Nørrebrogade
Aarhus, Denmark 8000

INTRODUCTION

Positron emission tomography of the exogeneous substrate for dopa decarboxylase 6-[^{18}F]fluoro-L-dopa ([^{18}F]fluorodopa) reveals time-dependent accumulation of radioactivity in the basal ganglia of non-human primates and humans.[1,2] Likewise, radioactivity accumulates in the basal ganglia of rat following injection with [^{3}H]dopa.[3,4] These accumulations *in vivo* are assumed to indicate the trapping of decarboxylated products in catecholamine terminals and so provide an index of the activity of dopa decarboxylase in catecholamine terminals of living brain. However, the isolation of a physiological parameter specifically related to dopa decarboxylase activity requires compartmental analysis of dynamic positron emission tomography studies. The radiochemical synthesis and metabolic pathway of [^{18}F]fluorodopa have been reviewed,[5,6] but no complete summary of the several approaches to the compartmental modeling of tracer dopa uptake is currently available. In this paper, we review the state of development of the methods of quantitation of the metabolism of [^{18}F]fluorodopa and other radiotracers for dopa decarboxylase, with special emphasis on current controversies and on applications of these methods for clinical studies.

The positron emission tomograph detects temporal changes in total radioactivity concentrations in a volume of brain tissue; the chemical composition of this radioactivity is unknown unless brain samples are also available for radiochemical fractionation. The [^{14}C]deoxyglucose method for quantifying regional cerebral glucose consumption in rat brain is based upon the analytic demonstration that deoxyglucose in blood is, with glucose, transferred across the blood–brain barrier, enters the pathway of anaerobic glycolysis, but is essentially trapped irreversibly after the hexokinase step. These observations validated the derivation of equations express-

[a] This work was supported by the MRC Canada (SP-30) and the MRC Denmark (12-1633 and 12-1634). P.D. is a recipient of the Jeanne Timmins Studentship.
[d] Address correspondence to Dr. Albert Gjedde at PET Centre in Aarhus, Denmark.

ing the rate of glucose utilization in rats in terms of activities measured in blood and brain *ex vivo*.[7] This method was then extended for [^{18}F]fluorodeoxyglucose studies of glucose consumption in human brain.[8-10] In contrast, qualitative positron emission tomographic studies of dopamine synthesis with [^{18}F]fluorodopa were first attempted prior to the invention of corresponding compartmental models. Efforts to arrive at quantitative analysis of dopa metabolism have subsequently led to models of tracer uptake which, in formal terms, resemble those describing glucose metabolism.[11,12] However, the modeling of dopa metabolism has proven to be more complex than for [^{18}F]fluorodeoxyglucose, requiring the addition of several physiological constraints for the separation of specific physiological parameters. The purpose of this review is to assess the extent to which physiological models of dopa decarboxylase activity are of heuristic value in measuring the relative rate of steps in dopamine synthesis, in a manner comparable to methods for *in vivo* assays of glucose consumption.

PATHWAY FOR DOPA METABOLISM

Pathways for the peripheral and central metabolism of [^{18}F]fluorodopa are summarized in FIGURE 1.[13] Corresponding steps define the pathway of metabolism of [^{3}H]dopa[14] and β-[^{11}C]dopa, but for the present we confine the discussion to [^{18}F]fluorodopa. In our nomenclature, the superscript indicates the substrate for each identified process or step.[15] [^{18}F]Fluorodopa in circulation is O-methylated by catechol-O-methyltransferase (COMT) at the apparent rate of k_0^{FDOPA} (min^{-1}). The product, O-methyl-6-[^{18}F]fluorodopa(O-methyl-[^{18}F]fluorodopa), is eliminated from circulation at the rate of k_{-1}^{OMFD} (min^{-1}). [^{18}F]Fluorodopa (along with other dopa decarboxylase substrates and O-methylated metabolites) are reversibly transferred across the blood–brain barrier by the common carrier of large neutral amino acids (K_1^{FDOPA}, mL g^{-1} min^{-1}; k_2^{FDOPA}, min^{-1}). The equilibrium partition volume of [^{18}F]fluorodopa is defined as K_1^{FDOPA}/k^{2FDOPA} (V_e^{FDOPA}, mL g^{-1}), whereas the vascular volume apparently occupied by the tracer in brain is expressed by V_0^{FDOPA} (mL g^{-1}). [^{18}F]Fluorodopa and other dopa analogues are potential substrates for O-methylation by catechol-O-methyltransferase within brain (k_5^{FDOPA}, min^{-1}).

[^{18}F]Fluorodopa in brain is decarboxylated at the rate of k_3^{FDOPA} (min^{-1}), corresponding to the relative activity of dopa decarboxylase in brain. The product [^{18}F]fluorodopamine, if not sequestered in vesicles (circle, FIG. 1), undergoes decomposition by monoamine oxidase at the rate of k_7^{FDA} (min^{-1}). The oxidative deamination of [^{18}F]fluorodopamine yields the acidic metabolites [^{18}F]fluorodihydroxyphenylacetic acid and [^{18}F]fluorohomovanillic acid. These acidic metabolites are eliminated from brain at the rate of k_9^{acids} (min^{-1}). Alternately, it can be assumed that [^{18}F]fluorodopamine and its acidic metabolites are eliminated from brain as a single compartment at rate constant $k_{cl}^{FDA+acids}$ (min^{-1}).

[^{18}F]Fluorodopa is a substrate *in vitro* for dopa decarboxylase obtained from rat striatum:[16] the major radiolabeled compounds formed in striatum of living rat are [^{18}F]fluorodopamine and its acidic metabolites.[17-20] The formation of 3-methoxytyramine, which occurs at a rate 5% that of the formation of dihydroxyphenylacetic acid in rat striatum,[21,22] is omitted in the present model: only traces of 6-[^{18}F]fluoro-3-methoxytyramine are detected in rat striatum.[17,18] However, the radiochemical fractionation of extracts from monkey brain likewise shows the major labeled compound to be O-methyl-[^{18}F]fluorodopa in cerebral cortex and cerebellum, whereas substantial amounts of [^{18}F]fluorodopamine and its acidic metabolites are

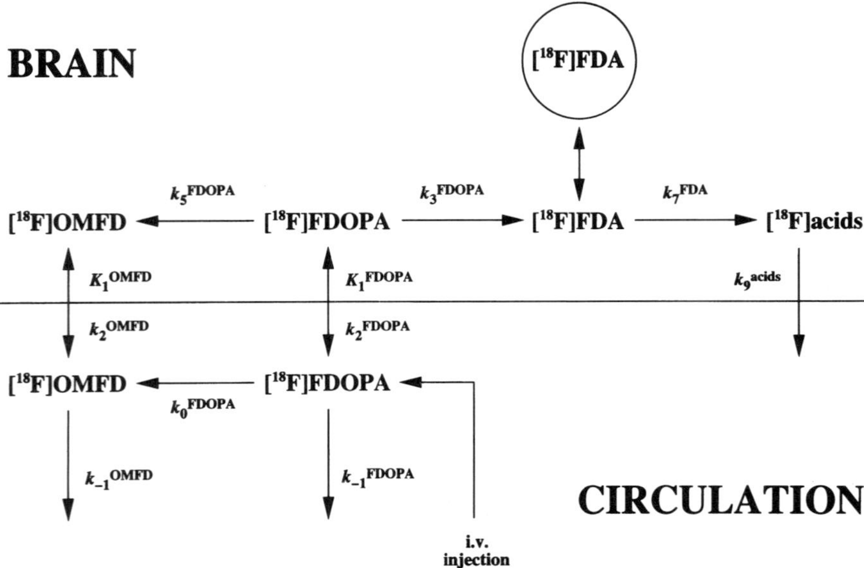

FIGURE 1. Schematic summaries of [¹⁸F]fluorodopa blood–brain transfer and metabolism, including the associated kinetic parameters, according to three different compartmental models (Models 1, 2, and 3). [¹⁸F]Fluorodopa in circulation is O-methylated (k_0^{FDOPA}) by catechol-O-methyltransferase to form O-methyl-[¹⁸F]fluorodopa (k_0^{FDOPA}). Both tracers are subsequently cleared from circulation by renal elimination (k_{-1}^{FDOPA} and k_{-1}^{OMFD}). Both tracers are transferred into brain (K_1^{FDOPA} and K_1^{OMFD} and out of brain (k_2^{FDOPA} and K_2^{OMFD}) by facilitated diffusion. [¹⁸F]Fluorodopa in brain is O-methylated (k_5^{FDOPA}) by catechol-O-methyltransferase to form O-methyl-[¹⁸F]fluorodopa. In brain regions containing dopa decarboxylase, [¹⁸F]fluorodopa is decarboxylated (k_3^{FDOPA}) to form [¹⁸F]fluorodopamine, most of which is rapidly sequestered in vesicles (*circle*) and so protected from oxidative deamination by monoamine oxidase. For Model 1, [¹⁸F]fluorodopamine is not metabolized or otherwise cleared from brain. For Model 2, [¹⁸F]fluorodopamine and its labeled acidic metabolites ([¹⁸F]acids) occupy the same compartment and are together cleared from brain ($k_1^{\text{FDA+acids}}$). For Model 3, [¹⁸F]fluorodopamine is not cleared from brain but is metabolized to form [¹⁸F]acids (k_7^{FDA}), which are subsequently cleared from brain into the cerebrospinal fluid and thence to blood (k_9^{acids}). The rates for these two latter processes are arbitrarily set to be equal.

present in caudate and putamen 60 min after [¹⁸F]fluorodopa administration.[23–25] An earlier report failing to detect O-methyl-[¹⁸F]fluorodopa in human blood[26] seems to have been based upon misidentification of radiochemical fractions in biological extracts.

The activity of cerebral dopa decarboxylase relative to [¹⁸F]fluorodopa and other substrates, defined as k_3^{FDOPA} (min⁻¹), is the fractional rate constant of dopa decarboxylase relative to its Michaelis-Menten constants ($V_{\text{max}}/[K_{\text{m}} + C]$). The half-saturation concentrations of dopa for its decarboxylase obtained from cat brain (7 μM),[27] rat brain (100 μM),[16] hog kidney (190 μM),[28] and human pheochromocytoma cells (50 μM)[29] are much greater than the endogenous substrate concentration in brain (<1 μM).[30] The temporal changes in the concentrations of labeled products and precursors in rat brain have been determined by high performance liquid chromatographic fractionation of extracts of plasma and brain. From these measurements we have calculated the activity of dopa decarboxylase in living rat striatum with respect to [^{18}F]fluorodopa (0.17 min^{-1}).[13] Similar estimates for the magnitude of dopa decarboxylase activity in rat striatum were obtained for [^{3}H]dopa (0.26 min^{-1}),[14] (0.20 min^{-1}),[31] and from data reported for β-[^{11}C]dopa (0.4 min^{-1}).[32] The Michaelis-Menten kinetics of [^{18}F]fluorodopa and [^{3}H]dopa for dopa decarboxylase from rat striatum *in vitro* are nearly identical.[16] Thus, [^{18}F]fluorodopa in rat brain is not biochemically distinguished from labeled DOPA in the irreversible decarboxylation step. However, 2-[^{18}F]fluorodopa is a relatively poor substrate for dopa decarboxylase from rat striatum; the K_m is 10-fold higher and the V_{max} lower than for 6-[^{18}F]fluorodopa.[16] Thus, the metabolism of ring-fluorinated dopa analogues is highly sensitive to position of substitution on the aromatic ring.

Decarboxylation of tracers in circulation is an alternate metabolic pathway omitted from the above schema. In the majority of *in vivo* autoradiographic studies with labeled dopa or [^{18}F]fluorodopa, experimental subjects and animals are pretreated with carbidopa, an inhibitor of dopa decarboxylase acting mainly in the periphery. This treatment increases the formation of labeled dopamine in striatum of the rat.[19] Carbidopa treatment of humans increases the area under the arterial curve for [^{18}F]fluorodopa and increases the specific striatal activity, but does not alter the magnitude of net tracer influx.[33] Recently, positron-emitting analogues of *meta*-tyrosine have become available.[34] These compounds are not substrates for catechol-*O*-methyltransferase in brain and in the periphery, but are readily decarboxylated in brain to yield *meta*-tyramines. In principle, the use of *meta*-tyrosines could greatly simplify the compartmental modeling of dopa decarboxylase activity.

In positron emission tomographic studies, cerebral concentrations of labeled dopa decarboxylase substrates and products are not measured directly, but must be construed from kinetic modeling of the observed total time-activity curves. The measured concentrations of [^{18}F]fluorodopa metabolites formed in rat striatum are in generally close agreement with concentrations predicted by compartmental modeling.[35] However, available estimates of dopa decarboxylase activity obtained by compartmental autoradiographic analysis of tracer dopa uptake in brain of rat, non-human primate, and human are nearly an order of magnitude lower than those obtained by high performance liquid chromatographic radiochemical fractionation of extracts from rat brain (TABLE 1). This discrepancy does not reflect a species difference: The magnitude of k_3^{FDOPA} is much higher in rat brain when obtained by chromatographic fractionation methods than by any of several compartmental models of a time series of autoradiograms from the same rats.[15] In liquid chromatographic studies of dopa decarboxylase tracer metabolism *ex vivo*, it is probable that consumption of dopa and other substrates by dopa decarboxylase is likely to continue for some minutes postmortem. This would alter the apparent relationship between labeled product and precursor in fractionated extracts, which would tend to increase the apparent magnitude of dopa decarboxylase activity. However, numerous other procedural differences exist between autoradiographic methods and analytic methods for the assay of dopa decarboxylase in living brain.[15] These factors have proven a formidable challenge in the development of positron emission tomographic methods for isolation of specific information of physiological interest, in particular the *in vivo* activity of dopa decarboxylase.

The acidic metabolites of dopamine, dihydroxyphenylacetic acid and homovanillic acid, and the corresponding metabolites of [^{18}F]fluorodopamine are eliminated from rat brain by a diffusion process at rates (min^{-1}) in the range 0.04–0.12.[13,14,22,31] Thus, the trapping in rat brain of radioactivity derived from [^{18}F]fluorodopa cannot be truly irreversible, but is determined by the rate of oxidative deamination of

[^{18}F]fluorodopamine *in vivo* and by the subsequent clearance rate of the acidic metabolites. Opinions currently differ as to whether or under which circumstances the elimination of acidic [^{18}F]fluorodopamine metabolites from brain can properly be omitted from compartmental models. Furthermore, the analysis of [^{18}F]fluorodopa uptake is hampered by the formation in blood of important amounts of *O*-methyl-[^{18}F]fluorodopa,[36] a brain-penetrating metabolite. In order to reduce the number of parameters in compartmental models, some groups have assumed a fixed ratio of blood–brain permeabilities for the tracer and its inert metabolite,[11,37,38] while others have proposed that the two permeabilities should be determined in separate experiments.[39] Several approaches for the determination of the tracer distribution volumes have been attempted. Finally, the consequences of partial volume effects on the estimation of kinetic parameters in compartmental models have not been addressed until recently.

PHYSIOLOGICAL SIGNIFICANCE OF DOPA DECARBOXYLASE ACTIVITY

The decarboxylation of [^{18}F]fluorodopa in living brain occurs in competition with at least two other processes (FIG. 1): the elimination rate from brain to blood (k_2^{FDOPA}) and, possibly, the rate of *O*-methylation in brain (k_5^{FDOPA}). We have demonstrated that the synthesis of [^{3}H]dopa from [^{3}H]tyrosine in living rat brain is not a committed step in cerebral [^{3}H]catecholamine synthesis because of the presence of pathways other than decarboxylation *in vivo*.[30] In this context, by determining the fraction of labeled dopa which is decarboxylated rather than eliminated by other processes, dopa decarboxylase activity can influence the synthesis of labeled dopamine in brain.[31,40,41]

A considerable body of evidence exists that dopa decarboxylase activity from rat striatum measured *ex vivo* is regulated by dopamine receptors[42,43] and by NMDA receptors.[44] The activity of dopa decarboxylase measured *in vivo* from the radiochemical fractionation of [^{3}H]dopa metabolites in cerebral extracts has now been found to be potentiated by acute treatment with neuroleptics and decreased by treatment with apomorphine, a dopamine receptor agonist.[31] Our earlier observation that dopa decarboxylase activity in rat brain is decreased after acute treatment with pargyline, an inhibitor of dopamine catabolism[14] may likewise indicate a certain regulation of dopa decarboxylase mediated by the occupation of autoreceptors by dopamine. Dopamine concentration in microdialysates from rat striatum, and presumably autoreceptor occupation, is elevated after acute treatment with pargyline.[21,22] It has been suggested that dopa is itself a dopamine autoreceptor antagonist,[45] possibly accounting for the activation in dopa decarboxylase activity observed in putamen of patients with advanced Parkinson's disease following infusion of dopa.[46]

COMPARTMENTAL MODELS OF DOPA METABOLISM

The plasma slope-intercept plot or multiple time graphical analysis[47,48] provides a linear graphical method for determination of net influx (K^{FDOPA}, mL g^{-1} min^{-1}) of [^{18}F]fluorodopa from blood into human brain.[49] The difference between radioactivity in the region of interest and in a reference region nearly devoid of dopamine innervation is assumed to be equal to the amount of decarboxylated product in the reference region. The distribution volume (V_d) of product relative to the plasma precursor concentration is plotted as a linear function of the normalized tracer circulation time (Θ, min), defined as the integral of the tracer concentration (corrected for peripheral metabolism) divided by the concentration at time T. The regression slope of the relation between V_d as a function of Θ is the net tracer clearance from blood to brain (K^{FDOPA}). The distribution volume of [^{18}F]fluorodopa in the human caudate and putamen as a function of the normalized tracer circulation is obviously linear, but tends to deviate from linearity at early times in the positron emission tomography experiment (FIG. 2). This deviation may reflect initially higher clearance of tracer into a reference region due to regional differences in the blood–brain transport of large neutral amino acids (see ref. 11).

The plasma slope method requires the correction of the total arterial input curves for the fractions of [^{18}F]fluorodopa and its *O*-methylated metabolite during the positron emission tomography experiment. Temporal changes in these fractions have been determined by solid-phase separations of plasma radioactivities based on the adsorption of [^{18}F]fluorodopa, but not *O*-methyl-[^{18}F]fluorodopa to basic alumina.[36,50] The solid-phase method, although perhaps more convenient, does not account for the presence of minor [^{18}F]fluorodopa metabolites occurring in radiochemical fractionations of arterial plasma of carbidopa-treated human subjects.[36,51] The presence of these metabolites is especially in evidence if the inhibition of peripheral dopa decarboxylase is incomplete.[51] Estimate of the net blood–brain clearance calculated relative to the plasma activity are listed in TABLE 2.

The tissue slope-intercept plot[52] has been used to measure the rate constant of trapping of dopa decarboxylase tracers relative to uptake in a reference region (k_3^{ref}, min^{-1}; TABLE 3), without requiring the arterial input curves.[53,54] However, this method is uncorrected for the presence in brain of the peripheral *O*-methylated metabolite. For this reason, the magnitude of the slope intercept plot relative to cortex, but not to plasma, is sensitive to experimental manipulation of the peripheral metabolism of [^{18}F]fluorodopa by catechol-*O*-methyltransferase.[55] The use of tissue slope-intercept plots may only be justified when it is certain that peripheral pharmacokinetics of the tracer is not an experimental variable. Furthermore, the rates of *O*-methylation of [^{18}F]fluorodopa in arterial circulation of normal human subjects vary over a twofold range.[51] Thus, individual differences in the peripheral pharmacokinetics of [^{18}F]fluorodopa could contribute to variance in estimates of the dopa decarboxylase activity by the tissue slope-intercept plot.

Both the plasma and the tissue slope-intercept methods yield transfer coefficients or rate constants proportional to the net blood–brain tracer clearance (K^{FDOPA}; TABLE 2), equal to $K_1^{FDOPA} k_3^{FDOPA}/(k_2^{FDOPA} + k_3^{FDOPA})$. The plasma and tissue slope intercept methods are roughly equivalent in their power to separate a group of six healthy voluntaeers and six patients with Parkinson's disease.[56] The reduced net clearance of [^{18}F]fluorodopa is more pronounced in the putamen than in the caudate of patients with Parkinson's disease (FIG. 2). The scan-rescan standard deviation of the K^{FDOPA} method in a series of 10 normal human subjects was 9% of the mean, whereas the between-subject standard deviation was 26%.[57] Head-placement is an additional factor in influencing the reproducibility of [^{18}F]fluorodopa studies, especially in studies on non-human primates. Thus, the standard deviation of separate estimates of K^{FDOPA} in cynomolgus monkeys was 14% if the two scans were carried out with the animal remaining in the scanner, but 34% when the two scans were performed on separate days.[58] However, these studies were carried out without registration of positron emission images to magnetic resonance images, and so are based upon regions of interest which were drawn by hand without reference to objective anatomical landmarks.

TABLE 1. Relative Activity of Cerebral Dopa Decarboxylase (k_3, min^{-1}) with respect to Some Radiolabeled Substrates *in Vivo*

Study	Method	k_3 Striatum	k_3 Other
[18F]fluorodopa, rat ($n = 45$)[13]	HPLC V_e and q independent	0.17 ± 0.02	
[3H]dopa, rat ($n = 13$)[14]	HPLC V_e and q independent	0.26 ± 0.06 (control) 0.13 ± 0.06 (pargyline)	0.02 ± 0.02 (neocortex)
[3H]dopa, rat ($n = 10$)[31]	HPLC V_e and q independent	0.20 ± 0.04 (control) 0.44 ± 0.06 (flupenthixol)	0.015 ± 0.003 (neocortex)
[3H]dopa, rat ($n = 13$) An autoradiographic study of right hemi- spheres from the same rats in above HPLC study.[15]	M1 (60 min) M1 (180 min) M2 (180 min) M3 (180 min) V_e and q fixed	0.025 ± 0.006 0.009 ± 0.002 0.06 ± 0.02 0.033 ± 0.009	0.008 ± 0.001 0.002 ± 0.001 0.017 ± 0.003 0.009 ± 0.002 (hippocampus)
β-[11C]dopa, rat ($n = 12$)[32]	HPLC V_e and q independent	0.4 ± 0.2	–
[18F]fluorodopa, rat ($n = 12$)[62]	M1 (140 min) q measured	0.01	–
[18F]fluorodopa, pig ($n = 8$)[138]	M1 V_e and q fixed	0.018 ± 0.002	0.002 ± 0.001 (cortex) 0.000 ± 0.001 (cerebellum)
[18F]fluorodopa, monkey ($n = 3$)[140]	M1 V_e measured, q fixed	0.015 ± 0.003	0 (cerebellum)
4-[18F]FMT, monkey ($n = 3$)[140]	M2 V_e measured, q fixed	0.03 ± 0.01	0.006 ± 0.004 (cerebellum)
6-[18F]FMT, monkey ($n = 3$)[140]	M2 V_e measured, q fixed	0.033 ± 0.004	0.006 ± 0.004 (cerebellum)
6-[18F]FMT, normal human ($n = 5$)[80]	M1	0.04 ± 0.01	0.0022 ± 0.0001 (cortex) 0.0013 ± 0.0001 (cerebellum)
[18F]fluorodopa, monkey ($n = 4$)[72]	M1 V_e and q fixed	0.06 ± 0.01 (control) 0.042 ± 0.007 (OR-611)	–
[18F]fluorodopa, normal human ($n = 4$)[60]	M1 M2 V_e floated, q fixed	0.012 ± 0.001 0.019 ± 0.001	–

[18F]fluorodopa, normal human ($n = 10$)[12]	M1 M2 V_e floated, q fixed	0.012 ± 0.004 0.04 ± 0.02	—
[18F]fluorodopa, normal human ($n = 12$)[37]	M1 (V_e fixed, q fixed) M1 (V_e floated, q fixed)	0.08 ± 0.02 (caudate, V_e fixed) 0.07 ± 0.01 (putamen, V_e fixed) 0.03 ± 0.01 (caudate, V_e floated) 0.03 ± 0.01 (putamen, V_e floated)	0.018 ± 0.007 0.017 ± 0.014 (amygdala)
[18F]fluorodopa, normal human ($n = 6$)[11]	M1 V_e and q fixed	0.032 ± 0.003 putamen	—
[18F]fluorodopa, Parkinson's disease, effect of COMT inhibition ($n = 6$)[59]	M1 V_e fixed, $q = 1.7$	0.04 ± 0.02 ($-$ OR 611) 0.02 ± 0.01 ($+$ OR 611)	—
[18F]fluorodopa, Parkinson's disease ($n = 16$)[143]	M1 V_e, q fixed	0.08 ± 0.05 (normal subjects, $n = 9$) 0.03 ± 0.02 (Parkinson's disease, $n = 16$)	
[18F]fluorodopa, Parkinson's disease ($n = 5$)[39]	M1 V_e floated, q fixed	0.02 ± 0.01 (normal subjects, $n = 3$) 0.007 ± 0.005 (Parkinson's disease, $n = 5$)	—
[18F]fluorodopa, Parkinson's disease ($n = 7$)[38]	M3 V_e and q fixed	0.08 ± 0.01 (putamen, control) 0.04 ± 0.01 (putamen, Parkinson's) 0.07 ± 0.02 (caudate, control) 0.05 ± 0.02 (caudate, Parkinson's)	0.010 ± 0.002 (control) 0.010 ± 0.006 (Parkinson's) (frontal cortex)
[18F]fluorodopa, psychosis ($n = 5$)[134]	M1 V_e and q fixed	0.075 ± 0.005 (caudate, control, $n = 13$) 0.10 ± 0.01 (caudate, psychosis, $n = 5$) 0.072 ± 0.004 (putamen, control, $n = 13$) 0.084 ± 0.008 (putamen, psychosis, $n = 5$)	—

NOTE: In some cases estimates are based upon time series of the concentrations of labeled dopamine and its acidic metabolites measured by chemical fractionation (HPLC) of extracts from rat brain. The kinetic models are: Model 1 (M1), in which labeled dopamine is irreversibly trapped in brain; Model 2 (M2), in which labeled dopamine and its metabolites occupy a single compartment and are cleared from brain at rate $k_{cl}^{DA+acids}$; and Model 3 (M3), which assumes that labeled dopamine is not diffusible, but is deaminated at rate k_7^{DA} yielding diffusible metabolites which are cleared at rate k_9^{acids}. We have constrained M3 such that the magnitudes of k_7^{DA} and k_9^{acids} were arbitrarily defined as equal. In most compartmental models the value of the blood–brain barrier permeability ratio for labeled dopa and its *O*-methylated metabolite (q) was fixed. The equilibrium distribution volume of labeled dopa decarboxylase substrate was either floated as an additional parameter, or fixed to the value obtained in a brain region devoid of dopa decarboxylase activity (Model 0). Each estimate is the mean $\pm$ SD of (n) separate determinations, or in the case of rat experiments, the best estimate $\pm$ 95% confidence intervals obtained within a population of (n) rats.

More extended compartmental models separate the net blood–brain transfer into at least three parameters: The distribution in brain of an inert tracer passively transferred across the blood–brain barrier is defined by the unidirectional blood–brain clearance (K_1^{FDOPA}, mL g^{-1} min^{-1}) and the equilibrium distribution volume (V_e^{FDOPA}, mL g^{-1}), plus a term describing the radioactivity in the vascular compartment (V_0^{FDOPA}, mL g^{-1}). In a region devoid of dopa decarboxylase activity, or for O-methyl-[18F]fluorodopa which is not a substrate for subsequent metabolism, the observed time activity curve may thus be described in terms of these three variables. We refer to this model as Model 0. The magnitudes of V_0^{FDOPA} and V_e^{FDOPA} can be first estimated by Model 0 in a reference region assumed to be devoid of significant dopa decarboxylase activity (i.e., occipital cortex), and then used as input parameters for the determination of relative dopa decarboxylase activity in a region of interest where the dopa decarboxylase activity is non-zero.[11,12] Alternately, one may attempt to determine separately the equilibrium distribution volume of [18F]fluorodopa in all regions[59,60] at the risk of imprecision due to overparameterization. We refer to the model in which the trapping of the decarboxylated product (e.g., tracer dopamine) is assumed to be irreversible in the time course of the positron emission tomographic experiment as Model 1.

ELIMINATION OF DECARBOXYLATED METABOLITES

[18F]Fluorohomovanillic acid accumulating in cerebrospinal fluid of monkey during positron emission tomography with [18F]fluorodopa appears to be derived from [18F]fluorodopamine formed within brain.[61] Thus, trapping of decarboxylated products in brain is not irreversible. We have calculated the activity of dopa decarboxylase relative to [3H]dopa in rat striatum by fitting our Model 1 to a time series of autoradiograms during 180 min after peripheral administration of tracer.[35] For circulation times longer than 60 min, the extrapolated radioactivity predicted in striatum by this model without clearance increasingly exceeds the measured radioactivities. Consequently, the magnitude of k_3^{FDOPA} determined by Model 1 was highly sensitive to the duration of the experiment (TABLE 1). The magnitude of k_3^{FDOPA} determined by fitting of Model 1 to dynamic time-activity data from a patient with Parkinson's disease and from a normal subject declined continuously as a function of tracer circulation time (FIG. 3). This phenomenon may account for the low value for k_3^{FDOPA} in rat striatum during 140 min of tracer circulation.[62] Thus, an expanded compartmental model is required to describe the further metabolism and eventual elimination of decarboxylated products formed in brain during extended tracer experiments.

The decarboxylated product [18F]fluorodopamine and its acidic metabolites formed with brain can be assumed to occupy a single compartment which is cleared from brain by a first order process ($k_{cl}^{FDA+acids}$, min^{-1}).[12] We refer to this as Model 2. We have shown elsewhere that the magnitude of $k_{cl}^{FDA+acids}$ changes as a function of tracer circulation time, and so properly cannot be called a rate constant.[15] However, the magnitude of $k_{cl}^{FDA+acids}$ becomes stable when the rates of formation and clearance of [18F]-labeled acidic metabolites approach secular equilibrium. The dopa decarboxylase activity measured in human brain is very sensitive to the use of Model 2 for [18F]fluorodopa studies lasting more than 60 min; the magnitude of k_3^{FDOPA} was increased severalfold when calculated by Model 2 rather than Model 1.[12,63] Therefore, use of Model 2 is likely to improve the accuracy of estimates of k_3^{FDOPA}, which tends to be underestimated by Model 1.

TABLE 2. Net Influx of [^{18}F]Fluorodopa (K^{FDOPA}) Calculated Relative to the Normalized Arterial Integral of [^{18}F]Fluorodopa

Study	Net Influx of [^{18}F]fluorodopa (K^{FDOPA}) (mL g^{-1} min^{-1} or mL striatum^{-1} min^{-1})
Monkey, mL g^{-1} min^{-1},[141]	0.010 ± 0.002 (untreated, $n = 4$) 0.010 ± 0.003 (carbidopa, 2.5 mg/kg, i.p., $n = 4$)
Monkey, effect of COMT inhibition, mL g^{-1} min^{-1},[67]	0.0030 ± 0.0002 (control, $n = 6$) 0.0041 ± 0.0006 (OR 462, $n = 6$)
Monkey, MPTP model of Parkinson's disease, mL g^{-1} min^{-1},[97]	0.008 ± 0.002 (right striatum, $n = 8$) 0.008 ± 0.002 (left striatum, $n = 8$) 0.002 ± 0.001 (1 month post-MPTP, $n = 4$) 0.0012 ± 0.0008 (5 months post-MPTP, $n = 4$) 0.0013 ± 0.0004 (9 months post-MPTP, $n = 4$)
Monkey, effect of amphetamine poisoning, mL g^{-1} min^{-1},[131]	0.009 ± 0.001 (control, $n = 6$) 0.0022 ± 0.0005 (<6 weeks post amphetamine, $n = 3$) 0.0042 ± 0.0005 (20 weeks post amphetamine, $n = 3$)
Normal human, effect of carbidopa, mL g^{-1} min^{-1},[33]	0.011 ± 0.002 (− carbidopa, $n = 3$) 0.010 ± 0.002 (+ carbidopa 250 mg, $n = 3$)
Normal human, mL g^{-1} min^{-1},[103]	0.012 ± 0.004 ($n = 19$) age = 52 ± 17 yr
Normal human, effect of aging, mL striatum^{-1} min^{-1},[49]	0.8 ± 0.2 (3rd–5th decades, $n = 5$) 0.6 ± 0.1 (6th–9th decades, $n = 5$)
Normal human, 3rd–8th decade, mL g^{-1} min^{-1},[102]	0.011 ± 0.003 (caudate, $n = 26$) 0.010 ± 0.002 (putamen, $n = 26$)
Normal aging of a kindred, mL striatum^{-1} min^{-1},[105]	0.26 ± 0.03 (control, age = 23 yr, $n = 12$) 0.22 ± 0.05 (control, age = 75 yr, $n = 12$)
Parkinson's disease, effect of COMT inhibition, mL g^{-1} min^{-1},[55]	0.011 ± 0.002 (control, − OR 611, $n = 5$) 0.011 ± 0.002 (control, + OR 611, $n = 5$) 0.007 ± 0.002 (Parkinson's disease, − OR-611, $n = 4$)
Parkinson's disease, effect of disease progression, mL g^{-1} min^{-1},[109]	0.013 ± 0.002 (control, $n = 12$) 0.007 ± 0.001 (Parkinson's disease, UPDRS < 15, $n = 6$) 0.006 ± 0.001 (Parkinson's disease, UPDRS > 15, $n = 6$)
Parkinson's disease, effect of disease progression, mL g^{-1} min^{-1},[104]	0.016 ± 0.005 (control caudate, $n = 5$) 0.011 ± 0.004 (Parkinson's disease caudate, $n = 9$) 0.010 ± 0.004 (several years later, $n = 9$) 0.015 ± 0.004 (control putamen, $n = 5$) 0.006 ± 0.002 (Parkinson's disease putamen, $n = 9$) 0.005 ± 0.002 (several years later, $n = 9$)
Parkinson's disease, effect of clinical severity, mL g^{-1} min^{-1},[107]	0.014 ± 0.004 (control, $n = 10$) 0.006 ± 0.002 (Hoehn and Yahr, I–II, $n = 10$) 0.005 ± 0.001 (Hoehn and Yahr III–IV, $n = 10$)
Familial Parkinson's disease, mL g^{-1} min^{-1},[110]	0.010 ± 0.001 (normal, $n = 33$) 0.005 ± 0.001 (sporadic Parkinson's disease, $n = 18$) 0.004 ± 0.001 (familial Parkinson's disease, $n = 10$) 0.008 ± 0.002 (unaffected members, $n = 32$)
Parkinson's disease, effect of grafting of fetal nigral neurons, mL g^{-1} min^{-1},[115]	0.008 ± 0.001 (putamen, pregraft, $n = 4$) 0.011 ± 0.001 (putamen, postgraft, $n = 4$) 0.014 ± 0.002 (caudate, pregraft, $n = 4$) 0.015 ± 0.003 (caudate, postgraft, $n = 4$)
Parkinsonism, Parkinson's disease, and dopa-responsive dystonia, mL striatum^{-1} min^{-1},[119]	0.30 ± 0.06 (normal, $n = 16$) 0.30 ± 0.05 (dopa-responsive dystonia, $n = 9$) 0.18 ± 0.02 (juvenile parkinsonism, $n = 3$) 0.15 ± 0.05 (young-onset parkinsonism, $n = 13$)

TABLE 2. (*Continued*)

Study	Net Influx of [^{18}F]fluorodopa (K^{FDOPA}) (mL g^{-1} min^{-1} or mL striatum^{-1} min^{-1})
Early hemiparkinsonism, mL g^{-1} min^{-1},[106]	0.012 ± 0.002 (normal, $n = 16$) 0.010 ± 0.002 (asymptomatic side, $n = 11$) 0.007 ± 0.001 (symptomatic side, $n = 11$)
Subjects from Guam, presenting mainly with either amyotrophic lateral sclerosis or Parkinson's disease, mL striatum^{-1} min^{-1},[116]	0.6 ± 0.2 (control, $n = 7$) 0.4 ± 0.2 (amyotrophic lateral sclerosis, $n = 4$) 0.17 ± 0.06 (Parkinson's disease, $n = 8$)
Petroleum waste ingestion, mL striatum^{-1} min^{-1},[133]	0.17 (acute poisoning, $n = 1$)
Progressive supranuclear palsy, mL striatum^{-1} min^{-1},[120]	0.7 ± 0.1 (control, $n = 13$) 0.2 ± 0.1 (progressive supranuclear palsy, $n = 9$)
Relatives from the pallido-ponto-nigral degeneration family, mL striatum^{-1} min^{-1},[118]	0.31 ± 0.03 (control, $n = 10$) 0.22 ± 0.02 (gene positive, asymptomatic, $n = 4$) 0.07 ± 0.05 (symptomatic, $n = 4$)
Wilson's disease, mL striatum^{-1} min^{-1},[124]	0.6 ± 0.1 (control, $n = 18$) 0.3 ± 0.1 (Wilson's disease, $n = 4$)

NOTE: Net influx has units of blood flow (mL g^{-1} min^{-1} or mL striatum min^{-1}). The effects of treatment with inhibitors of catechol-O-methyltransferase (COMT) inhibitors (OR 462, OR 611) are reported. Results of clinical investigations of movement disorders are summarized. In studies of the progression of Parkinson's disease, clinical severity is assessed by Hoehn and Yahr or the Unified Parkinson's Disease Rating Scale (UPDRS) scores. Each estimate is the mean ± SD of (n) determinations.

Alternately, the decarboxylated product and its acidic metabolites can be assumed to occupy separate compartments in brain. In this model, which we define as Model 3, the decarboxylated compound in brain, assumed to be nondiffusible, is further metabolized to diffusible metabolites at rate constant k_7^{FDA} (min^{-1}). The diffusible acidic metabolites leave brain at the rate of k_9^{acids} (min^{-1}). This system is soluble when k_7^{FDA} and k_9^{acids} are assumed to be of equal magnitude ($k_7^{\text{FDA}} = k_9^{\text{acids}}$).[64] Although the equality is arbitrary, the rate constants for the deamination of [^{18}F]fluorodopamine (0.055 min^{-1})[13] and [^{3}H]dopamine (0.013 min^{-1})[14] formed in striatum of living rat falls within the same order of magnitude of the corresponding rate constants for the elimination of the acidic metabolites (0.12 min^{-1} [ref. 13]; 0.04 min^{-1} [refs. 14, 22, 31]).

We have fitted Model 3 to time-activity curves obtained by quantitative autoradiography of rat brain during 180 min of [^{3}H]dopa circulation.[15] In the rat basal ganglia, the magnitude of k_3^{DOPA} calculated for the 180-min experiments was higher when calculated by Models 2 or 3 than by Model 1, which assumes irreversible trapping in brain. However, inclusion of the additional terms increased k_3^{DOPA} by only 20% when only the first 60 min of the time-activity curves were considered. Thus, Model 1 provides a satisfactory model for the behavior of [^{3}H]dopa in rat brain when circulation time is relatively brief, albeit with a systematic underestimation of dopa decarboxylase activity. Omission of the elimination of labeled dopamine from the compartmental model results in lower estimates of k_3^{DOPA} in rats[15] and of k_3^{DOPA} in normal human subjects (TABLE 1).[60] Fitting of Model 3 to dynamic positron emission tomography data from a patient with Parkinson's disease and a normal subject (FIG. 3) results in estimates of k_3^{DOPA} that are systematically greater than when Model 1 is fitted to the same data. Furthermore, the magnitude of the estimate of k_3^{FDOPA} is relatively stable for circulation times between 45 and 90 min, as expected

TABLE 3. Activity of Dopa Decarboxylase in Caudate/Putamen (k_3^{ref}, min^{-1}) of Monkey and Human for a Variety of Labeled Substrates[a]

Study	Relative Dopa Decarboxylase Activity
5-hydroxy-[^{11}C]tryptophan, normal monkey[77]	0.007 ± 0.001 ($n = 4$)
5-hydroxy-[^{11}C]tryptophan, monkey, effect of the dopa decarboxylase cofactor pyridoxine[79]	0.008 ± 0.002 (control, $n = 7$) 0.009 ± 0.003 (pyridoxine 10 mg kg^{-1}, $n = 5$)
β-[^{11}C]dopa, monkey, effect of COMT inhibition with Ro 40-7592[74]	0.011 ± 0.001 (control, $n = 4$) 0.011 ± 0.002 (Ro 40-7592, $n = 4$)
6-fluoro-[^{11}C]dopa, monkey, effect of COMT inhibition with Ro 40-7592[74]	0.0057 ± 0.0006 (control, $n = 4$) 0.009 ± 0.002 (Ro 40-7592, $n = 4$)
β-[^{11}C]DOPA, normal monkey[75]	0.012 ± 0.001 ($n = 10$)
β-[^{18}F]fluoromethylene-D, L-*meta*-tyrosine, normal monkey[81]	0.009 ± 0.001 ($n = 3$)
2-[^{18}F]fluoro-*meta*-L-tyrosine, normal monkey[81]	0.007 ± 0.001 ($n = 2$)
β-[^{11}C]DOPA, normal human[54]	0.015 ± 0.007 ($n = 8$)
β-[^{11}C]dopa, Parkinson's disease[142]	0.012 ± 0.005 (control, $n = 8$) 0.008 ± 0.001 (Parkinson's disease, $n = 8$)
[^{18}F]fluorodopa, Parkinson's disease as a function of clinical staging[108]	0.016 ± 0.003 (caudate, control, $n = 8$) 0.012 ± 0.002 (caudate, Hoehn and Yahr 1, $n = 7$) 0.010 ± 0.003 (caudate, Hoehn and Yahr 2–4, $n = 13$) 0.016 ± 0.002 (putamen, control, $n = 8$) 0.010 ± 0.003 (putamen, Hoehn and Yahr 2–4, $n = 7$) 0.006 ± 0.003 (putamen, Hoehn and Yahr 2–4, $n = 13$)
β-[^{11}C]dopa, Parkinson's disease as function of clinical severity, on and off dopa states, ($n = 5$)[46]	0.012 ± 0.002 (caudate, early disease, off dopa) 0.012 ± 0.002 (caudate, early disease, on dopa) 0.017 ± 0.003 (caudate, advanced disease off dopa) 0.016 ± 0.002 (caudate, advanced disease, on dopa) 0.006 ± 0.003 (putamen, advanced disease, off dopa) 0.008 ± 0.003 (putamen, advanced disease, on dopa) 0.011 ± 0.004 (putamen, early disease, off dopa) 0.009 ± 0.004 (putamen, early disease, on dopa)
[^{18}F]fluorodopa, olivopontocerebellar atrophy[117]	0.011 ± 0.002 (caudate, controls, $n = 27$) 0.010 ± 0.001 (caudate, patients, $n = 10$) 0.010 ± 0.001 (putamen, controls, $n = 27$) 0.007 ± 0.002 (putamen, patients, $n = 10$)
[^{18}F]fluorodopa, corticobasal degeneration (cerebellar input)[130]	0.020 ± 0.005 (caudate, controls, $n = 10$) 0.007 ± 0.003 (caudate, patients, affected side, $n = 4$) 0.020 ± 0.004 (putamen, controls, $n = 10$) 0.007 ± 0.002 (putamen, patients, affected side, $n = 4$)

[a] Calculated relative to uptake measured in a reference region devoid of dopa decarboxylase activity. Radiotracer experiments were carried out with 5-hydroxy-[^{11}C]tryptophan, β-[^{11}C]dopa, 6-fluoro-[^{11}C]dopa, 2-[^{18}F]fluoro-*meta*-L-tyrosine, [^{18}F]fluoro-*meta*-L-tyrosine, β-[^{18}F]fluoromethylene-D,L-*meta*-tyrosine[^{18}F], or [^{18}F]fluorodopa. Each estimate is the mean $\pm$ SD of (n) determinations.

for a model incorporating the formation and clearance of acidic metabolites. We note that the precision of the estimate of k_3^{FDOPA} is systematically greater for fitting of Model 1 than for Model 3 (FIG. 3), but tends to become better for Model 3 as a function of increasing tracer circulation time. Thus, the precision sacrificed by incorporation of an additional kinetic term is compensated by the improved accuracy for experiments lasting longer than 60 min.

The available estimates of the rate constant for elimination of dopa decarboxyl-

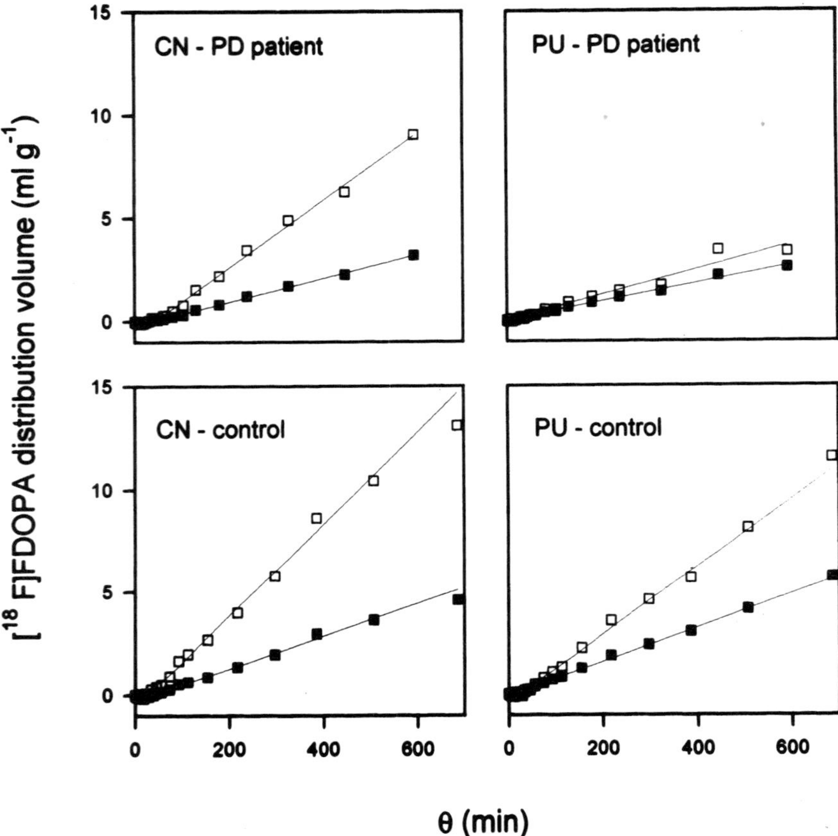

θ (min)

FIGURE 2. The distribution volume of [18F]fluorodopa (V_d^{FDOPA}, mL g^{-1}) as a function of the normalized time-concentration integral of metabolite-corrected plasma [18F]fluorodopa activity [$\Theta = \int C_a^{FDOPA}(t)\,dt / C_a^{FDOPA}(T)$, min] in the caudate nucleus (CN, *left*) and the putamen (PU, *right*) of a patient with Parkinson's disease (*upper*) and a normal control subject (*lower*). The measured data (■) and the data after correction for partial volume effects (□) are illustrated. Magnetic resonance images were registered to the dynamic positron emission tomographic data and were obtained with the Scanditronix PC 2048 tomograph. Corrected time-activity curves were calculated by simulation. The regression slopes of the linear portions represent the net tracer influx (K^{FDOPA}, mL g^{-1} min^{-1}). Partial volume corrections were performed by Dr. Olivier Rousset.

ase products *in vivo* indicate a half-life for [18F]fluorodopamine and [18F]fluorotyramines of 1–2 h^{-1} in brain of living primates (TABLE 4), close to estimates obtained earlier for endogenous dopamine in rat brain.[14] The magnitude of $k_7^{FDA} = k_9^{acids}$ for [18F]fluorodopamine in human brain, also 0.01 min^{-1} is increased twofold in patients with Parkinson's disease.[64] Likewise, $k_{cl}^{FDA+acids}$ was increased severalfold in partially dopamine-denervated striatum of monkeys lesioned with the neurotoxin MPTP.[65] These results are consistent with a more rapid utilization of the residual dopamine in the partially dopamine-depleted striatum. The estimation of net clearance of

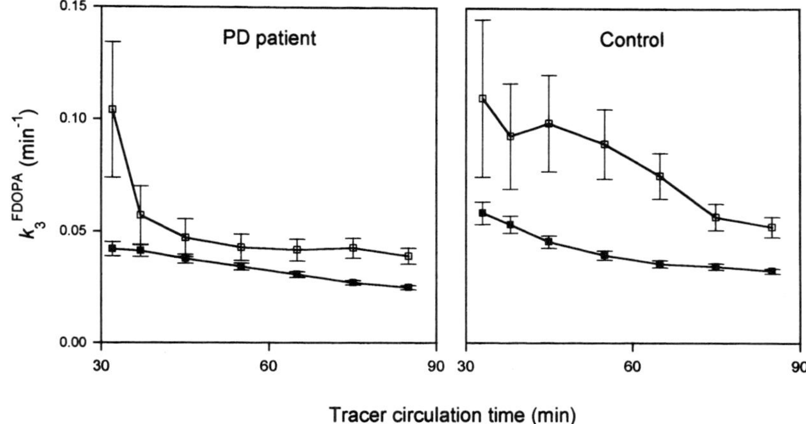

FIGURE 3. Estimates of relative dopa decarboxylase activity (k_3^{DOPA}, min^{-1}) in the putamen as a function of tracer circulation time according to compartmental Model 1(■), which assumes that [18F]fluorodopamine is irreversibly trapped in brain, and Model 3 (□), which incorporates terms for the formation and elimination of [18F]fluorodopamine metabolites in putamen of a patient with Parkinson's disease (*left*) and a normal subject (*right*). For each successive frame between 30 and 90 min the magnitude of the distribution volume was first determined in cortex, and then used as an input parameter for estimation of the dopa decarboxylase activity. Error bars represent 95% confidence intervals in estimates of k_3^{DOPA}.

tracer into brain may be especially difficult in patients with Parkinson's disease, and in others manifesting accelerated turnover of cerebral dopamine if accelerated tracer metabolism in brain results in early deviation of cerebral activity from that predicted by linear models of tracer uptake. However, present data do not suggest that elimination from brain of metabolites has greatly altered the apparent distribution volume in human striatum before 90 min of tracer circulation (FIG. 2).

THE PRESENCE IN CIRCULATION OF BRAIN PENETRATING METABOLITES

In the circulation [18F]fluorodopa is rapidly metabolized by catechol-*O*-methyltransferase, yielding *O*-methyl-[18F]fluorodopa in rat,[13,17,18,66] monkey,[23,24,67] and human.[12,36,51] The tracers [3H]dopa[4,14] and β-[11C]dopa[68] are also extensively *O*-methylated in circulation. Omission of carbidopa-pretreatment results in increased metabolism of [18F]fluorodopa in human circulation by peripheral decarboxylation.[51] There is evidence that ring-fluorination favors the peripheral *O*-methylation of labeled dopa *in vivo.*[66]

In compartmental analysis when an *O*-methylated metabolite is present in arterial plasma, total cerebral radioactivity in a region devoid of dopa decarboxylase activity must be described as the sum of the concentrations of two brain-penetrating tracers, calculated from their respective arterial curves in terms of a single measured permeability and a distribution volume. The estimation of the unidirectional blood–brain clearance K_1^{FDOPA} is then weighted almost entirely to initial blood–brain tracer clearance occurring prior to substantial peripheral metabolism. However,

TABLE 4. Rate Constants (min^{-1}) for the Elimination of Radiolabeled Dopamine Analogues and Their Acidic Metabolites Formed in Brain

Study	Method	Rate Constant for Elimination from Striatum
[^{3}H]dopa, rat (n = 13)[14]	HPLC	k_7^{DA} = 0.013 ± 0.002 k_9^{acids} = 0.037 ± 0.003
[^{3}H]dopa, rat (n = 10)[31]	HPLC	k_9^{acids} = 0.03 ± 0.01 (control) k_9^{acids} = 0.10 ± 0.02 (flupenthixol)
[^{3}H]dopa, rat (n = 13)[15]	M2 M3	$k_{cl}^{DA+acids}$ = 0.017 ± 0.003 k_7^{DA} = k_9^{acids} = 0.029 ± 0.004
[^{18}F]fluorodopa, rat (n = 45)[13]	HPLC	k_7^{DA} = 0.06 ± 0.02 k_9^{acids} = 0.12 ± 0.04
4-[^{18}F]fluoro-*meta*-L-tyrosine, monkey (n = 3)[140]	M2	$k_{cl}^{DA+acids}$ = 0.0005 ± 0.0009
6-[^{18}F]fluoro-*meta*-L-tyrosine, monkey (n = 3)[140]	M2	$k_{cl}^{DA+acids}$ = 0.001 ± 0.001
[^{18}F]fluorodopa, monkey (n = 2)[65]	M2	$k_{cl}^{DA+acids}$ = 0.005 ± 0.001 (control) $k_{cl}^{DA+acids}$ = 0.024 ± 0.002 (MPTP)
[^{18}F]fluorodopa, normal human (n = 10)[12]	M2	$k_{cl}^{DA+acids}$ = 0.004 ± 0.002
[^{18}F]fluorodopa, normal human (n = 2)[60]	M2	$k_{cl}^{DA+acids}$ = 0.0010 ± 0.0006
[^{18}F]fluorodopa, Parkinson's disease[64]	M3	k_7^{DA} = k_9^{acids} 0.011 ± 0.003 (caudate, control, n = 11) 0.016 ± 0.004 (caudate, Parkinson's disease, n = 3) 0.013 ± 0.002 (putamen, control, n = 11) 0.025 ± 0.007 (putamen, Parkinson's disease, n = 3)

NOTE: Radiotracer experiments were carried out with dopa decarboxylase substrates [^{3}H]dopa, [^{18}F]fluorodopa, 6-[^{18}F]fluoro-*meta*-L-tyrosine, and 4-[^{18}F]fluoro-*meta*-L-tyrosine. In some cases estimates are based upon time series of the concentrations of labeled dopamine analogues and their acidic metabolites determined by chemical fractionation (HPLC) of rat brain extracts. In these experiments, the rate constant for the deamination of labeled dopamine analogues in brain (k_7^{DA}) and for the elimination of acidic metabolites from brain (k_9^{acids}) could be separately determined. The compartmental kinetic models are Model 2 (M2), in which labeled dopamine analogues and their acidic metabolites occupy a single compartment and are cleared from brain at rate $k_{cl}^{DA+acids}$, and Model 3 (M3), in which labeled dopamine analogues are not diffusible, but are deaminated at rate k_7^{DA} yielding diffusible metabolites which are cleared at rate k_9^{acids}. It is necessary to constrain M3 such that the magnitudes of k_7^{DA} and k_9^{acids} are arbitrarily defined as equal. Each estimate is the mean ± SD of (n) determinations, or in the case of rat experiments, the best estimate ± 95% confidence intervals obtained in a population of (n) rats.

the estimation of equilibrium distribution volume is weighted heavily towards O-methyl-[^{18}F]fluorodopa, which is the predominant species in circulation and in cerebral cortex at late times. It can be plausibly asserted that the unidirectional blood–brain clearances of [^{18}F]fluorodopa and its O-methylated metabolite, both substrates for the common carrier of large neutral amino acids, should be in constant proportion, to be measured by experiment. Thus, we include in our models a constant of proportionality, q, describing the ratio of the permeabilities of O-methyl-[^{18}F]fluorodopa and [^{18}F]fluorodopa (K_1^{OMFD}/K_1^{FDOPA}).[11]

The magnitude of the permeability ratio q has been measured in the rat using [^{18}F]fluorodopa and its O-methylated metabolite (q = 2.3),[62] and has been also measured in human brain by positron emission tomography (q = 1.9,[39] q = 1.7,[12] q = 1.1.[60] The definitive experiment, in which the uptake of O-methyl-[^{18}F]fluorodopa and, in a separate experiment, that of [^{18}F]fluorodopa during complete blockade of catechol-O-methyltransferase, were measured in the same individuals has not been performed. It would also be necessary to correct for possible fluctuations in the concentrations of other large neutral amino acids in plasma. For the present, we propose using $q = 1.6$, the mean of three available determinations of q in human brain. We find that the estimate of k_3^{DOPA} calculated by Model 3 is insensitive to the magnitude of q in the range 0.5–3.0.[15]

There is no evidence that the equilibrium distribution volumes of [18F]fluorodopa (TABLE 5) and O-methyl-[18F]fluorodopa (TABLE 6) are significantly different in brain of rat, monkey, or human. This observation tends to validate the use of distribution of tracer at a late time, when O-methyl-[18F]fluorodopa is the major labeled species in blood, as a means of constraining the equilibrium distribution of [18F]fluorodopa in compartmental models. However, the equilibrium distribution of O-methyl-[18F]fluorodopa in human brain may not be entirely homogenous: the value of V_e^{OMFD} is 1.04 ± 0.11 in striatum and 0.92 ± 0.12 in cerebellum.[69] Indeed, the striatum visibly accumulated more radioactivity than surrounding cortex in that study. The specific activity of dopa decarboxylase purified to homogeneity from human pheochromocytoma is 1 mmol dopa per gram of dopa decarboxylase enzyme per minute.[29] The activity of dopa decarboxylase from normal human postmortem caudate is 10 nmol dopa per gram of brain per minute.[70] From the molecular mass of dopa decarboxylase $(50,000 \text{ Da})$[29] we can therefore calculate the concentration of enzyme to be about 200 nM in human caudate. The intrinsic affinity of dopa decarboxylase to dopa, and presumably also the O-methylated metabolite, is 100 μM.[16] According to this calculation, the binding potential of O-methyl-[18F]fluoro-dopa in human caudate (B_{max}/K_d) is therefore expected to be about 0.002 mL g^{-1}, which could account for the slight accumulation of O-methyl-[18F]fluorodopa observed in human caudate during positron emission tomography.

The presence of the brain-penetrating O-methylated metabolite could, in principle, be avoided by means of pharmacological blockade of catechol-O-methyltransferase activity. Partial inhibition of this enzyme with the competitive inhibitor U 0521 increased the formation of [18F]fluorodopamine in striatum of living rat.[18] In several qualitative positron emission tomographic studies with [18F]fluorodopa, more potent catechol-O-methyltransferase inhibitors increased the contrast between striatum and surrounding tissue.[71–73] Pretreatment with the catechol-O-methyltransferase inhibitor Ro 40-7592 did not alter the magnitude of k_3^{ref} for β-[11C]dopa in monkey brain calculated by the tissue-slope intercept method.[74] However, the use of another catechol-O-methyltransferase inhibitor OR 611 decreased the magnitude of k_3^{FDOPA} in monkey brain by 35%,[72] and by 50% in brain of patients with Parkinson's disease,[63] suggesting that some catechol-O-methyltransferase inhibitors may interfere with dopa decarboxylase activity in brain. Administration of Ro 40-7592 in conjunction with benserazide, an inhibitor of dopa decarboxylase supposed to act only in the periphery, resulted in decreased estimates of dopa decarboxylase activity in monkey putamen calculated relative to cortical uptake (k_3^{ref}; TABLE 3); this was presumably due to a potentiation of the weak central action of benserazide which is also O-methylated.[75] However, in a study of normal subjects and patients with Parkinson's disease, the magnitude of [18F]fluorodopa influx relative to plasma was unaffected by pretreatment with OR 611.[55] The improvement in images obtained with catechol-O-methyltransferase inhibition is qualitative; in available studies the variance in kinetic estimates has not been reduced by catechol-O-methyltransferase inhibition.[55] In the same study, the dopa decarboxylase activity calculated relative to uptake in a reference tissue was much higher after catechol-O-methyltransferase inhibition. Thus, the tissue reference uptake method may be sensitive to the fraction of [18F]fluorodopa and its O-methylated metabolite in brain.

TABLE 5. Unidirectional Blood–Brain Clearance (K_1, mL^{-1} g^{-1} min^{-1}) and the Equilibrium Distribution Volume (V_e, mL g^{-1}) of Some Radiolabeled Substrates for Dopa Decarboxylase

Study	K_1 Striatum	V_e Striatum	K_1 Cortex	V_e Cortex	K_1 Cerebellum	V_e Cerebellum
[3H]dopa, rat ($n = 16$)[14]	0.046 ± 0.015	1.0 ± 0.2	0.063 ± 0.004	0.8 ± 0.2	–	–
[3H]dopa, rat ($n = 3$)[66]	0.038 ± 0.006	–	0.022 ± 0.007	–	0.027 ± 0.008	
[18F]fluorodopa, rat ($n = 3$)[66]	0.049 ± 0.005	–	0.044 ± 0.007	–	0.048 ± 0.007	–
[18F]fluorodopa, rat ($n = 12$)[62]	0.03 ± 0.02	–	0.03 ± 0.02	–	–	–
[18F]fluorodopa, pig ($n = 8$)[138]	0.029 ± 0.003	–	0.032 ± 0.001	–	0.026 ± 0.003	0.63 ± 0.06
[18F]fluorodopa, monkey ($n = 3$)[140]	0.033 ± 0.003	0.5 ± 0.1	–	–	0.038 ± 0.001	0.42 ± 0.05
4-[18F]FMT, monkey ($n = 3$)[140]	0.043 ± 0.005	1.0 ± 0.1	–	–	0.03 ± 0.01	0.5 ± 0.3
6-[18F]FMT, monkey ($n = 3$)[140]	0.044 ± 0.008	0.9 ± 0.3	–	–	0.04 ± 0.01	0.5 ± 0.1
[18F]fluorodopa, monkey ($n = 4$)[72]	0.050 ± 0.007	–	–	–	–	–
6-[18F]FMT, normal human ($n = 5$)[80]	0.08 ± 0.01	2.7 ± 0.1	0.08 ± 0.01	1.4 ± 0.1	0.09 ± 0.01	1.3 ± 0.1
[18F]fluorodopa, normal human ($n = 4$)[60]	0.04 ± 0.02	1.3 ± 0.5	–	–	–	–
[18F]fluorodopa, normal human ($n = 10$)[12]	0.031 ± 0.006	0.4 ± 0.1	–	–	–	0.6 ± 0.1
[18F]fluorodopa, normal human ($n = 6$)[11]	0.035 ± 0.006	–	0.026 ± 0.002	–	–	–
[18F]fluorodopa, normal human ($n = 12$)[37]	0.04 ± 0.02	1.05 ± 0.04	0.04 ± 0.02	0.6 ± 0.2	–	–
[18F]fluorodopa, normal human ($n = 3$)[39]	0.042 ± 0.007	1.2 ± 0.4	0.039 ± 0.007	0.7 ± 0.2	–	–
[18F]fluorodopa, Parkinson's disease ($n = 5$)[39]	0.04 ± 0.01	1.0 ± 0.2	0.041 ± 0.005	0.8 ± 0.2	–	–

NOTE: Dynamic time-activity data from rat, monkey, and human were obtained by radiochemical fractionation of brain activity (rat) or quantitative positron emission tomography (monkey and human) following intravenous administration of [3H]dopa, 6-[18F]fluoro-L-dopa ([18F]fluorodopa), 6-[18F]fluoro-*meta*-L-tyrosine (6-[18F]FMT), or 4-[18F]fluoro-*meta*-L-tyrosine (4[18F]FMT). Kinetic parameters were calculated by linear and nonlinear regression of activities measured in brain and in arterial plasma. Each estimate is the mean ± SD of (n) determinations, or in the case of rat experiments, the estimate obtained for a population of (n) rats.

TABLE 6. Unidirectional Blood–Brain Clearance (K_1, mL^{-1} g^{-1} min^{-1}) and the Equilibrium Distribution Volume (V_e, mL g^{-1}) of the Brain-penetrating Tracer Metabolites O-methyl-[³H]dopa and O-methyl-[¹⁸F]fluorodopa

Study	K_1 Striatum	V_e Striatum	K_1 Cortex	V_e Cortex	K_1 Cerebellum	V_e Cerebellum
O-methyl-[³H]dopa, rat (n = 13)[14]	0.04 ± 0.01	0.8 ± 0.2	0.08 ± 0.03	0.9 ± 0.3	–	–
O-methyl-[¹⁸F]fluorodopa, rat (n = 12)[62]	0.08 ± 0.01	–	0.09 ± 0.01	–	–	–
O-methyl-[¹⁸F]fluorodopa, monkey (n = 4)[139]	0.04 ± 0.01	1.0 ± 0.1	0.037 ± 0.005	0.93 ± 0.03	0.047 ± 0.006	1.0 ± 0.1
O-methyl-[¹⁸F]fluorodopa, normal human (n = 5)[69]	0.04 ± 0.01	1.0 ± 0.1	0.04 ± 0.01	0.9 ± 0.1	–	–
O-methyl-[¹⁸F]fluorodopa, normal human (n = 3)[39]	0.03 ± 0.01	0.8 ± 0.1	0.033 ± 0.002	0.7 ± 0.1	–	–
O-methyl-[¹⁸F]fluorodopa, Parkinson's disease (n = 5)[39]	0.05 ± 0.01	1.0 ± 0.2	0.06 ± 0.02	0.9 ± 0.2	–	–

NOTE: Dynamic time-activity data from rat, monkey and human were obtained by radiochemical fractionation of plasma and brain activity after intravenous injection of [³H]dopa (rat[14]) or O-methyl-[¹⁸F]fluorodopa, (rat[62]), or quantitative positron emission tomography (monkey and human) following intravenous administration of O-methyl-[¹⁸F]fluorodopa. Kinetic parameters were calculated by linear and nonlinear regression of activities measured in brain and in arterial plasma. Each estimate is the mean ± SD of (n) determinations, or in the case of rat experiments, the estimate obtained for a population of (n) rats.

CEREBRAL ACTIVITY OF CATECHOL-O-METHYLTRANSFERASE

The distributions of [^{18}F]fluorodopa and its O-methylated metabolite in a brain region devoid of dopa decarboxylase activity (Model 0) are assumed to be determined in terms of three parameters, K_1^{FDOPA}, V_e^{FDOPA}, and q. In Model 0, the rate of the O-methylation of [^{18}F]fluorodopa within brain (k_5^{FDOPA}) is assumed to be zero. At 90 min after [^{18}F]fluorodopa injection, the distribution volume of unmetabolized tracer in rat cerebellum was 0.14 mL g^{-1}, whereas that of the O-methylated metabolite was 0.62 mL g^{-1},[16-18] suggesting that some additional process of comparable magnitude to k_2^{FDOPA} is removing [^{18}F]fluorodopa from cerebellum. This process is unrelated to dopa decarboxylase because only traces of decarboxylated metabolites were found in cerebellar extracts. The activity of catechol-O-methyltransferase with respect to [^{3}H]dopa (k_5^{DOPA}) in rat brain has been calculated indirectly to be 0.06 min^{-1}.[13] The published Michaelis-Menten constants for catechol-O-methyltransferase from rat brain[76] predict that k_5^{DOPA} should have a magnitude close to 0.02 min^{-1}. Thus, the available evidence indicates that the assumption that k_5^{FDOPA} equals zero probably is incorrect. What are the consequences of underestimating the catechol-O-methyltransferase activity of cerebral parenchyma on the estimates of [^{18}F]fluorodopa metabolism?

Were the magnitude of k_5^{FDOPA} greater than zero, the concentration of [^{18}F]fluorodopa in brain would be reduced by an unknown amount, in proportion to the synthesis of the O-methylated metabolite in the brain parenchyma. This error would be without great effect on the apparent magnitude of V_e^{FDOPA}, assuming both amino acids to be subject to facilitated diffusion across the blood–brain barrier. However, were k_5^{FDOPA} greater than zero in a region of dopa decarboxylase activity, the true brain concentrations of substrate for decarboxylation would be lower than predicted; the magnitude of k_3^{FDOPA} calculated from overestimated [^{18}F]fluorodopa concentrations would thus be underestimated. Brain-penetrating catechol-O-methyltransferase inhibitors would also block k_5^{FDOPA}, which would be expected to increase the magnitude of k_3^{FDOPA}. However, in tissue slope-intercept studies with [^{18}F]fluorodopa, treatment with Ro 40-7592, a brain-penetrating catechol-O-methyltransferase inhibitor,[22] was without effect on the magnitude of k_3^{ref} in monkey striatum.[77]

To investigate the effect of underestimating cerebral catechol-O-methyltransferase activity on kinetic parameter estimation, we fitted Model 3 to autoradiographic data obtained in the rat nucleus accumbens during 180 min of circulation of [^{3}H]dopa.[15] The magnitude of k_5^{DOPA} was varied in the range 0 to 0.15 min^{-1} as an input parameter. Other input parameters for these analyses were $V_e^{DOPA} = 0.75$ mL g^{-1} (estimated in cingulate cortex where k_3^{DOPA} is negligible), $q = 1.5$,[14] and V_0^{FDOPA} is assumed to be equal to 0 mL g^{-1} (since the autoradiographic sections were devoid of blood). We found that K_1^{DOPA} and k_7^{DA} were relatively unaffected by the magnitude of k_5^{DOPA}, with coefficients of variation of 1% and 3%, respectively. However, k_3^{DOPA} increases with k_5^{DOPA} with a slope of 0.63 (Fig. 4). The near perfect linearity in the k_3^{DOPA}/k_5^{DOPA} relationship (r > 0.999) is likely model-based as opposed to physiological. Thus, we conclude that the presence of unknown amounts of catechol-O-methyltransferase activity in brain may plausibly result in a significant and systematic underestimation of the magnitude of k_3^{FDOPA}.

OTHER DOPA DECARBOXYLASE SUBSTRATES FOR *IN VIVO* STUDIES

The dopa decarboxylase substrate 5-hydroxy-L-β-[^{11}C]tryptophan (5-hydroxy-[^{11}C]tryptophan) accumulates in monkey brain as a function of dopa decarboxylase

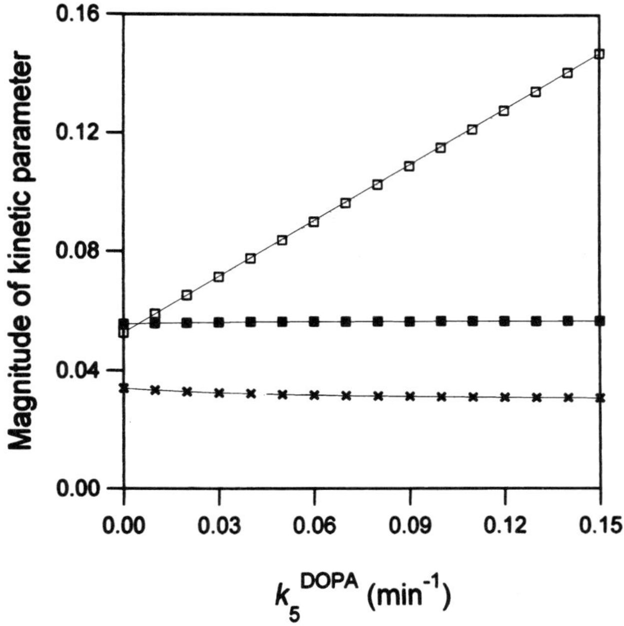

FIGURE 4. Estimates of the unidirectional blood–brain clearance ($\blacksquare$, K_1^{DOPA}, mL g^{-1} min^{-1}) dopa decarboxylase activity ($\square$, k_3^{DOPA}, min^{-1}), and the rate constant for the catabolism and elimination of [^{18}F]fluorodopamine (X, k_7^{DA}, min^{-1}) as a function of the cerebral activity of catechol-*O*-methyltransferase (k_5^{DOPA}, min^{-1}) in the rat nucleus accumbens body, calculated according to compartmental Model 3. A time series of autoradiograms during 180 min of [^{3}H]dopa circulation was used to generate a time-activity curve in the region of interest. After normalization of brain activities to common arterial curves for [^{3}H]dopa and its *O*-methylated metabolite, the compartmental model was fitted to the data set by nonlinear regression.

activity. The rate constant is somewhat lower than for β-[^{11}C]dopa in the same animals,[77] suggesting that dopa is the preferred substrate *in vivo*, as it is *in vitro*.[28] Furthermore, the decarboxylation of 5-hydroxy-[^{11}C]tryptophan was more sensitive to competition from "cold" 5-hydroxytryptophan (3–10 mg kg^{-1}), than from dopa (4–30 mg kg^{-1}), consistent with a signal arising from decarboxylation of radiolabeled 5-hydroxytryptophan preferentially in serotonin terminals. However, 5-hydroxy-[^{11}C]tryptophan uptake was also reduced in monkeys treated with the selective neurotoxin MPTP,[77] indicating that the nigrostriatal dopamine innervation plays a role in the decarboxylation of this tracer. The converse may not be true: selective destruction of the serotonin innervation did not substantially alter the *in vivo* synthesis of [^{3}H]dopamine from [^{3}H]dopa in living rat striatum.[78] However, synthesis of [^{3}H]dopamine in olfactory tubercle and amygdala, where the serotonin innervation is more dense than is the dopamine innervation, was sensitive to destruction of serotonin fibers. A stimulation of striatal dopa decarboxylase activity with respect to 5-hydroxy-[^{11}C]tryptophan is reported in monkeys treated with pyridoxine, the dopa decarboxylase cofactor,[79] but we did not find that this effect reached statistical significance (TABLE 3).

Non-indolamine tracers of dopa decarboxylase, which are not recognized by catechol-O-methyltransferase, would obviate the need to incorporate several physiological constraints into models of dopamine synthesis.[34,80] The fluoro-*meta*-L-tyrosines have blood–brain permeabilities and distribution volumes in brain comparable to those of [^{18}F]fluorodopa (TABLE 5) and O-methyl-[^{18}F]fluorodopa (TABLE 6). The rate constants for the decarboxylation of 6-[^{18}F]fluoro-*meta*-L-tyrosine in brain of monkey, calculated by a linear plot relative to occipital cortex (k_3^{ref}), was twofold higher than that for [^{18}F]fluorodopa.[81] The rate constants for dopa decarboxylase activity (k_3^{FDOPA}) relative to 4-[^{18}F]fluoro-*meta*-L-tyrosine and 6-[^{18}F]fluoro-*meta*-L-tyrosine in monkey and human brain are also within the range of values obtained for [^{18}F]fluorodopa (TABLE 1). The estimates of dopa decarboxylase activity for 4- and 6-[^{18}F]fluoro-*meta*-L-tyrosine in monkey brain (0.03 min^{-1}) were higher than the value obtained by the same group for [^{18}F]fluorodopa (0.015 min^{-1}). However, dopa decarboxylase activity relative to 4- and 6-[^{18}F]fluoro-*meta*-L-tyrosine (k_3^{4FT}, k_3^{6FT}) was corrected for elimination of decarboxylated metabolites (Model 2), whereas k_3^{FDOPA} was calculated by a procedure neglecting decarboxylated metabolites (Model 1). We have seen above that omission of the elimination of tracer dopamine from the compartmental model results in lower values for k_3^{FDOPA} (TABLE 1; refs. 15 and 60). Therefore, it cannot be concluded from available data that the [^{18}F]fluoro-*meta*-L-tyrosines are better *in vivo* dopa decarboxylase substrates than is [^{18}F]fluorodopa.

The near absence of brain-penetrating plasma metabolites simplifies modeling of *meta*-tyrosine uptake considerably. At 30 min after injection of 6-[^{18}F]fluoro-*meta*-L-tyrosine, the only major metabolite in plasma from monkeys (not treated with carbidopa) was the deaminated compound 6-[^{18}F]fluoro-*meta*-hydroxyphenylacetic acid.[80] However, the dispositions of the decarboxylated metabolites of 4- and 6-[^{18}F]fluoro-*meta*-L-tyrosine formed in brain is currently uncertain. At 30 min after injection of 4-[^{18}F]fluoro-*meta*-L-tyrosine, the predominant labeled compound in rat striatum was 4-[^{18}F]fluoro-3-methylphenylacetic acid;[34] the available data suggest that the corresponding labeled tyramines are more rapidly deaminated in living brain than is labeled dopamine or [^{18}F]fluorodopamine.[13,14] Indeed, endogenous tyramines are normally present at very low concentrations in mammalian brain, but rapidly increase by as much as 100-fold after blockade of monoamine oxidase, indicative of very rapid turnover in the absence of vesicular storage.[82] Thus, it is unlikely that 4- or 6-[^{18}F]fluoro-*meta*-tyramine formed in brain are stored in synaptic vesicles. Indeed, [^{18}F]fluoro-*meta*-tyramine is a relatively poor substrate for the plasma membrane dopamine transporter and the vesicular monoamine transporter.[83] The mechanism by which the corresponding deaminated species should be retained in brain is uncertain, but diffusion rates for these compounds may be very slow relative to the duration of the positron emission study.

The dopa decarboxylase substrate fluoro-β-methylene-*meta*-tyrosine yields a product which is a suicide substrate for monoamine oxidase in catecholaminergic neurons.[84] The [^{18}F]-labeled L-enantiomer of this compound accumulates in striatum of living mouse and monkey.[85] The D,L raceimate of this compound and [^{18}F]fluorodopa have similar net blood–brain clearances in monkey brain. Suicide substrates for dopa decarboxylase such as monofluoromethyldopa,[86] or the corresponding *meta*-tyrosine, may also have potential as tracers for dopa decarboxylase activity, although the binding potential, calculated above, may be low.

PARTIAL VOLUME EFFECTS

In all positron emission tomographic studies the measured radioactivity in a volume of brain is altered by spillover from and into adjacent tissues, phenomena which are known as partial volume effects (PVE). Time-activity curves measured in regions of interest smaller than the intrinsic resolution of the tomograph are especially sensitive to degradation by partial volume. The [18F]fluorodeoxyglucose estimates of regional glucose consumption in brain of patients with Alzheimer's disease sensitive to partial volume, especially in the presence of cortical atrophy.[87] The density of dopamine transporters measured *in vivo* are also sensitive to partial volume.[88] The volume of the normal human caudate is reported to decline by 0.4% per annum,[89] indicating that normal atrophy of aging may result in changes in the recovery of the signal from [18F]fluorodopa. The small size of the caudate-putamen in non-human primates is certain to compound the signal loss due to the partial volume effect, although the use of new high-resolution tomographs[90] may improve matters. The preponderance of evidence indicates that estimates of net tracer influx (TABLE 2) and dopa decarboxylase activity (TABLE 1) are lower in non-human primate and pig than in normal humans. This is consistent with more extensive spillover from the striatum of smaller-brained species.

The consequences of partial volume effects for compartmental analysis of [18F]fluorodopa have only recently been investigated systematically. After registration of magnetic resonance images to positron emission tomographic data, the brain is segmented into four tissue types, assumed to be homogeneous with respect to tracer uptake (caudate, putamen, white matter, cortical grey matter). The corrected time-activity curves are then generated for each tissue volume by simulation.[91] Preliminary results of this correction on time-activity curves measured in human cortex and caudate in a normal subject and a patient with Parkinson's disease are illustrated in FIGURE 5. Dynamic data were acquired with the Scanditronix PC 2048 tomograph (axial resolution 6 mm) during 90 min of [18F]fluorodopa circulation. After correction for partial volume, radioactivity increased by about 40% in cerebral cortex, resulting in an increase in the magnitude of the unidirectional blood–brain clearance K_1^{FDOPA}, and consequently the equilibrium distribution volume V_e^{FDOPA}. Time-activity curves for caudate nucleus were much greater after correction for spillover (FIG. 5). Fitting of Model 3 to the corrected data produced great increases in the magnitude of k_3^{FDOPA}, which suggests that the compartmental model is unstable. The net tracer influx was also increased by partial volume correction (FIG. 2). Thus, the degradation of signal due to spillover is a major factor in the underestimation of dopa decarboxylase activity with existing positron emission tomographs. This may be especially important in clinical [18F]fluorodopa studies in which spillover may vary as a function of pathological atrophy or normal aging.

CLINICAL STUDIES OF PARKINSON'S DISEASE AND RELATED DISORDERS

The neurochemical pathology of Parkinson's disease and other movement disorders have been extensively investigated by means of positron emission tomography. The majority of these studies have employed linear methods for the determination of net tracer influx. In MPTP-poisoned cynomolgus monkeys, a model of idiopathic Parkinson's disease, the magnitude of K^{FDOPA} on the side of the lesion correlated well with the size and number of dopamine neurons in the ipsilateral substantia nigra.[92] Likewise, the decreased K^{FDOPA} in idiopathic Parkinson's disease correlated with the postmortem cell counts in the substantia nigra.[93] In a limited series of patients with Parkinson's disease, the reduced [18F]fluorodopa uptake in caudate and putamen seemed to correlate with reduced binding of the dopamine uptake

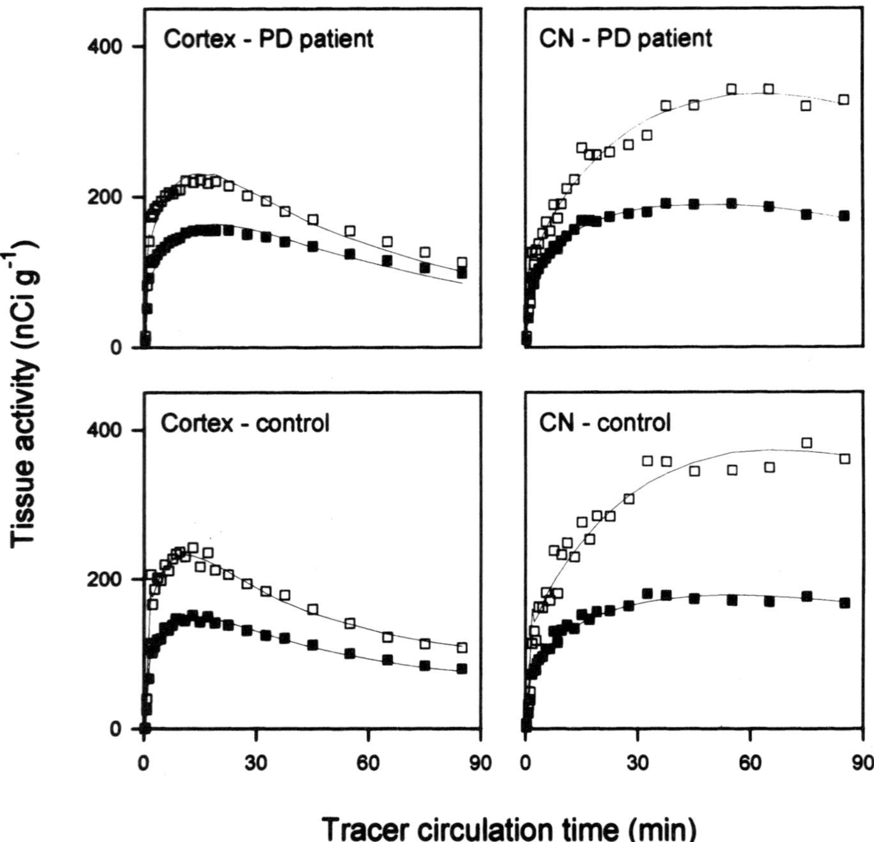

FIGURE 5. Observed (■) and partial volume-corrected (□) time-activity data in (*left*) occipital cortex and caudate nucleus (CN, *right*) of a Parkinson's disease (PD) patient (*upper*) and a normal control subject (*lower*) during 90 min after administration of [^{18}F]fluorodopa. Magnetic resonance images were registered to the dynamic positron emission tomographic data and were acquired using the Scanditronix PC 2048 tomograph. Corrected time-activity curves were calculated by simulation (Dr. Olivier Rousset). The smooth curves indicate the fitting of Model 3 to the observed data and to the data corrected for partial volume effects.

site ligand [^{11}C]nomifensine.[94] The binding *in vitro* of radioligands for dopamine uptake sites is reduced by 80% in the parkinsonian basal ganglia.[95,96] Furthermore, MPTP administration to monkeys producing 75% decreases in K^{FDOPA} resulted in 98% decreases in striatal dopamine content.[97] The net uptake of [^{18}F]fluorodopa in striatum provides an index of the reduced integrity of the dopamine innervation in Parkinson's disease, but does not seem to decline as markedly as do the dopamine reuptake sites. In rat striatum there is about 20% residual dopa decarboxylase activity when the striatal tyrosine hydroxylase activity has been totally abolished by lesions with 6-hydroxydopamine; the remaining enzyme activity was reported to be in a non-neuronal compartment resistant to kainic acid.[98] Thus, reductions in

K^{FDOPA} need not bear a simple relation to the magnitude of the dopamine lesion, possibly due to the presence of dopa decarboxylase in other compartments unaffected by the disease.

The interpretation of [^{18}F]fluorodopa studies of Parkinson's disease is potentially confounded by possible declines in the functional state of the dopamine innervation of the putamen in the course of normal aging. For example, the concentration of dopa decarboxylase protein in postmortem caudate from neurologically normal subjects declined by 20% between the third and eight decade of life; the enzyme concentration was unchanged in the putamen.[99] The concentration of dopamine in human postmortem striatum of neurologically normal humans declined substantially (-60% in putamen) between the third and eighth decades of life.[100] Likewise, the density of vesicular binding sites labeled *in vitro* with tritiated α-dihydrotetrabenazine declined with a half-life of 40 years in caudate nucleus from elderly control subjects, while binding site density declined as a function of Parkinson's disease duration with a half-life of only 10 years,[101] suggesting a pre-morbid disease process lasting 10 years.

Striatal [^{18}F]fluorodopa influx declined by 20% between the third and eighth decades of life in a group of 10 normal subjects,[49] but did not change in 26[102] or 19 normal subjects[103] in the same range of ages, and did not decline in normal subjects scanned twice at intervals several years apart.[104] Neither was there any great discernible difference in K^{FDOPA} measured in young adults and in their healthy grandparents.[105] Thus, the available methods fail to detect a decline in K^{FDOPA} associated with normal human aging. Current methods may not be sufficiently sensitive to detect decreases in dopa decarboxylase activity in living brain associated with normal aging. The apparent dissociation between dopamine concentration and other *in vitro* markers and dopa decarboxylase activity measured *in vivo* in normal aging has led to the suggestion that senile denervation of the striatum may result in up-regulation of the activity of dopa decarboxylase in human brain.[98]

The magnitude of K^{FDOPA} was normal on the asymptomatic side of patients with early hemiparkinsonism, but was reduced by 50% on the symptomatic side.[106] Reduced influx of [^{18}F]fluorodopa is more marked in the putamen than in the caudate of patients with Parkinson's disease (FIG. 2). The putaminal [^{18}F]fluorodopa net influx was slightly more affected in a group of patients with Hoehn and Yahr clinical staging III–IV than in a less affected group[107,108] and was slightly less in patients with clinical score less than 15 by the unified Parkinson's disease rating scale, than in a group with clinical score greater than 15.[109] Declines in putaminal [^{18}F]fluorodopa uptake correlated strongly with locomotor disability, while (less marked) declines in uptake in the caudate nucleus correlated more with impairment in a memory task.[108] The [^{18}F]fluorodopa influx constant was reduced by 52% in the putamen and 28% in the caudate in a large group ($n = 18$) of patients with sporadic Parkinson's disease,[109] further evidence that the disease preferentially affects the putamen. The dorsal putamen may be affected early in the disease and the ventral putamen in more advanced cases of Parkinson's disease.[104] Spillover effects would tend to exaggerate the reduced influx in the caudate nucleus, which is smaller in some profiles than is the putamen. However, after correction for partial volume effects, the influx of [^{18}F]fluorodopa was nearly normal in parkinsonian caudate nucleus (FIG. 2). Likewise, the postmortem dopamine concentrations are likewise more reduced in putamen (-98%) than in caudate nucleus (-81%) of patients dying with Parkinson's disease.[111]

K^{FDOPA} readily detects the dopamine depletion in Parkinson's disease but fails to discriminate between clinical measures of disease severity (TABLE 3). However, the net tracer influx correlated with the akinesia score and was more evident in caudate nucleus than in putamen, and is reported to decline at a rate of about 10% per year in a group of patients with Parkinson's disease.[104] In a qualitative study the contrast between striatum and cortex declined five times more rapidly in patients with Parkinson's disease than in age-matched control subjects.[112] Both groups speculated that the declines were suggestive that the remaining dopamine innervation is highly susceptible to an ongoing disease process, a finding consistent with some postmortem studies.[101] However, the magnitude of K^{FDOPA} reflects the composite of blood–brain transfer of [^{18}F]fluorodopa, which is unlikely to be substantially altered in the disease state, and dopa decarboxylase activity, which is the physiological variable presumed to be altered by the disease. Let us assume that K_1^{FDOPA} and k_2^{FDOPA} were constant with age, whereas k_3^{FDOPA} declined by 10% of its initial value with each decade of aging of normals. From the definition of K^{FDOPA} [$K_1^{FDOPA}k_3^{FDOPA}/(k_2^{FDOPA} + k_3^{FDOPA})$], it is clear that the magnitude of K^{FDOPA} would be initially stable but would then decline precipitously with advanced age. Thus, the concept of K^{FDOPA} as a linear function of age, or as a linear function of disease duration or staging, is almost meaningless.

Intrastriatal grafting of fetal nigrostriatal neurons is a promising technique for the treatment of Parkinson's disease. Dopa decarboxylase assays have the potential to provide an objective assessment of the efficacy of efforts to replace the dopamine innervation. In the limited studies available to date, grafts resulting in significant improvement in several measures of clinical status were not associated with notable concomitant increases in K^{FDOPA}.[113,114] This may reflect the inability of existing methods to detect small increases in K^{FDOPA} (less than 20%), which might, nonetheless, impart a certain clinical improvement. More recently, six months after bilateral transplantations of fetal nigral neurons in the postcommissural putamen, the magnitude of K^{FDOPA} in the putamen was increased by 20–30%.[115] These changes were associated with substantial declines in the Unified Parkinson's Disease Rating Score, in percentage "off time," and the "on time" with dyskinesia.

The ratio of [^{18}F]fluorohomovanillic acid to [^{18}F]fluorodopamine was much higher in extracts of striatum of monkeys on the side of MPTP-lesions.[25] Possibly the rate of metabolism of [^{18}F]fluorodopamine in striaum is also highly accelerated in late Parkinson's disease when vesicular storage is highly compromised. As discussed above, results obtained with linear methods assuming irreversible trapping in brain are problematic in conditions where dopamine metabolism is accelerated. Using an extended compartmental model of [^{18}F]fluorodopa metabolism, we have observed increased clearance of [^{18}F]fluorodopamine from caudate and putamen of a group of patients with Parkinson's disease.[63]

OTHER DISORDERS OF THE BASAL GANGLIA

A complex of neurological disorders with aspects of Parkinson's disease and motor neuron disease has been endemic among Chamorro aboriginals of the Island of Guam. The net uptake of [^{18}F]fluorodopa (K^{FDOPA}) in whole striatum was extremely low in parkinsonian patients from Guam as compared to age-matched normal subjects from Guam. However, Guamanians with the amyotrophic lateral sclerosis form of the disease had intermediate uptake.[116] The magnitude of k_3^{ref} relative to occipital cortex was reduced in putamen, but normal in caudate of patients with multiple system atrophy. This decline correlated with decreased binding of the opioid receptor ligand [^{11}C]diprenorphine to striatonigral projection neurons in the putamen.[117]

Asymptomatic patients with linkage to the gene for hereditary pallido-ponto-nigral degeneration had reduced [^{18}F]fluorodopa influx.[118] [^{18}F]Fluorodopa influx to striatum in cases of juvenile-onset parkinsonism was in the range of typical values for Parkinson's disease.[119] [^{18}F]Fluorodopa influx is substantially reduced in cases of progressive supranuclear palsy,[120] in two patients with Shy-Drager syndrome,[121] in affected individuals in a pedigree with autosomal dominant parkinsonism,[122] in patients with advanced amyotrophic lateral sclerosis,[123] and in subjects with symptomatic Wilson's disease,[124] but was normal in a group of three patients with dopa-responsive dystonia[125] and in a single patient with hereditary progressive dystonia (Segawa's disease).[126] Dopa-responsive dystonia is now understood to result from a mutation in the gene for tyrosine hydroxylase.[127]

A decrease in [^{18}F]fluorodopa influx in patients with the hereditary disorder neuroacanthocytosis was restricted to the posterior putamen, whereas the anterior and posterior putamen were equally affected in Parkinson's disease.[128] In a qualitative study, [^{18}F]fluorodopa accumulation was reduced in patients with Lesch-Nyhan disease.[129] The uptake of [^{18}F]fluorodopa in the caudate and putamen was substantially reduced (-66%) in a series of four patients with corticobasal degeneration, while the metabolic rate measured with [^{18}F]fluorodeoxyglucose was also reduced on the basal ganglia on the affected side.[130] In contrast, [^{18}F]fluorodeoxyglucose uptake was entirely normal in a group of patients with Parkinson's disease.[108] Together, these results indicate that reduced [^{18}F]fluorodopa uptake occurs in many disorders of the basal ganglia, sometimes in association with altered postsynaptic markers.

In a group of monkeys with chronic amphetamine poisoning, an initial 75% decline in the magnitude of K^{FDOPA} in striatum occurred, which was partially reversed six months later.[131] In postmortem brain from chronic human users of methamphetamine, dopa decarboxylase enzyme (μg/g protein) was unaltered, whereas dopamine content and dopamine transporter density were reduced by half.[132] However, quantitative Western blotting is uninformative of the activity state of dopa decarboxylase enzyme *in vivo*. In a single case study, accidental ingestion of a mixture of petroleum hydrocarbons resulted in a transitory parkinsonian syndrome lasting several months.[133] [^{18}F]fluorodopa uptake was substantially reduced several months after poisoning, but later normalized as the symptoms largely resolved.

NEUROPSYCHIATRIC DISORDERS

The dopa decarboxylase activity with respect to [^{18}F]fluorodopa in caudate and putamen was significantly elevated in a group of five patients with psychosis and in 13 patients with complex partial seizures and interictal psychosis.[134] The net influx constant for [^{18}F]fluorodopa was increased by 20% in putamen of a series of seven unmedicated patients with schizophrenia.[135] One of the schizophrenic subjects of Hietala *et al.*[135] had a value of K^{FDOPA} lower than any of the control subjects, suggesting that schizophrenia may be heterogenous with respect to DOPA decarboxylase activity in putamen. The net influx of [^{18}F]fluorodopa is substantially increased in medial prefrontal cortex, insular cortex, hypothalamus, amygdala, and the tail of the caudate of a group of three male severe stutterers without other neuropsychiatric history,[136] although the units appear to be semiquantitative. In a qualitative study, the cerebral uptake of 5-hydroxy-[^{11}C]tryptophan is reported to be decreased in patients with major depression,[137] perhaps indicative of reduced cerebral serotonin synthesis in that condition.

CONCLUSIONS

The assay of *in vivo* dopa decarboxylase activity from compartmental modeling of time series of autoradiograms is a formidable problem. However, the presence of brain-penetrating metabolites is not an insurmountable barrier to the analysis of dynamic positron emission tomographic studies; the magnitude of k_3^{FDOPA} is nearly insensitive to the estimate of q, the permeability ratio. The formation of *O*-methyl-[^{18}F]fluorodopa *in situ* is, however, a factor likely resulting in the systematic underestimation of dopa decarboxylase activity. The availability of positron-emitting derivatives of *meta*-tyrosine is likely to obviate the need to consider the magnitudes of q and k_5^{FDOPA} in compartmental models. Whereas labeled dopamine is retained in vesicles, labeled tyramines are rapidly decomposed in brain by monoamine oxidase. The mechanism by which the deaminated compounds derived from *meta*-tyrosines are retained in brain must be clarified. For all tracers investigated, the elimination of decarboxylated metabolites from brain can be neglected when tracer circulation is less than 60 min. However, in extended dopa decarboxylase tracer experiments, neglecting the elimination of cerebral metabolites results in significant underestimation of cerebral enzyme activity. The magnitude of dopa decarboxylase activity tends to be lower when V_e^{FDOPA} is determined as a separate parameter rather than constrained by cortical values. Compartmental modeling of dopa decarboxylase activity is very sensitive to partial volume effects. Higher resolution positron emission tomographs and routine application of partial volume corrections are required to arrive at more accurate estimates of dopa decarboxylase activity *in vivo*. The relationship between dopa decarboxylase activity measured *in vivo* and *in vitro* with other markers of dopamine transmission remains to be fully elucidated. Nonetheless, the utility of dopa decarboxylase tracers for investigations of dopamine transmission in living brain is substantially validated; an index of the functional state of the biochemical pathway for dopamine synthesis can be assayed in living brain.

REFERENCES

1. GARNETT, E. S., G. FIRNAU, C. NAHMIAS & R. CHIRAKAL. 1983. Striatal dopamine metabolism in living monkeys examined by positron emission tomography. Brain Res. **280:** 169–171.
2. GARNETT, E. S., G. FIRNAU & C. NAHMIAS. 1983. Dopamine visualized in the basal ganglia of living man. Nature **305:** 137–138.
3. HORNE, M. K., C. H. CHENG & G. W. WOOTEN. 1984. The cerebral metabolism of L-dihydroxyphenylalanine: An autoradiographic and biochemical study. Pharmacology **28:** 12–26.
4. LISKOWSKY, D. R. & L. T. POTTER. 1985. A pre-positron emission tomography study of L-3,4-dihydroxy-[^{3}H]phenylalanine distribution in the rat. Neurosci. Lett. **53:** 161–167.
5. LUXEN, A., M. GUILLAUME, W. P. MELEGA, V. W. PIKE, O. SOLIN & R. WAGNER. 1992. Production of 6-[^{18}F]fluoro-L-DOPA and its metabolism in vivo—A critical review. Nucl. Med. Biol. **19:** 149–158.
6. VOLKOW, N. D., J. S. FOWLER, S. J. GATLEY, J. LOGAN, G.-J. WANG, Y.-S. DING & S. DEWEY. 1996. PET evaluation of the dopamine system of the human brain. J. Nucl. Med. **37:** 1242–1256.
7. SOKOLOFF, L., M. REIVICH, C. KENNEDY, M. H. DES ROSSIERS, C. S. PATLAK, K. D. PETTIGREW, O. SAKURADA & M. SHINOHARA. 1977. The [^{14}C]deoxyglucose method for the measurement of local cerebral glucose utilization: Theory, procedure, and normal values in the consious and anesthetized albino rat. J. Neurochem. **28:** 897–916.
8. PHELPS, M. E., S. C. HUANG, E. J. HOFFMAN, C. SELIN, L. SOKOLOFF & D. E. KOHL.

1979. Tomographic measurement of local cerebral glucose metabolic rate in humans with (F-18)2-fluoro-2-deoxy-D-glucose: Validation of method. Ann. Neurol. **6:** 371–388.

9. REIVICH, M., D. KUHL, A. WOLF, J. GREENBERG, M. PHELPS, T. IDO, V. CASELLA, J. FOWLER, E. HOFFMAN, A. ALAVI, P. SOM & L. SOKOLOFF. 1979. The [^{18}F]fluorodeoxyglucose method for the measurement of local cerebral glucose metabolism in man. Circ. Res. **44:** 127–137.

10. GJEDDE, A. 1982. Calculation of glucose phosphorylation from brain uptake of glucose analogues in vivo: A re-examination. Brain Res. Rev. **4:** 237–274.

11. GJEDDE, A., J. REITH, S. DYVE, G. LÉGER, M. GUTTMAN, M. DIKSIC, A. EVANS & H. KUWABARA. 1991. Dopa decarboxylase activity of the living human brain. Proc. Natl. Acad. Sci. USA **88:** 2721–2725.

12. HUANG, S.-C., D.-C. YU, J. R. BARRIO, S. GRAFTON, W. P. MELEGA, J. M. HOFFMAN, N. SATYAMURTHY, J. C. MAZZIOTTA & M. E. PHELPS. 1991. Kinetics and modeling of L-6-[^{18}F]fluoro-DOPA in human positron emission tomographic studies. J. Cereb. Blood Flow Metab. **11:** 898–913.

13. CUMMING, P., H. KUWABARA & A. GJEDDE. 1994. A kinetic analysis of 6-[^{18}F]fluoro-L-dihydroxyphenylalanine metabolism in the rat. J. Neurochem. **63:** 1675–1682.

14. CUMMING, P., H. KUWABARA, A. ASE & A. GJEDDE. 1995. Regulation of DOPA decarboxylase activity in brain of living rat. J. Neurochem. **65:** 1381–1390.

15. DEEP, P., H. KUWABARA, A. GJEDDE & P. CUMMING. 1997. Modelling the cerebral kinetics of [^{3}H]DOPA in rat by compartmental analyses of autoradiograms. J. Neurosci. Methods. In press.

16. CUMMING, P., M. HÄUSSER, W. R. W. MARTIN, J. GRIERSON, M. ADAM, T. RUTH & E. G. McGEER. 1988. Kinetics of the in vitro decarboxylation and the in vivo metabolism of 2-[^{18}F]- and 6-[^{18}F]-fluorodopa in the hooded rat. Biochem. Pharmacol. **37:** 247–250.

17. CUMMING, P., B. E. BOYES, W. R. W. MARTIN, M. ADAM, J. GRIERSON, T. RUTH & E. G. McGEER. 1987. The metabolism of [^{18}F]-6-fluoro-L-3,4-dihydroxyphenylalanine in the hooded rat. J. Neurochem. **48:** 601–608.

18. CUMMING, P., B. E. BOYES, W. R. W. MARTIN, M. ADAM, T. RUTH & E. G. McGEER. 1987. Altered metabolism of [^{18}F]-6-fluorodopa in the hooded rat following inhibition of catechol-*O*-methyltransferase with U-0521. Biochem. Pharmacol. **36:** 2527–2531.

19. MELEGA, W. P., J. H. HOFFMAN, A. LUXEN, C. H. K. NISSENSON, M. E. PHELPS & J. R. BARRIO. 1990. The effects of carbidopa on the metabolism of 6-[^{18}F]fluoro-L-dopa in rats, monkeys and humans. Life Sci **47:** 149–157.

20. MELEGA, W. P., A. LUXEN, M. M. PERLMUTTER, C. H. K. NISSENSON, M. E. PHELPS & J. R. BARRIO. 1990. Comparative in vivo metabolism of 6-[^{18}F]fluoro-L-DOPA and [^{3}H]L-DOPA in rats. Biochem. Pharmacol. **39:** 1853–1860.

21. WOOD, P. L. & C. A. ALTAR. 1988. Dopamine release in vivo from nigrostriatal, mesolimbic, and mesocortical neurons: Utility of 3-methoxytryamine measurements. Pharmacol. Rev. **40:** 163–187.

22. CUMMING, P., E. BROWN, G. DAMSMA & H. C. FIBIGER. 1992. Formation and clearance of interstitial metabolites of dopamine and serotonin in rat striatum: An in vivo microdialysis study. J. Neurochem. **59:** 1905–1914.

23. FIRNAU, G., S. SOOD, R. CHIRAKAL, C. NAHMIAS & E. S. GARNETT. 1987. Cerebral metabolism of 6-[^{18}F]fluoro-L-3,4-dihydroxyphenylalanine in the primate. J. Neurochem. **48:** 1077–1082.

24. MELEGA, W. P., S. T. GRAFTON, S.-C. HUANG, N. SATYAMURTHY, M. E. PHELPS & J. R. BARRIO. 1991. L-6-[^{18}F]Fluoro-DOPA metabolism in monkeys and humans: Biochemical parameters for the formulation of tracer kinetic models with positron emission tomography. J. Cereb. Blood Flow Metab. **11:** 890–897.

25. MELEGA, W. P., J. M. HOFFMAN, J. S. SCHNEIDER, M. E. PHELPS & J. R. BARRIO. 1991. 6-[^{18}F]Fluoro-L-DOPA metabolism in MPTP-treated monkeys: Assessment of tracer methodologies for positron emission tomography. Brain Res. **543:** 271–276.

26. FIRNAU, G., S. SOOD, R. CHIRAKAL, C. NAHMIAS & E. S. GARNETT. 1988. Metabolites of 6-[^{18}F]fluoro-L-DOPA in human blood. J. Nucl. Med. **29:** 363–369.

27. BOUCHARD, S. & A. G. ROBERGE. 1979. Biochemical properties and kinetic parameters

of dihydroxphenylalanine-5-hydroxytryptophan decarboxylase in brain, liver, and adrenals of cat. Can. J. Biochem. **57:** 1014–1018.

28. CHRISTENSON, J. G., W. DAIRMAN & S. UDENFRIEND. 1970. Preparation and properties of a homogeneous aromatic L-amino acid decarboxylase from hog kidney. Arch. Biochem. Biophys. **141:** 356–367.

29. ICHINOSE, H., K. KOJIMA, A. TOGARI, Y. KATO, S. PARVEZ, H. PARVEZ & T. NAGATSU. 1985. Simple purification of aromatic L-amino acid decarboxylase from human pheochromocytoma using high performance liquid chromatography. Anal. Biochem. **150:** 408–414.

30. CUMMING, P., A. ASE, H. KUWABARA & A. GJEDDE. 1997. [³H]DOPA formed from [³H]tyrosine in brain of living rat is not committed to dopamine synthesis. J. Cereb. Blood Flow Metab. In press.

31. CUMMING, P., A. ASE, C. LALIBERTÉ, H. KUWABARA & A. GJEDDE. 1997. In vivo regulation of DOPA decarboxylase by dopamine receptors in rat brain. J. Cereb. Blood Flow Metab. In press.

32. MIWA, S., P.-G. GILLBERG, P. BJURLING, N. YUMOTO, I. ODANO, Y. WATANABE & B. LÅNGSTRÖM. 1992. Assessment of dopamine and its metabolites in the intracellular and extracellular compartments of the rat striatum after peripheral administration of L-[¹¹C]DOPA. Brain Res. **578:** 122–128.

33. HOFFMAN, J. M., W. P. MELEGA, T. C. HAWK, S. C. GRAFTON, A. LUXEN, D. K. MAHONEY, J. R. BARRIO, S.-C. HUANG, J. C. MAZZIOTTA & M. E. PHELPS. 1992. The effects of carbidopa administration on 6-[¹⁸F]fluoro-L-DOPA kinetics in positron emission tomography. J. Nucl. Med. **33:** 1472–1477.

34. MELEGA, W. P., M. M. PERLMUTTER, A. LUXEN, C. H. K. NISSENSON, S. T. GRAFTON, S.-C. HUANG, M. E. PHELPS & J. R. BARRIO. 1989. 4-[¹⁸F]Fluoro-L-m-tyrosine: An L-3,4-dihydroxyphenylalanine analog for probing presynaptic dopaminergic function with positron emission tomography. J. Neurochem. **53:** 311–314.

35. DEEP, P., A. GJEDDE & P. CUMMING. 1997. Evaluating the accuracy of a tracer DOPA compartmental model. J. Neurosci. Methods. In press.

36. BOYES, B. E., P. CUMMING, W. R. W. MARTIN & E. G. MCGEER. 1986. Determination of plasma [¹⁸F]-6-fluorodopa during positron emission tomography: Elimination and metabolism in carbidopa treated subjects. Life Sci. **39:** 2243–2252.

37. KUWABARA, H., P. CUMMING, J. REITH, G. C. LÉGER, M. DIKSIC, A. C. EVANS & A. H. GJEDDE. 1993. Human striatal L-DOPA decarboxylase estimated in vivo using 6-[¹⁸F]fluoro-DOPA and positron emission tomography: Error analysis and application to normal subjects. J. Cereb. Blood Flow Metab. **13:** 43–56.

38. KUWABARA, H., P. CUMMING, Y. YASUHARA, G. C. LÉGER, M. GUTTMAN, M. DIKSIC, A. C. EVANS & A. H. GJEDDE. 1995. Regional striatal DOPA transport and decarboxylase activity in Parkinson's disease. J. Nucl. Med. **36:** 1226–1231.

39. DHAWAN, V., T. ISHIKAWA, C. PATLAK, T. CHALY, W. ROBESON, A. BELAKHLEF, C. MARGOULEFF, F. MANDEL & D. EIDELBERG. 1996. Combined FDOPA and 3OMFD PET studies in Parkinson's disease. J. Nucl. Med. **37:** 209–216.

40. GJEDDE, A., G. C. LÉGER, P. CUMMING, Y. YASUHARA, A. C. EVANS, M. GUTTMAN & H. KUWABARA. 1993. Striatal L-DOPA decarboxylase activity in Parkinson's disease in vivo: Implications for the regulation of dopamine synthesis. J. Neurochem. **61:** 1538–1541.

41. OPACKA-JUFFRY, J. & D. C. BROOKS. 1995. L-Dihydroxyphenylalanine and its decarboxylase: New ideas on their neuroregulatory roles (Review). Move. Disord. **10:** 241–249.

42. ZHU, M. Y., A. V. JUORIO, I. A. PATERSON & A. A. BOULTON. 1992. Regulation of the aromatic L-amino acid decarboxylase by dopamine receptors in rat brain. J. Neurochem. **58:** 636–641.

43. HADJICONSTANTINOU, W., T. A. WEMLINGER, C. SILVIA, D. KRAJNC & N. H. NEFF. 1993. Aromatic L-amino acid decarboxylase of mouse striatum is modulated via dopamine receptors. J. Neurochem. **60:** 2175–2180.

44. HADJICONSTANTINOU, M., Z. L. ROSSETTI, T. M. WEMLINGER & N. H. NEFF. 1995. Dizocilpine enhances striatal tyrosine hydroxylase and aromatic L-amino acid decarboxylase activity. Eur. J. Pharmacol. **289:** 97–101.

45. TEDROFF, J., R. TORSTENSON, P. HARTVIG, K. J. LINDNER, Y. WATANABE, P. BJURLING, G. WESTERBERG & B. LÅNGSTRÖM. 1997. L-DOPA modulates striatal dopaminergic function in vivo. Evidence from PET investigations in non-human primates. Synapse **25:** 56–61.

46. TORSTENSON, R., P. HARTVIG, B. LÅNGSTRÖM, G. WESTERBERG & J. TEDROFF. 1997. Differential effects of levodopa on dopaminergic function in early and advanced Parkinson's disease. Ann. Neurol. **41:** 334–340.

47. GJEDDE, A. 1981. High- and low-affinity transport of D-glucose from blood to brain. J. Neurochem. **36:** 1463–1471.

48. PATLAK, C. S., R. G. BLASBERG & J. D. FENSTERMACHER. 1983. Graphical evaluation of blood-to-brain transfer constants from multiple-time uptake data. J. Cereb. Blood Flow Metab. **3:** 1–7.

49. MARTIN, W. R. W., M. R. PALMER, C. S. PATLAK & D. B. CALNE. 1989. Nigrostriatal function in humans studied with positron emission tomography. Ann. Neurol. **26:** 535–542.

50. CHAN, G. L.-Y., K. S. MORRISON, J. E. HOLDEN & T. J. RUTH. 1992. Plasma L-[^{18}F]6-fluorodopa input function: A simplified method. J. Cereb. Blood Flow Metab. **12:** 881–884.

51. CUMMING, P., G. LÉGER, H. KUWABARA & A. GJEDDE. 1993. Pharmacokinetics of plasma 6-[^{18}F]fluoro-L-3,4-dihydroxyphenylalanine ([^{18}F]DOPA) in humans. J. Cereb. Blood Flow Metab. **13:** 668–675.

52. PATLAK, C. S. & R. G. BLASBERG. 1985. Graphical evaluation of blood-to-brain transfer constants from multiple-time uptake data: Generalizations. J. Cereb. Blood Flow Metab. **5:** 584–590.

53. BROOKS, D. J., E. P. SALMON, C. J. MATHIAS, N. QUINN, K. L. LEENDERS, R. BANNISTER, C. D. MARSDEN & R. S. J. FRACKOWIAK. 1990. The relationship between locomotor disability, autonomic dysfunction, and the integrity of the striatal dopaminergic system in patients with multisystem atrophy, pure autonomic failure, and Parkinson's disease, studied with PET. Brain **113:** 1539–1552.

54. HARTVIG, P., H. ÅGREN, L. REIBRING, J. TEDROFF, P. BJURLING, T. KIHLBERG & B. LÅNGSTROM. 1991. Brain kinetics of L-β-[^{11}C]DOPA in humans studied by positron emission tomography. J. Neural Transm. **86:** 25–41.

55. SAWLE, G. V., D. J. BURN, P. K. MORRISH, A. A. LAMMERTSMA, B. J. SNOW, S. LUTHRA, S. OSMAN & D. J. BROOKS. 1994. The effect of entacapone (OR-611) on brain [^{18}F]-6-fluorodopa metabolism: Implications for levodopa therapy of Parkinson's disease. Neurology **44:** 1292–1297.

56. HOSHI, H., H. KUWABARA, G. LÉGER, P. CUMMING, M. GUTTMAN & A. GJEDDE. 1993. 6-[^{18}F]fluoro-L-DOPA metabolism in living human brain: A comparison of six analytical methods. J. Cereb. Blood Flow Metab. **13:** 57–69.

57. VINGERHOETS, F. J. G., B. J. SNOW, M. SCHULZER, S. MORRISON, T. J. RUTH, J. E. HOLDEN, S. COOPER & D. B. CALNE. 1994. Reproducibility of fluorine-18-6-fluorodopa positron emission tomography in normal human subjects. J. Nucl. Med. **35:** 18–26.

58. PATE, B. D., B. J. SNOW, K. A. HEWITT, K. S. MORRISON, T. J. RUTH & D. B. CALNE. 1991. The reproducibility of striatal uptake data obtained with positron emission tomography and fluorine-18-L-6-fluorodopa tracer in non-human primates. J. Nucl. Med. **32:** 1246–1251.

59. ISHIKAWA, T., V. DHAWAN, T. CHALY, W. ROBESON, A. BELAKHEF, F. MANDEL, R. DAHL, C. MARGOULEFF & D. EIDELBERG. 1996. Fluorodopa positron emission tomography with an inhibitor of catechol-*O*-methyltransferase: Effect of the plasma 3-*O*-methyldopa on data analysis. J. Cereb. Blood Flow Metab. **16:** 854–863.

60. WAHL, L. & C. NAHMIAS. 1996. Modeling of fluorine-18-6-fluoro-L-dopa in humans. J. Nucl. Med. **37:** 432–437.

61. HAMMERSTAD, J. P., B. D. PATE, K. A. HEWITT, G. L.-Y. CHAN, T. J. RUTH & D. B. CALNE. 1993. The transport of L-6-fluorodopa and its metabolites from blood to cerebrospinal fluid and brain. Ann. Neurol. **34:** 603–608.

62. REITH, J., S. DYVE, H. KUWABARA, M. GUTTMAN, M. DIKSIC & A. GJEDDE. 1990.

Blood-brain transfer and metabolism of 6-[^{18}F]fluoro-L-DOPA in rat. J. Cereb. Blood Flow Metab. **10:** 707–719.

63. ISHIKAWA, T., V. DHAWAN, T. CHALY, W. ROBESON, A. BELAKHEF, F. MANDEL, R. DAHL, C. MARGOULEFF & D. EIDELBERG. 1996. Fluorodopa positron emission tomography with an inhibitor of catechol-methyltransferase: Effect on the plasma 3-O-methyldopa on data analysis. J. Cereb. Blood Flow Metab. **16:** 854–863.

64. KUWABARA, H., P. CUMMING, G. LÉGER, M. GUTTMAN, S. RAJAGOPAL & A. GJEDDE. 1993. Dopamine turnover is increased in striatum of patients with Parkinson's disease. Brain 93, May 22–28. Sendai, Japan.

65. BARRIO, J. R., S. C. HUANG, W. P. MELEGA, D. C. YU, J. M. HOFFMAN, J. S. SCHNEIDER, N. SATYAMURTHY, J. C. MAZZIOTTA & M. E. PHELPS. 1990. 6-[^{18}F]Fluoro-L-DOPA probes dopamine turnover rates in central dopaminergic structures. J. Neurosci. Res. **27:** 487–493.

66. CUMMING, P., A. ASE, M. DIKSIC, J. HARRISON, D. JOLLY, H. KUWABARA, C. LALIBERTÉ & A. GJEDDE. 1995. Metabolism and blood-brain clearance of L-3,4-dihydroxy-[^{3}H]phenylalanine ([^{3}H]DOPA) and 6-[^{18}F]fluoro-L-DOPA ([^{18}F]FDOPA) in the rat. Biochem. Pharmacol. **50:** 943–946.

67. MILETICH, R. S., G. COMI, K. BANKIEWICZ, R. PLUNKETT, R. ADAMS, G. DI CHIRO & I. J. KOPIN. 1993. 6-[^{18}F]Fluoro-L-dihydroxyphenylalanine metabolism and positron emission tomography after catechol-O-methyltransferase inhibition in normal and hemiparkinsonian monkeys. Brain Res. **626:** 1–13.

68. TSUKADA, H., K.-J. LINDNER, P. HARTVIG, Y. TANI, P. BJURLING, T. KIHLBERG, G. WESTERBERG, Y. WATANABE & B. LÅNGSTRÖM. 1994. Effect of 6R-L-erythro-5,6,7,8-tetrahydrobiopterin on in vivo L-[β-^{11}C]DOPA turnover in rat striatum with infusion of L-tyrosine. J. Neural Transm. **95:** 1–15.

69. WAHL, L., R. CHIRAKAL, G. FIRNAU, E. S. GARNETT & C. NAHMIAS. 1994. The distribution and kinetics of [^{18}F]6-fluoro-3-O-methyl-L-dopa in the human brain. J. Cereb. Blood Flow Metab. **14:** 664–670.

70. MACKAY, A. V. P., P. DAVIES, A. J. DEWAR & C. M. YATES. 1978. Regional distribution of enzymes associated with neurotransmission by monoamines, acetylcholine and GABA in human brain. J. Neurochem. **30:** 827–839.

71. LAIHINEN, A., J. O. RINNE, U. K. RINNE, M. HAAEPARANTA, U. RUOTSALAINEN, J. BERGMAN & O. SOLIN. 1992. [^{18}F]-6-fluorodopa PET scanning in Parkinson's disease after selective COMT inhibition with nitecapone (OR-462). Neurology **42:** 199–203.

72. GUTTMAN, M., G. LÉGER, A. RECHES, A. EVANS, H. KUWABARA, J. M. CEDARBAUM & A. GJEDDE. 1993. Administration of the new COMT inhibitor OR-611 increases striatal uptake of fluorodopa. Move. Disord. **8:** 298–304.

73. PAUWELS, T., S. DETHY, S. GOLDMAN, M. MONCLUS & A. LUXEN. 1994. Effect of catechol-O-methyltransferase inhibition on peripheral and central metabolism of 6-[^{18}F]fluoro-L-DOPA. Eur. J. Pharmacol. **257:** 53–58.

74. HARTVIG, P., K. J. LINDNER, J. TEDROFF, P. BJURLING, K. HÖRNFEL & B. LÅNGSTROM. 1992. Regional brain kinetics of 6-fluoro-(β-^{11}C)-L-dopa and (β-^{11}C)-L-dopa following COMT inhibition: A study in vivo using positron emission tomography. J. Neural Transm. **87:** 15–22.

75. TEDROFF, I., P. HARTVIG, P. BJURLING, Y. ANDERSSON, G. ANTONI & B. LÅNGSTRÖM. 1991. Central action of benserazide after COMT inhibition demonstrated in vivo by PET. J. Neural Transm. **87:** 15–22.

76. ROTH, J. A. 1992. Membrane-bound catechol-O-methyltransferase: A reevaluation of its role in the O-methylation of catecholamine neurotransmitters (Review). Rev. Physiol. Biochem. Pharmacol. **257:** 53–58.

77. HARTVIG, P., K. J. LINDNER, J. TEDROFF, Y. ANDERSSON, P. BJURLING & B. LÅNGSTRÖM. 1992. Brain kinetics of ^{11}C-labelled tryptophan and 5-hydroxy-L-tryptophan in the Rhesus monkey: A study using positron emission tomography. J. Neural Transm. **88:** 1–10.

78. CUMMING, P., V. LJUBIC-THIBAL, C. LALIBERTÉ & M. DIKSIC. 1997. The effect of unilateral neurotoxic lesions to serotonin fibres in the medial forebrain bundle on the metabolism of [^{3}H]DOPA in the telencephalon of the living rat. Brain Res. **747:** 60–69.

79. HARTVIG, P., K. J. LINDNER, B. LÅNGSTRÖM & J. TEDROFF. 1995. Pyridoxine effect on synthesis rate of serotonin in the monkey brain measured with positron emission tomography. J. Neural Transm. **102:** 91–97.

80. NAHMIAS, C., L. WAHL, R. CHIRAKAL, G. FIRNAU & E. S. GARNETT. 1995. A probe for intracerebral aromatic amino-acid decarboxylase activity: Distribution and kinetics of [^{18}F]6-fluoro-L-m-tyrosine in the human brain. Move. Disord. **10:** 298–304.

81. DEJESUS, O. T., C. J. ENDRES, S. E. SHELTON, J. NICKLES & J. E. HOLDEN. 1997. Evaluation of fluorinated m-tyrosine analogs as PET imaging agents of dopamine nerve terminals: Comparison with 6-fluorodopa. J. Nucl. Med. **38:** 630–636.

82. BAKER, G. B., A. J. NAZARALI, R. T. COUTTS, R. G. MICETICH & T. W. HALL. 1984. Brain levels of 5-hydroxytryptamine, tryptamine and 2-phenylethylamine in the rat after administration of N-cyanoethyltranylcypromine. Prog. Neuro. Psychopharmacol. & Biol. Psychiatry **18:** 793–802.

83. ENDRES, C. J., S. SWAMINATHAN, O. T. DEJESUS, M. SIEVER, A. E. RUOHO & D. MURALI. 1997. Affinities of dopamine analogs for monoamine granular and plasma membrane transporters: Implication for PET dopamine studies. Life Sci. **60:** 2399–2406.

84. PALFREYMAN, M. G., I. A. MCDONALD, J. R. FOZARD, Y. MELY, A. J. SLEIGHT, M. ZREIKA, J. WAGNER, P. BEY & P. J. LEWIS. 1985. Inhibition of monoamine oxidase selectively in brain monoamine nerves using the bioprecursor (E)β-fluoromethylene-m-tyrosine (MDL 72394), a substrate for aromatic L-amino acid decarboxylase. J. Neurochem. **45:** 1850–1860.

85. DEJESUS, P. T., J. E. HOLDEN, C. ENDRES, D. MURALI, T. R. OAKES, S. SHELTON, H. UNO, D. HOUSER, L. FREUND, S. B. PERLMAN & R. J. NICKLES. 1992. Visualization of dopamine nerve terminals by positron emission tomography using [^{18}F]fluoro-β-fluoromethylene-m-tyrosine. Brain Res. **597:** 151–154.

86. DYKE, L. E. 1987. Effect of monofluoromethyldopa (MFMD) on trace amine levels. Life Sci. **40:** 571–575.

87. MELTZER, C. C., J. K. ZUBIETA, F. J. BRAND, L. E. TUNE, H. S. MAYBERG & J. J. FROST. 1996. Regional hypometabolism in Alzheimer's disease as measured by PET after correction for effects of partial volume averaging. Neurology **47:** 454–461.

88. WONG, D. F., J. C. HARRIS, S. NAIDU, F. YOKOI, S. MARENCO, R. F. DANNALS, H. T. RAVERT, M. YASTER, A. EVANS, O. ROUSSET, R. N. BRYAN, A. GJEDDE, M. J. KUHAR & G. R. BREESE. 1996. Dopamine transporters are markedly reduced in Lesch-Nyhan disease in vivo. Proc. Natl. Acad. Sci. **93:** 5539–5543.

89. MURPHY, D. G. M., C. DECARLI, M. B. SCHAPIRO, S. I. RAPOPORT & B. HORWITZ. 1992. Age-related differences in volumes of subcortical nuclei, brain matter, and cerebrospinal fluid in healthy men measured with magnetic resonance imaging. Arch. Neurol. **49:** 839–845.

90. HUME, S. P., A. A. LAMMERTSMA, R. MYERS, S. RAJESWARAN, P. M. BLOOMFIELD, S. ASHWORTH, R. A. FRICKER, E. M. TORRES, A. WATSON & T. JONES. 1996. The potential of high-resolution positron emission tomography to monitor striatal dopaminergic function in rat models of disease. J. Neurosci. Methods **76:** 103–112.

91. ROUSSET, O. G., Y. MA, G. LÉGER, A. GJEDDE & A. EVANS. 1993. Corrections for partial volume effects in PET using MRI-based 3D simulations of individual human brain metabolism. *In* Quantification of Brain Function. Tracer Kinetics and Image Analysis in Brain PET. K. Uemmura *et al.*, Eds.: 113–120. Elsevier. New York.

92. PATE, B. D., T. KAWAMATA, T. YAMADA, E. G. MCGEER, K. A. HEWITT, B. J. SNOW, T. J. RUTH & D. B. CALNE. 1993. Correlation of striatal fluorodopa, uptake in the MPTP monkey with dopaminergic indices. Ann. Neurol. **34:** 331–338.

93. SNOW, B. J., I. TOOYAMA, E. G. MCGEER, T. YAMADA, D. B. CALNE, H. TAKAHASHI & H. KIMURA. 1993. Human positron emission tomographic [^{18}F]fluorodopa studies correlate with dopamine cell counts and levels. Ann. Neurol. **34:** 324–330.

94. TEDROFF, J., S.-M. AQUILONIUS, A. LAIHINEN, U. RINNE, P. HARTVIG, J. ANDERSON, H. LUNDQVIST, M. HAARPARANTA, O. SOLIN, G. ANTONI, A. D. GEE, J. ULIN & B. LÅNGSTRÖM. 1990. Striatal kinetics of [^{11}C]-(+)-nomifensine and 6-[^{18}F]fluoro-L-dopa in Parkinson's disease measured with positron emission tomography. Acta Neurol. Scand. **81:** 24–30.

95. CHANAGLIA, G., F. J. ALVAREZ, A. PROBST & J. M. PALACIOS. 1992. Mesostriatal and mesolimbic dopamine uptake binding sites are decreased in Parkinson's disease and progressive supranuclear palsy: A quantitative autoradiographic study using [^{3}H]mazindol. Neuroscience **49:** 317–327.

96. WEIHMULLER, F. B., J. ULAS, L. NGUYEN, C. M. COTMAN & J. M. MARSHALL. 1992. Elevated NMDA receptors in parkinsonian striatum. Neuroreport **3:** 977–980.

97. MELEGA, W. P., M. J. RALEIGH, D. B. STOUT, A. A. DESALLES, S. R. CHERRY, M. BLURTON-JONES, G. G. MORTON, S.-C. HUANG & M. E. PHELPS. 1996. Longitudinal behavioural and 6-[^{18}F]fluoro-L-DOPA/PET: Assessment in MPTP-hemiparkinsonian monkeys. Exp. Neurol. **141:** 318–329.

98. MELAMED, E., F. HEFTI, D. J. PETTIBONE, J. LIEBMAN & R. J. WURTMAN. 1981. Aromatic L-amino-acid decarboxylase in rat corpus striatum: Implications for action of L-dopa in parkinsonism. Neurology **31:** 651–655.

99. KISH, S. J., X. H. ZHONG, O. HORNYKIEWICZ & J. W. HAYCOCK. 1995. Striatal 3,4-dihydroxyphenylalanine decarboxylase in aging: Disparity between postmortem and positron emission tomography studies? Ann. Neurol. **38:** 260–264.

100. KISH, S. J., K. SHANNAK, A. RAJPUT, J. H. N. DECK & O. HORNYKIEWICZ. 1992. Aging produces a specific pattern of striatal dopamine loss: Implications for the etiology of idiopathic Parkinson's disease. J. Neurochem. **58:** 642–648.

101. SCHERMAN, D., C. DESNOS, F. DARCHEN, P. POLLAK, F. JAVOY-AGID & Y. AGID. 1989. Striatal dopamine deficiency in Parkinson's disease: Role of aging. Ann. Neurol. **26:** 551–557.

102. SAWLE, G. V., J. G. COLEBATCH, A. SHAH, D. J. BROOKS, C. D. MARSDEN & R. S. J. FRACKOWIAK. 1990. Striatal function in normal aging: Implications for Parkinson's disease. Ann. Neurol. **28:** 799–804.

103. EIDELBERG, D., S. TAKIKAWA, V. DHAWAN, T. CHALY, W. ROBESON, R. DAHL, D. MARGOULEFF, J. R. MOELLER, C. S. PATLAK & S. FAHN. 1993. Striatal ^{18}F-DOPA uptake: Absence of an aging effect. J. Cereb. Blood Flow Metab. **13:** 881–888.

104. MORRISH, P. K., G. V. SAWLE & D. J. BROOKS. 1996. An [^{18}F]dopa-PET and clinical study of the rate of progression in Parkinson's disease. Brain **119:** 585–591.

105. CORDES, M., B. J. SNOW, S. COOPER, M. SCHULZER, B. D. PATE, T. J. RUTH & D. B. CALNE. 1994. Age-dependent decline of nigrostriatal dopaminergic function: A positron emission tomographic study of grandparents and their grandchildren. Ann. Neurol. **36:** 667–670.

106. MORRISH, P. K., G. V. SAWLE & D. J. BROOKS. 1995. Clinical and [^{18}F]dopa PET findings in early Parkinson's disease. J. Neurol. Neurosurg. Psychiatry **59:** 597–600.

107. ANTONINI, A., P. VONTOBEL, M. PSYLLA, I. GÜNTHER, P. R. MAGUIRE, J. MISSIMER & K. L. LEENDERS. 1995. Complementary positron emission tomographic studies of the striatal dopaminergic system in Parkinson's disease. Arch. Neurol. **52:** 1183–1190.

108. HOLTHOFF-DETTO, V. A., J. KESSLER, K. HERHOLZ, H. BÖNNER, U. PIETRZYK, M. WÜRKER, M. GHAEMI, K. WIENHARD, R. WAGNER & W.-D. HEISS. 1997. Functional effects of striatal dysfunction in Parkinson's disease. Arch. Neurol. **54:** 145–150.

109. TAKIKAWA, S., V. DHAWAN, T. CHALY, W. ROBESON, R. DAHL, I. ZANZI, F. MANDEL, P. SPETSIERIS & E. EIDELBERG. 1994. Input functions for 6-[Fluorine-18]fluorodopa quantitation in Parkinsonism: Comparative studies and clinical correlations. J. Nucl. Med. **35:** 955–963.

110. PICCINI, P., P. K. MORRISH, N. TURJANSKI, G. V. SAWLE, D. J. BURN, R. A. WEEKS, M. H. MARK, D. M. MARAGANORE, A. J. LEES & D. J. BROOKS. 1997. Dopaminergic function in familial Parkinson's disease: A clinical and ^{18}F-dopa positron emission tomography study. Ann. Neurol. **41:** 222–229.

111. KISH, S. J., K. SHANNAK & O. HORNYKIEWICZ. 1988. Uneven patterns of dopamine loss in the striatum of patients with idiopathic Parkinson's disease. N. Engl. J. Med. **318:** 876–880.

112. VINGERHOETS, F. J. G., B. J. SNOW, C. S. LEE, M. SCHULZER, E. MAK & D. B. CALNE. 1994. Longitudinal fluorodopa positron emission tomographic studies of the evolution of idiopathic parkinsonism. Ann. Neurol. **36:** 759–764.

113. FREED, C. R., R. E. BREEZE, N. L. ROSENBERG, S. A. SCHNECK, E. KRIEK, J.-X. QI,

T. LONE, Y.-B. ZHANG, J. A. SNYDER, T. H. WELLS, L. O. RAMIG, L. THOMPSON, J. C. MAZZIOTA, S. C. HUANG, S. T. GRAFTON, D. BROOKS, G. SAWLE, G. SCHROTER & A. A. ANSARI. 1992. Survival of implanted fetal dopamine cells and neurologic improvement 12 to 46 months after transplantation for Parkinson's disease. N. Engl. J. Med. **327:** 1549–1555.

114. SAWLE, G. V., P. M. BLOOMFIELD, A. BJÖRKLUND, D. J. BROOKS, P. BRUNDIN, K. L. LEENDERS, O. LINDVALL, C. D. MARSDEN, S. REHNCRONA, H. WIDNER & R. S. J. FRACKOWIAK. 1992. Transplantation of fetal dopamine neurons in Parkinson's disease: PET [^{18}F]6-L-fluorodopa studies in two patients with putaminal implants. Ann. Neurol. **31:** 166–173.

115. FREEMAN, T. B., C. W. OLANOW, R. A. HAUSER, G. M. NAUERT, D. A. SMITH, C. V. BORLONGAN, P. R. SANBERG, D. A. HOLT, J. H. KORDOWER, F. J. G. VINGERHOETS, B. J. SNOW, D. CALNE & L. L. GAUGER. 1995. Bilateral fetal nigral transplantation into the postcommissural putament in Parkinson's disease. Ann. Neurol. **38:** 379–388.

116. SNOW, B. J., R. F. PEPPARD, M. GUTTMAN, J. OKADA, W. R. W. MARTIN, J. STEELE, A. EISEN, G. CARR, B. SHOENBERG & D. B. CALNE. 1990. Positron emission tomographic scanning demonstrates a presynaptic dopaminergic lesion in Lytico-Bodig. Arch. Neurol. **47:** 870–874.

117. RINNE, J. O., D. J. BURN, C. J. MATHIAS, N. P. QUINN, C. D. MARSDEN & D. J. BROOKS. 1995. Positron emission tomography studies on the dopaminergic system and striatal opioid binding in the olivopontocerebellar atrophy variant of multiple system atrophy. Ann. Neurol. **37:** 568–573.

118. KISHORE, A., Z. K. WSZOLEK, B. J. SNOW, R. DE LA FUENTE-FERNANDEZ, F. ARWERT, M. WIJKER, M. SCHULZER, D. B. CALNE & F. J. G. VINGERHOETS. 1996. Presynaptic nigrostriatal function in genetically tested asymptomatic relatives from the pallido-ponto-nigral degeneration family. Neurology **47:** 1588–1590.

119. SNOW, B. J., T. G. NYGAARD, H. TAKAHASHI & D. B. CALNE. 1993. Positron emission tomographic studies of dopa-responsive dystonia and early-onset idiopathic parkinsonism. Ann. Neurol. **34:** 733–738.

120. CORDES, M., B. J. SNOW, S. MORRISON, V. SOSSI, T. J. RUTH & D. B. CALNE. 1993. Parametric imaging of the rate constant K_i using [^{18}F]Fluoro-L-dopa positron emission tomography in progressive supranuclear palsy. Neuroradiology **35:** 404–409.

121. BHATT, M. H., B. J. SNOW, W. R. W. MARTIN, S. COOPER & D. B. CALNE. 1990. Positron emission tomography in Shy-Drager syndrome. Ann. Neurol. **28:** 101–103.

122. WSZOLEK, Z. K., R. F. PFEIFFER, M. H. BHATT, R. L. SCHELPER, M. CORDE, B. J. SNOW, R. L. RODNITZKY, E. C. WOLTERS, F. ARWERT & D. B. CALNE. 1992. Rapidly progressive autosomal dominant parkinsonism and dementia with pallido-ponto-nigral degeneration. Ann. Neurol. **32:** 312–320.

123. TAKAHASHI, H., B. J. SNOW, M. H. BHATT, R. PEPPARD, A. EISEN & D. B. CALNE. 1993. Evidence for dopaminergic deficit in sporadic amyotrophic lateral sclerosis on positron emission scanning. Lancet **342:** 1016–1018.

124. SNOW, B. J., M. BHATT, W. R. W. MARTIN & D. B. CALNE. 1991. The nigrostriatal dopaminergic pathway in Wilson's disease studied with positron emission tomography. J. Neurol. Neurosurg. Psychiatry **54:** 12–17.

125. TAKAHASHI, H., B. J. SNOW, T. G. NYGAARD & D. B. CALNE. 1993. Clinical heterogeneity of dopa-responsive dystonia: PET observations. *In* Advances in Neurology, Vol. 60. H. Narabayashi *et al.*, Eds.: 586–590. Raven Press. New York.

126. OKADA, A., K. NAKAMURA, B. J. SNOW, M. H. BHATT, M. NOMOTO, M. OSAME & D. B. CALNE. 1993. PET scan study on the dopaminergic system in a Japanese patient with hereditary progressive dystonia (Segawa's disease) (Case Report). *In* Advances in Neurology, Vol. 60. H. Narabayashi *et al.*, Eds.: 691–694. Raven Press. New York.

127. LÜDECKE, B., P. M. KNAPPSKOG, P. T. CLAYTON, R. A. H. SURTEES, J. D. CLELLAND, S. J. R. HEALES, M. P. BRAND, K. BARTHOLOMÉ & T. FLATMARK. 1996. Recessively inherited L-DOPA-responsive parkinsonism in infancy caused by a point mutation (L205P) in the tyrosine hydroxylase gene. Hum. Mol. Genet. **5:** 1023–1028.

128. BROOKS, D. J., V. IBANEZ, E. D. PLAYFORD, G. V. SAWLE, P. N. LEIGH, R. S. KOCEN, A. E. HARDING & C. D. MARSDEN. 1991. Presynaptic and postsynaptic striatal

dopaminergic function in neuroacanthocytosis: A positron emission tomographic study. Ann. Neurol. **30:** 166–171.

129. ERNST, M., A. J. ZAMETKIN, J. A. MATOCHIK, D. PASCUALVACA, P. H. JONS, K. HARDY, J. G. HANKERSON, D. J. DOUDET & R. M. COHEN. 1996. Presynaptic dopaminergic deficits in Lesch-Nyhan disease. N. Engl. J. Med. **334:** 1568–1572.

130. NAGASAWA, H., H. TANJI, H. NOMURA, H. SAITO, Y. ITOYAMA, I. KIMURA, S. TUJI, T. FUJIWARA, R. IWATA, M. ITOH & T. IDO. 1996. PET study of cerebral glucose metabolism and fluorodopa uptake in patients with corticobasal degeneration. J. Neurol. Sci. **139:** 21–217.

131. MELEGA, W. P., J. QUINTANA, M. J. RALEIGH, D. B. STOUT, D.-C. YU, K.-P. LIN, S.-C. HUANG & M. E. PHELPS. 1996. 6-[^{18}F]Fluoro-L-DOPA-PET studies show partial reversal of long-term effects of chronic amphetamine in monkeys. Synapse **22:** 63–69.

132. WILSON, J. M., K. S. KALASINSKY, A. I. LEVEY, C. BERGERON, G. REIBER, R. M. ANTHONY, G. A. SCHMUNK, K. SHANNAK, J. W. HAYCOCK & S. J. KISH. 1996. Striatal dopamine nerve terminal markers in human chronic methamphetamine users. Nature Med. **2:** 699–703.

133. TETRUD, J. W., W. LANGSTON, I. IRWIN & B. SNOW. 1994. Parkinsonism caused by petroleum waste ingestion. Neurology **44:** 1051–1054.

134. REITH, J., C. BENKELFAT, A. SHERWIN, Y. YASUHARA, H. KUWABARA, F. ANDERMANN, S. BACHNEFF, P. CUMMING, M. DIKSIC, S. E. DYVE, P. ÉTIENNE, A. C. EVANS, S. LAL, M. SHEVELL, G. SAVARD, D. F. WONG, G. CHOUINARD & A. GJEDDE. 1994. Elevated dopa decarboxylase activity in living brain of patients with psychosis. Proc. Natl. Acad. Sci. USA **91:** 11651–11654.

135. HIETALA, J., E. SYVÄLAHTI, K. VUORIO, V. RÄKKÖLÄINEN, J. BERGMAN, M. HAARPARANTA, O. SOLIN, M. KUOPPAMÄKI, O. KIRVELÄ, U. RUOTSALEINEN & R. SALOKANGAS. 1995. Presynaptic dopamine function in striatum of neuroleptic-naive schizophrenic patients. Lancet **346:** 1130–1131.

136. WU, J. C., G. MAGUIRE, G. RILEY, A. LEE, D. KEATOR, C. TANG, J. FALLON & A. NAJAFI. 1997. Increased dopamine activity associated with stuttering. Neuroreport **8:** 767–770.

137. ÅGREN, H., L. REIBRING, P. HARTVIG, J. TEDROFF, P. BJURLING, K. HÖRNFELDT, Y. ANDERSSON, H. LUNDQVIST & B. LÅNGSTRÖM. 1991. Low brain uptake of L-[^{11}C]5-hydroxytryptophan in major depression: A positron emission tomography study on patients and healthy volunteers. Acta Psychiatr. Scand. **83:** 449–455.

138. DANIELSEN, E. H., D. F. SMITH, A. D. GEE, T. K. VENKATACHALAM, S. B. HANSEN & A. GJEDDE. 1997. The metabolism of [^{18}F]-DOPA in pigs estimated by PET (Abstract). BrainPET 97, Washington, D.C.

139. DOUDET, D., C. A. MCLELLAN, R. CARSON, H. R. ADAMS, H. MIYAKE, T. G. AIGNER, R. T. FINN & R. M. COHEN. 1991. Distribution and kinetics of 3-O-methyl-6-[^{18}F]fluoro-L-DOPA in the rhesus monkey brain. J. Cereb. Blood Flow Metab. **11:** 726–734.

140. BARRIO, J. R., S.-C. HUANG, D.-C. YU, W. P. MELEGA, J. QUINTANA, S. R. CHERRY, A. JACOBSON, M. NAMAVARI, N. SATYAMURTHY & M. E. PHELPS. 1996. Radiofluorinated L-m-tyrosines: New in-vivo probes for central dopamine biochemistry. J. Cereb. Blood Flow Metab. **16:** 667–678.

141. CHAN, G. L.-Y., D. J. DOUDET, T. DOBKO, K. A. HEWITT, P. SCHOFIELD, B. D. PATE & T. J. RUTH. 1995. Routes of administration and effect of carbidopa pretreatment on 6-[^{18}F]fluoro-L-DOPA scans in non-human primates. Life Sci. **56:** 1759–1766.

142. TEDROFF, J., S.-M. AQUILONIUS, P. HARTVIG, E. BREDBERG & P. BJURLING. 1992. Cerebral uptake and utilization of therapeutic [beta-11C]-L-DOPA in Parkinson's disease measured by positron emission tomography. Acta Neurol. Scand. **85:** 95–102.

143. ISHIKAWA, T., V. DHAWAN, T. CHALY, C. MARGOULEFF, W. ROBESON, J. R. DAHL, F. MANDEL, P. SPETSIERIS & D. EIDELBERG. 1996. Clinical significance of striatal DOPA decarboxylase activity in Parkinson's disease. J. Nucl. Med. **37:** 216–222.

Role of Apoptotic Proteins in Ischemic Hippocampal Damage

JAMES N. DAVIS[a] AND FRANCIS J. ANTONAWICH

Department of Neurology
State University at New York at Stony Brook
Stony Brook, New York 11794-8124
and
The Northport DVA Medical Center
Northport, New York 11768

WHAT IS APOPTOSIS?

Classic View

Wylie and co-workers[1] proposed that cells died in two ways, apoptosis or necrosis. They viewed non-necrotic cell deaths as having the following characteristics developed from work using lymphocytes and thymocytes. Such cells have a characteristic morphological appearance as they undergo apoptosis. Initially, the nuclear chromatin becomes dispersed at the edge of the nuclear membrane, and an increase in protein synthesis can be seen as an increase in endoplasmic reticulum density. The cell then "packages" itself into membrane-bound subcellular particles termed aposomes. Thus, the characteristic ultramicroscopic appearance is a major criterion. Wylie also showed that protein synthesis inhibition could prevent apoptosis, leading to the hypothesis that the cell actively evoked its own death by producing "suicide" proteins. Finally, a third criterion is the appearance of DNA fragmentation in a characteristic pattern caused by internucleosmal cleavage of chromatin. When the fragmented cellular DNA is subjected to agarose electrophoresis, it forms a characteristic "stepladder" appearance. The stepladder conforms to multiples of approximately 180 kb, the length of DNA bound to a single nucleosome. In the past five years, a histochemical technique has been developed to detect cells undergoing this form of DNA fragmentation, the TUNEL procedure.[2] This procedure relies on the specificity of terminal transferase to attach nucleotides to fragmented DNA. By use of labeled nucleotides, cells with fragmented DNA can be detected.

Thus, in the classic view, apoptosis had three characteristics: a special electron microscopic appearance, prevention by protein synthesis inhibition, and a distinctive stepladder appearance to the DNA. TABLE 1 lists some forms of apoptotic cell death that seem to fit these criteria.

Forms of Apoptosis

In the past decade, it has been recognized that not all forms of apoptosis use the same molecular mechanisms. Although the above criteria have been used to

[a] Address correspondence to James N. Davis, Department of Neurology, HSC T12, Room 020, Stony Brook, NY 11794-8121. E-mail: jdavis@neuro.som.sunysb.edu

TABLE 1. Forms of Apoptotic Cell Death

Examples	Biological Events
Normal tissue turnover	Wound healing
Normal embryonic development	Maturing fetus
Metamorphosis	Insect changing from larva to adult
Hormone-induced atrophy	Menstruation
Cell-mediated immune killing	Natural killer cells
X-radiation	Treatment of cancer

define apoptotic cells, clear examples now exist of non-necrotic cell death that differ from "classic" apoptosis. For example, in macrophages apoptosis is accelerated by protein synthesis inhibition. DNA fragmentation is a late event in some apoptotic neurons[3] and does not occur in others. TUNEL staining can be detected in necrotic areas of tissues when nuclear membrane integrity is lost.[4–6] In part this recognition of different forms of apoptosis is inevitable as the molecular mechanisms underlying this form of cell death are better understood. To understand neuronal ischemic death, it seems logical to study what is known about apoptosis in neuronal systems.

C. elegans

Among the most compelling work in apoptosis is the study of the nervous system of *C. elegans*, a small worm. This microscopic animal has a life span of little more than two days and a simple, well-characterized genetic background. Mutant *C. elegans* that do not undergo programmed neuronal death during development have been identified and the genes responsible characterized.[7–9] More than 10 genes appear to participate in apoptosis in *C. elegans*. Most of these are involved in removal of apoptotic cells, but at least two seem to play important roles in the genesis of the nervous system, ced-3 and ced-9. Ced-9 is analogous to the mammalian protein, *bcl-2*.[10] *Bcl-2* is found in lymphoma cells where its overexpression may be an important event in the unfettered division of the cancerous cell.[11–13] Ced-9 is required for cell survival during neuronal development in *C. elegans*, supporting the idea that *bcl-2* is an "anti-apoptotic" protein.

Ced-3[14] is analogous to the mammalian protease, interleukin-1β converting enzyme (ICE). Originally thought to be solely the rate-controlling enzyme in the production of interleukin from its protein precursor, ICE is now recognized as a member of a family of proteases that appears to be the final common steps in various forms of programmed cell death.

Cultured Neurons

Another very useful system for studying apoptosis has been the sympathetic ganglia when trophic factors have been removed. Sympathetic neurons grow well in tissue culture in the presence of nerve growth factor. When nerve growth factor is removed, sympathetic neurons undergo apoptosis without DNA fragmentation.[15] The earliest change is an elevation in c-*fos*, an immediate early gene (IEG). Ganglia overexpressing *bcl-2* do not undergo apoptosis,[16] and ICE inhibitors also prevent its development.[17] Thus, both cultured neurons and *C. elegans* neurons share some

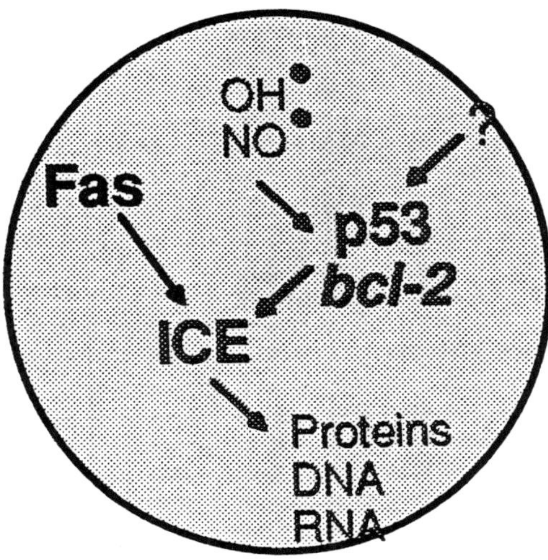

FIGURE 1. Apoptosis: Two pathways in programmed cell death.

analogous apoptotic proteins during programmed cell death. Other proteins important in apoptosis have been identified from studies of lymphocytes and thymocytes. In these a membrane protein called FAS seems to trigger apoptosis.[2] Hormones and a variety of stimuli can elicit cell death. The FAS protein shares a "death domain" with other membrane receptors and interacts with specific cytoplasmic proteins that appear to activate directly the ICE family of proteases. Thus, there appears to be at least two pathways, one through activation of FAS and the other involving *bcl*-2 (FIG. 1). Both pathways involve the ICE family of proteases, but different members of the family may service the two pathways.

SELECTIVE ISCHEMIC NEURONAL DEATH

The purpose of this review is to discuss recent work being carried out in our laboratory and that of others in which some of the apoptotic proteins have been implicated in ischemic cell death.

Ischemic cell death occurs in both focal and transient cerebral ischemia. In focal ischemia, the central area of the ischemic insult undergoes a necrotic cell death, characterized by mitochondrial swelling, breakdown of plasma and nuclear membranes, and cellular lysis, while the penumbra, the region surrounding this area, shows evidence of selective cell death. This selective cell death has been most intensively studied in the hippocampal formation. Hippocampal CA1 neurons die after a brief episode of transient forebrain ischemia, whereas adjacent CA3 neurons do not. Furthermore, the CA1 neurons die after a delay of several hours. They appear to function in a grossly normal fashion after brief ischemic exposure, but then begin to show a variety of behaviors that culminate in cell death between two

TABLE 2. Models of Ischemia: Histological Events Associated with Transient Ischemic Death in CA1 Neurons of the Hippocampus

Time	Event
5 min	Dendritic and reversible mitochondrial swelling
3 h	Decline in total mRNA
6–12 h	Silver degeneration appears
12–24 h	Dendritic cytoplasmic swelling
	Dendritic microvacuolation and loss of microtubules (tubulin and MAP)
	Endoplasmic reticulum swelling
	Polyribosomal disaggregation
24 h	Endoplasmic reticulum cisterns massively proliferate
	Fragmentary endoplasmic reticulum membranes and lysosomes around nucleus
	Nuclear chromatin slightly clumped
24 h–3 days	Loss of cytoplasmic RNA, dendritic degeneration, structural damage, DNA fragmentation and cell death

and four days after the ischemia. TABLE 2 summarizes published studies of CA1 death in the gerbil after transient ischemia.[18–25] Although the microscopic appearance of CA1 death is not one of classic apoptosis or necrosis, the fact that death occurs hours after the insult without early disruption of the plasma membrane suggests that CA1 cell death may share features of apoptosis. We and others have spent considerable time comparing CA1 death to apoptosis as it occurs in thymocytes and lymphocytes. We are convinced that ischemic cell death does not involve an early DNase activation and is not prevented by protein synthesis inhibition. We are intrigued by recent observations in neuronal cell death from either removal of trophic factor or the naturally occurring cell death seen during development; we feel that ischemic cell death may more closely follow these forms of cell death.

CA1 Damage Depends on Temperature, Glucose, and Glucocorticoids

The adrenal steroid, glucocorticoid, has a profound effect on delayed ischemic CA1 cell death in the hippocampus. Immediate administration of glucocorticoids following transient ischemia exacerbate ischemic neuronal damage, whereas either immediate adrenalectomy or adrenalectomy 24 h after ischemia is associated with partial protection.[26,27] Protection from delayed neuronal death also occurs when stress-induced glucocorticoid release is prevented by administering metyrapone, a synthesis inhibitor,[28] and following administration of the glucocorticoid receptor blocker RU-38486.[29] The extent of ischemic pyramidal cell death is also highly sensitive to brain temperature.[30–32] Maintenance of brain temperature during the ischemic and post-ischemic periods is of critical importance following transient ischemia.[33–35] Hypothermia is a positive regulator of CA1 pyramidal damage. Decreases in brain temperature of as little as 1.5 to 2.0 °C are sufficient to prevent CA1 cell death. The extent of neuroprotection varies based on when cooling is initiated, its duration, and degree.[34] Hypothermia is believed to provide beneficial effects by saving high-energy phosphates, maintaining high intracellular pH levels, and attenuating glutamate release via modulation of protein kinase C levels.[36,37] One complication of studying changes in glucocorticoids is that these hormones participate in the regulation of body temperature. Following both adrenalectomy and metyrapone administration, a drop in body and brain temperature occurs which may contribute to the attenuation of CA1 cell death.[38]

Both the acute and chronic administration of glucocorticoids is associated with elevated plasma glucose levels.[39] Glucocorticoid-impaired utilization of glucose appears to play a role in ischemic pyramidal cell death by limiting available intracellular glucose. Sapolsky[40] has shown that providing alternate fuels such as mannose or β-hydroxybutyrate to animals partially protects them from the damaging effects of glucocorticoids and various metabolic insults such as kainic acid or 3-acetylpyridine administration. It has been postulated that this stress-induced adrenal steroid acts by inhibiting glucose transport into vulnerable hippocampal neurons and glia.[41] Furthermore, these high plasma glucose concentrations during ischemia can worsen neuronal damage presumably by increasing·the formation of lactic acid.[42]

ISCHEMIC CELL DEATH IS NOT CLASSIC APOPTOSIS

Studies of DNA Fragmentation

We examined whether DNA fragmentation does indeed occur in CA1 neurons.[3] At no time point were we able to detect DNA fragmentation on ethidium bromide-treated gels of DNA extracted from the CA1 pyramidal layer after 5 min of bilateral carotid occlusion. Because of reports of DNA fragmentation in focal ischemia, we examined gerbil DNA from infarcted cerebral hemispheres at various times after ligation of the ipsilateral carotid artery. Beginning at 48 h and extending through to 54 h after carotid occlusion, we were able to identify the characteristic stepladder appearance in DNA. We have concluded that DNA fragmentation is a late event in ischemic cell death and that it may occur in some forms of necrotic cell death. We speculated that breakdown of the nuclear membrane might be responsible, allowing endonucleases from lysosomes or the cytoplasm to attack remaining pieces of chromatin. If this is true, then only when DNA fragmentation is an early event in cell death can it be used as specific evidence of apoptosis.

Involvement of Apoptotic Proteins

We believe that an orderly temporal sequence of events leads to ischemic cell death (FIG. 2). The first time period is characterized by an initial oxidative stress associated with the elevated Ca^{2+} and restoration of the circulation. This stress evokes a second period characterized by an expression of immediate early genes and heat shock proteins. Associated with the expression of heat shock proteins is the activation of p53. p53 moves from the cytoplasm to the nucleus leading to a third period where a family of proteins, the *bcl*-2 family, interacts. That interaction then leads to the final period where the irreversible expression of nonspecific proteases, such as ICE, leads to cell destruction.

Immediate Early Genes

Cells respond to changes in their environments in a complex manner consisting of short- and long-term responses. The long-term responses occur after a delay and usually are the result of fundamental changes in cell function. A group of genes

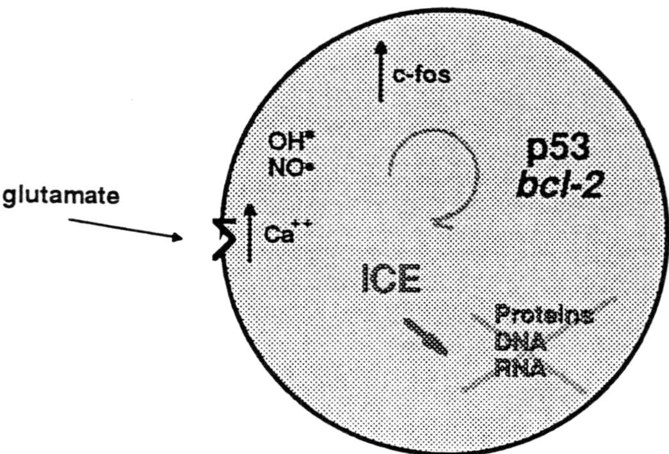

FIGURE 2. Ischemic cell death.

has been found that may well serve the role of carrying information to the cell's DNA and altering transcription, the IEGs.[43] The best studied IEGs are the products of c-fos and c-jun activation, the Fos and Jun proteins. These proteins can form heterodimeric combinations through a leucine zipper and act as a transcription factor, AP-1. One mechanism for the expression of IEGs is an increase of intracellular Ca^{2+}, calmodulin binding, and subsequent phosphorylation of one or more transcription factors leading to IEG expression. Another route of IEG expression involves alterations in the oxidative state of the cell influencing a highly conserved cysteine in the leucine zipper of Fos and Jun proteins.[44] In recent cell studies, antisense mRNA to c-fos has been able to modulate programmed cell death suggesting an important role for c-fos in apoptosis. Nonetheless, studies in intact animals suggest that c-fos expression may be a late event in cell death. IEG activation in rats and gerbils after transient ischemia has been studied.[43] There appears to be an early activation of these genes in most areas of brain (including neurons which will go on to death and those that are resistant to transient ischemia). The later effects are more complex and vary with the IEG being studied. c-fos is expressed again in vulnerable cells as they begin to show signs of cell death. Thus, the early activation may be a response to elevated intracellular Ca^{2+} while the later, more complicated responses could be part of a sequence of events that underlie ischemic cell death.

p53

Alterations in the p53 molecule have been linked with various forms of cancer.[45–47] It appears as though p53 is activated and translocates to the nucleus when a cell's DNA is damaged. There p53 appears to act as a transcription factor binding to DNA and preventing cell replication by arresting it in the G_1 phase. It is this ability to arrest cell growth that led to the discovery that p53 overexpression may lead to cell death. p53 has been implicated in programmed cell death in thymocyte, lymphocyte, and other cell types. The molecule and many of its mutations are well

TABLE 3. *bcl-2* Protein Family

	Good	Bad
	bcl-2	bax
	bcl-x$_l$	bcl-x$_s$
	mcl-1	bak
	bag	bad
		blk
		bip-1

characterized. It is known that the N terminus is required for activation and the C terminus for tetramer formation. p53 appears to be active as a tetramer. Our approach at elucidating the role of p53 in ischemia has led us to a collaborative effort with Dr. Peter Tegtmeyer at the State University of New York at Stony Brook. His laboratory has been active in studying the role of p53 in transforming cells. They have constructed a truncated fragment of p53 containing amino acids 315–390 of the C terminus. This fragment serves to bind native p53, but prevents tetramer formation and p53 action[48,49] and therefore may provide a means in which ischemic cell death may be regulated. Although p53 malfunction leads to the formation of tumors, overexpression of p53 can cause a programmed cell death. The exact mechanism by which p53 elicits apoptosis is not understood. It may involve an interaction with cell cycle proteins, but p53 is known to stimulate the production of *bax*, one of the family of *bcl-2* proteins important in cell death.[50,51] This stimulation of *bax* appears to turn on the production of proteases leading to the destruction of the cell.

bcl-2 *Family of Proteins*

The B-cell lymphoma-2 gene (*bcl-2*) was first identified at the t(14:18) translocation site common to non-Hodgkin's follicular lymphomas[11] (TABLE 3). Both the message and protein expression of *bcl-2* are widespread in the developing nervous system, although in the adult rodent there is a significant decrease in immunoreactivity. Protein expression in the adult has been limited to areas believed to continue neurogenesis, such as the hippocampal dentate gyrus and cerebellar granule cells. In contrast, the adult distribution pattern of *bcl-2* messenger RNA resembles that found in development, with the dentate gyrus, as well as the subiculum and CA1–CA3 regions of the hippocampus expressing *bcl-2* message.[52,53] Thus it seems logical to explore the role of *bcl-2* in ischemic cell death. The role of *bcl-2* in programmed cell death is complicated. In a neural cell line, *bcl-2* expression was associated with modulation of reactive oxygen species and cell glutathione levels,[12,54] which might be the indirect effects of other *bcl-2* actions. Transfer of *bcl-2* expression vectors is associated with cell survival after trophic factors are removed. Microinjection of *bcl-2* messages has been shown to protect sympathetic neurons from apoptosis following nerve growth factor removal.[55,56] Recently, overexpression of *bcl-2* in transgenic mice demonstrated protection from naturally occurring cell death and focal ischemic damage.[57] This is encouraging because delayed neuronal death following transient global ischemia is comparable to developmental cell death.

TABLE 4. Dimer Forms of *bcl-2* Proteins

	Good	Bad
bcl-2	bcl-2	bax
	bag	bad
		bak
		bcl-x$_s$
bcl-x$_l$	bcl-x$_l$	bad
		bax
		bak
		bcl-x$_s$

Other proteins in the *bcl-2* family have recently been described (TABLE 4). Bax is a protein homologous to *bcl-2* which forms a dimer with it and prevents the actions of *bcl-2*.[58] Overexpression of bax counters the death repressor effects of *bcl-2*. One particularly interesting *bcl-2* related protein is *bcl-x*. Although neuronal *bcl-2* levels decrease with age, *bcl-x* expression is retained in the adult system.[59] *Bcl-x* is 74% homologous to *bcl-2* and it also promotes cell survival. *Bcl-x* encodes two proteins, *bcl-x$_l$* and *bcl-x$_s$*, with opposing functions. The L form promotes survival whereas the S form is an inhibitor of *bcl-2*/*bcl-x* function.[60] Of particular interest is the fact that while *bcl-x$_s$* is expressed at high levels in cells undergoing a rapid rate of turnover, *bcl-x$_l$* is found in long-lived postmitotic cells, such as the adult brain.[61] Our data suggest that while hippocampal *bcl-2* levels are quite low, *bcl-x$_l$*, which is primarily found in postmitotic cells, serves as the major hippocampal neuroprotective member. Furthermore, the protein band obtained for *bcl-x$_l$* in the gerbil is quite different from that of the mouse. It occurs as a triplicate comprising bands that are 28, 30, and 32 kDa in size.[62] This is most probably a result of alternate splicing, which is common in this family of protooncogenes.[11]

The exact mechanism by which *bcl-2* influences cell survival is not known. It is now believed that there may be a *bax*/*bcl-2* ratio of expression that is essential for cell survival. Following a focal ischemic insult, both *bax* and *bcl-2* mRNA levels are reported to increase in the peripheral region of a cerebral infarct. However, bax protein levels demonstrate a moderate increase whereas *bcl-2* demonstrates a very low increase.[63] Other evidence has suggested an increase in bax immunohisto-chemical staining as compared to *bcl-2* following transient ischemia in rats.[60] Our immunoprecipitation studies suggest that initially there is an excess of *bcl-x$_l$* compared to bax in the hippocampus, and with the presence of more ischemia-induced bax protein additional interactions become possible. This heterodimerization formed with *bax* may disrupt a more favorable *bcl-x$_l$* dimerization paradigm.[62] The net effect is a shift in the balance of expression from a *bcl-2* to a *bax* dominance,[64] resulting in protease activation and an increase in cell death. This shift in the balance may be influenced by the tumor suppressor gene p53, which is induced following ischemia. Although *bcl-2* blocks p53 dependent apoptosis,[65] ischemic induction of p53 expression negatively regulates *bcl-2* and positively regulates *bax*,[66] suggesting that *bcl-2* is the critical regulator of ischemic cell death.

Proteases

In programmed cell death, the end result is the destruction of cell contents. Such destruction must involve degradative enzymes. There are two general groups of these enzymes: those in lysosomes dealing with externally ingested materials, and those in other cell compartments that regulate the normal turnover and replacement of cell constituents. It is this latter group that seems most likely involved in programmed cell death. ICE is a nonspecific cysteine protease which demonstrates a cleavage site (Asp-X, where X is a small hydrophobic residue) atypical of eukaryotic proteases. The findings that mutations in the ced-3 gene, which is similar to ICE, prevent neuronal death in *C. elegans* has focused attention on this enzyme in mammalian systems.

ICE family members found in the brain include ICE, Nedd2, CPP32, and ICH-1. One member of this family, the Nedd2 gene, may be of particular importance in rodents. It is believed to be the predominant ICE homologue in the gerbil central nervous system.[67] There is growing evidence that ICE or a similar protease(s) may be important in ischemia. Transgenic mice making an ICE inhibitory protein have smaller cerebral infarcts than wild-type littermates.[68] A second study reported that mRNA for Nedd2 was increased in an ischemic infarct 8 h after occlusion of the middle cerebral artery in a rat.[69] In the same study, mRNA for the expression of CPP32, another member of the ICE family of proteases, was measured and found to be increased from 16 to 24 h after occlusion while mRNA for ICE did not change.[69] These studies were all carried out in rats with focal ischemia and may not be applicable to the transient global ischemic cell death described above.

SUMMARY

In this review, we have presented evidence that apoptotic proteins may be involved in ischemic cell death. We tried to keep in mind that focal and global ischemia almost certainly produces different forms of cell death. For example, necrotic cell death is clearly part of a focal cerebral infarct, although it is not seen in brief global insults. We also tried to make the point that not all apoptosis is the same and that various forms of non-necrotic cell death, including ischemic cell death after global ischemia, may share some of the same molecular mechanisms as classic forms of apoptosis. Finally, we wish to leave the reader with the clear impression that all the evidence is not in hand. More work needs to be done in animals to define the role of apoptotic proteins. For example, glial cells probably are important in necrosis and may play a role in ischemic cell death after transient global ischemia. Yet it is likely that glial cells die from injury in a different manner than neurons. A better understanding of these processes should lead to new therapeutic approaches that may make possible the salvaging of neurons well after an ischemic insult.

REFERENCES

1. FURUKAWA, S., Y. FURUKAWA, E. SATOYOSHI & K. HAYASHI. 1987. Synthesis/secretion of nerve growth factor is associated with cell growth in cultured mouse astroglial cells. Biochem. Biophys. Res. Commun. **142:** 395–402.
2. NAGATA, S. 1996. Fas-mediated apoptosis (Review). Adv. in Exp. Med. Biol. **406:** 119–124.
3. WU, P. & J. N. DAVIS. 1994. DNA fragmentation is NOT an early event in ischemic neuronal death. Soc. Neurosci. Abstr. **20:** 1044 (Abstr.).
4. IWAI, T., A. HARA, M. NIWA, M. NOZAKI, T. UEMATSU, N. SAKAI & H. YAMADA. 1995. Temporal profile of nuclear DNA fragmentation in situ in gerbil hippocampus following transient forebrain ischemia. Brain Res. **671:** 305–308.

5. LI, Y., M. CHOPP, N. JIANG, F. YAO & C. ZALOGA. 1995. Temporal profile of in situ DNA fragmentation after transient middle cerebral artery occlusion in the rat. J. Cereb. Blood Metab. **15:** 389–397.

6. LI, Y., M. CHOPP, N. JIANG, Z. G. ZHANG & C. ZALOGA. 1995. Induction of DNA fragmentation after 10 to 120 minutes of focal cerebral ischemia in rats. Stroke **26:** 1252–1258.

7. ELLIS, H. M. & H. R. HORVITZ. 1986. Genetic control of programmed cell death in the nematode *C. elegans.* Cell **44:** 817–829.

8. HORVITZ, H. R., P. W. STERNBERG, I. S. GREENWALD, W. FIXSEN & H. M. ELLIS. 1983. Mutations that affect neural cell lineages and cell fates during the development of the nematode *Caenorhabditis elegans.* Cold Spring Harbor Symp. Quant. Biol. **48:** 453–463.

9. FESUS, L. 1993. Biochemical events in naturally occurring forms of cell death. FEBS **328:** 1–5.

10. HENGARTNER, M. O. & H. R. HORVITZ. 1994. *C. elegans* cell survival gene ced-9 encodes a functional homolog of the mammalian proto-oncogene bcl-2. Cell **76:** 665–676.

11. REED, J. C. 1994. Bcl-2 and the regulation of programmed cell death. J. Cell Biol. **124:** 1–6.

12. HOCKENBERY, D. M., Z. N. OLTVAI, X. YIN, C. L. MILLIMAN & S. J. KORSMEYER. 1993. Bcl-2 functions in an anti-oxidant pathway to prevent apoptosis. Cell **75:** 241–251.

13. HANADA, M., C. AIME-SEMPE, T. SATO & J. C. REED. 1995. Structure-function analysis of bcl-2 protein. J. Biol. Chem. **270:** 11962–11969.

14. YUAN, J., S. SHAHAM, S. LEDOUX, H. M. ELLIS & H. R. HORVITZ. 1993. The *C. elegans* cell death gene ced-3 encodes a protein similar to mammalian interleukin-1 beta-converting enzyme. Cell **75:** 641–652.

15. DECKWERTH, T. L. & E. M. JOHNSON, JR. 1993. Temporal analysis of events associated with programmed cell death (apoptosis) of sympathetic neurons deprived of nerve growth factor. J. Cell Biol. **123:** 1207–1222.

16. GREENLUND, L. J., S. J. KORSMEYER & E. M. JOHNSON, JR. 1995. Role of BCL-2 in the survival and function of developing and mature sympathetic neurons. Neuron **15:** 649–661.

17. DESHMUKH, M., J. VASILAKOS, T. L. DECKWERTH, P. A. LAMPE, B. D. SHIVERS & E. M. JOHNSON, JR. 1996. Genetic and metabolic status of NGF-deprived sympathetic neurons saved by an inhibitor of ICE family proteases. J. Cell Biol. **135:** 1341–1354.

18. CRAIN, B. J., W. D. WESTERDAM, A. H. HARRISON & J. V. NADLER. 1988. Selective neuronal death after transient forebrain ischemia in the Mongolian gerbil: A silver impregnation study. Neuroscience **27:** 387–402.

19. DESHPANDE, J., K. BERGSTEDT, T. LINDEN, H. KALIMO & T. WIELOCH. 1992. Ultrastructural changes in the hippocampal CA1 region following transient cerebral ischemia: Evidence against programmed cell death. Exp. Brain Res. **88:** 91–105.

20. KIRINO, T. 1982. Delayed neuronal death in the gerbil hippocampus following ischemia. Brain Res. **239:** 57–69.

21. KIRINO, T. & K. SANO. 1984. Selective vulnerability in the gerbil hippocampus following transient ischemia. Acta Neuropathol. **62:** 201–208.

22. KIRINO, T. & K. SANO. 1984. Fine structural nature of delayed neuronal death following ischemia in the gerbil hippocampus. Acta Neuropathol. **62:** 209–218.

23. KIRINO, T., A. TAMURA & K. SANO. 1984. Delayed neuronal death in the rat hippocampus following transient forebrain ischemia. Acta Neuropathol. **64:** 139–147.

24. YAMAMOTO, K., K. MORIMOTO & T. YANAGIHARA. 1986. Cerebral ischemia in the gerbil: Transmission electron microscopic and immunoelectron microscopic investigation. Brain Res. **384:** 1–10.

25. YANAGIHARA, T., J. M. BRENGMAN & E. MUSHYNSKI. 1990. Differential vulnerability of microtubule components in cerebral ischemia. Acta Neuropathol. **80:** 499–505.

26. SAPOLSKY, R. M. & W. A. PULSINELLI. 1985. Glucocorticoids potentiate ischemic injuries to neurons: Therapeutic implications. Science **229:** 1397–1400.

27. MORSE, J. K. & J. N. DAVIS. 1990. Regulation of ischemic hippocampal damage by adrenal steroids in the gerbil: Adrenalectomy alters the rate of pyramidal cell death. Exp. Neurol. **110:** 86–92.

28. MORSE, J. K. & J. N. DAVIS. 1989. Chemical adrenalectomy decreases CNS temperature and protects hippocampal cells following ischemia. Pharmacologist **31:** 183 (Abstr.).

29. ANTONAWICH, F. J., P. WU & J. N. DAVIS. 1997. Regulation of ischemic cell death by glucocorticoids and ACTH. (Unpublished data.)

30. BUSTO, R., W. D. DIETRICH, M. Y. T. GLOBUS, I. VALDES, P. SCHEINBERG & M. D. GINSBERG. 1987. Small differences in intraischemic brain temperature critically determine the extent of ischemic neuronal injury. J. Cereb. Blood Flow Metab. **7:** 729–738.

31. BUSTO, R., W. D. DIETRICH, M. Y. T. GLOBUS & M. D. GINSBERG. 1989. The importance of brain temperature in cerebral ischemic injury. Stroke **20:** 1113–1114.

32. COLBOURNE, F., S. M. NURSE & D. CORBETT. 1993. Temperature changes associated with forebrain ischemia in the gerbil. Brain Res. **602:** 264–267.

33. BUSTO, R., W. D. DIETRICH, Y. T. GLOBUS & M. D. GINSBERG. 1989. Postischemic moderate hypothermia inhibits CA1 hippocampal ischemic neuronal injury. Neurosci. Lett. **101:** 299–304.

34. COLBOURNE, F. & D. CORBETT. 1995. Delayed postischemic hypothermia: A six-month survival study using behavioral and histological assessments of neuroprotection. J. Neurosci. **15:** 7250–7260.

35. COLBOURNE, F. & D. CORBETT. 1994. Delayed and prolonged post-ischemic hypothermia is neuroprotective in the gerbil. Brain Res. **654:** 265–272.

36. MIZUHARA, A. 1996. The protective effects of hypothermia in a new transient cerebral ischemic model of the rat—A ^{31}P magnetic resonance spectroscopy *in vivo* study. J. Jpn. Assoc. Thorac. Surg. **44:** 1–8.

37. BUSTO, R., M. Y. T. GLOBUS, J. T. NEARY & M. D. GINSBERG. 1994. Regional alterations of protein kinase C activity following transient cerebral ischemia: Effects of intraischemic brain temperature modulation. J. Neurochem. **63:** 1095–1103.

38. MORSE, J. K. & J. N. DAVIS. 1990. Adrenalectomy affects brain temperature and further delays hippocampal damage following transient ischemia. Stroke **21:** 177 (Abstr.).

39. KOIDE, T., T. W. WIELOCH & B. K. SIESJO. 1986. Chronic dexamethasone pretreatment aggravates ischemic neuronal necrosis. J. Cereb. Blood Flow Metab. **6:** 395–404.

40. SAPOLSKY, R. M. 1986. Glucocorticoid toxicity in the hippocampus: Reversal by supplementation with brain fuels. J. Neurosci. **6:** 2240–2244.

41. SAPOLSKY, R. M. 1993. Potential behavioral modifications of glucocorticoid damage to the hippocampus. Behav. Brain Res. **57:** 175–182.

42. SIESJO, B. K., M. SMITH & D. S. WARNER. 1987. Acidosis and ischemic brain damage. *In* Cerebrovascular Diseases. W. J. Powers & M. E. Raichle, Eds.: 83–94. Raven Press. New York.

43. VENDRELL, M., T. CURRAN & J. I. MORGAN. 1993. Glutamate, immediate-early genes, and cell death in the nervous system. Ann. N. Y. Acad. Sci. **679:** 132–141.

44. ABATE, C., L. PATEL, F. J. I. RAUSCHER & T. CURRAN. 1990. Redox regulation of fos and jun DNA-binding activity in vitro. Science **249:** 1157–1161.

45. LEONARD, C. J., C. E. CANMAN & M. B. KASTAN. 1995. The role of p53 in cell-cycle control and apoptosis: Implications for cancer. *In* Important Advances in Oncology. 11th edit. V. T. DeVita, Jr., S. Hellman & S. A. Rosenberg, Eds.: 33–42. J. B. Lippincott. Philadelphia, PA.

46. HAINAUT, P. 1995. The tumor suppressor protein p53: A receptor to genotoxic stress that controls cell growth and survival. Curr. Opin. Oncol. **7:** 76–82.

47. OREN, M. 1994. Relationship of p53 to the control of apoptotic cell death. Semin. Cancer Biol. **5:** 221–227.

48. WANG, P., M. REED, Y. WANG, G. MAYR, J. E. STENGER, M. E. ANDERSON, J. F. SCHWEDES & P. TEGTMEYER. 1996. P53 domains: Oligomerization and transformation. Mol. Cell. Biol. **14:** 5182–5191.

49. REED, M., Y. WANG, G. MAYR, M. E. ANDERSON, J. F. SCHWEDES & P. TEGTMEYER. 1993. p53 Domains: Suppression, transformation, and transactivation. Gene Expression **3:** 95–107.

50. MIYASHITA, T., S. KRAJEWSKI, M. KRAJEWSKA, H. G. WANG, H. K. LIN, D. LIEBERMANN, B. HOFFMAN & J. C. REED. 1995. Tumor suppressor p53 is a regulator of bcl-2 and bax gene expression in vitro and in vivo. Oncogene. **9:** 1799–1805.

51. MIYASHITA, T. & J. C. REED. 1995. Tumor suppressor p53 is a direct transcriptional activator of the human bax gene. Cell **80:** 293–299.
52. CASTREN, E., Y. OHGA, M. P. BERZAGHI, G. TZIMAGIOGIS, H. THOENEN & D. LINDHOLM. 1994. Bcl-2 messenger RNA is localized in neurons of the developing and adult rat brain. Neuroscience **61:** 165–177.
53. MERRY, D. E., D. J. VEIS, W. F. HICKEY & S. J. KORSMEYER. 1994. Bcl-2 protein expression is widespread in the developing nervous system and retained in the adult PNS. Development **120:** 301–311.
54. KANE, D. J., T. A. SARAFIAN, R. ANTON, H. HAHN, E. B. GRALLA, J. S. VALENTINE, T. ORD & D. E. GREDESEN. 1993. Bcl-2 inhibition of neural death: Decreased generation of reactive oxygen species. Science **262:** 1274–1277.
55. ALLSOPP, T. E., S. WYATT, H. F. PATTERSON & A. M. DAVIES. 1993. The proto-oncogene bcl-2 can selectively rescue neurotrophic factor-dependent neurons from apoptosis. Cell **73:** 295–307.
56. GARCIA, I., I. MARTINOU, Y. TSUJIMOTO & J. D. MARTINOU. 1992. Prevention of programmed cell death of sympathetic neurons by the *bcl*-2-proto-oncogene. Science **258:** 302–304.
57. MARTINOU, J. D., M. DUBOIS-DAUPHIN, J. K. STAPLE, I. RODRIQUEZ, H. FRANKOWSKI, M. MISSOTTEN, P. ALBERTINI, D. TALABOT, S. CATSICAS, C. PIETRA & J. HUARTE. 1994. Overexpression of BCL-2 in transgenic mice protects neurons from naturally occurring cell death and experimental ischemia. Neuron **13:** 1017–1030.
58. KORSMEYER, S. J., J. R. SHUTTER, D. J. VEIS, D. E. MERRY & Z. N. OLTVAI. 1993. Bcl-2/bax: A rheostat that regulates an anti-oxidant pathway and cell death. Cancer Biol. **4:** 327–332.
59. GONZALEZ-GARCIA, M., I. GARCIA, L. DING, S. O'SHEA, L. H. BOISE, C. B. THOMPSON & G. NUNEZ. 1995. Bcl-x is expressed in embryonic and postnatal neural tissues and functions to prevent neuronal cell death. Proc. Natl. Acad. Sci. USA **92:** 4304–4308.
60. KRAJEWSKI, S., J. K. MAI, M. KRAJEWSKA, M. SIKORSKA, M. MOSSAKOWSKI & J. C. REED. 1995. Upregulation of bax protein levels in neurons following cerebral ischemia. J. Neurosci. **15:** 6364–6376.
61. BOISE, L. H., M. GONZALEZ-GARCIA, C. E. POSTEMA, L. DING, T. LINDSTEN, L. A. TURKA, X. MAO, G. NUNEZ & C. B. THOMPSON. 1993. Bcl-x, a bcl-2-related gene that functions as a dominant regulator of apoptotic cell death. Cell **74:** 597–608.
62. ANTONAWICH, F. J., H. J. FEDEROFF, S. KRAJEWSKI, J. C. REED & J. N. DAVIS. 1996. Ischemic CA1 hippocampal neurons express bax and can be rescued by bcl-2 induction with a herpes simplex virus (HSV) amplicon. Soc. Neurosci. Abstr. **22:** 1179 (Abstr.).
63. SIMON, R. P., J. CHEN, R. L. ZHU, J. O. LAN, D. A. GREENBERG & S. H. GRAHAM. 1995. Alteration in anti-apoptotic gene expression associated with induction of tolerance to focal ischemia. Soc. Neurosci. Abstr. **21:** 512 (Abstr.).
64. ZHANG, L. X., M. A. SMITH, J. C. REED, M. CLARK, A. N. FELDMAN, D. R. RUBINOW & R. M. POST. 1995. Ratio of Bcl-2 and Bax expression during development and apoptosis of neurons in the CNS. Soc. Neurosci. Abstr. **21:** 559 (Abstr.).
65. CHIOU, S., Y. RAO & E. WHITE. 1994. Bcl-2 blocks p53 dependent apoptosis. Mol. Cell. Biol. **14:** 2556–2563.
66. MCGAHAN, L., G. S. ROBERTSON & A. M. HAKIM. 1995. Expression of *myc* and p53 following transient global ischemia. Soc. Neurosci. Abstr. **21:** 1300 (Abstr.).
67. SIMAN, R., S. TRUSKO, R. DIROCCO, V. R. MARCY & R. SCOTT. 1995. Localization of ICE-like proteases and enzymes associated with apoptosis in the mammalian CNS. Soc. Neurosci. Abstr. **21:** 2021 (Abstr.).
68. HARA, H., K. FINK, M. ENDRES, R. M. FREDLANDER, V. GAGLIARDINI, J. YUAN & M. A. MOSKOWITZ. 1997. Attenuation of transient focal cerebral ischemic injury in transgenic mice expressing a mutant ICE inhibitory protein. J. Cereb. Blood Metab. **17:** 370–375.
69. ASAHI, M., M. HOSHIMARU, Y. UEMURA, T. TOKIME, M. KOJIMA, T. OHTSUKA, N. MATSUURA, T. AOKI, K. SHIBAHARA & H. KIKUCHI. 1997. Expression of interleukin-1b converting enzyme gene family and *bcl-2* gene family in the rat brain following permanent occlusion of the middle cerebral artery. J. Cereb. Blood Metab. **17:** 11–18.

Neurological Aspects of the Conscious and Unconscious Mind

ORRIN DEVINSKY

Department of Neurology
Hospital for Joint Diseases
New York University School of Medicine
301 East 17th Street
New York, New York 10003

This paper reviews data supporting a modular, parallel distributed system of consciousness using the visual system as a model, considers the neurological mechanisms underlying the unity of consciousness, and suggests that the right hemisphere is dominant for a sense of self, an individual's consciousness of himself in relation to body and environment, and as an emotional and psychical being.

CONSCIOUSNESS

Consciousness escapes a satisfying definition. Simplistically, consciousness is the subjective awareness of something, extending from a percept to a repertoire of directed cognitive faculties.[1-3] The object of awareness may be an environmental or bodily stimulus, an emotional feeling, mental imagery, an abstract thought, inner speech, a memory, a volitional act, or a plan.

Consciousness is relatively selective because the active contents of conscious awareness are limited by effort, the amount of information, organizational skills, and the difficulty of keeping data segregated.[4] Most mental processes and knowledge, such as color perception, constancy, understanding spoken speech, and walking, are nonconscious. When information about our personal past (episodic memory) or about the world (semantic memory) is needed, retrieval brings it from long-term memory into working memory, accessible to and coexistent with consciousness. Consciousness has limited awareness of processes; it perceives the products of cognition.[5] We are better at reporting on processes that manipulate information of which we are consciously aware.[6]

CEREBRAL PROCESSING OF VISUAL INPUT

The landmark studies of Hubel and Wiesel[7] supported the hierarchical model of visual processing in the brain, which dominated twentieth century neuroscience. Visual input is processed as it moves from the retina to the geniculate cortex to the striate cortex to visual association areas, and more complex features are recognized at each subsequent (higher) level. Hierarchical processing of visual input is supported by progressive delays in the latency of the neuronal response and increasing receptive field size as input moves from V1 to visual association cortices. This serial model is correct but incomplete. The additional concepts of two visual processing systems, parallel processing, data feedback from "higher" to "lower" centers, the nonreplicated role of "lower" centers for detailed analysis, synchrony, and awareness (consciousness) must also be considered.

Two Visual Processing Systems

Visual input to the striate cortex is processed by two primary systems: a ventral system involving the temporal lobe for object discrimination and recognition, and a dorsal system involving the parietal lobe for spatial perception, landmark recognition, and visuomotor performance.[8]

Parallel Processing of Visual Input

The nonhierarchical, parallel model of central visual processing was only recently conceptualized. Cases supporting this model were reported more than a century ago, but were not accepted because they lacked a theoretical framework. Independent extracalcarine visual areas mediating color and motion perception were documented by clinical and neuropathological studies in the late nineteenth century.[9–12] However, Henschen[13] and Holmes[14] dismissed evidence for color or motion areas. Reports of isolated loss of motion (akinetopsia) and color (achromatopsia) vision were vanquished from neurology for more than 50 years.

The theoretical structure for acceptance of the clinical data was built by anatomical and physiological studies of visual cortex in monkeys showing that multiple visual association areas (V3–V5) contain independent retinal representations.[15–18] Each of these areas has a neuronal receptive field larger than that in V1; each area is smaller than V1. Rather than being redundant, these specialized areas receive different inputs from V1 and V2. The connections between V3, V4, and V5 strongly support a primarily parallel network.

Parallel outputs are a consistent feature of cortical connectivity.[19,20] Cortical areas contain functionally distinct cell groups with common properties. The groups have parallel outputs to other cortical and subcortical areas. Each cortical area parcels different output signals to different areas, segregating multiple operations.[18] Cortical connections are usually between areas with similar functions. Thus, portions of V1 and V2 that segregate color input have strong connections to V4, the cortical color vision area in the fusiform gyrus.

Feedback Connections and the Role of V1 and V2

The hierarchical model views visual input as traveling down a one-way path toward a more complex and integrated visual image. However, robust connections go from association to primary visual cortices. While the forward connections from V1 to V2 are modality specific, the feedback connections from V3–V5 to V1–2 are diffuse.[21] For example, the feedback from cortical units in V4 is not limited to cells in V1 and V2 that project to V4, but also includes cells in V1 and V2 that project to V3 and V5. These feedback fibers may contribute to several functions[18] including access to the detailed visual field map (benefits of selective recognition, e.g., color, are balanced by losses in topographical detail, allowing feedback fibers to gain access to data in V1 and "zoom in"); linking and activating one visual modality from another, and integrating the visual image by providing pathways for joining of form, color, and motion.[18]

Neuronal Synchrony and Integration of the Visual Image

How is the visual image integrated by the brain? The multiple specialized cortical visual areas "see" different aspects of the world, such as orientation, depth, form, motion, and color. These areas do not provide convergent input to a "visual integration center" that "sees the whole picture," but instead are connected in parallel with each other and reciprocally with V1 and V2. When two specialized visual areas project to a common cortical area, their inputs are largely distinct. Local circuits could integrate these inputs, but the results would be multiple local circuits in separate areas. Synchronous neuronal firing can perform integration.

Synchrony in neuronal populations depends on neuronal groups interconnected by mutually excitatory and inhibitory synaptic connections.[22] Synchronous activity occurs in multiple neurons in the visual cortex[23,24] as well as in other areas such as the hippocampus[25] and auditory cortex.[26] Further, following stimulation, cells in the retina, lateral geniculate cortex, and visual cortex respond in repetitive oscillatory bursts with frequencies in the 40–60 Hz band.[23,27] With a continuous stimulus, cells in different visual areas and hemispheres can synchronize their responses to stimuli sharing particular features, such as the same orientation or direction of motion.[28,29] With visual experience, cells in the visual cortex can link with other cells sharing certain properties. As cell repertories or groups become synchronously activated over time, their connections may selectively compete for space on other cells.[30] The stability of groups is increased if the probability of their synchronous firing is high.

Synthesis of the visual image may depend on simultaneous and synchronous activity in nonspecialized (V1 and V2) and specialized (V3–V6) visual areas.[18] Perceptual awareness (consciousness) of visual input may rely on synchronously linked activity in multiple areas.

LEVELS OF CONSCIOUSNESS

Cognitive Perspective

Boundaries between conscious and nonconscious knowledge and behaviors can be discrete or continuous. Some components of nonconscious behavior are fully unconscious (i.e., inaccessible to consciousness). Instincts, the process but not the product of sensory perception, irretrievable memories, and much procedural knowledge lie beyond introspective awareness. Complex innate and overlearned behaviors can utilize declarative memories, despite being inaccessible to consciousness.[31]

Preconscious stimuli such as subliminal percepts and implicit memories (i.e., nonconscious perceptual and mnemonic data, respectively) can influence thought and behavior, but remain below the threshold of conscious awareness. Other percepts and memories lie beyond conscious view, but can be activated into consciousness with various degrees of attention, persistence, and effort. Peripheral awareness includes percepts, thoughts, and memories situated at the fringe of awareness. Directing awareness toward them brings them into consciousness. Primary consciousness is the experience, or awareness, of percepts, feelings, memories, and thoughts. Reflective consciousness is awareness of one's own primary consciousness (i.e., making one's conscious experience the focus of thought).

Neurological Perspective

Neurological levels of the conscious-nonconscious mind focus on levels of alertness and arousal and the contents of perceptual, cognitive, emotional, and motor systems.[32] Consciousness is absent during coma and tonic-clonic seizures. In the persistent vegetative state following coma, sleep-wake cycles return and the patient may briefly fixate on an object or blink to threat, but consciousness is profoundly impaired.[33] Akinetic mutism almost completely eliminates spontaneous motor and verbal behavior,[34] severely restricting consciousness. One month after a left mesial frontal infarct, a woman recalled that, while akinetic and mute, "she did not talk because she had nothing to say." Her mind was "empty." "Nothing mattered."[35]

Complex partial seizures (CPS) and absence seizures cause various defects in cognition, awareness, and consciousness. Preserved verbal or nonverbal responsiveness and recall during the event distinguish simple partial seizures from CPS.[36] During absence seizures and CPS, patients may fail to respond to a question but blink reflexively to a loud clap or sit if led toward a chair. When asked during a CPS, "Are you a zebra?" patients may respond. "Uh huh." They comprehend the raised voice and expectation of a response, but not the semantic content. The boundary separating simple and complex partial seizures is often vague. Patients may recall hearing "everything that was said, but not tuning in," or "hearing the sounds but not understanding words."

Focal cortical disorders do not suggest that there is a region mediating consciousness. Consciousness is impaired when seizures involve a zone of cortical or subcortical areas. The critical anatomical areas and cortical volumes involved during ictally impaired consciousness are incompletely defined. During CPS discharges on invasively recorded EEGs may be limited to one temporal lobe, bilateral mesial temporal areas, bifrontal mesial areas, and generalized spike and slow wave discharges arising in the thalamus. However, because ictal sampling of cortical and subcortical areas is limited, spread patterns and volumetric area are imprecise. Further, on some invasively recorded EEGs, the ictal discharge remains limited to one lobe, but ipsilateral and contralateral lobes may show prominent slowing. The application of computerized volumetrics and on-line neuropsychological testing may help to solve this problem.

UNITY OF CONSCIOUSNESS

A Modular Model

The greatest challenge to understanding consciousness is its unity, otherwise called the "binding problem." How do we experience existence through this unified sense of self that seamlessly joins external and internal stimuli, memory, plans, emotions, and reflective thought? The search for a cortical area, possibly heteromodal association cortex, that unifies consciousness, linking together cortical areas and pointing the "flashlight," has failed. No such area exists. Rather, modules and networks subserve various cognitive functions and work in parallel to accomplish independent but coordinated behavioral patterns.

The modular model of mind provides an anatomical and physiological foundation for parallel processing.[37] In this model, the mind consists of hardwired, innate, domain-specific cognitive modules processing and interpreting information in auditory and visual perception, language, memory, and other areas. Parallel distributed processing (PDP; connectionism) may dominate information processing in the brain.[37–39] The PDP model postulates multiple independent processing units performing simple and complex functions. The various networks are anatomically and functionally distinct with different programming rules and modulating influences. The parallel processing is nonconscious, although when steady state is reached, conscious awareness of information is possible. The PDP model was initially applied to sensory-perceptual processing, but is likely relevant for attention, memory, and language.

Consciousness and working memory may more heavily rely on the slower sequential processing mode than nonconscious PDP processes. Consciousness has access to the products of PDP processes, but cannot introspectively report on how the information was obtained. Working memory mediates consciousness by activated representations of the organism and its current goals while accessing relevant data from long-term memory. Instead of working memory solving the binding problem in consciousness, PDP (and thalamic synchronization, see below) better fulfills the unification process by massive parallel processes that are independent but interactive. Just as there is no one visual association cortex that "sees" the world, no association cortex mediates consciousness.

Conscious Unity: A Paradox

Consciousness relies on parallel processing, but mainly operates through serial processing. Just as the visual system has no cortical or subcortical site that "puts the picture together" from V1–V6 inputs, the brain contains no integrator that mediates consciousness. Conscious experience focuses (on the percepts, thoughts, plans, and actions) like a flashlight beam that is visible to our mind. The light's beam illuminates only a limited surface of cognitive space. The light requires random access memory (RAM). The greater the automatization, the less the RAM. Consciousness and self-consciousness are considered pinnacles of cerebral activity. However, automatization to accomplish tasks without working memory is a basic mechanism of brain function.

Synchronization

Massive parallel connections and synchronization may unify conscious behavior. A subcortical pacemaker, the intralaminar thalamic nucleus, may synchronize subcortical and cortical activity. A proposed model of thalamocortical circuitry has two resonant loops, one between specific thalamic nuclei and the other between nonspecific thalamic nuclei and the cortex.[40,41] The thalamic reticular nucleus and cortical 40-Hz interneurons synchronize oscillations in both loops. Specific thalamic nuclei project to layer IV interneurons, which synchronize pyramidal cells in layers V and VI to the 40-Hz oscillation. These pyramidal cells project back to the thalamus: layer VI to specific nuclei, layer V to intralaminar nonspecific nuclei, and both layers to the reticular nucleus.

The intralaminar nonspecific nucleus, projecting throughout the neocortex, provides the anatomical connections for diffuse but near simultaneous neocortical stimulation.[41,42] Analogous loops may link basal ganglia with the cortex, thalamus, and brain stem; the thalamus may be the pacemaker. Similarly, within the cortex, discrete channel-specific synchronous connections underlie the content of consciousness whereas nonspecific loops temporally unite conscious experience.[41] Macroscopic 40-Hz waves may sweep the cortex from frontal to occipital regions, binding related sensory inputs by temporal coincidence.[41] This 40-Hz rhythm is widespread in the central nervous system, ranging from sensory end organs such as the retina[43] to thalamic and neocortical levels.[41,44]

Consciousness can be conceived as a unified group of modules with strongly connected cortical and subcortical components. Parallel connections link related modular components at cortical and subcortical levels. Sensory, cognitive, and motor modules comprise the principal module prototypes, each with many modules. The scanning 40-Hz rostrocaudal neocortical wave may link perceptual, cognitive, and motor modules related to the same percept or task. This wave may join related conscious and nonconscious processes.

What are the implications of this subcortical pacemaker and the scanning 40-Hz wave for neurology? Destruction of the thalamic pacemaker nuclei causes coma or profoundly impairs alertness and awareness. Involvement of these thalamic nuclei may account for the impaired consciousness in absence seizures. Impairment of the scanning wave function may contribute to psychomotor slowing from metabolic disorders and intoxicating drugs.

Commissurotomy

Intuitively, disconnecting the right and left hemispheres should profoundly disrupt the unity of consciousness. It does not, although the corpus callosum is the largest fiber bundle in the human brain. After commissurotomy, most patients are remarkably unchanged in their personality, humor, language, and intelligence. Patients' behavior is spontaneous, and they maintain a coherent stream of thought during conversation and in relating stories.[45] The preserved unit of consciousness is usually explained as the language-dominant hemisphere directing thought and behavior while subcortical systems link the two hemispheres.[46]

The right hemisphere, operating independently and isolated from the left hemisphere, shows intelligence: it can perceive, analyze, remember, perform complex reasoning, emotionally respond, demonstrate cultural knowledge, and behaviorally adapt to environmental situations with creative responses.[47-50] Using the criterion of intelligence, Sperry[51] posited two independent spheres of consciousness following commissurotomy.

THE RIGHT HEMISPHERE AND SELF

The right hemisphere may dominate awareness and image of self and the relation of self, visuospatially and psychically, to the environment. Acute lesions of the right hemisphere more severely disrupt the sense of self than left-sided lesions. Right-hemisphere lesions can result in failure to recognize profound deficits, such as cortical blindness or left-sided hemiplegia (anosognosia), respond appropriately to recognized deficits (anosodiaphoria), or attend to the left half of extrapersonal and personal space. They can also cause the delusional belief that duplicate persons are impersonating well-known persons (Capgras syndrome) or delusional reduplications,[52-54] impairments in episodic (self-referential) memories,[55] and conversion symptoms. Social disinhibition can follow right frontal lesions (verbal dysdecorum),[57,58] and experiential phenomena can occur during right temporal lobe seizures, evoking the emotion of familiarity (déjà vu).[59,60]

The right hemisphere may dominate our sense of self. Lesions of the right parietal lobe can impair our body image. Left-sided neglect, anosognosia, and anosodiaphoria can be explained by destruction of the module controlling body image and physical relation of self to environment. Right parietotemporal lesions can impair our topographic orientation—our relation of body to environmental location. Right temporal disorders can affect our sense of familiar and foreign, evoke fear and mania, and evoke experiential phenomena. Right frontal lesions can profoundly alter our social behavior, impairing our relation of self to others, our social self. Linguistic consciousness is a function of the left hemisphere. Consciousness of the corporeal and emotional, and possibly much of our social and psychical self, may be a function of the right hemisphere.

REFERENCES

1. NATSUOLAS, T. 1978. Consciousness. Am. Psychol. **33:** 906–914.
2. FARTHING, G. W. 1992. The Psychology of Consciousness. Prentice Hall. Englewood Cliffs, NJ.
3. FARBER, I. B. & P. S. CHURCHLAND. 1995. Consciousness and the neurosciences. *In* The Cognitive Neurosciences. M. S. Gazzanniga, Ed.: 1295–1306. MIT Press. Cambridge, MA.
4. HIRST, W. & D. KALMAR. 1987. Characterizing attentional resources. J. Exp. Psychol. **116:** 68–81.
5. NSIBETT, R. E. & T. D. WILSON. 1977. Telling more than we can know: Verbal reports on mental processes. Psychol. Rev. **84:** 231–259.
6. ERICSSON, K. A. & H. A. SIMON. 1984. Protocol Analysis. MIT Press. Cambridge, MA.
7. HUBEL, D. H. & T. N. WIESEL. 1969. Anatomical demonstration of columns in the monkey striate cortex. Nature **221:** 747–750.
8. UNGERLEIDER, L. G. & M. MISHKIN. 1982. Two cortical visual systems. *In* Analysis of Visual Behavior. D. J. Ingle, M. A. Goodale & R. J. W. Mansfield, Eds.: 549–586. MIT Press. Cambridge, MA.
9. WILBRAND, H. 1884. Ophthalmiatrische Beitrage zur Diagnostik der Gehirkrankheiten. J. F. Bergmann. Wiesbaden.
10. MACKAY. G. 1888. A discussion on a contribution to the study of hemianopsia, with special reference to acquired colour-blindness. Br. Med. J. **2:** 1033–1037.
11. MACKAY, G. & J. C. DUNLOP. 1899. The cerebral lesions in a case of complete acquired colour-blindness. Scott. Med. Surg. **5:** 503–512.
12. RIDDOCH, G. 1917. Dissociation of visual perception due to occipital injuries, with especial reference to appreciation of movement. Brain **40:** 15–57.
13. HENSCHEN, S. E. 1893. On the visual path and centre. Brain **16:** 170–180.
14. HOLMES, G. 1945. The Ferrier Lecture: The organization of the visual cortex in man. Proc. R. Soc. Lond. B **132:** 348–361.
15. ZEKI, S. M. 1969. Representation of central visual fields in prestriate cortex of monkey. Brain Res. **14:** 271–291.
16. CRAGG, B. J. 1969. The topography of the afferent projections in the circumstriate visual cortex of the monkey studied by the Nauta method. Vision Res. **93:** 733–747.
17. ALLMAN, J. M. & J. H. KAAS. 1971. A representation of the visual field in the caudal third of the middle temporal gyrus of the owl monkey (*Aotus trivirgatus*). Brain Res. **31:** 85–105.
18. ZEKI, S. 1993. A Vision of the Brain. Blackwell. Oxford, England.
19. GOLDMAN-RAKIC, P. 1984. Modular organization of prefrontal cortex. Trends Neurosci. **7:** 419–429.

20. ZEKI, S. & S. SHIP. 1988. The functional logic of cortical connections. Nature **335:** 311–316.

21. PERKEL, D. J., J. BULLIER & H. KENNEDY. 1986. Topography of the afferent connectivity of area 17 in the macaque monkey: A double-labelling study. J. Comp. Neurol. **253:** 374–402.

22. NUNEZ, P. L. 1995. Neocortical Dynamics and Human EEG Rhythms. Oxford University Press. New York.

23. GRAY, C. M., P. KONIG, A. K. ENGEL & W. SINGER. 1989. Oscillatory responses in cat visual cortex exhibit inter-columnar synchronization which reflects global stimulus properties. Nature **338B:** 334–337.

24. ENGEL, A. K., P. KONIG, C. M. GRAY & W. SINGER. 1990. Stimulus-dependent neuronal activity in cat visual cortex: Inter-columnar interaction as indicated by cross-correlation analysis. Exp. Neurol. **6:** 12–29.

25. HOROWITZ, J. M. 1972. Evoked activity of single units and neural populations in the hippocampus of the cat. Electroencephalogr. Clin. Neurophysiol. **32:** 227–240.

26. ABELES, M. & G. L. GERSTEIN. 1988. Detecting spatiotemporal firing patterns among simultaneously recorded single neurons. J. Neurophysiol. **60:** 909–924.

27. LAUFER, M. & M. VERZEANO. 1967. Periodic activity in the visual system of the cat. Vision Res. **7:** 215–229.

28. SINGER, W. 1990. Search for coherence: A basic principle of cortical self-organization. Concepts Neurosci. **1:** 1–26.

29. ENGEL, A. K., P. KONIG, A. K. KREITER & W. SINGER. 1991. Interhemispheric synchronization of oscillatory neuronal responses in cat visual cortex. Science **252:** 1177–1179.

30. EDELMAN, G. 1987. Neural Darwinism: The Theory of Neuronal Group Selection. Basic Books. New York.

31. KIHLSTROM, J. F. 1987. The cognitive unconscious. Science **237:** 1445–1452.

32. PLUM, F. & J. D. POSNER. 1980. The Diagnosis of Stupor and Coma. F. A. Davis. Philadelphia, PA.

33. JENNETT, B. & F. PLUM. 1972. Persistent vegetative state after brain damage. Lancet **1:** 734–737.

34. CAIRNS, H., R. C. OLDFIELD, J. B. PENNYBACKER, *et al.* 1941. Akinetic mutism with an epidermoid cyst of the third ventricle. Brain **64:** 273–290.

35. DAMASIO, A. R. & G. W. VAN HOESEN. 1983. Focal lesions of the limbic frontal lobe. *In* Neuropsychology of Human Emotion. K. M. Heilman & P. Satz, Eds.: 85–110. Guilford Press. New York.

36. DEVINSKY, O., K. KELLEY, R. J. PORTER & W. H. THEODORE. 1988. Clinical and electroencephalographic features of simple partial seizures. Neurology **38:** 1347–1352.

37. FODOR, J. 1983. The Modularity of Mind. MIT/Bradford Press. Cambridge, MA.

38. HINTON, G. E. & J. A. ANDERSON, Eds. 1981. Parallel Models of Associative Memory. Erlbaum, Hillsdale, NJ.

39. RUMELHART, D. E., J. L. MCCLELLAND & PDP RESEARCH GROUP. 1986. Parallel Distributed Processing: Explorations in the Microstructures of Cognition. MIT Press. Cambridge, MA.

40. LLINAS, R., U. RIBARY, M. JOLIOT & X.-J. WANG. 1994. Content and context in temporal thalamocortical binding. *In* Temporal Coding in the Brain. G. Buzaski *et al.*, Eds.: 251–272. Springer-Verlag. Berlin.

41. LLINAS, R. & U. RIBARY. 1992. Oscillations in CNS neurons: A possible role for cortical interneurons in the generation of 40-Hz oscillations. *In* Induced Rhythms in the Brain. E. Basar & T. Bullock, Eds.: 147–154. Birkhauser, Boston, MA.

42. CUNNINGHAM, E. T. & S. LEVAY. 1986. Laminar and synaptic organization of the projection from the thalamic nucleus centralis to primary visual cortex in the cat. J. Comp. Neurol. **254:** 65–77.

43. GHOSE, G. M. & R. D. FREEMAN. 1992. Oscillatory discharge in the visual system: Does it have a functional role? J. Neurophysiol. **68:** 1558–1574.

44. LLINAS, R., A. A. GRACE & Y. YAROM. 1991. In vitro neurons in mammalian cortical layer 4 exhibit intrinsic oscillatory activity in the 10 to 50 Hz frequency range. Proc. Natl. Acad. Sci. USA **88:** 897–901.

45. ZAIDEL, D. W. 1994. A view of the world from a split-brain perspective. *In* The Neurological Boundaries of Reality. E. Critchley, Ed.: 161–174. Farrand Publication. London.
46. GAZZANIGA, M. S. 1988. Brain modularity: Toward a philosophy of conscious experience. *In* Consciousness in Contemporary Science. A. J. Marcel & F. Bisiach, Eds.: 218–238. Oxford University Press. Oxford, England.
47. SPERRY, R. W. 1966. Brain bisection and mechanisms of consciousness. *In* Brain and Conscious Experience. J. C. Eccles, Ed.: 298–313. Springer, New York.
48. SPERRY, R. W., E. ZAIDEL & D. ZAIDEL. 1979. Self-recognition and social awareness in the disconnected minor hemisphere. Neuropsychologia **17:** 153–166.
49. BOGEN, J. E. & G. M. BOGEN. 1969. The other side of the brain. 3. The corpus callosum and creativity. Bull. Los. Angel. Neurol. Soc. **34:** 191–220.
50. ZAIDEL, E. 1983. A response to Gazzaniga: Language in the right hemisphere, convergent perspectives. Am. Psychol. **38:** 542–546.
51. SPERRY, R. W. 1976. Mental phenomena as causal determinants in brain function. *In* Consciousness and the Brain: A Scientific and Philosophical Inquiry. G. G. Globus, G. Maxwell & I. Savodnik, Eds.: 163–177. Plenum. New York.
52. MALLOY, P., C. CIMINO & R. WESTLAKE. 1992. Differential diagnosis of primary and secondary Capgras delusions. Neuropsychiatry Neuropsychol. Behav. Neurol. **5:** 83–96.
53. RUFF, R. L. & B. T. VOLPE. 1981. Environmental reduplication associated with right frontal and parietal lobe injury. J. Neurol. Neurosurg. Psychiatry **44:** 382–386.
54. SIGNER, S. F. 1992. Psychosis in neurologic diseases: Capgras symptom and delusions of reduplication in neurologic disorders. Neuropsychiatry Neuropsychol. Behav. Neurol. **5:** 138–143.
55. MARKOWITSCH, H. J. 1996. Organic and psychogenic retrograde amnesia: Two sides of the same coin? Neurocase **2/4:** 357–371.
56. CHANDARANA, P., G. B. YOUNG, D. R. MACDONALD, *et al.* 1992. Unusual neuropsychiatric symptoms as a manifestation of a frontotemporal tumor. Neuropsychiatry Neuropsychol. Behav. Neurol. **5:** 53–55.
57. ALEXANDER, M. P., D. F. BENSON & D. T. STUSS. 1989. Frontal lobes and language. Brain Lang. **37:** 656–691.
58. BENSON, D. F. 1994. The Neurology of Thinking. : 163–164. Oxford University Press. New York.
59. MULLAN, S. & W. PENFIELD. 1959. Illusions of comparative interpretation and emotion. Arch. Neurol. Psychiatry **81:** 269–284.
60. COLE, M. & O. L. ZANGWILL. 1963. Deja vu in temporal lobe epilepsy. J. Neurol. Neurosurg. Psychiatry **26:** 37–38.

Sensory Coding in Cortical Neurons

Recent Results and Speculations[a]

JONATHAN D. VICTOR[b] AND KEITH P. PURPURA

Department of Neurology and Neuroscience
Cornell University Medical College
1300 York Avenue
New York, New York 10021

INTRODUCTION

What would a satisfactory theory of higher brain function look like? At one level of detail, one would want to know how properties of neurons are determined by their connections and ion channels, and how the properties of these ion channels are in turn determined by their molecular structure. However, although an understanding at this level of detail is certainly required, it is far from sufficient. To account for higher brain function, one needs a way to link function on a cellular and molecular level to perception, behavior, and consciousness.

Consider an attempt to understand the properties of a gas from the physics of individual atoms. Although one may be convinced that the macroscopic properties ultimately depend on the properties of their atomic constituents, it is not satisfying simply to state that one can simulate a gas by modeling a large number of atoms. Even if it were a computational practicality to keep track of the detailed state of each atom, the exercise would provide little, if any, understanding. Rather, through the use of a theory (in this case, statistical thermodynamics), one can deduce that only certain population statistics (i.e., temperature and pressure) are needed to describe the state of the gas. These macroscopic state variables suffice to account for how the gas behaves, and the macroscopic state variables depend in precise manner on the state variables of the constituents. Defining this dependence provides the crucial link between microscopic and macroscopic behavior.

In some ways, our current understanding of brain function is analogous to what our understanding of a gas would be, in the absence of a theory of statistical thermodynamics. A detailed understanding of the function of the cellular and molecular elements of the brain is available. There is a recognized need[1] to connect this understanding with more macroscopic levels, but little is known about the linkage. The number of macroscopic state variables will certainly be far fewer than the number of microscopic state variables needed to describe the states of each ion channel, synaptic vesicle, etc., but it is unclear whether macroscopic state variables should correspond to average activity in specific neural populations, or alternatively, whether more complex statistics (such as correlation structure) would ultimately lead to a more concise description.

How can one proceed? In order to define the problem more precisely, we focus

[a] This work was supported by National Institutes of Health grants EY9314 (J.D.V.) and NS01677 (K.P.P.), The McDonnell-Pew Foundation (K.P.P.), The Revson Foundation (K.P.P.), and The Hirschl Trust (J.D.V.).
[b] Corresponding author. E-mail: jdvicto@med.cornell.edu

on the relationship between the firing pattern of individual neurons and the visual sensory information that these neurons represent. It is well-known that cortical neurons exhibit a high degree of variability, both across neurons within a sensory area, and across responses elicited by a single neuron to repetitive presentations of the same stimulus. It is not known, however, whether visual information is represented primarily in the average activity of a population, or whether the details of individual firing patterns are significant. More generally, our goal is to attempt to determine which statistical aspects of a neuron's firing pattern (the microscopic state) are relevant to the visual percept (the macroscopic state)—that is, how do neurons code sensory information?

Before introducing our approach, we emphasize that one should not anticipate a simple answer. Rather, mounting evidence not only in the visual system,[2-9] but also in the auditory[10-12] and olfactory[13,14] systems, indicates that subtle aspects of the neural discharge are crucial for sensory processing. Furthermore, one should not assume that neural coding is best analyzed with techniques that have been developed for other (e.g., engineering) purposes. A neural discharge is a sequence of discrete events, often sparse in time, and not a continuous signal. The domains to be represented (objects, sensations, behaviors, or even colors[14,15]) do not have a Euclidean vector space structure, so it would be unwise to force such a formalism on spike trains.

Approach to Analysis of Neural Coding

Our approach to the analysis of neural coding was designed to reduce the implicit assumptions concerning the nature of the coding to a bare minimum, and to motivate these few assumptions by neurobiological principles. Although we certainly do not know how a sensory stimulus is represented in the discharge pattern of a cortical neuron, we make the assumption that sensory stimuli which are similar to each other will be represented by firing patterns which are similar, whereas distinct sensory stimuli will be represented by firing patterns which are different. However, what is not at all clear is how the terms "similar" or "different" should be interpreted when applied to neural discharges. In many respects, this is the crux of the matter: it determines which aspects of a spike discharge are relevant to perception (or even, to the next stage in neural processing), and which aspects are irrelevant.

For example, one might imagine that the only relevant aspect of a spike train is the number of impulses it contains. In this view, the details of the timing of individual neurons do not convey any information and would be considered to be a source of "noise." Another view is that the timing of individual impulses (in addition to the number of impulses) conveys information. This idea is motivated by the notion that a neuron can act as a coincidence detector[16-20]: the effect of an impulse train on such a neuron depends crucially on exactly when (with a level of precision determined by the dynamics of the coincidence detector[17]) the impulses occur. A third view is that intervals between impulses are critical. The rationale behind this idea is that, presumably as a consequence of properties of the NMDA receptor and Ca^{2+} channels, the effect of an action potential can depend critically on the length of the intervals since the previous potentials. This dependence can result in both short-term and long-term potentiation,[21] both of which are sensitive to the pattern of interspike intervals.[21-23]

As we will show below, these candidate hypotheses for notions of similarity can be formalized within a uniform framework. Furthermore, we can use the postulate that similar stimuli should elicit similar responses, whereas different stimuli should elicit different responses, to test whether the kinds of temporal structure that are implicit in these hypotheses are relevant to coding by real cortical neurons. Recent studies[24–26] based on these ideas have demonstrated the prominence of temporal coding in primate visual cortex, and have begun to characterize the nature of these codes. A striking finding of these studies[25] is that the temporal coding may be sufficiently rich so as to allow a single spike train to carry information about multiple stimulus attributes. The purpose of this paper is to review these recent results, to present some preliminary studies which focus on the possibility of multidimensional encoding, and to advance some speculations concerning their larger implications.

BACKGROUND AND METHODS

Mathematical Essentials

We will formalize the notions of similar and different, as applied to neural discharges, by the mathematical construct of a "metric" (distance) between spike trains. More details concerning this approach may be found elsewhere.[25,26] Fundamentally, a metric D is a way of assigning a non-negative number to a pair of spike trains S_a and S_b, which expresses the distance between these spike trains in an abstract space. For example, under the assumption that the only relevant aspect of a spike train is the number of spikes it contains, then the corresponding metric, which we will call D^{count}, is one which sets the distance $D^{count}(S_a, S_b)$ equal to the difference in the number of spikes in S_a and S_b.

However, D^{count} is insensitive to the temporal pattern of the impulses. To add sensitivity to temporal pattern, we introduce other, somewhat more complex, notions of distance. These distances are defined in terms of a set of allowed elementary transformations of spike trains, each of which have an associated "cost." Given a set of allowed steps, we will define the distance between two spike trains S_a and S_b as the minimum total cost of a sequence of elementary transformations that takes S_a to S_b. For all of the distances we will consider, we assume that inserting a spike into a train has unit cost, and deleting a spike from a train has unit cost. The other kinds of allowed steps determine the kind of temporal structure to which the distance is sensitive.

The first such family of metrics we will consider is sensitive to the absolute timing of individual spikes. These metrics will be denoted $D^{spike}[q]$, where q is a parameter (with units cost/s^{-1}) which determines the degree of temporal sensitivity. For the metric $D^{spike}[q]$, we add an elementary step of moving an individual spike by an amount ΔT; the cost associated with this step is asserted to be $q\Delta T$. That is, for the metric $D^{spike}[q]$, the distance between two spike trains S_a and S_b is the minimal cost of transforming S_a to S_b by a sequence of spike insertions, spike deletions, and shifts in time of individual spikes, with the costs of these transformations as defined above. One such sequence of transformations is shown in FIGURE 1.

To gain an intuitive understanding of $D^{spike}[q]$, it helps to consider two limiting cases. First, consider a cost/s q which is zero. In this regime, shifting the time of a spike is free; a unit cost is assessed only for adding or deleting spikes. That is, the distance between these two spike trains is the difference in the number of spikes— just as in D^{count}.

The other extreme is that the cost/s to move a spike, q, is very large. Consider two spike trains, each of which consist of only a single spike, but which occur at times that differ by an amount ΔT. One candidate path between these trains consists of moving the solitary spike; this path has a cost $q\Delta T$. Another candidate path

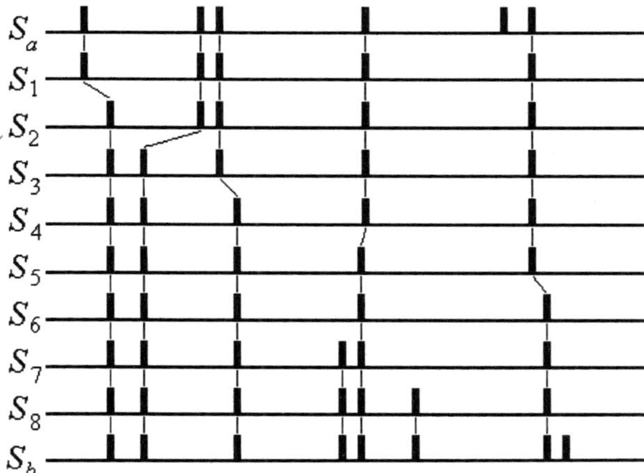

FIGURE 1. A minimal-cost path of elementary steps associated with $D^{\text{spike}}[q]$ that transforms spike train S_a to spike train S_b. (From Victor & Purpura.[25] Reprinted with permission from the *Journal of Neurophysiology*.)

consists of deleting the spike from S_a and then inserting a spike into S_b. This two-step path has a cost of 2. The definition of the metric $D^{\text{spike}}[q]$ states that the distance between these two spike trains is the minimum of these two quantities. That is, if the two spikes are separated by an amount ΔT which is less than $2/q$, the distance between them is $q\Delta T$ (it is cheaper to move the spike); if they are separated by an amount which is $2/q$ or more, the distance between them is 2 (it is cheaper to remove the spike from S_a and then reinsert it into S_b at the correct time). Both of these spike trains have a distance of 1 from the "null" (empty) spike train (via the step of deleting a spike). Thus, the two spike trains are regarded as lying at a greater distance from each other than either lies from the null train, unless their spikes are synchronized to within $1/q$.

In essence, $D^{\text{spike}}[0] = D^{\text{count}}$ measures distances between spike trains in a manner that is independent of the time of occurrence of the spikes. $D^{\text{spike}}[q]$, for a $q > 0$, formalizes a kind of temporal coding in which spikes, whose times match to within $1/q$, are regarded as having similar import, and spikes whose times are more separated and regarded as unrelated. Should we find that the metrics $D^{\text{spike}}[q]$ provide for substantial stimulus-dependent clustering of responses, we will have identified a qualitative feature of temporal coding. Furthermore, the value of q which maximizes this clustering can be regarded as a measure of the precision of the temporal coding.

We will also consider a second family of metrics, denoted $D^{\text{interval}}[q]$, which is sensitive not to the absolute timing of individual spikes, but rather to the lengths of the interspike intervals. Similar to $D^{\text{spike}}[q]$, $D^{\text{interval}}[q]$ is defined as the minimum cost to transform one spike train into another via certain allowed elementary transformations. The allowed transformations consist of adding a spike (at unit cost), deleting a spike (at unit cost), and changing the length of an interspike interval by an amount ΔT (at cost $q\Delta T$). Note that an essential difference exists between a transformation that changes the length of an interspike interval and one that shifts the time of occurrence of a single spike: stretching an interspike interval delays all subsequent spikes by a fixed amount, whereas changing the time of occurrence of a single spike stretches one interspike interval (the one preceding the spike in question) and shortens another (the one following the spike in question). A striking example of the qualitative difference between $D^{\text{interval}}[q]$ and $D^{\text{spike}}[q]$ is that $D^{\text{interval}}[q]$ can distinguish a neuron whose firing pattern is driven by a chaotic nonlinear recursion from one whose firing pattern is determined by a renewal process with equal interval statistics,[26] whereas $D^{\text{spike}}[q]$ cannot.

For the metrics $D^{\text{spike}}[q]$ and $D^{\text{interval}}[q]$, efficient algorithms[25,26] may be constructed which allow rapid calculation of the minimal-cost path, and hence the distance, between pairs of spike trains. These algorithms are closely related to the algorithms developed by Sellers[27,28] for the quantification of homology between sequences of amino acids and nucleotides. It is also possible to define many other families of metrics,[26] including metrics that are sensitive to patterns of bursts and motifs of spikes (as might be suggested by the work of Abeles)[10] and metrics appropriate to multichannel analysis.

In the cortical recordings we consider, previous analysis[25] has shown that the "nontrivial" metrics $D^{\text{spike}}[q]$ and $D^{\text{interval}}[q]$ provide a greater degree of stimulus-dependent clustering (i.e., a higher value of H, as described below) than the spike count metric D^{count}. This is strong evidence that in early cortical visual processing, the temporal pattern of impulses is important in transmitting sensory information. We also found that the optimal value of q depends systematically on the stimulus modality under consideration. Encoding of contrast was strongest for $D^{\text{spike}}[q]$ for values of q near 100; encoding of texture was strongest for values of q near 10, and the optimal value of q for other modalities was between these extremes. In principle, this suggests that temporal coding can be used to represent information on more than one stimulus attribute within a single spike train. It is this possibility of multidimensional representation that we focus on in this paper.

Physiological Methods

We analyze neural discharges recorded in visual areas V1 and V2 of two awake rhesus monkeys[25] and seven anesthetized, paralyzed cynomolgus monkeys. All procedures involving the animals were performed in accordance with National Institutes of Health guidelines for the care and use of laboratory animals.

Procedures for recordings in the awake monkey are described in more detail elsewhere.[25] Briefly, animals were trained to perform a fixation task; eye position was monitored with implanted search coils,[29–32] and extracellular recording was performed as previously described.[33,34] The times of extracellularly recorded action potentials (to the nearest millisecond) and the monkey's eye position were recorded by a program running under a real-time UNIX-based operating system,[35] which also controlled presentation of the visual stimuli by a separate microcomputer and reward delivery. A successful trial consisted of stable eye position maintained within 0.5 deg of the fixation point during stimulus presentation.

Data were recorded from one hemisphere of each monkey. Of the 25 recording sites, histological reconstruction and receptive field mapping[36] verified that six were in V1, nine were in V2, four (not analyzed here) were in V3, and the remaining six sites were either in V1 or V2. Ten recording sites yielded single-unit recordings, and the remainder yielded multiunit recordings from two or three neurons. In the analysis of the latter data sets, the neuron of origin for each spike was not identified.

Procedures for recordings in the anesthetized, paralyzed monkey are described in more detail elsewhere.[37] Briefly, anesthesia was induced with ketamine 15 mg/

kg i.m. potentiated by xylazine 2 mg/kg i.m., surgical procedures were performed with supplemental methohexital 1–2 mg/kg i.v., and recordings were carried out under anesthesia with sufentanil 1–6 μg/kg/h i.v. or urethane (400 mg/kg i.v. loading, 200 mg/ kg i.v. every 12 h). Pupils were dilated with atropine 1%. Flurbiprofen 2.5% (Ocufen, Allergan, Irvine, CA) was instilled as prophylaxis against ocular inflammation, and contact lenses were used to protect the corneas. Blood pressure, EKG, oxygen saturation, and core temperature were continuously monitored. Prior to physiological recording but following all surgical procedures, paralysis was induced and maintained with pancuronium bromide 0.3 mg/kg i.v. bolus, 0.3 mg/kg/h i.v. Ventilator settings were adjusted to maintain an end-expiratory CO_2 at 30–35 mmHg. Dexamethasone 1 mg/kg i.v. was given daily to reduce cerebral edema. Procaine penicillin G 25,000 U/ kg i.m. and benzathine penicillin G 25,000 U/kg i.m. was administered as prophylaxis against surgical infection, with gentamicin (5 mg/kg i.m. daily) added on subsequent days if indications of respiratory infection were present. Local antibiotic (bacitracin, neomycin, and polymyxin B ointment) was applied if a conjunctival discharge was present. Animals maintained in this fashion generally remained in good physiologic condition and retained excellent optics for 72 h.

Extracellular single-unit recordings were obtained with tungsten-in-glass Ainsworth microelectrodes (typical resistance 1–2 MΩ), followed by amplification, filtering, and waveform discrimination by height or by a hoop discriminator (Tucker-Davis Technologies, Gainesville, FL). Identification of electrolytically placed lesions (5 μA for 5 s) provided laminar identification of the recording site in most cases. Refraction was optimized for the viewing distance of 114 cm with trial lenses as determined by retinoscopy and from optimizing the responses of isolated single units. The visual display was presented on a Tektronix 608 monitor, mean luminance 150 cd/m^2, whose control signals were generated by specialized hardware (modified from ref.[38]) interfaced to a DEC 11/93 computer, which recorded spike times with a resolution of 3.70 ms (three monkeys, 9 units) or 1.23 ms (four monkeys, 13 units).

Stimuli consisted of stationary sinusoidal luminance gratings. For the recordings in the awake monkeys, stimuli were varied in contrast, orientation, and spatial frequency. For recordings in the anesthetized monkeys, stimuli were also varied in spatial phase. Contrast $[(L_{max} - L_{min})/(L_{max} + L_{min})]$ was varied in two (0.5, 1.0) to eight (0.04, 0.08, 0.12, 0.16, 0.24, 0.32, 0.64, 0.96) steps. Orientation was varied in three to eight equally spaced in steps of 11.25 or 22.5 deg. Spatial frequency was varied in two to seven values spaced by factors of two, which included the optimal spatial frequency. Spatial phase was varied in steps of 0.0625 of a cycle. Data sets consisted of 15–40 responses (in the awake animal) or 16–64 responses (in the anesthetized animal) to each stimulus, obtained in block-randomized order.

Data Analysis

As described recently,[25] the aim of the initial stage of data analysis was to determine, for each candidate metric, to what extent the distances between neural responses depended systematically on the stimulus. The spike count metric D^{count} and members of each of the two families of metrics $D^{spike}[q]$ and $D^{interval}[q]$ were considered in turn, with values of q ranging from 1 to 256. For each metric, the degree of clustering was measured by an information-theoretic quantity H, which expresses the certainty with which a hypothetical "observer" could determine which stimulus led to each observed response. To classify responses, the observer used a decision rule based solely on the pairwise distances between spike trains (relative to the metric under consideration). In essence, the decision rule examines the average distance from each spike train to the cloud of spike trains generated by each stimulus, and classifies it as belonging to the stimulus that corresponds to the nearest cloud. The rationale for this approach is that if a metric induced nearly perfect clustering (i.e., the responses to each stimulus were near to each other, and responses to distinct stimuli were distant from each other), then the reliability of this hypothetical observer would be high, and H would be near-maximal. Conversely, if the metric were insensitive to the aspects of spike trains that signal stimulus attributes, spike trains would not cluster in a systematic fashion, and distances between responses to repeated presentations of identical stimuli would be no different than distances between responses to distinct stimuli. In this case, the performance of the observer, and the quantity H, would be at chance levels.

The reader is cautioned on three fronts. First, there are well-known technical pitfalls associated with attempting to estimate information from finite data sets. Some of these pitfalls (i.e., sparse filling of bins[11,39]) are avoided by our approach, which circumvents binning procedures, but others (the upward bias of information due to small sample sizes[40,41]) are not. Hence, our measured values of H must always be compared with an estimate H_0 of this bias, which is calculated from resampled data sets.[25,26,42,43] (All values quoted below for H are significant by this criterion, and within a data set, H_0 has only a minor dependence on the choice of metric.) Second, although our measure is derived from classical information–theoretical considerations,[44] we do not mean to imply that the calculated value of H represents the actual amount of information that the nervous system extracts from a particular spike train: there is no pretense that the scheme we have used to derive H reflects neural processes. Finally, the primary motivation of this approach is that it avoids certain a priori assumptions as to the nature of the distance between spike trains (such as whether or not it is Euclidean), and as to the nature of the variability of responses (i.e., the shape of the "clouds" corresponding to particular response classes). No pretense is made that this approach yields the largest possible value of H. On the contrary, it is known to be suboptimal (in comparison with other classifier-based methods)[45] in certain situations, but this is the trade-off for limiting assumptions concerning the nature of the coding.

To focus on the possibility of encoding of multiple stimulus attributes through temporal structure, the final stage of data analysis consisted of a visualization of the geometry of the spike trains, as defined by a metric (typically $D^{spike}[q]$) which provided significant clustering. To do this, we used multidimensional scaling.[46,47] This technique embeds the spike trains into a Euclidean space, in a manner in which the natural Euclidean distance best approximates the distances yielded by the metric under consideration. Because the metrics we have considered are not Euclidean, this embedding can only be approximate. Nevertheless, it provides a vivid understanding of the relationships between neural responses to stimuli that vary in two or three attributes, and whether these relationships are consistent with our a priori notions of the stimulus dimensions (e.g., contrast, spatial frequency, and orientation), which are relevant to early vision.

RESULTS

The first data set we consider (FIG. 2) was obtained from a small multiunit cluster recorded in visual area V1 of an awake, fixating macaque. FIGURE 2 shows 16 responses to each of 40 stimuli: gratings presented in each of eight orientations (equally spaced at 22.5° intervals) and each of five spatial frequencies (1, 3, 5, 11,

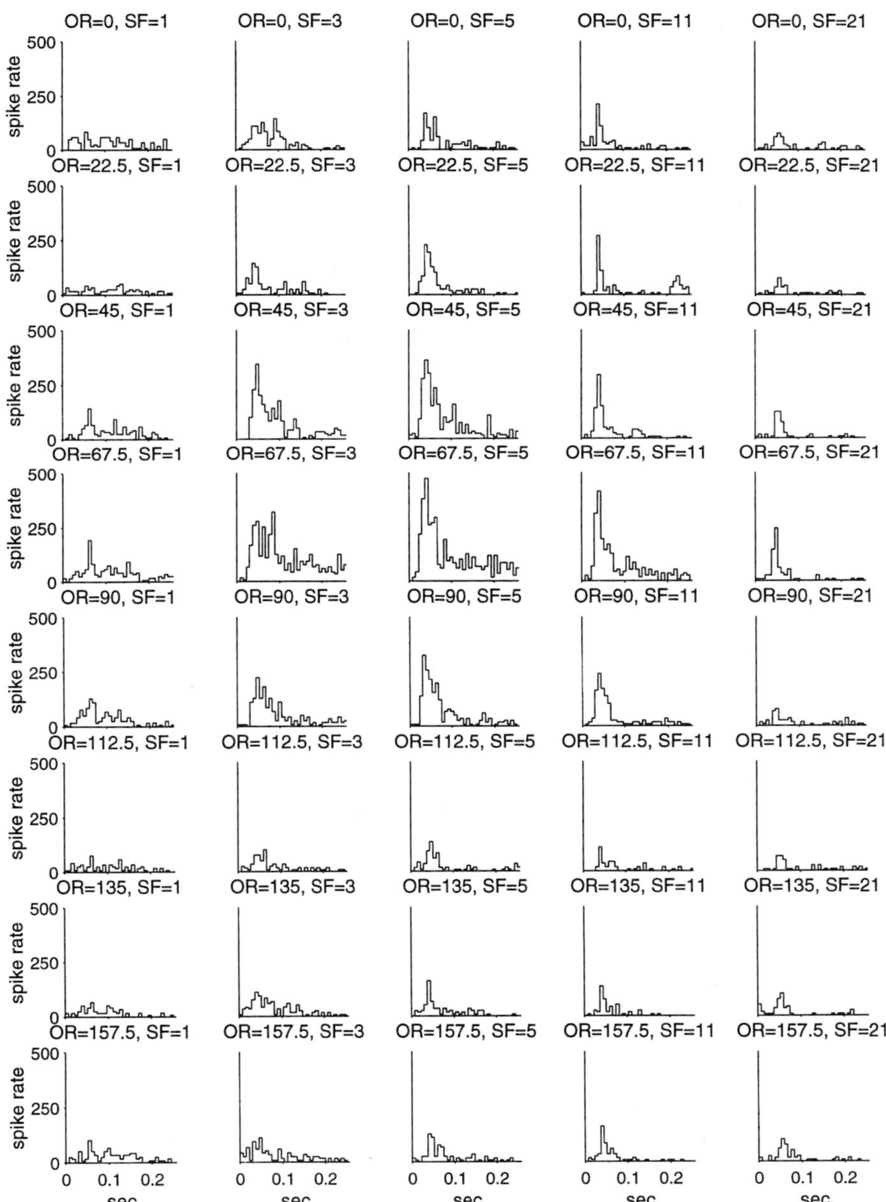

FIGURE 2. Response histograms recorded in macaque primary visual cortex elicited by 40 stimuli, consisting of grating patches presented at five spatial frequencies (*columns*) and eight orientations (*rows*). Contrast: 1.0. Sixteen responses to each of the stimuli were recorded. Recording H30011.

and 21 cycles/degree [c/deg]), covering the range of sensitivity of the neuron. The histograms show a maximal response in the midrange of spatial frequencies, and an orientation tuning that peaks at 67.5 deg. A formal analysis of response clustering reveals that this tuning is not just manifest in the spike count, but also in the temporal pattern of the impulses: the information-theoretical measure of clustering, H, was 1.10 for D^{count}, 1.76 for D^{spike} (maximal at $q = 16$), and 1.65 for $D^{interval}$ (maximal at $q = 8$). Analysis of subsets of these data (rows and columns of FIG. 2, corresponding to restriction to a single orientation or a single spatial frequency) also revealed the largest value of H for D^{spike}, the next largest for $D^{interval}$, and the smallest for D^{count}. Across these "slices," optimal values of q scattered substantially, from 4 to 256. No clear difference was found in the range of optimal values of q for the separation of responses to the series of orientations (at a given spatial frequency) or for the separation of responses to the series of spatial frequencies (at a given orientation). We therefore chose D^{spike} with an intermediate value of q, 64, to analyze the geometrical structure of the entire set of responses to the 40 stimuli. For $D^{spike}[64]$, H was 1.56.

We applied multidimensional scaling to the distances between pairs of individual responses, as determined by $D^{spike}[64]$. This provided an embedding of the spike trains into a vector space, in which the distances between individual spike trains are approximated by the ordinary (Euclidean) distances between the corresponding points in the vector space. For each stimulus, we then found the centroid of the points that corresponded to the set of spike trains it elicited, by averaging their coordinates in the vector-space embedding. Two views of the results of this procedure are shown in FIGURE 3. The 40 centroids arrange themselves in a highly systematic fashion. To a first approximation, the responses to each orientation (represented in color) sweep out separate arcs. Along each arc, responses to lower spatial frequencies (thicker lines) lie along corresponding positions. This is clearest for the orientations to which responses were largest (large arcs, in greens and yellows), but is also true for orientations which led to smaller responses (small arcs, in reds and blues).

As seen from FIGURE 3, the response space induced by $D^{spike}[64]$ has substantial geometrical complexity. One measure of this complexity is a "dimension index,"[26] defined from the eigenvalues that emerge from the multidimensional scaling procedure. For this data set, the dimension index is 2.8, which indicates that several dimensions are required to provide a reasonable approximation to the distance $D^{spike}[64]$. Furthermore, some of the eigenvalues that emerge from multidimensional scaling are negative, which suggests that a Euclidean geometry (of any dimension) may not be even qualitatively appropriate.[26] A priori, perhaps one might have expected that joint representation of orientation and spatial frequency might correspond to the Fourier plane (e.g., spatial frequency and orientation corresponding to polar coordinates). Clearly, such a simple picture is not recovered. Nevertheless, we see that distance $D^{spike}[64]$ places the observed responses into an abstract space in which the two stimulus parameters are represented in a largely independent fashion.

FIGURE 4 shows a similar analysis of recordings from a supragranular complex cell in V1 of an anesthetized, paralyzed macaque. Sixty-four responses were obtained to each of 15 stimuli: gratings presented in each of five contrasts (0.0625 to 1.0 in octave steps) and three spatial frequencies (0.5, 2, and 4 c/deg). On successive presentations, the grating stimulus was positioned in a pseudorandomly chosen spatial phase. The response histograms (FIG. 4) show only modest responses, primarily at the two highest contrasts and the two highest spatial frequencies. However, the clustering analysis again reveals clear evidence of temporal coding: H was 0.16 for D^{count}, 0.25 for D^{spike} (maximal at $q = 32$), and 0.24 for $D^{interval}$ (maximal at $q = 64$).

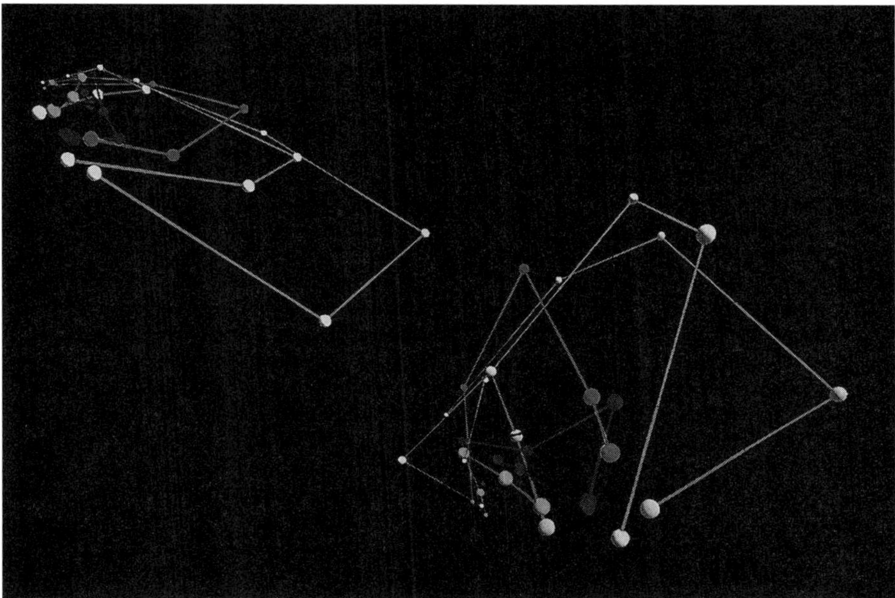

FIGURE 3. Two views of multidimensional scaling of the data of FIGURE 2 for $D^{\text{spike}}[64]$. Each point corresponds to the centroid of the locus of responses for one of the 40 stimuli. Stimulus orientation is rendered by color (red = 0 deg, orange = 22.5 deg, yellow = 45 deg, yellow-green = 67.5 deg, green = 90 deg, cyan = 112.5 deg, blue = 135 deg, violet = 157.5 deg), and spatial frequency (1, 3, 5, 11, and 21 c/deg) is rendered by line thickness and sphere size (thick lines and large spheres for lowest spatial frequency).

Multidimensional scaling, carried out as above with $D^{\text{spike}}[64]$, again revealed a systematic mapping of the two-parameter stimulus set into the abstract response space. As shown in the left-hand view in FIGURE 5, each spatial frequency occupies a different sector of the space. To a first approximation, the trajectories corresponding to each spatial frequency are rotations of each other. Thus, as in FIGURE 3, we see that the distance $D^{\text{spike}}[64]$ defines a response space in which the two stimulus parameters are independently represented, albeit in a distorted manner. The dimension index for this embedding is 3.2.

FIGURE 6 shows the analysis of a three-parameter data set recorded in V2 of an awake, fixating macaque. Stimuli varied in contrast (0.5 and 1.0), spatial frequency (3, 5, and 11 c/deg), and orientation (three steps of 22.5 deg). Response histograms (FIG. 6) typically have a transient and a sustained component. Inspection of the response histograms suggests that responses to the higher contrast have a larger transient component. However, neither the sustained nor the transient component provides an obvious separation of spatial frequency and orientation. For this data set, H was 0.36 for D^{count}, 0.43 for D^{spike} (maximal at $q = 64$), and not significant for D^{interval}. With multidimensional scaling (FIG. 7, left half), the separation of response loci is not nearly as clear here as in the previous two examples. Correspondingly, the dimension index for this embedding is 7.5, also significantly higher than in the two previous examples. Nevertheless, in the two views of the representation

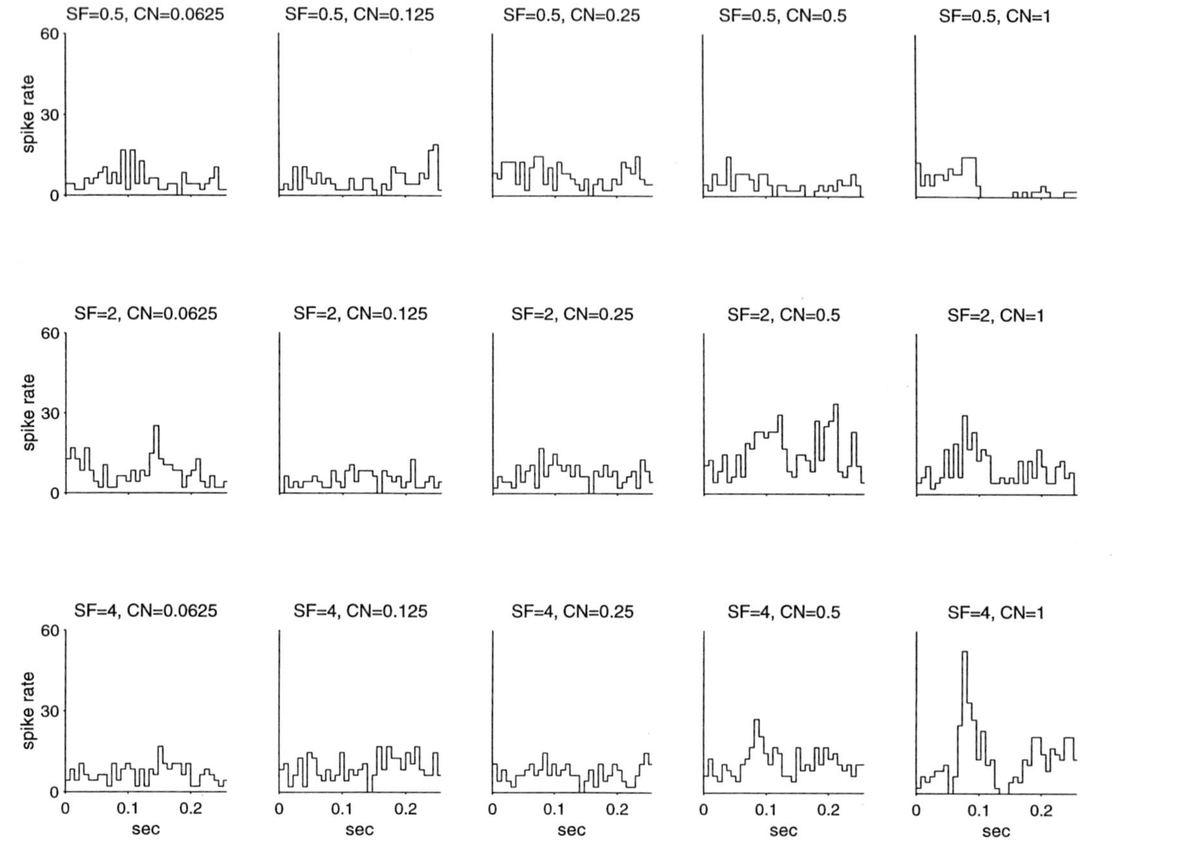

FIGURE 4. Response histograms recorded in macaque primary visual cortex elicted by 15 stimuli, consisting of grating patches presented at five contrasts (*columns*) and three spatial frequencies (*rows*). The orientation was optimal for the cell. Sixty-four responses to each of the stimuli were recorded. Recording 19/12.

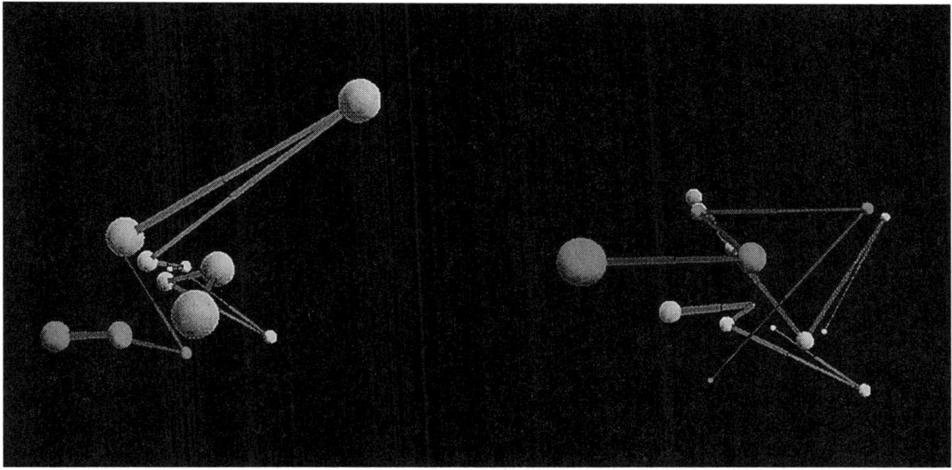

FIGURE 5. Two views of multidimensional scaling of the data of FIGURE 4 for $D^{\text{spike}}[64]$. Each point corresponds to the centroid of the locus of responses for one of the 15 stimuli. Stimulus contrast (0.0625, 0.125, 0.25, 0.5, and 1.0) is rendered by line thickness and sphere size (thick lines and large spheres for highest contrast), and spatial frequency is rendered by color (blue = 0.5 c/deg, green = 2 c/deg, orange = 4 c/deg).

of the loci of the centroids, it is clear that the three attributes of contrast (rendered as brightness), spatial frequency (rendered as sphere size), and orientation (rendered as color) are arrayed in distinct, but interpenetrating, patterns.

Representing the set of responses to a stimulus by the position of the centroid of the individual responses is a convenient way to visualize the location of a cloud of responses. However, there is no guarantee that this averaging procedure corresponds to a midpoint in the abstract space defined by the metrics we have considered, or even that such a midpoint exists. For this reason, we have explored a different way of reducing the set of responses to each stimulus to a single "point" in the abstract representation space (i.e., a single spike train). For each set of responses, we attempted to identify a "consensus spike train"—a spike train for which the mean squared distance (in the sense of $D^{\text{spike}}[q]$) to each of the observed responses is minimized. The results of this calculation, as applied to each of the individual responses, are shown in FIGURE 8. Of note, the consensus spike trains (for $D^{\text{spike}}[64]$) have fewer spikes (average 11.4) than the individually measured responses (average 13.4). This indicates that some, but not all, of the spikes present in the raw data are present at reproducible times within the response. In this context, reproducible means that the jitter of occurrence times is within the window of $1/q$ (here, $1/64 \approx$ 16 ms) that corresponds to $D^{\text{spike}}[q]$.

Finally, we applied multidimensional scaling to the individual consensus spike trains of FIGURE 8. This results in the embedding illustrated in FIGURE 7 (right half). The separate representation of the three stimulus attributes is somewhat clearer when the consensus process, as opposed to a vectorial average, is used to identify a "typical" response. However, this apparent improvement is difficult to quantify, and arguably may result from a fortuitous choice of the projection of the embeddings (the dimension index of the average embedding is 7.5; the dimension

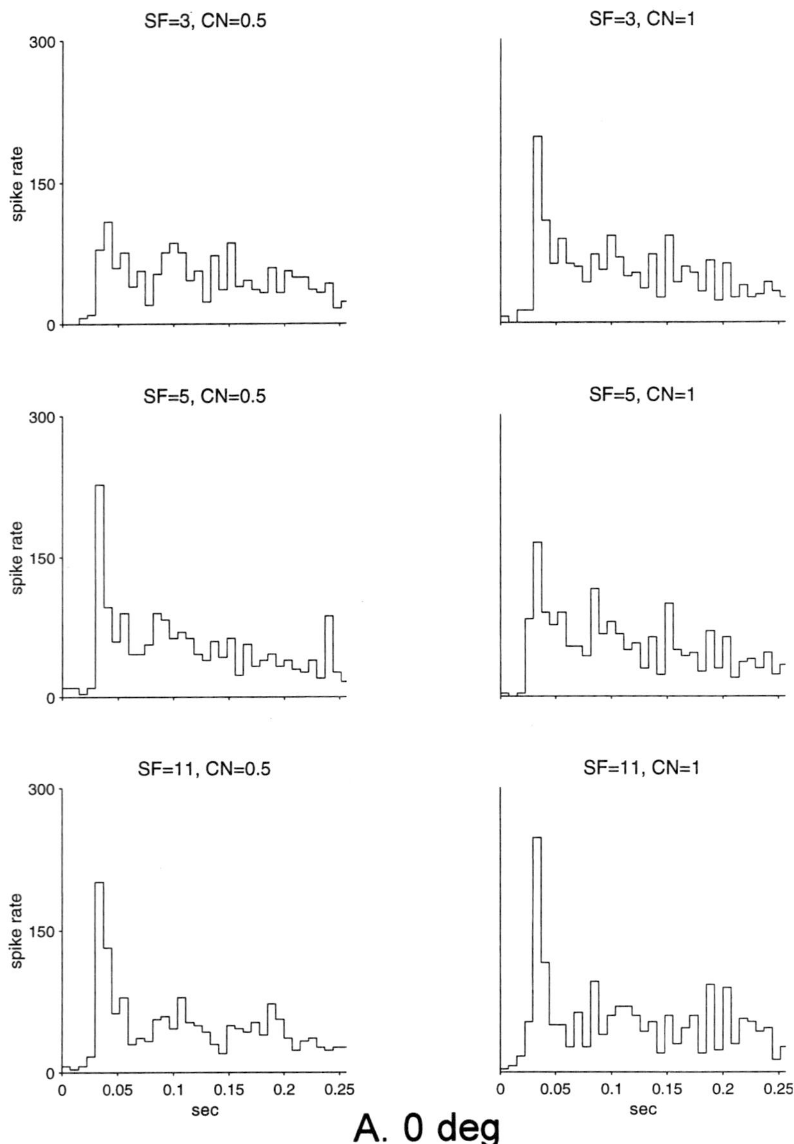

FIGURE 6. Response histograms recorded in macaque area V2 elicited by 18 stimuli, consisting of grating patches presented at two contrasts (*columns*), three spatial frequencies (*rows*), and three orientations (**panels A:** 0 deg; **B:** 22.5 deg; **C:** 45 deg). Forty-two responses to each of the stimuli were recorded. Recording H21131.

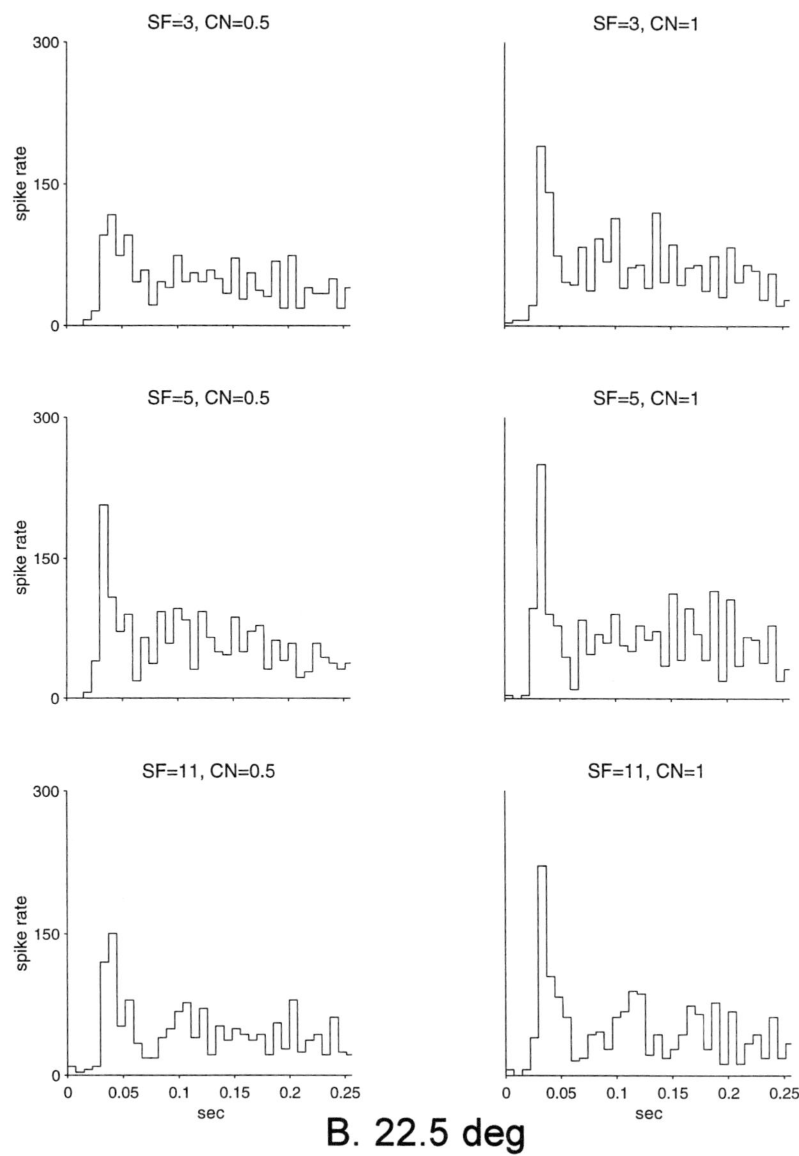

FIGURE 6. (*Continued*)

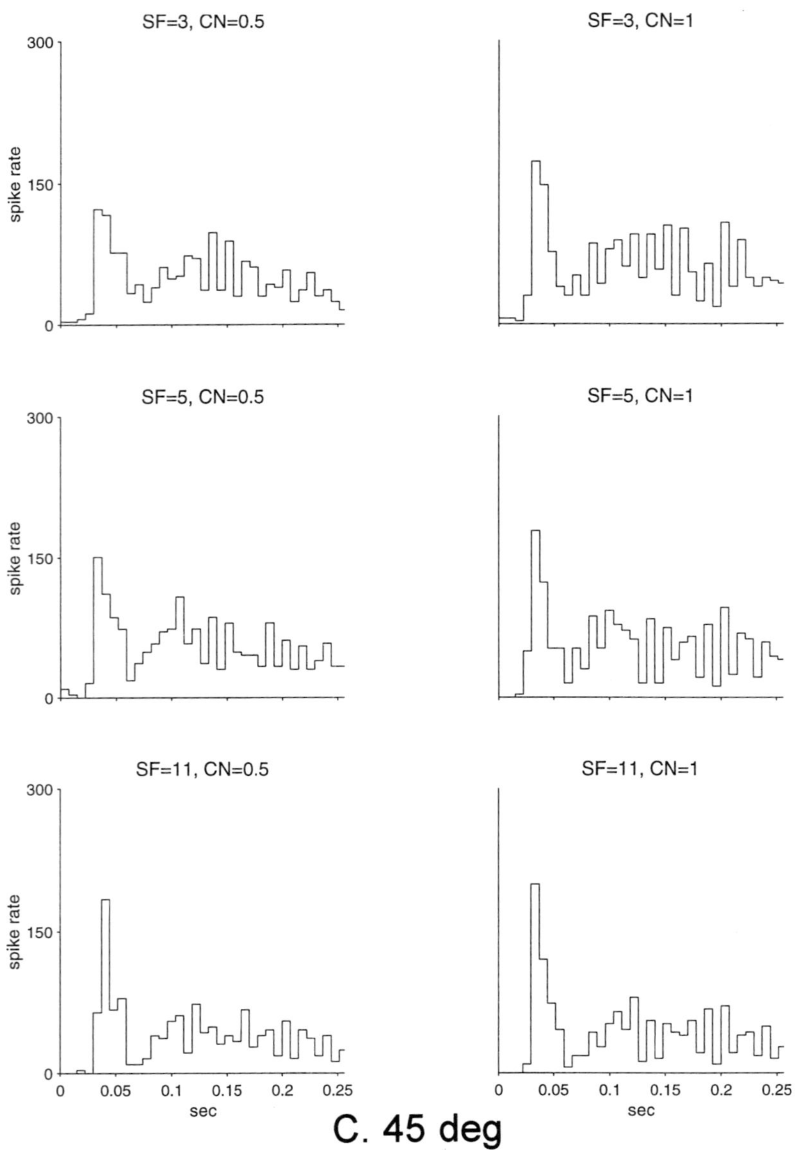

FIGURE 6. (*Continued*)

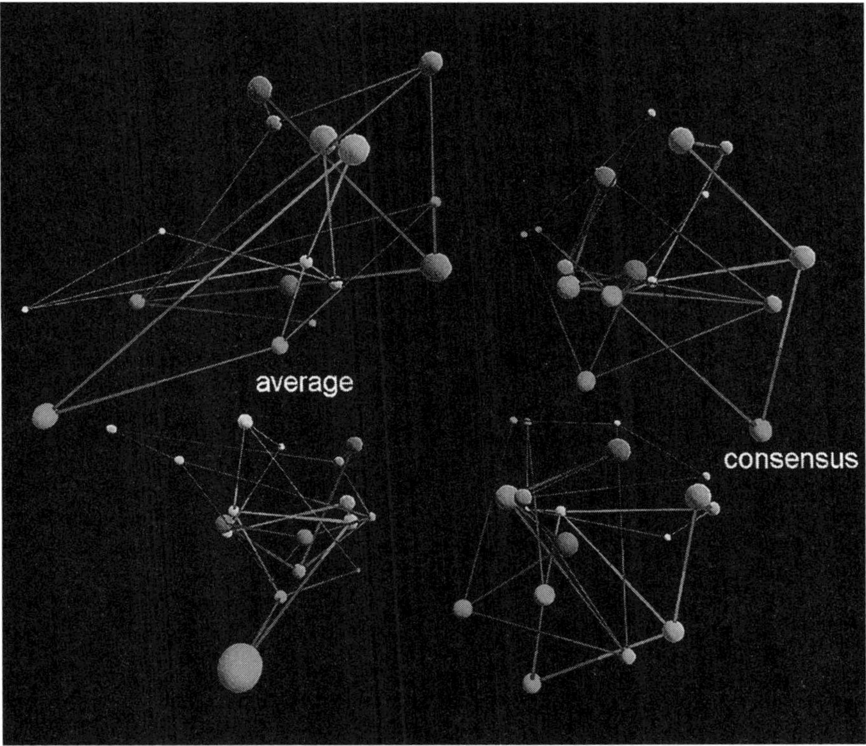

FIGURE 7. (*Left, labeled average*) Two views of multidimensional scaling of the data of FIGURE 6 for D^{spike}[64]. Each point corresponds to the centroid of the locus of responses for one of the 18 stimuli. Stimulus contrast (0.5 and 1.0) is rendered by brightness (bright spheres for higher contrast), spatial frequency (3, 5, and 11 c/deg) is rendered by line thickness and sphere size (thick lines and large spheres for lowest spatial frequency), and orientation is rendered by color (orange = 0 deg, green = 22.5 deg, blue = 45 deg). (*Right, labeled consensus*) Multidimensional scaling of the corresponding consensus response sequences (FIG. 8).

index of the consensus embedding is 6.5). What is more striking is that the embedding based on single consensus spike trains (FIG. 7, right half), with fewer spikes, retains much of the complexity of the centroid embedding (FIG. 7, left half)—consistent with the notion that only the spikes whose times of occurrence were reproducible were carrying visual information.

DISCUSSION

We have presented a new theoretical approach to the analysis of how visual information is encoded in impulse trains. Rather than adapt general-purpose methods of analysis that have been developed for continuous signals, our strategy exploits the fact that spike trains are sequences of discrete events. Two neurobiological

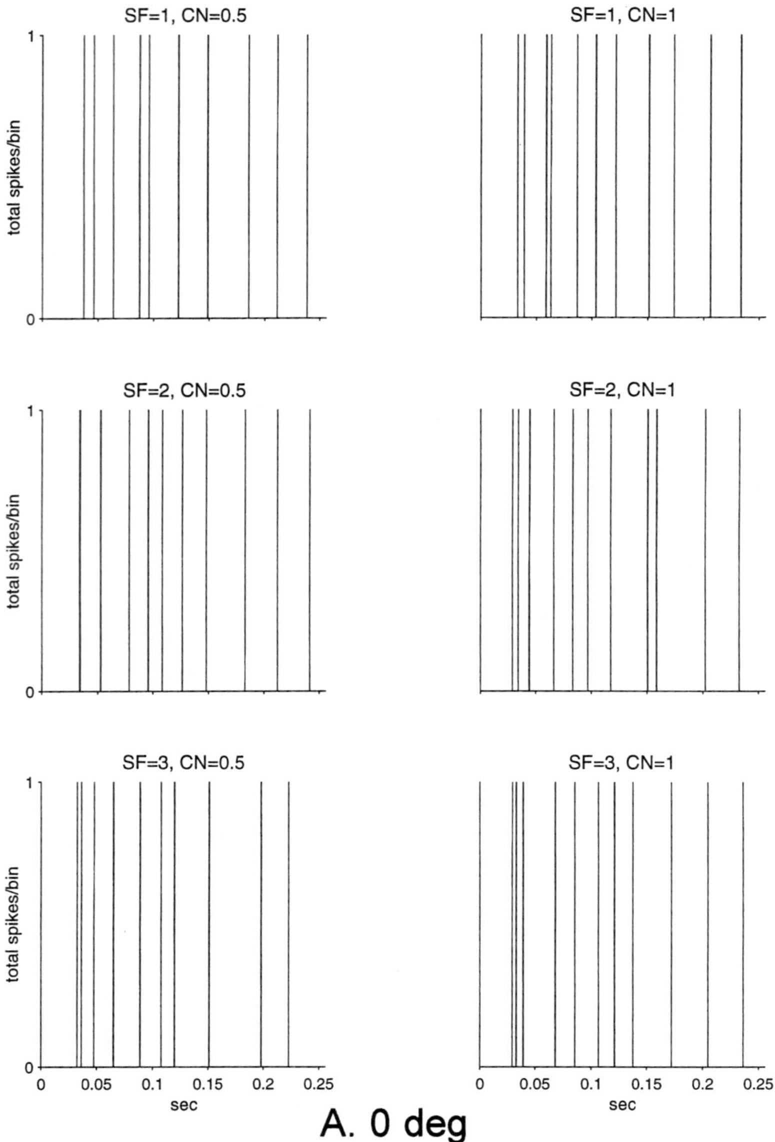

FIGURE 8. The consensus spike trains corresponding to the recordings of FIGURE 6 and $D^{\text{spike}}[64]$. Layout of contrast (*columns*), spatial frequency (*rows*), and orientation (**panels A:** 0 deg; **B:** 22.5 deg; **C:** 45 deg) as in FIGURE 6.

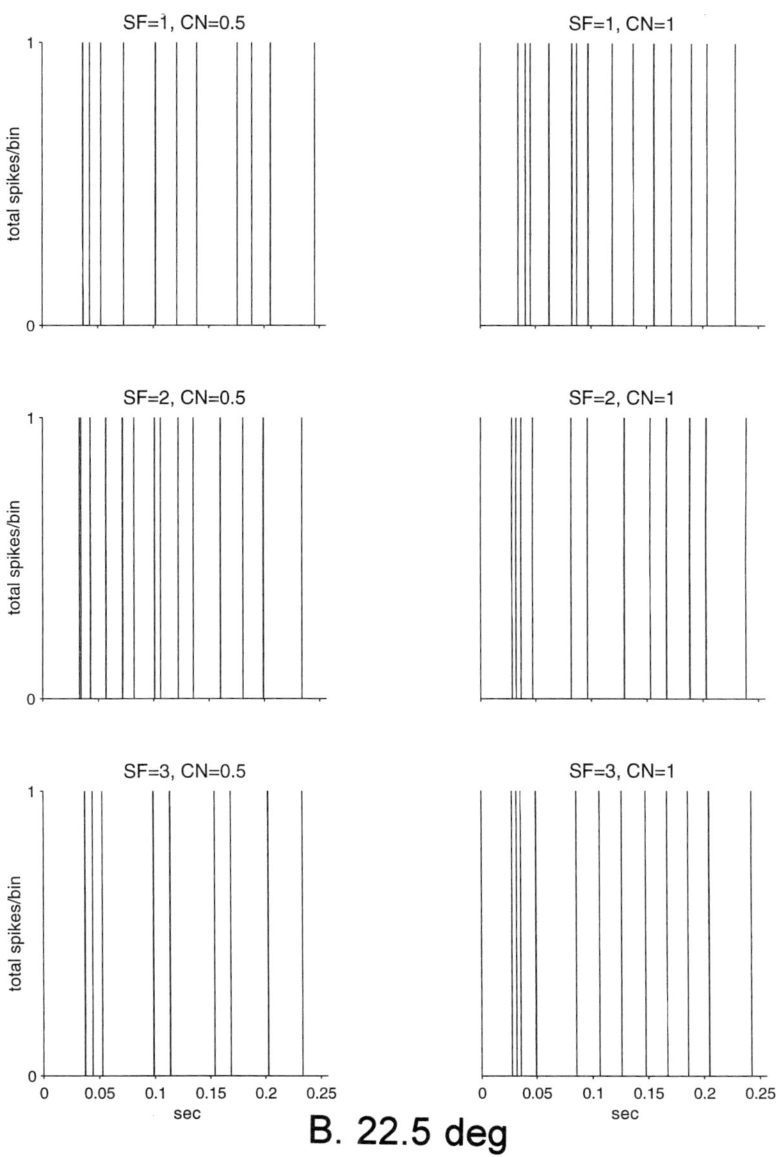

FIGURE 8. (*Continued*)

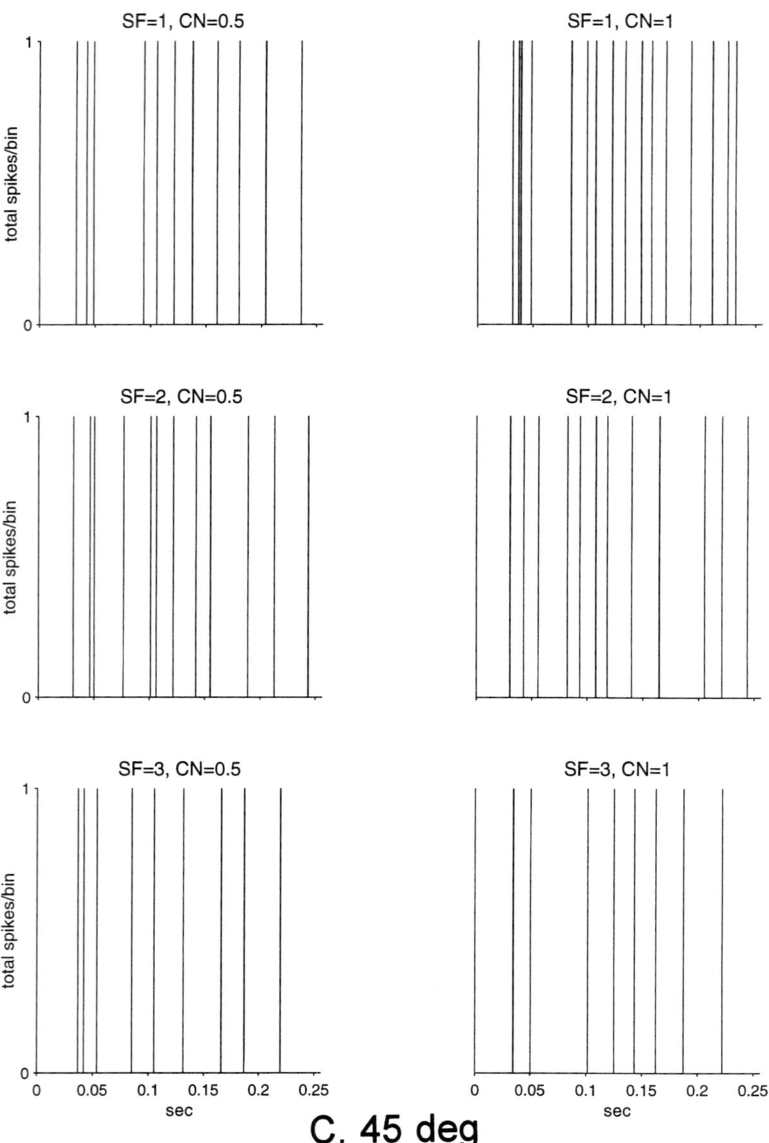

FIGURE 8. (*Continued*)

heuristics form the main motivation of the approach. One is the notion that neurons act as coincidence detectors; to the extent that this is true, inputs that have similar spike times will have similar postsynaptic effects. The second heuristic is that in some neurons, potentiation, habituation, and other effects of voltage- and time-dependent conductances are crucial; for these neurons, inputs that have similar spike intervals will have similar postsynaptic effects.

These considerations lead directly to notions of distances, or metrics, between spike trains, considered as points in an abstract space. For each candidate notion of distance, we can determine whether responses to visual stimuli that differ in some particular attribute (such as contrast or spatial frequency) tend to be more widely separated than stimuli which are similar in this attribute. This has led to the demonstration that for neurons in macaque V1 and V2, temporal coding is quite prominent, and that this encoding is primarily in terms of absolute spike times.[25,26] Moreover, there is a clear tendency for contrast to be coded with high temporal precision, texture type with low temporal precision, and other attributes (orientation and spatial frequency) to be coded with an intermediate precision.[25] The observation that multiple visual attributes may be encoded on separate time scales gains support from other approaches, both at the single-unit level[8,48,49] and the population level.[37] This provides a way for the temporal structure of a spike train to contain multiplexed information concerning more than one stimulus attribute.[48]

Here, we pursue this idea one step further. We demonstrate that the spike time distance suffices to define a map from a stimulus attribute space to a response space, in which the two- or three-dimensional array of stimulus responses map unambiguously into separate and orderly trajectories. At the level of the lateral geniculate, such temporal multiplexing also occurs,[4] but is most likely due to Poisson firing within an envelope whose shape is determined by a spatiotemporally inseparable receptive field.[50] Although such behavior may well play a role in the multidimensional cortical coding we have observed, more subtle processes must be at work as well: we have shown that the temporal structure in the response of a cortical visual neuron is not simply that of Poisson firing within an envelope.[25]

In FIGURE 7, we have shown that the neural representation of a three-parameter stimulus set is fully preserved in single artificial spike trains, each of which is the consensus of the observed neural responses to a stimulus. Indeed, our preliminary results suggest that the consensus spike trains may provide a cleaner representation of the stimulus space than the standard average response. Should this finding be further substantiated, it would have at least two important implications. Because only a subset of the spikes in a response would be required to convey information concerning the parameters we have studied, the remaining spikes would be available to convey other information. More importantly, it would indicate that coincidences of spike times (to within a resolution of ≈ 16 ms) across neurons conveying overlapping information might serve to identify the "informative" spikes.[51]

It is important to point out that several caveats exist concerning this approach. First, the metrics that we have considered were chosen for their simplicity and their ability to focus on two caricatures of neural processing; no claim is made that any of the metrics considered are optimal ones (either for the purpose of extracting information, or for the purpose of multidimensional scaling), or that a single universal metric (independent of sensory modality, brain region, etc.) exists. Perhaps a neural code, common to all sensory modalities, exists at some final stage of object recognition, but a comparison[26] of coding in visual and auditory cortices[12] suggests that there are significant differences between specific sensory areas. Most likely, coding will use general features of neurons already recognized, including coincidence detection[17] and sensitivity to interval patterns.[21-23] However, we have only considered caricatures of neurons, rather than biophysically realistic models of how temporal codes might be set up and processed.

Finally, although we have demonstrated that temporal codes can carry information concerning multiple stimulus attributes within a single discharge, we can hardly claim that coding *across* neurons can be neglected. Indeed, recognition of even simple visual stimuli requires disambiguation and analysis of far more than two or three attributes. The substantial variability of individual responses, and the low absolute amounts of information,[25] imply that coding across neurons must play a large role. Theoretical considerations[52] support our contention that analysis of such coding will require a mathematical formalism more general than vector spaces. As we have seen here, the discrete nature of spike trains naturally leads to such a formalism, which readily generalizes[26] to the analysis of populations of neurons. Coding at the population level must be at least as complex as coding at the level of the single unit. Our results thus suggest that population coding is likely to make fundamental use of the discrete and temporally precise nature of neural impulses. That is, in a theory of higher brain function, the macroscopic state of a population of neurons must take into account not only the total number of neurons that are firing, but also their temporal relationships.

SUMMARY

We described a novel approach to the study of how spike trains encode sensory information. This approach emphasizes the idea that spike trains are sequences of discrete events, rather than approximations to continuous signals. Aided by some simple heuristics, such as a caricature of neurons as coincidence detectors, we constructed candidate notions of "distances" between spike trains, considered as points in an abstract space. Each candidate distance was evaluated for relevance to biological encoding by determining whether it led to systematic, stimulus-dependent, clustering of the neural responses. We showed here that these distances can also be used to construct a "response space" for the neuron. The response space, which is typically not Euclidean, can represent two or three stimulus attributes. We also introduced the notion of a "consensus spike train," defined as the spike train with minimum average distance from a set of observed responses. For the distances we considered, the consensus spike train (for a particular stimulus) contained only those spikes that were present at consistent times across the observed responses to that stimulus, and thus contained fewer spikes than the typical observed responses. Nevertheless, these consensus spike trains provided an equivalent (or even superior) representation of the stimulus array.

ACKNOWLEDGMENTS

We thank Aaron Hoffman and Matthew Tepel for assistance in developing and implementing the consensus algorithm, and Annemarie Canel for additional software development.

REFERENCES

1. CHURCHLAND, P. S. & T. J. SEJNOWSKI. 1988. Pespectives on cognitive neuroscience. Science **242:** 741–745.

2. BIALEK, W., F. RIEKE, R. R. DE RUYTER VAN STEVENINCK & D. WARLAND. 1991. Reading a neural code. Science **252:** 1854–1857.

3. DAYHOFF, J. E. & G. L. GERSTEIN. 1983. Favored patterns in spike trains. II. Application. J. Neurophysiol. **49:** 1347–1363.

4. GAWNE, T. J., J. W. MCCLURKIN, B. J. RICHMOND & L. M. OPTICAN. 1991. Lateral geniculate neurons in behaving primates. III. Response predictions of a channel model with multiple spatial-to-temporal filters. J. Neurophysiol. **66:** 809–823.

5. HELLER, J., J. A. HERTZ T. W. KJAER & B. J. RICHMOND. 1995. Information flow and temporal coding in primate pattern vision. J. Computat. Neurosci. **2:** 175–193.

6. MCCLURKIN, J. W., T. J. GAWNE, L. M. OPTICAN & B. J. RICHMOND. 1991. Lateral geniculate neurons in behaving primates. II. Encoding information in the temporal shape of the response. J. Neurophysiol. **66:** 794–808.

7. OPTICAN, L. M. & B. J. RICHMOND. 1987. Temporal encoding of two-dimensional patterns by single units in primate inferior temporal cortex. III. Information theoretic analysis. J. Neurophysiol. **57:** 162–178.

8. PURPURA, K., M. N. CHEE-ORTS & L. M. OPTICAN. 1993. Temporal encoding of texture properties in visual cortex of awake monkey. Soc. Neurosci. Abstr. **19:** 771.

9. RICHMOND, B. J., L. M. OPTICAN, M. PODELL & H. SPITZER. 1987. Temporal encoding of two-dimensional patterns by single units in primate inferior temporal cortex. I. Response characteristics. J. Neurophysiol. **57:** 132–146.

10. ABELES, M. 1982. Local Cortical Circuits, an Electrophysiological Study. Springer. Berlin.

11. GEISLER, W. S., D. G. ALBRECHT, R. J. SALVI & S. S. SAUNDERS. 1991. Discrimination performance of single neurons: Rate and temporal-pattern information. J. Neurophysiol. **66:** 334–362.

12. MIDDLEBROOKS, J. C., A. E. CLOCK, L. XU & D. M. GREEN. 1994. A panoramic code for sound location by cortical neurons. Science **264:** 842–844.

13. LAURENT, G., M. WEHR & H. DAVIDOWITZ. 1996. Temporal representations of odors in an olfactory network. J. Neurosci. **16:** 3837–3847.

14. SKARDA, C. A. & W. J. FREEMAN. 1987. How brains make chaos to make sense of the world. Behav. Brain Sci. **10:** 161–195.

15. WUERGER, S., L. T. MALONEY & J. KRAUSKOPF. 1995. Proximity judgments in color space: Tests of a Euclidean color geometry. Vision Res. **35:** 827–835.

16. ABELES, M. 1982. Role of the cortical neuron: Integrator or coincidence detector? Isr. J. Med. Sci. **18:** 83–92.

17. BOURNE, H. R. & R. NICOLL. 1993. Molecular machines integrate coincident synaptic signals. Cell 72/Neuron 10(Suppl.): 65–85.

18. MEL, B. W. 1993. Synaptic integration in an excitable dendritic tree. J. Neurophysiol. **70:** 1086–1101.

19. SOFTKY, W. R. & C. KOCH. 1993. The highly irregular firing of cortical cells is inconsistent with temporal integration of random EPSP's. J. Neurosci. **13:** 334–350.

20. SOFTKY, W. R. 1995. Simple codes versus efficient codes. Curr. Opinion Neurobiol. **5:** 239–247.

21. BLISS, T. V. P. & G. L. COLLINGRIDGE. 1993. A synaptic model of memory: Long-term potentiation in the hippocampus. Nature **361:** 31–39.

22. LARSON, J., D. WONG & G. LYNCH. 1986. Patterned stimulation at the theta frequency is optimal for the induction of hippocampal long-term potentiation. Brain Res. **368:** 347–350.

23. ROSE, G. M. & T. V. DUNWIDDIE. 1986. Induction of hippocampal long-term potentiation using physiologically patterned stimulation. Neurosci. Lett. **69:** 244–248.

24. VICTOR, J. D. & K. PURPURA. 1994. A new approach to the analysis of spike discharges: Cost-based metrics. Soc. Neurosci. Abstr. **20:** 315.

25. VICTOR, J. D. & K. PURPURA. 1996. Nature and precision of temporal coding in visual cortex: A metric-space analysis. J. Neurophysiol. **76:** 1310–1326.

26. VICTOR, J. D. & K. PURPURA. 1997. Metric-space analysis of spike trains: Theory, algorithms, and application. Network **8:** 127–164.

27. SELLERS, P. H. 1974. On the theory and computation of evolutionary distances. SIAM J. Appl. Math. **26:** 787–793.

28. SELLERS, P. H. 1979. Combinatorial complexes. SIAM J. Appl. Math. **26:** 787–793.
29. JUDGE, S. J., B. J. RICHMOND & F. C. CHU. 1980. Implantation of magnetic search coils for measurement of eye position: An improved method. Vision Res. **20:** 535–538.
30. RICHMOND, B. J., R. H. WURTZ & T. SATO. 1983. Visual responses of inferior temporal neurons in the awake rhesus monkey. J. Neurophysiol. **50:** 1415–1432.
31. ROBINSON, D. A. 1963. A method of measuring eye movement using a scleral search coil in a magnetic field. IEEE Trans. Biomed. Eng. **10:** 137–145.
32. WURTZ, R. H. 1969. Visual receptive fields of striate cortex neurons in awake monkeys. J. Neurophysiol. **32:** 727–742.
33. CRIST, C. F., D. S. G. YAMASAKI, H. KOMATSU & R. H. WURTZ. 1988. A grid system and a microsyringe for single cell recording. J. Neurosci. Methods **26:** 117–122.
34. MCCLURKIN, J. W., T. J. GAWNE, B. J. RICHMOND, L. M. OPTICAN & D. L. ROBINSON. 1991. Lateral geniculate neurons in behaving primates. I. Responses to two-dimensional stimuli. J. Neurophysiol. **66:** 777–793.
35. HAYS, A. V., B. J. RICHMOND & F. C. CHU. 1982. A Unix-based multiple process real-time data acquisition and control. Wescon Conference Proceedings **2/1:** 1–10.
36. GATTAS, R., A. P. B. SOUSA & C. G. GROSS. 1988. Visuotopic organization and extent of V3 and V4 of the macaque. J. Neurosci. **8:** 1831–1845.
37. VICTOR, J. D., K. PURPURA, E. KATZ & B. MAO. 1994. Population encoding of spatial frequency, orientation, and color in macaque V1. J. Neurophysiol. **72:** 2151–2166.
38. MILKMAN, N., G. SCHICK, M. ROSSETTO, F. RATLIFF, R. SHAPLEY & J. D. VICTOR. 1980. A two-dimensional computer-controlled visual stimulator. Behav. Res. Methods Instrum. **12:** 283–292.
39. CHEE-ORTS, M. N. & L. M. OPTICAN. 1993. Cluster method for analysis of transmitted information in multivariate neuronal data. Biol. Cybern. **69:** 29–35.
40. CARLTON, A. G. 1969. On the bias of information estimates. Psychol. Bull. **71:** 108–109.
41. TREVES, A. & S. PANZERI. 1995. The upward bias in measures of information derived from limited data samples. Neural Computation **7:** 399–407.
42. FAGEN, R. M. 1978. Information measures: Statistical confidence limits and inference. J. Theor. Biol. **73:** 61–79.
43. OPTICAN, L. M., T. J. GAWNE, B. J. RICHMOND & P. J. JOSEPH. 1991. Unbiased measures of transmitted information and channel capacity from multivariate neuronal data. Biol. Cybern. **65:** 305–310.
44. ABRAMSON, N. 1963. Information Theory and Coding. McGraw-Hill. New York.
45. GOLOMB, D., J. HERTZ, S. PANZERI, A. TREVES & B. RICHMOND. 1997. How well can we estimate the information carried in neuronal responses from limited samples? Neural Computation **9:** 649–665.
46. GREEN, P. E. 1978. Analyzing Multivariate Data. Dryden Press. Hinsdale, IL.
47. KRUSKAL, J. B. & M. WISH. 1978. Multidimensional Scaling. Sage Publications. Beverly Hills, CA.
48. MCCLURKIN, J. W., L. M. OPTICAN, B. J. RICHMOND & T. J. GAWNE. 1991. Concurrent processing and complexity of temporally coded messages in visual perception. Science **253:** 675–677.
49. VOLGUSHEV, M., T. R. VIDYASAGAR & X. PEI. 1995. Dynamics of the orientation tuning of postsynaptic potentials in the cat visual cortex. Visual Neurosci. **12:** 621–628.
50. GOLOMB, D., D. KLEINFELD, R. C. REID, R. M. SHAPLEY & B. I. SHRAIMAN. 1994. On temporal codes and the spatiotemporal response of neurons in the lateral geniculate nucleus. J. Neurophysiol. **72:** 2990–3003.
51. MEISTER, M., L. LAGNADO & D. A. BAYLOR. 1995. Concerted signaling by retinal ganglion cells. Science **270:** 1207–1210.
52. HOPFIELD, J. J. 1995. Pattern recognition computation using action potential timing for stimulus representation. Nature **376:** 33–36.

Transforming Sensory Perceptions into Motor Commands: Evidence from Programming of Eye Movements[a]

R. JOHN LEIGH,[b] KLAUS G. ROTTACH,[c]
AND VALLABH E. DAS

Department of Neurology
Veterans Affairs Medical Center
and
University Hospitals
Case Western Reserve University
Cleveland, Ohio 44106

INTRODUCTION

In his teachings and writings, Fred Plum has promoted an approach to solving neurological problems that is based on understanding pathological physiology.[1] One additional benefit of this strategy is that it may also contribute to a better understanding of normal brain functions. Consider, for example, the ways that the brain detects a sensory stimulus and then programs a motor response to it; either step may be separately affected by disease, producing quite different disturbances of function. At least part of this difference may reflect the way in which the neural signal is encoded. Although a direct approach to elucidate such behavior is to record the activity of neurons, studying disturbances of behavior due to lesions may afford insights, provided that a clear relationship between behavior and neuronal activity is established. The study of the control of eye movements meets this criterion, because the extraocular muscles have no functional stretch reflex,[2] and it is therefore possible to relate their relatively simple range of movements (three degrees of rotational freedom) to the discharge of ocular motoneurons using simple, linear, differential equations.[3,4] Thus, hypotheses that have been formulated from electrophysiological data can be tested by measuring the changes of responses due to lesions of the nervous system. This brief review attempts to illustrate how this approach has been applied to investigate the way that the brain programs a shift of gaze to view a novel visual target. Specifically, we will examine how saccades—rapid, conjugate eye movements—shift the line of sight so that an image detected in the retinal periphery is brought to the fovea, where it can be seen best.

[a] This work was supported by U.S. Public Health Service grant EY06717, the Medical Research Service of the Department of Veterans Affairs, and the Evenor Armington Fund (to R.J.L.), and Deutsche Forschungsgemeinschaft (to K.G.R.).

[b] Address correspondence to: R. John Leigh, M.D., Department of Neurology, University Hospitals, 11100 Euclid Avenue, Cleveland, Ohio 44106-5000. E-mail: rj14@po.cwru.edu
[c] Current address: Department of Neurology, Zentralklinikum, 86156 Augsburg, Germany.

DIFFERENCES BETWEEN THE INITIAL CODING OF THE VISUAL STIMULUS AND THE FINAL MOTOR COMMAND

In primary visual cortex (Brodmann area 17, V1), the responses to *visual stimuli*—such as the target for a saccade—are organized in a *retinotopic map*. Indeed, this map serves as the basis for testing the integrity of occipital cortex during conventional visual field testing.[5] Thus, the location of visual stimuli is represented by the distribution of activity across the cortical map.

The *motor command* for the eye movement response arises from the motoneurons of the third, fourth, and sixth cranial nerves, which lie in the brain stem. Unlike neurons in visual cortex, the ocular motoneurons encode the characteristics of the saccade in terms of their *temporal discharge*; the eye movement is proportional to the total number of discharge spikes.[3,6] Thus, an important issue to be resolved is: How does the brain transform the stimulus, which is encoded in terms of the location of active neurons within visual cortex (i.e., "place coded") into the saccadic command on ocular motoneurons, which is encoded in terms of discharge frequency and duration (i.e., "temporally coded")?

One obvious approach is to look at intermediate stages in the programming of saccades and, in this regard, a structure that has attracted considerable recent interest is the superior colliculus.[7-9] Although the superior colliculus is not essential for programming all types of saccades,[10] it does seem necessary for generation of saccades at short latency to visual stimuli (so-called express saccades).[11] The dorsal layers of the superior colliculus are visual in terms of function and connections, and contain a retinotopic "place-map" in which the fovea is represented anteriorly and the visual periphery posteriorly, with the upper fields on the medial border and the lower fields on the lateral border.[12] Both these dorsal layers and cortical areas project visual signals to the ventral layers of the superior colliculus,[7,13] which contain a "motor map" that is in polar coordinates.[14] Stimulation of the ventral layers causes saccades with a contralateral horizontal component; the direction and size of the saccade is a function of the *site* of stimulation, not the strength of stimulation (i.e., a motor place-map).[14] Saccades of similar magnitude correspond to lines running medial-to-lateral (largest with stimulation caudally), and saccades of similar direction correspond to lines running anterior to posterior. Thus, the motor map of the ventral superior colliculus encodes the saccadic *desired displacement vector*. The ventral layers of superior colliculus are known to project to the reticular burst neurons that generate the premotor command for saccades, and which, in turn, project monosynaptically to the ocular motoneurons. Thus, the reticular burst neurons also play a crucial role in the spatial-temporal transformation of the programs for saccades.

ELECTROPHYSIOLOGICAL PROPERTIES OF SACCADIC BURST NEURONS OF THE BRAIN-STEM RETICULAR FORMATION

The ocular motoneurons receive the command for horizontal saccadic eye movements from burst neurons in the paramedian pontine reticular formation (PPRF) and the command for vertical saccades from burst neurons in the rostral interstitial nucleus of the medial longitudinal fasciculus (riMLF), which lies in the prerubral fields of the rostral midbrain.[15-17] The burst neurons are so called because of their high-frequency discharge, which occurs just before and during a saccade. The signal for a saccade is temporally encoded: the peak velocity of the saccade is related to the maximal rate of the burst (in spikes/second), and the size of the eye movement is related to the total number of spikes discharged. Except during saccades, both sets of burst neurons are held silent by monosynaptic projections from omnipause neurons that lie in the nucleus raphe interpositus of the pons.[18,19] The omnipause neurons are so called because they pause their inhibitory discharge for *all* saccades, horizontal, vertical, or oblique.

The motor layers of the superior colliculus project to burst neurons, and so a spatial-to-temporal transformation of neural signals must occur at this level. Another issue is whether the *polar* place-map of the superior colliculus is transformed to Cartesian mapping in the two set of burst neurons. In other words, how independent are the two populations in the PPRF and riMLF? This becomes an issue during programming of oblique saccades, when the activity of the two separate populations of neurons needs to be coordinated. A key point is that the duration of a saccade is related to the size of the movement—bigger movements take longer.

In one view of the way that oblique saccades are programmed—the "common source" model—the command from the burst neurons is specified in polar coordinates: an oblique (radial) velocity at angle Θ.[20] Then, neural circuitry converts this into a signal multiplied by cosineΘ for the horizontal motoneurons and a signal multiplied by sineΘ for the vertical motoneurons. Important predictions of this model are (1) the horizontal and vertical components of oblique saccades may have different durations than when similar sized movements are made as purely horizontal or vertical saccades; (2) the horizontal and vertical components will have synchronous onset and offset; and (3) the trajectory of the oblique saccade will be straight. An alternative hypothesis—the Cartesian coordinate model—proposes that the central command for the oblique saccade is broken down into horizontal and vertical components before being sent to the horizontal and vertical burst neurons.[21,22] The critical predictions of this model are (1) the horizontal and vertical saccadic components of oblique saccades will have the same duration as when made as purely horizontal or vertical saccades; (2) although the horizontal and vertical components of oblique saccades will have a synchronous onset, they may end at different times; and (3) the trajectory of oblique saccades could be curved. The nature of coding in the motor map of the superior colliculus (polar coordinates) might be interpreted as favoring the common-source model. Another observation supporting the common source model is that, at least in monkey, the duration of the smaller component of an oblique saccade is prolonged (i.e., slowed down) so that the trajectory of the saccade is straight.

TESTS OF MODELS FOR OBLIQUE SACCADE GENERATION

Recently, we have studied oblique saccades in three patients with Niemann-Pick type C disease.[23] All showed a selective defect of vertical saccades, which were slow and hypometric. Horizontal saccades were similar in velocity and accuracy to age-matched control subjects. Furthermore, horizontal and vertical pursuit and vestibular eye movements were normal. The initial movement of oblique saccades was mainly horizontal and most of the vertical component occurred after the horizontal component ended; this resulted in strongly curved trajectories compared with control subjects (FIG. 1A and B). After completion of the horizontal component of an oblique saccade, the eyes oscillated horizontally at 10–20 Hz until the vertical component ended (FIG. 1C). We postulated that the omnipause neurons were silent until the vertical component was completed and that the horizontal oscillations

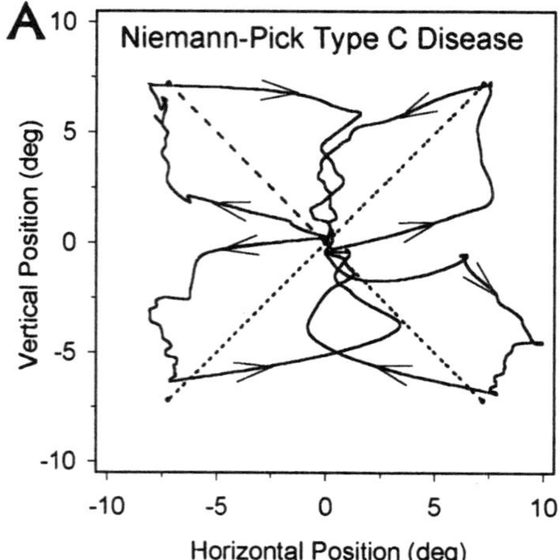

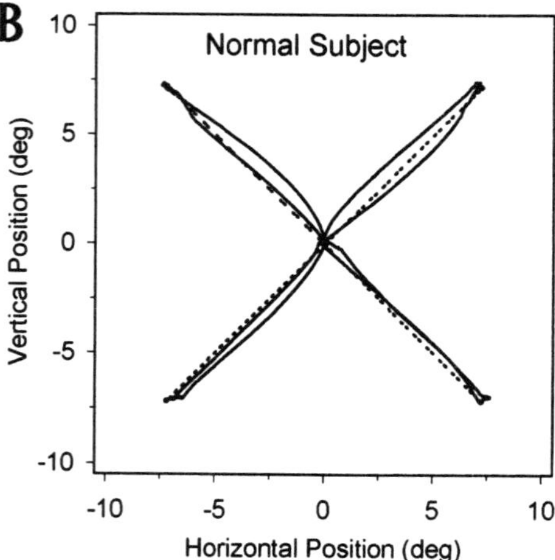

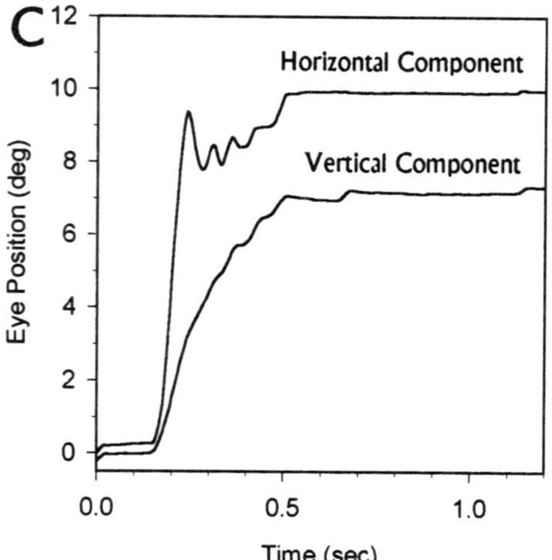

FIGURE 1. Tests of models for generation of oblique saccades. (**A**) Comparison of trajectories of oblique saccades made to and from four target positions starting at primary position in a patient with Niemann-Pick type C disease and (**B**) in an age-matched control subject. Arrowheads indicate the direction of eye movement. The trajectory of the target jump is shown as a dotted line. The trajectories of the patient's saccades are strongly curved, reflecting the initial, faster, horizontal component and the later, slower, vertical component. (**C**) Time plot comparing horizontal and vertical components of an oblique saccade made by a patient with Niemann-Pick type C disease. Horizontal oscillations occurred after the horizontal component had ended, but while the vertical component was still going on.

reflected the known instability of burst neurons.[17,24] Taken together, these data strongly support the Cartesian coordinate model.

Nichols and Sparks have also tested these two models by electrically stimulating the superior colliculus during oblique saccades. They produced perturbations of trajectory that supported the Cartesian coordinate model.[25] To resolve the issue of how oblique saccades may have a straight trajectory in monkeys, they propose that prolongation of the smaller component is achieved downstream from the colliculus, by cross-coupling between the horizontal and vertical burst neurons.[21,22,25]

THE POSSIBLE ROLE OF LOCAL FEEDBACK IN THE GENERATION OF SACCADES

Up until this point, we have considered the control of visually guided saccades as an "open-loop" process: the eye movement is programmed to move the image of the target from its position in the retinal periphery to the fovea (FIG. 2A). In other words, the saccade size is driven by desired change in eye position, which is computed from "retinal error." Certainly, the substantial delays inherent in the visual system (> 100 ms) prevent visual correction of errors sensed during the saccade itself (< 100 ms). However, several lines of experimental evidence suggested that the brain takes into account current eye position during a saccade and led D. A. Robinson to propose that the generation of saccades was under local feedback control in the brain stem.[26] The evidence for such local feedback rests on several observations:

1. If a saccade is transiently stopped in mid-flight by electrically stimulating the omnipause neurons, then immediately afterwards the saccade recommences its trajectory at a latency much shorter than could be accounted for by responding to the visual consequences of the arrested movements.[27]
2. If a target is briefly flashed on the fovea during a saccade made in darkness, an eye movement can be made back to that target, even though the visual information does not specify its position.[28]
3. If the eye is driven off-target during a saccade by electrically stimulating the superior colliculus, an appropriate compensatory movement is made, even without visual stimuli.[29]

In Robinson's scheme, the motor signal is continuously compared with an internal representation of the desired movement to determine how far the eye has moved compared with how far it needs to go. Recent evidence[30] suggests that the superior colliculus may be the site of this comparison (FIG. 2B). However, as pointed out above, the representation of the desired eye movement in the ventral layers of the superior colliculus and the motor signal for the saccade on the burst neurons are quite different. This raises one additional problem: How can the brain compare signals with such different representations?

POSSIBLE ROLE OF THE SUPERIOR COLLICULUS IN THE FEEDBACK CONTROL OF SACCADES

The case for suggesting that the superior colliculus contributes to feedback control of saccades rests on the demonstration that certain populations of its neurons

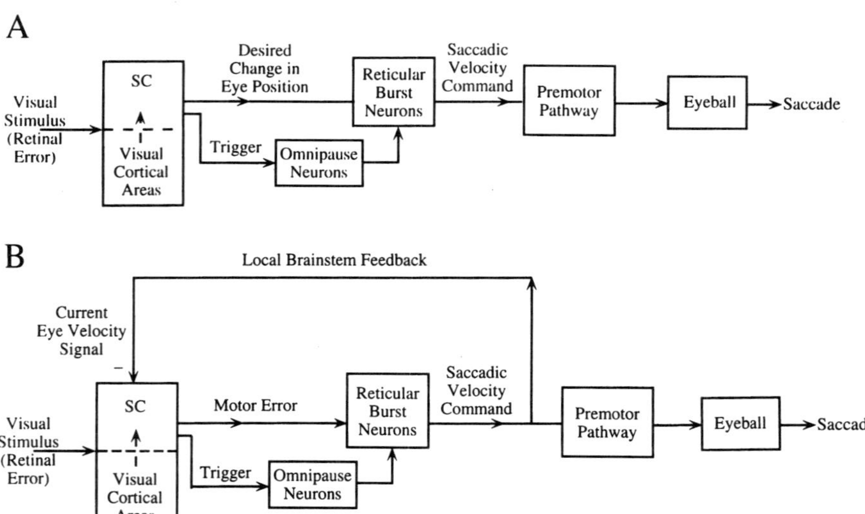

FIGURE 2. Simplified models for generation of visually guided saccades. (**A**). In this "open-loop" scheme, the visual stimulus for the saccade is retinal error (change in target position minus current eye position). This visual stimulus for the saccade is encoded in place maps in visual cortical areas and the superior colliculus (SC). The ventral layers of the SC provide a signal for desired change in eye position, and also the trigger signal that turns omnipause neurons off and allows reticular burst neurons to commence discharge. The burst neurons generate a saccadic velocity command, which is temporally encoded and which projects both directly and indirectly to ocular motoneurons (premotor pathway) to move the eye in a saccade. (**B**). In this scheme, a current eye velocity signal (temporally encoded) is continuously fed back and compared with the desired change in eye position (spatially encoded) to compute motor error. The superior colliculus is shown as the site at which the temporal-spatial transformations and computation of motor error occur. Similar schemes[30] and alternatives[32,33] for the role of the superior colliculus in the feedback control of saccades are discussed in the text.

encode signals that imply a continuous comparison between how far the eye has moved compared with how far it needs to go. The difference between current eye displacement and desired eye displacement is called the "motor error." Within the motor map of the ventral layers of the superior colliculus lie "collicular-burst" neurons. The location on the motor map at which collicular-burst cells are active remains the same throughout the eye movement, and is determined by the size of the saccade. It has been suggested that the discharge of collicular-burst neurons, which progressively declines throughout the saccade, might encode motor error.[30] However, further studies have suggested that these collicular-burst neurons are more likely to encode desired change in eye position.[27,31]

Lying more ventral to the collicular-burst neurons are cells with quite different electrophysiological properties: fixation neurons and build-up neurons.[8,9] The fixation neurons lie at the rostral pole of the superior colliculus and may suppress saccades via projections to omnipause neurons and by inhibiting collicular-burst neurons. Thus, cessation of activity of the fixation cells in superior colliculus plays a key role in the generation of express saccades. When a visual stimulus becomes the target for a saccade, build-up neurons start to discharge at a site on the motor map related to the amplitude and direction of the upcoming saccade. Subsequently, the activity of fixation neurons starts to decline, and a rostral spread of activity of build-up neurons occurs from the initial site of activity (corresponding to the size and direction of the upcoming saccade) towards the fixation zone (i.e., no saccade).[9] It has been postulated that this spread of activity may contribute to the transformations of signals that are required before motor error can be computed.[32,33] In support of this scheme, selective inactivation of the rostral pole of the superior colliculus causes disruption of steady fixation by saccadic intrusions.[34] On the other hand, pharmacological inactivation of the more caudal portions of the superior colliculus with muscimol causes impaired initiation of saccades, which are hypometric and slow.[35]

Optican has extended this scheme for feedback control of saccades by the superior colliculus, drawing attention to nonlinear relationships ("warping") between the visual field and collicular place-maps.[32,33] He has proposed that the superior colliculus provides two separate signals: the collicular-burst cells provide the reticular burst neurons with a signal encoding *desired* change in eye position. On the other hand, the build-up layer of neurons provide the reticular burst neurons with a signal encoding *current* change in eye position. These two signals undergo a spatial-to-temporal transformation before they are compared by reticular neurons to compute motor error. Note that the build-up layer receives a temporally encoded eye velocity command from the reticular burst neurons. In this scheme, the rostrally spreading wave of activity in the build-up layers acts as a spatial integrator within the local feedback loop controlling saccade generation. Thus, it is the distribution of activity across the map, rather than the average discharge rate of the population of neurons, that enacts the integration required to calculate current change in eye position. Thus, in this scheme, the superior colliculus carries out three distinctly different functions: (1) the fixation neurons control the trigger for saccade onset through their projections to omnipause neurons; (2) the collicular-burst neurons encode the desired change in eye position that the saccade must achieve; and (3) the build-up neurons contribute to feedback control of the saccades by computing current change in eye position. This model is currently being tested by the techniques of pharmacological inactivation and microstimulation during saccades.

Lesions restricted to the superior colliculus in humans are rare; however, disease often involves the adjacent mesencephalic reticular formation, in which lie "long-lead" reticular burst neurons that may provide the build-up neurons of the superior colliculus with the current eye velocity signal.[36] It has been shown that lesions in the mesencephalic reticular formation cause both slow and hypometric saccades (both horizontally and vertically), and cause inappropriate saccades that intrude on steady fixation ("square wave jerks");[37,38] this constellation of findings is typical of certain parkinsonian disorders, especially progressive supranuclear palsy.[39]

SUMMARY

The visual stimulus for a saccadic eye movement is encoded in place-coded maps in cerebral cortex and the dorsal superior colliculus. In contrast, the motor command for the saccade is encoded by the temporal discharge properties of ocular motoneurons and premotor burst neurons in the brain-stem reticular formation. Thus, there is need for a spatial-temporal transformation of neural signals, and recent findings suggest that the superior colliculus might contribute to this process. The ventral, output layers of the superior colliculus encode the metric of the desired saccade in polar coordinates. However, premotor neurons in the pontine and mesencephalic reticular formation are organized to generate horizontal and vertical saccades, respectively. Studies of oblique saccades in patients with slow vertical components—due to Niemann-Pick type C disease—support the interpretation that the saccadic command from the reticular formation is encoded in Cartesian coordinates. Currently, saccades are thought to be generated under local, brain-stem feedback control in which current eye displacement is continuously subtracted from desired eye displacement to compute motor error—the remaining movement required for the eye to acquire the target. If the superior colliculus is positioned in the feedback loop, then there is a need for transformation of premotor signals back into a place-coded version of motor error. Recent studies suggest that, during the saccade, this might be achieved by a wave of activity spreading rostrally, which traverses the collicular map in a direction corresponding to progressively smaller movements and finally activates a group of neurons concerned with fixation. These new hypotheses are ripe for testing by basic and clinical studies. By confronting the issue of what signal transformations are required to program visually guided saccades, new experimental approaches have emerged. Such computational approaches offer insights into how the brain controls behavior not just by measuring stimulus and response, but by asking what "currency" is being used by interacting populations of neurons at any stage in the process.

ACKNOWLEDGMENTS

We are grateful to Lance M. Optican, Ph.D., for helpful advice and Adriana Kori, M.D., for critically reading the manuscript.

REFERENCES

1. PLUM, F. & J. B. POSNER. 1981. Diagnosis of stupor and coma. 3rd edit. F. A. Davis. Philadelphia, PA.
2. KELLER, E. L. & D. A. ROBINSON. 1971. Absence of a stretch reflex in extraocular muscles of the monkey. J. Neurophysiol. **34:** 908–919.
3. ROBINSON, D. A. & E. L. KELLER. 1972. The behavior of eye movement motoneurons in the alert monkey. Bibl. Ophthalmol. **82:** 7–16.
4. LEIGH, R. J. & D. S. ZEE. 1991. The Neurology of Eye Movements. 2nd edit. F. A. Davis. Philadelphia. PA.
5. HORTON, J. C. & W. F. HOYT. 1991. The representation of the visual field in human striate cortex. A revision of the classic Holmes map. Arch. Ophthalmol. **109:** 816–824.
6. FUCHS, A. F., C. A. SCUDDER & C. R. S. KANEKO. 1988. Discharge patterns and recruitment order of identified motoneurons and internuclear neurons in the monkey abducens nucleus. J. Neurophysiol. **60:** 1874–1895.
7. SPARKS, D. L. & R. HARTWICH-YOUNG. 1989. The deep layers of the superior colliculus. *In* The Neurobiology of Saccadic Eye Movements. R. H. Wurtz & M. E. Goldberg, Eds: 213–255. Elsevier. Amsterdam.
8. MUNOZ, D. P. & R. H. WURTZ. 1995. Saccade-related activity in monkey superior colliculus. I. Characteristics of burst and buildup cells. J. Neurophysiol. **73:** 2313–2333.
9. MUNOZ, D. P. & R. H. WURTZ. 1995. Saccade-related activity in monkey superior colliculus. II. Spread of activity during saccades. J. Neurophysiol. **73:** 2334–2348.
10. SCHILLER, P. H., S. D. TRUE & J. L. CONWAY. 1980. Deficits in eye movements following frontal eye-field and superior colliculus ablations. J. Neurophysiol. **44:** 1175–1189.
11. SCHILLER, P. H., J. H. SANDELL & J. H. R. MAUNSELL. 1987. The effect of frontal eye

field and superior colliculus lesions on saccadic latencies in the rhesus monkey. J. Neurophysiol. **57:** 1033–1049.

12. CYNADER, M. & N. BERMAN. 1972. Receptive-field organization of monkey superior colliculus. J. Neurophysiol. **35:** 187–200.

13. MOSCHOVAKIS, A. K. & S. M. HIGHSTEIN. 1994. The anatomy and physiology of primate neurons that control rapid eye movements. Annu. Rev. Neurosci. **17:** 465–488.

14. ROBINSON, D. A. 1972. Eye movements evoked by collicular stimulation in the alert monkey. Vision Res. **12:** 1795–1808.

15. BÜTTNER-ENNEVER, J. A. & U. BÜTTNER. 1988. The reticular formation. *In* Neuroanatomy of the Oculomotor System. Reviews of Oculomotor Research. J. A. Büttner-Ennever, Ed. Vol. 2: 119–176. Elsevier. Amsterdam.

16. HEPP, K., V. HENN, T. VILIS & B. COHEN. 1989. Brainstem regions related to saccade generation. *In* The Neurobiology of Saccadic Eye Movements. R. H. Wurtz & M. E. Goldberg, Eds: 105–212. Elsevier. Amsterdam.

17. VAN GISBERGEN, J. A. M., D. A. ROBINSON & S. GIELEN. 1981. A quantitative analysis of generation of saccadic eye movements by burst neurons. J. Neurophysiol. **45:** 417–442.

18. LANGER, T. & C. R. S. KANEKO. 1990. Brainstem afferents to the oculomotor omnipause neurons in monkey. J. Comp. Neurol. **295:** 413–427.

19. BÜTTNER-ENNEVER, J. A., B. COHEN, M. PAUSE & W. FRIES. 1988. Raphe nucleus of the pons containing omnipause neurons of the oculomotor system in the monkey, and its homologue in man. J. Comp. Neurol. **267:** 307–321.

20. VAN GISBERGEN, J. A. M, A. J. VAN OOPSTAL & J. J. M. SCHOENMAKERS. 1985. Experimental test of two models for the generation of oblique saccades. Exp. Brain Res. **57:** 321–336.

21. GROSSMAN, G. E. & D. A. ROBINSON. 1988. Ambivalence in modelling oblique saccades. Biol. Cybern. **58:** 13–18.

22. BECKER, W. & R. JÜRGENS. 1990. Human oblique saccades: Quantitative analysis of the relation between horizontal and vertical components. Vision Res. **30:** 893–920.

23. ROTTACH, K. G., R. D. VON MAYDELL, V. E. DAS, A. Z. ZIVOTOFSKY, A. O. DISCENNA, J. L. GORDON, D. M. D. LANDIS & R. J. LEIGH. 1996. Evidence for independent feedback control of horizontal and vertical saccades from Neimann-Pick type C disease. Vision Res. In press.

24. ZEE, D. S. & D. A. ROBINSON. 1979. A hypothetical explanation of saccadic oscillations. Ann. Neurol **5:** 405–414.

25. NICHOLS, M. J. & D. L. SPARKS. 1995. Component stretching during oblique stimulation-evoked saccades: The role of the superior colliculus. J. Neurophysiol. **76:** 582–600.

26. ROBINSON, D. A. 1975. Oculomotor control signals. *In* Basic Mechanisms of Ocular Motility and their Clinical Implications. G. Lennerstrand & P. Bach-y-Rita, Eds.: 337–374. Pergamon Press. Oxford.

27. KELLER, E. L. & J. A. EDELMAN. 1994. Use of interrupted saccade paradigm to study spatial and temporal dynamics of saccadic burst cells in superior colliculus in monkey. J. Neurophysiol. **72:** 2754–2770.

28. HALLETT, P. E. & A. D. LIGHTSTONE. 1976. Saccadic eye movements to flashed targets. Vision Res. **16:** 107–114.

29. SPARKS, D. L. & L. E. MAYS. 1983. Spatial localization of saccade targets. I. Compensation for stimulation induced perturbations in eye position. J. Neurophysiol. **49:** 45–63.

30. WAITZMAN, D. M., T. P. MA, L. M. OPTICAN & R. H. WURTZ. 1991. Superior colliculus neurons mediate the dynamic characteristics of saccades. J. Neurophysiol. **66:** 1716–1737.

31. MUNOZ, P., D. M. WAITZMAN & R. H. WURTZ. 1996. Activity of neurons in monkey superior colliculus during interrupted saccades. J. Neurophysiol. **75:** 2562–2580.

32. OPTICAN, L. M. 1995. A field theory of saccade generation: Temporal-to-spatial transform in the superior colliculus. Vision Res. **35:** 3313–3320.

33. OPTICAN, L. M. 1994. Control of saccade trajectory by the superior colliculus. *In* Contemporary Ocular Motor and Vestibular Research. A Tribute to David A. Robinson.

A. F. Fuchs, Th. Brandt, U. Büttner & D. S. Zee, Eds.: 98–105. Thieme Verlag. Stuttgart.

34. MUNOZ, D. P. & R. H. WURTZ. 1993. Fixation cells in monkey superior colliculus. II. Reversible activation and deactivation. J. Neurophysiol. **70:** 576–589.

35. HIKOSAKA, O. & R. H. WURTZ. 1985. Modification of saccadic eye movements by GABA-related substances. I. Effect of muscimol and bicuculline in monkey superior colliculus. J. Neurophysiol. **53:** 266–291.

36. WAITZMAN, D. M., V. L. SILAKOV & B. COHEN. 1996. Central mesencephalic reticular formation (cMRF) neurons discharging before and during eye movements. J. Neurophysiol. **75:** 1546–1572.

37. SILAKOV, V. L. & D. M. WAITZMAN. 1996. Changes of remembered saccades and fixation during temporary inactivation of the mesencephalic reticular formation (MRF). Soc. Neurosci. Abstr. **22:** 665.

38. WAITZMAN, D. M. & V. L. SILAKOV. 1996. Effects of ibotenic acid (IBO) lesions of the mesencephalic reticular formation (MRF) on primate saccades. Soc. Neurosci. Abstr. **22:** 665.

39. ROTTACH, K. G., D. E. RILEY, A. O. DiSCENNA, A. Z. ZIVOTOFSKY & R. J. LEIGH. 1996. Dynamic properties of horizontal and vertical eye movements in parkinsonian syndromes. Ann. Neurol. **39:** 368–377.

A Pivotal Role of Nitric Oxide in Migraine Pain

LARS LYKKE THOMSEN[a] AND JES OLESEN

Department of Neurology
Glostrup Hospital
University of Copenhagen
Glostrup, Denmark

INTRODUCTION

In 1980 Furchgott and Zawadzki reported that vasodilatation induced by acetylcholine depends on the presence of intact endothelium.[1] The mediator of this endothelium-dependent vasodilatation was identified some years later as nitric oxide (NO), which previously was considered merely to be an atmospheric pollutant.[2] Since then the biology of this small and short-lived messenger molecule has been increasingly and very intensively investigated. Today a vast amount of knowledge is available regarding the biology of NO, and an increasing volume of evidence suggests that nitric oxide plays a pivotal role in migraine pain (for reviews see refs. 3–5). The present review focuses on this new knowledge.

BIOLOGY OF NITRIC OXIDE RELEVANT TO MIGRAINE

The highly reactive free radical NO is a lipophilic gas of formula $\cdot N = O$.[6] The half-life of NO is reported to be very short, in the range of 5–30 s under bioassay conditions.[2,6] NO is rapidly converted to nitrogen dioxide (NO_2), which again rapidly forms the more stable metabolites nitrite (NO_2^-) and nitrate (NO_3^-).[7] NO is generated from the terminal guanidino nitrogen of L-arginine. The family of enzymes catalyzing NO synthesis is known as NO synthases (NOS) (for review see ref. 8). NOS activity has been reported in many tissues including endothelium, brain, peripheral nerves, vascular smooth muscle, myocardium, macrophages, neutrophils, and microglia of several species (for review see ref. 6). Purification and cloning of NOS has revealed the existence of at least three isoforms.[8] Two of these are constitutive, Ca^{2+}/calmodulin dependent (cNOS) and release NO from, for example, endothelium (eNOS) and neurons (nNOS). This release is accelerated in response to stimulation of several specific membrane-bound receptors by, for example, glutamate, bradykinin, 5-HT, acetylcholine, histamine, endothelin-1, substance P, and probably calcitonin-gene-related peptide (CGRP)[9–15] (FIG. 1). Increased flow velocity and the subsequent increase of shear stress in endothelial cells may also stimulate eNOS.[9] Another NO synthase is inducible and Ca^{2+} independent (iNOS). iNOS generates NO for long periods and in large amounts in response to endotoxins and cytokines.[16–18] Most physiological actions of NO are mediated via activation of

---

[a] Address correspondence to Lars Lykke Thomsen, M.D., Ph.D., Department of Neurology, Glostrup Hospital, Ndr Ringvej 57, DK-2600 Glostrup, Denmark.

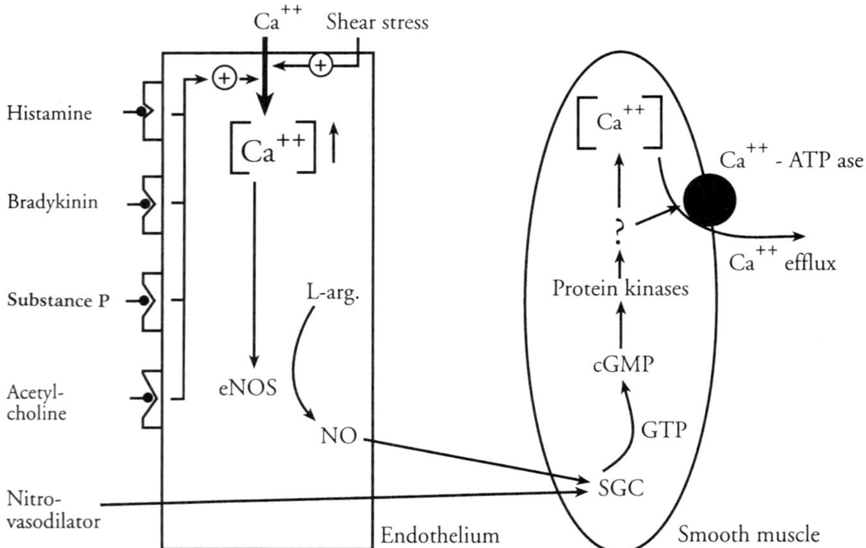

FIGURE 1. Molecular events in the nitric oxide (NO) pathway illustrated by endothelium-derived synthesis of NO. Endothelium NO synthase (eNOS) is stimulated by an increase in intracellular calcium. NO diffuses from endothelial cells to smooth muscle cells and activates the soluble guanylate cyclase (cGC). This in turn leads to an increase in cyclic guanosine monophosphate (cGMP) and via activation of protein kinases and subsequent poorly understood intermediary processes stimulates the membrane bound Ca^{2+} ATPase. Ca^{2+} then diffuses out of the cell, eventually leading to smooth muscle relaxation and vasodilatation. Nitrovasodilators act as NO donors and activate the same pathway.

soluble guanylate cyclase (sGC) and a consequent increase in cyclic guanosine monophosphate (cGMP), eventually leading to a decrease in intracellular Ca^{2+} in target cells (for reviews see refs. 19 and 20).

Nitric oxide has an amazing number of physiological effects throughout the body of which several, theoretically, may be implicated in the pathophysiology of migraine. Thus, endothelium-dependent vasodilatation is of importance in cerebrovascular regulation, and in addition neurogenic vasodilatation may be mediated via perivascular nerves, which operate through NO (nonadrenergic, noncholinergic nerves). Furthermore, NO mediates neurotransmission in the central nervous system, which is important for pain perception (hyperalgesia). NO may also contribute to sensory transmission in peripheral nerves. Moreover, NO contributes to the control of platelets and, when produced in large amounts, NO contributes to host defense reactions important in nonspecific immunity and neurotoxicity (for review see ref. 19). Finally, NO may release CGRP from perivascular nerve endings and may thus play a role in neurogenic inflammatory reactions.[21]

EXPERIMENTAL MODELS OF HUMAN HEADACHE SUITABLE FOR THE STUDY OF NITRIC OXIDE MECHANISMS IN MIGRAINE

Histamine and glyceryl trinitrate (GTN) are substances that reliably and dose dependently produce headache in normal volunteers and migraine sufferers.[22–24]

GTN itself has no known action in the human body but acts to liberate NO and is thus generally regarded as an NO donor.[25–27] GTN is the most suitable substance for experimental studies of NO-induced headache because it is well tolerated and diffuses freely across membranes due to its lipid solubility. It may thus deliver NO to several tissues including those protected by the blood–brain barrier.

The following observations support that GTN induces headache by liberating NO:

- GTN-induced headache in normal controls is very short-lived and is therefore unlikely to be caused by metabolites other than NO, because these have a longer half-life.[23]
- The long-acting nitrate 5-isosorbide-mononitrate (5-ISMN) induces a dose-dependent headache and arterial dilatation but its metabolites, apart from NO, are different from those of GTN.[28]
- N-Acetylcysteine, which augments GTN effects in the heart by increasing the formation of NO or by enhancing the effect of NO itself, also augments the headache response to GTN and prolongs GTN-induced arterial dilatation of the superficial temporal artery, but not of the radial arteries.[29]

Histamine also seems to induce headache via NO. Thus, in human cerebral blood vessels histamine stimulates an endothelial H_1 receptor, which activates nitric oxide synthase (NOS).[12,13,30] Histamine thus stimulates the endogenous formation of NO whereas GTN delivers NO directly. The next question is how relevant are these observations for migraine?

NITRIC OXIDE SUPERSENSITIVITY IN MIGRAINE

Previous studies have suggested that migraine patients experience a migraine-like headache in association with nitroglycerin administration more often than do non-migraineurs.[31] Most recently it has been confirmed in controlled double-blind trials that migraineurs with a time-delay of several hours (peak intensity 5.5 h after nitroglycerin infusion) actually develop a genuine migraine attack after nitroglycerin infusion[24,32] (FIG. 2). This migraine headache is preceded by an immediate headache response during the infusion, resembling but not fulfilling diagnostic criteria for migraine without aura (International Headache Society [IHS] criteria).

The immediate headache response, which also is seen in non-migraineurs, is more severe in migraineurs[24] (FIG. 3). Thus, migraineurs are hypersensitive to nitroglycerin-induced headache and most likely therefore to nitric oxide. An increased headache response could, however, reflect a greater general sensitivity to pain, or it could be due to increased physiological sensitivity to NO. It is well known that nitroglycerin dilates the middle cerebral artery via NO without affecting cerebral blood flow and thereby the arterioles.[33,34] Applying the ultrasound technique transcranial Doppler,[35] which provides an indirect measure of large intracranial artery diameters in situations of unchanged blood flow,[33,34,36,37] we examined whether the increased sensitivity to the NO donor was reflected not only in increased headache in migraineurs but also in increased dilatation of the middle cerebral artery. Indeed, migraineurs were found to be more sensitive in this aspect as well. During a 3-h observation period, the time profile of the nitroglycerin-induced middle cerebral artery dilatation corresponded with the headache response.[32,38] Furthermore, a decreased aggregation of platelets to collagen in combination with increased

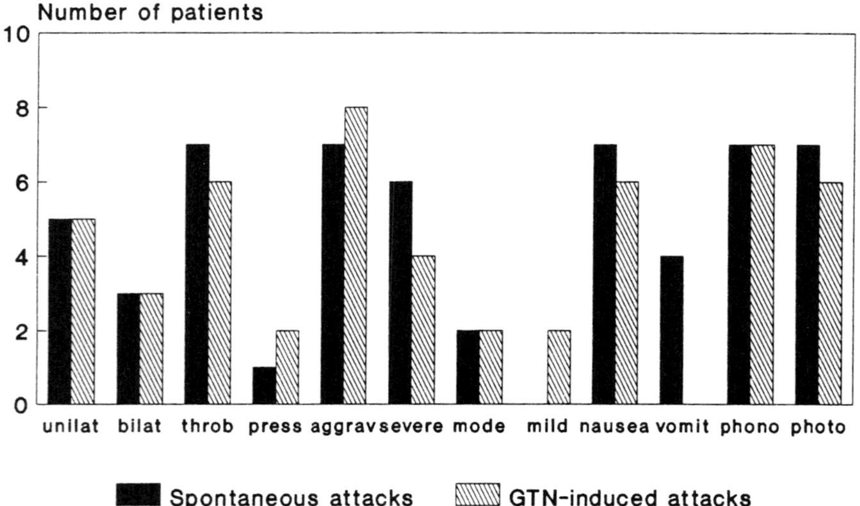

FIGURE 2. Clinical characteristics of glyceryl trinitrate (GTN)-induced migraines. A comparison between spontaneous and GTN-induced migraine in 8 out of 10 migraine patients who developed migraine after GTN infusion (0.5 μg/kg/min, for 20 min) is illustrated. The peak intensity of GTN-induced migraine occurred on average 5.5 h after the start of infusion. (Data from Thomsen *et al.*[32]) *Abbreviations*: Unilat, unilateral; bilat, bilateral; throb, throbbing; aggrav, aggravation by physical activity; mode, moderate; phono, phonophobia; photo, photophobia.

platelet arginine levels in migraineurs support that migraineurs are supersensitive to physiological effects of NO.[39]

Moreover, migraineurs have been found to be hypersensitive to histamine regarding headache development in controlled trials.[22,40] The headache induced during histamine infusion was almost completely blocked by the histamine H_1-blocker, mepyramine, whereas the H_2-blocker, cimetidine, only had a small effect.[22] In a recent double-blind controlled trial, migraineurs were randomized to pretreatment with either mepyramine or placebo before histamine infusion. One-half of the patients pretreated with placebo developed, besides the immediate headache during the histamine infusion, a delayed migraine attack fulfilling the IHS criteria for migraine without aura. The peak intensity of this histamine-induced migraine attack was reached 5.1 h after the infusion. The patients pretreated with mepyramine only developed a very mild headache, if any.[41] It is highly interesting that the temporal profile of the induced headache was exactly the same as that after the infusion of GTN. As mentioned above, activation of endothelial H_1-receptors induce the formation of endogenous nitric oxide.[12,13] Thus, the increased sensitivity to histamine in migraineurs may also be explained by hypersensitivity to activation of the NO pathway, and activation of this pathway is likely to be a final common pathway for the headache and arterial dilatation induced by both histamine and GTN. Further evidence for the latter has recently been supplied by the finding that GTN-induced headache could not be prevented by histamine H_1-receptor blocking, indicating that the final common mechanism of histamine- and GTN-induced headache is not explained by histamine release after GTN infusion.[42]

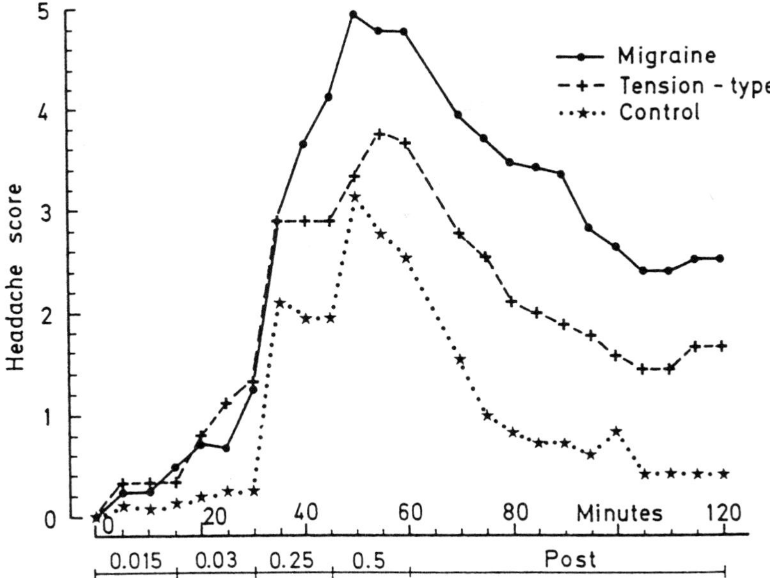

FIGURE 3. Headache intensity over time during four different doses of nitroglycerin. Comparison between responses in migraineurs ($n = 17$), tension-type headache sufferers ($n = 9$), and healthy subjects ($n = 17$). During doses above 0.015 μg/kg/min migraine patients experienced significantly more headaches than did controls ($p < 0.05$ Kruskal Wallis and multiple range test). (From Olesen et al.[24] Reprinted with permission from *Neuroreport*.)

NITRIC OXIDE, A FINAL COMMON PATHWAY FOR SEVERAL MIGRAINE TRIGGERS

In addition to GTN and histamine, other substances, which have been shown to reliably cause more headache than placebo in single-dose experiments including reserpine, metachlorophenyl-piperazine (mCPP), postacyclin and hypoxia, may cause headache via NO.[5] The best-known example of hypoxic headache is high altitude headache. However, no formal study of the effects of hypoxia in migraine sufferers is available. Recently, it was shown that persons living at high altitudes had a huge increase in the prevalence of migraine.[43] Hypoxia increases longevity of NO whereas pure oxygen acts as a NO scavenger reducing the lifetime and thereby the effect of NO.[44] Hypoxic vascular headache and hypoxia-induced migraine may thus be due to increased spontaneous NO concentration. In one study prostacyclin has been shown to cause headache in migraineurs.[45] Prostacyclin is a vasodilatator and may act directly on smooth muscle receptors but, in cerebral vessels protected by the blood–brain barrier, it is more likely to act through endothelial receptors by liberating NO.[9]

In migraineurs reserpine has been shown to cause headache with some migrainous features.[46] Reserpine depletes not only platelets but also presynaptic nerve terminals of their content of monoamines. Substances released include 5-HT. The 5-HT$_{2c}$ (formerly called 5-HT$_{1c}$) receptor has recently been suggested to play a crucial role in the initiation of migraine attacks.[47] 5-HT caused an endothelium-dependent relaxing response in a number of vessels from different species, and this effect was mediated through the 5-HT_{2c} receptor. The vascular response to 5-HT_{2c} activation, at least in the pig, is primarily a consequence of the release of NO.[14] mCPP is a direct agonist at the 5-HT_{2c} receptor and, therefore, is likely to cause vascular headache via NO synthesis.[47] We concluded that NO is a likely common denominator for headaches induced by GTN, histamine, reserpine, mCPP, prostacyclin, and hypoxia.[5]

POTENTIAL MECHANISMS OF NITRIC OXIDE-INDUCED MIGRAINE

At present it is not known in greater detail where and how activation of the NO pathway causes experimental migraine headache and how this trigger mechanism may be related to "natural" migraine triggers. Regarding the latter, natural triggers such as hormones, alcohol, and chocolate may elicit fluctuations in neurotransmitter concentrations both in brain and blood, which in turn may stimulate the formation of NO in brain neurons and arterial endothelium and may possibly also interact with NOS-containing nerve terminals.[9,19,48] Formation of NO may also be elicited by pathological reactions such as spreading depression of Leao, which is the proposed mechanism of the migraine aura.[49] In relation to the site where NO-mediated triggering events may be set up, speculations concerning histamine-induced migraines may be more helpful than speculations concerning GTN. Thus, whereas GTN diffuses freely across biological membranes, histamine does not cross the blood–brain barrier[50] and when administered systemically most likely works on endothelial receptors. Moreover, histamine only causes headache when injected into the internal, but not into the external, carotid artery.[51] Because of its short half-life, NO can only diffuse very short distances ($150\text{--}160~\mu\text{m}$ from a single cell).[52] If histamine-induced migraine headache is set up by H_1 activated liberation of NO, this is, therefore, likely to involve processes initiated within or just around the intracranial vasculature. Interestingly, human cerebral arteries are pain-sensitive structures. More than 50 years ago Ray and Wolff[53] described that in man the proximal parts of the large intracranial arteries composing the circle of Willis were sensitive to mechanical stimulation. These arteries became less sensitive over the hemispheric convexities. The quality of the induced pain was described as deep, intense, dull, and aching. The pain became throbbing when the stimulus was repeated, and when the stimulus was prolonged the pain was described to be associated with nausea.[53] More recently, Nichols et al.[54] showed that mechanical dilatation of human large cerebral arteries during balloon angioplasty in local anesthesia gave rise to pain referred to areas where migraine pain is most often experienced (FIG. 4). Thus, both the quality and location of pain elicited from the large intracranial arteries is similar to the clinical features during migraine headache. It is therefore interesting that NO is a powerful vasodilator and that dilatation of the large cranial arteries has been reported during spontaneous migraine headache.[37,55,56]

Another theoretical possibility is that central pain modulating effects of nitric oxide are involved. Animal studies suggest that NO plays a role in central modulation of nociception and produces hyperalgesia.[57,58] In man the role of NO in nociceptive modulation is largely unknown. A recent study examining the influence of intravenous infusion of four increasing doses of the NO-donor GTN on the perception of noxious stimulations in man did not clarify this issue but seemed to have ruled out that central hyperalgesia elicited by NO is involved in GTN-induced headaches. Thus, relative to placebo, GTN altered the measured pressure pain thresholds only

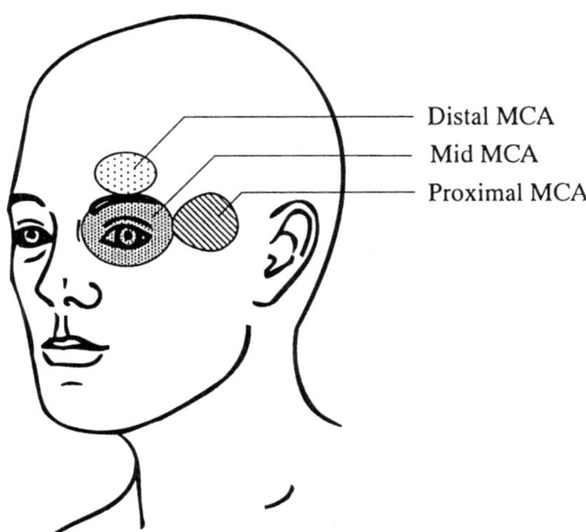

FIGURE 4. Areas of referred pain during middle cerebral artery (MCA) dilatation. Dilatation of large intracranial arteries is likely to be involved in spontaneous and NO-induced migraines. Shown are areas where pain is experienced during mechanical dilatation of the MCA. (Modified from Nichols *et al.*[54])

in one of three stimulated regions, and a response isolated to one of three stimulated regions suggests other mechanisms.

Direct activation of perivascular sensory nerve fibers[59] by NO may provide other possibilities. Experimental studies in rats have shown alterations in vascular permeability and ultrastructural changes in the dura mater as part of a so-called neurogenic inflammation induced by stimulation of the trigeminal ganglion. Based on the effect of several antimigraine drugs in this animal model, perivascular neurogenic inflammation has been hypothesized to play a key role in migraine.[59] Trigeminal ganglion stimulation has been shown to be associated with a release of CGRP and substance P also in man.[60] Interestingly, increased levels of CGRP from the external jugular vein has been demonstrated during migraine attacks.[61] Furthermore, sumatriptan returns the increased levels of CGRP during attacks to normal.[62] Animal studies have suggested that GTN—and therefore most likely also NO—may release CGRP from perivascular nerves at least around cerebral arterioles.[21] It is tempting to propose an increased sensitivity to such effects of NO in migraineurs, perhaps as part of a neurogenic inflammation around intracranial arteries. The release of involved peptides may in turn cause (1) prolonged vasodilatation, (2) sensitization of perivascular nociceptors, and (3) further release of NO from either perivascular nerve endings or endothelium (mediated by, for example, substance P). A circulus vitiosus may thus develop over time eventually leading to the fully developed migraine attack. The elucidation of whichever of the above hypotheses that turn out to be true represents fascinating challenges for the future that likely will provide new therapeutic approaches to migraine.

REFERENCES

1. FURCHGOTT R. F. & J. V. ZAWADZKI. 1980. The obligatory role of endothelial cells in the relaxation of arterial smooth muscle by acetylcholine. Nature **288:** 373–376.
2. PALMER, R. M. J., A. G. FERRIGE & S. MONCADA. 1987. Nitric oxide release accounts for the biological activity of endothelium-derived relaxing factor. Nature **327:** 524–526.

3. OLESEN, J., L. L. THOMSEN & H. K. IVERSEN. 1994. Nitric oxide is a key molecule in migraine and other vascular headaches. Trends Pharmacol. Sci. **15:** 149–153.

4. THOMSEN, L. L., H. K. IVERSEN, L. H. LASSEN & J. OLESEN. 1994. The role of nitric oxide in migraine pain: Therapeutic implications. CNS Drugs **2:** 417–422.

5. OLESEN, J., L. L. THOMSEN, L. H. LASSEN & I. JANSEN-OLESEN. 1995. The nitric oxide hypothesis of migraine and other vascular headaches. Cephalalgia **15:** 94–100.

6. KIECHLE, F. L. & T. MALINSKI. 1993. Nitric oxide biochemistry, pathophysiology and detection. Am. J. Clin. Pathol. **100:** 567–575.

7. WENNMALM, Å. & A PETERSON. 1991. Analysis of nitrite as a marker for endothelium-derived relaxing factor in bilogical fluids using electron paramagnetic resonance spectrometry. J. Cardiovasc. Pharmacol. **17:** s34–s40.

8. KNOWLES, R. G. & S. MONCADA. 1994. Nitric oxide synthases in mammals. Biochem. J. **298:** 249–258.

9. LÜSCHER, T. F. & P. M. VANHOUTTE. 1990. The endothelium: Modulator of cardiovascular functions. CRC Press. Boca Raton, FL.

10. GARTHWAITE, J. 1993. Nitric oxide signalling in the nervous system. The Neurosciences **5:** 171–180.

11. GRAY, D. W. & I. MARSHALL. 1992. Human alpha-calcitonin gene-related peptide stimulates adenylate cyclase and guanylate cyclase and relaxes rat thoracic aorta by releasing nitric oxide. Br. J. Pharmacol. **107:** 691–696.

12. TODA, N. 1990. Mechanism underlying responses to histamine of isolated monkey and human cerebral arteries. Am. J. Physiol. **258:** H311–H317.

13. AYAJIKI, K., T. OKAMURA & N. TODA. 1992. Involvement of nitric oxide in endothelium-dependent, phasic relaxation caused by histamine in monkey cerebral arteries. Jpn. J. Pharmacol. **60:** 357–362.

14. GLUSA, E. & M. RICHTER. 1993. Endothelium-dependent relaxation of porcine pulmonary arteries via 5-HT$_{1c}$-like receptors. Naunyn-Schmiedeberg's Arch. Pharmakol. **347:** 471–477.

15. DE NUCCI, G., R. THOMAS, P. D'ORLEANS-JUSTE, E. ANTUNES, C. WALDER, T. D. WARNER & J. R. VANE. 1988. Pressor effects of circulating endothelin are limited by its removal in the pulmonary circulation and by the release of prostacyclin and endothelium derived relaxing factor. Proc. Natl. Acad. Sci. USA **85:** 9797–9800.

16. STUEHR, D. J., H. J. CHO, N. S. KWON, M. F. WEISE & C. F. NATHAN. 1991. Purification and characterization of the cytokine-induced macrophage nitric oxide synthase: An FAD- and FMN-containing flavoprotein. Proc. Natl. Acad. Sci. USA **88:** 7773–7777.

17. BUSSE, R. & A. MÜLSCH. 1990. Induction of nitric oxide synthase by cytokines in vascular smooth muscle cells. FEBS Lett. **275:** 87–90.

18. WALLACE, M. N. & S. K. BISLAND. 1994. NADPH-diaphorase activity in activated astrocytes represents inducible nitric oxide synthase. Neuroscience **59:** 905–919.

19. MONCADA, S., R. M. J. PALMER & E. A. HIGGS. 1991. Nitric oxide: Physiology, pathophysiology and pharmacology. Pharmacol. Rev. **43:** 109–142.

20. MAYER B. 1994. Regulation of nitric oxide synthase and soluble guanylyl cyclase. Cell Biochem. Funct. **12:** 167–177.

21. WEI, E. P., M. A. MOSKOWITZ, P. BACCALINI & H. A. KONTOS. 1992. Calcitonon gene related peptide mediates nitroglycerin and sodium nitroprusside induced vasodilation in feline cerebral arterioles. Circ. Res. **70:** 1313–1319.

22. KRABBE, A. E. & J. OLESEN. 1980. Headache provocation by continuous intravenous infusion of histamine. Clinical results and receptor mechanisms. Pain **8:** 253–259.

23. IVERSEN, H. K., J. OLESEN & P. TFELT-HANSEN. 1989. Intravenous nitroglycerin as an experimental model of vascular headache. Basic Characteristics. Pain **38:** 17–24.

24. OLESEN, J., H. K. IVERSEN & L. L. THOMSEN. 1993. Nitric oxide supersensitivity. A possible molecular mechanism of migraine pain. Neuroreport **4:** 1027–1030.

25. GRUETTER, C. A., P. J. KADOWITZ & L. J. IGNARRO. 1981. Methylene blue inhibits coronary arterial relaxation and guanylate cyclase activation by nitroglycerin, sodium nitrate and amyl nitrate. Can. J. Physiol. Pharmacol. **59:** 150–156.

26. IGNARRO, L. J., H. LIPTON, J. C. EDWARDS, W. H. BARICOS, A. L. HYMAN, P. J. KADOWITZ & C. A. GRUETTER. 1981. Mechanisms of vascular smooth muscle relaxation

by organic nitrates, nitrites, nitroprusside and nitric oxide: Evidence for the involvement of S-nitrosothiols as active intermediates. J. Pharmacol. Exp. Ther. **218:** 739–749.

27. FEELISCH, M. & E. A. NOACK. 1987. Correlation between nitric oxide formation during degradation of organic nitrates and activation of guanylate cyclase. Eur. J. Pharmacol. **139:** 19–30.

28. IVERSEN, H. K., T. H. NIELSEN, K. GARRE, P. TFELT-HANSEN & J. OLESEN. 1992. Dose-dependent headache response and dilatation of limb and extracranial arteries after three doses of 5-isosorbide-mononitrate. Eur. J. Clin. Pharmacol. **42:** 31–35.

29. IVERSEN, H. K. 1992. N-acetylcysteine enhances nitroglycerin-induced headache and cranial arterial responses. Clin. Pharmacol. Ther. **52:** 125–133.

30. OTTOSEN, A. L. P., I. JANSEN, M. LANGEMARK, J. OLESEN & L. EDVINSSON. 1991. Histamine receptors in the isolated human middle meningeal artery. A comparison with cerebral and temporal arteries. Cephalalgia **11:** 183–188.

31. SICUTERI, F., E. DEL BENE, M. POGGIONI & A. BONAZZI. 1987. Unmasking latent dysnociception in healthy subjects. Headache **27:** 180–185.

32. THOMSEN, L. L., C. KRUUSE, H. K. IVERSEN & J. OLESEN. 1994. A nitric oxide donor (nitroglycerin) triggers genuine migraine attacks. Eur. J. Neurol. **1:** 73–80.

33. DAHL, A., D. RUSSELL, R. NYBERG-HANSEN & K. ROOTWELL. 1989. Effect of nitroglycerin on cerebral circulation measured by transcranial Doppler and SPECT. Stroke **20:** 1733–1736.

34. IVERSEN, H. K., S. HOLM & L. FRIBERG. 1989. Intracranial hemodynamics during intravenous nitroglycerin infusion. Cephalalgia **9(Suppl. 10):** 84–85.

35. THOMSEN, L. L. & H. K. IVERSEN. 1993. Experimental and biological variation of three dimensional transcranial doppler measurements. J. Appl. Physiol. **75:** 2805–2810.

36. BUSIJA, D. W., D. D. HEISTAD & M. L. MARCUS. 1981. Continuous measurements of cerebral blood flow in anesthetized cats and dogs. Am. J. Physiol. **241:** H228–H234.

37. FRIBERG, L., J. OLESEN, H. K. IVERSEN & B. SPERLING. 1991. Migraine pain associated with middle cerebral artery dilatation: Reversal by sumatriptan. Lancet **338:** 13–17.

38. THOMSEN, L. L., H. K. IVERSEN, T. A. BRINCK & J. OLESEN. 1993. Arterial supersensitivity to nitric oxide (nitroglycerin) in migraine sufferers. Cephalalgia **13:** 395–399.

39. D'ANDREA, G., A. R. CANANZI, F. FERINI, F. ALECCI, L. ZAMBERLAN, L. HASSELMARK & K. M. A. WELCH. 1994. Decreased collagen-induced platelet aggregation and increased arginine levels in migraine: A possible link with the NO pathway. Cephalalgia **14:** 352–357.

40. DE MARINIS, M., M. FELICIANI, L. JANIRI, R. CERBO & A. AGNOLI. 1990. Increased reactivity to a met-enkephalin analog in the control of autonomic responses in migraine patients. Clin. Neuropharmacol. **13:** 507–521.

41. LASSEN, L. H., L. L. THOMSEN & J. OLESEN. 1995. Histamine induces migraine via the H_1-receptor. Support for the no hypothesis of migraine. Neuroreport. In press.

42. IVERSEN, H. K. & J. OLESEN. 1994. Nitroglycerin-induced headache is not dependent on histamine release. Support for a direct nociceptive action of nitric oxide. Cephalalgia **14:** 437–442.

43. ARREGUI, A., J. CARERA, F. LEON-VELARDE, S. PAREDES, D. VISCARRA & D. ARBAIZA. 1991. High prevalence of migraine in high-altitude population. Neurology **41:** 1668–1669.

44. RENGASAMY, A. & R. A. JOHNS. 1991. Characterization of endothelium-derived relaxing factor/nitric oxide synthase from bovine cerebellum and mechanism of modulation by high and low oxygen tensions. J. Pharmacol. Exp. Ther. **259:** 310–316.

45. PEATFIELD, R. C., M. J. GAWEL & F. C. ROSE. 1981. The effect of infused prostacyclin in migraine and cluster headache. Headache **21:** 190–195.

46. LANCE, J. W. 1991. 5-Hydroxytryptamine and its role in migraine. Eur. Neurol. **31:** 279–281.

47. FOZARD, J. R. & H. O. KALKMAN. 1994. 5-Hydroxytryptamine (5-HT) and the initiation of migraine: New perspectives. Naunyn-Schmiedebergs Arch. Pharmakol. **350:** 225–229.

48. GARTHWAITE, J., S. L. CHARLES & R. CHESS-WILLIAMS. 1988. Endothelium-derived

relaxing factor release on activation of NMDA receptors suggests a role as intercellular messenger in the brain. Nature **336:** 385–388.

49. GOADSBY, P. J., H. KAUBE & K. L. HOSKIN. 1992. Nitric oxide synthesis couples cerebral blood flow and metabolism. Brain Res. **595:** 167–170.

50. OLDENDORF, W. H. 1971. Brain uptake of radiolabeled aminoacids, amines and hexoses after arterial injection. Am. J. Physiol. **221:** 1629–1639.

51. NORTHFIELD, D. W. C. 1938. Some observations on headache. Brain **61:** 133–162.

52. LEONE, A. M., V. W. FURST, S. CELLECK, N. P. WIKLUND & S. MONCADA. 1995. Visualizing the cellular release of nitric oxide. Endothelium **3(Suppl):** s5 (Abstr. 19).

53. RAY, B. S. & H. G. WOLFF. 1940. Experimental studies on headache. Pain sensitive structures of the head and their significance in headache. Arch. Surg. **41:** 813–856.

54. NICHOLS, F. T., III, M. MAWAD, J. P. MOHR, B. STEIN, S. HILAL & J. MICHELSEN. 1990. Focal headache during balloon inflation in the internal carotid and middle cerebral arteries. Stroke **21:** 555–559.

55. IVERSEN, H. K., T. H. NIELSEN, J. OLESEN & P. TFELT-HANSEN. 1990. Arterial responses during migraine headache. Lancet **336:** 837–839.

56. THOMSEN, L. L., H. K. IVERSEN & J. OLESEN. 1995. Cerebral blood flow velocities are reduced during attacks of unilateral migraine without aura. Cephalalgia **15:** 109–116.

57. MCMAHON, S. B., G. R. LEWIN & P. D. WALL. 1993. Central hyperexcitability triggered by noxious inputs. Curr. Opin. Neurobiol. **3:** 602–610.

58. MELLER, S. T. & G. F. GEBHART. 1993. Nitric oxide (NO) and nociceptive processing in the spinal cord. Pain **52:** 127–136.

59. MOSKOWITZ, M. A. 1993. Neurogenic inflammation in the pathophysiology and treatment of migraine. Neurology **43(Suppl. 3):** S16–S20.

60. GOADSBY, P. J., L. EDVINSSON & R. EKMAN. 1988. Release of vasoactive peptides in the extracerebral circulation of humans and the cat during activation of the trigeminovascular system. Ann. Neurol. **23:** 193–196.

61. GOADSBY, P. J., L. EDVINSSON & R. EKMAN. 1990. Vasoactive peptide release in the extracerebral circulation of humans during migraine headache. Ann. Neurol. **28:** 183–187.

62. GOADSBY, P. J. & L. EDVINSSON. 1991. Sumatriptan reverses the changes in calcitonin gene-related peptide seen in the headache phase of migraine. Cephalalgia **11(Suppl. 11):**3–4.

Food For Thought

The Metabolic and Circulatory Requirements
of Cognition

MARCUS E. RAICHLE[a]

Washington University School of Medicine
4525 Scott Avenue
St. Louis, Missouri 63110

INTRODUCTION

Over the past 10 years the field of cognitive neuroscience has emerged as a very important growth area in neuroscience. Cognitive neuroscience combines the experimental strategies of cognitive psychology with various techniques to actually examine how brain function supports mental activities. At the forefront of this research in normal humans are the new techniques of functional brain imaging: positron emission tomography (PET) and magnetic resonance imaging (MRI). The signals used by PET and functional MRI, or fMRI as it is now called, are based on the fact that changes in the cellular activity of the brain of normal, awake humans and laboratory animals are accompanied almost invariably by changes in local blood flow. This robust, empirical relationship has fascinated scientists for well over 100 years, but its cellular basis remains largely unexplained despite considerable research. Also, the accompanying metabolic changes do not appear to follow exactly the time-honored notion of a close coupling between blood flow and the oxidative metabolism of glucose.[1,2]

On the occasion of this celebration of the career of Fred Plum, it seems especially appropriate to review both the history and the current status of the relationship between blood flow and brain function in the context of functional brain imaging. Over many years Plum and his colleagues have contributed substantially to our understanding of brain circulation and metabolism in both health and disease. Many of his students, including me, have worked to carry on that tradition in our own research.

HISTORICAL BACKGROUND

The quest for an understanding of the functional organization of the normal human brain, using techniques that assess changes in brain circulation, has occupied mankind for more than a century. One has only to consult William James's monumental two-volume text Principles of Psychology (ref. 3, p. 97) to find reference to changes in brain blood flow during mental activities. He references primarily the work of the Italian physiologist Angelo Mosso[4] who recorded the pulsations of the human cortex in patients with skull defects. Mosso showed that these pulsations

[a] E-mail: marc@npg.wustl.edu

increased regionally during mental activity and concluded—correctly we now know—that brain circulation changes selectively with neuronal activity.

No less a figure than Paul Broca was also interested in the circulatory changes associated with mental activities as manifested by changes in brain temperature.[5] While best known for his seminal observations on the effect of lesions of the left frontal operculum on language function, Broca also studied the effect of various mental activities, especially language, on the localized temperature of the scalp of medical students.[6] Although such measurements might seem unlikely to yield any useful information, the reported observations, unbiased by preconceived notions of the functional anatomy of the cortex, were remarkably perceptive. Also active in the study of brain temperature and brain function in normal humans were Angelo Mosso[7] and Hans Berger.[8] Berger later abandoned his efforts in this area in favor of the development of the electroencephalogram.

Despite a promising beginning, including the seminal experimental observations of Roy and Sherrington,[1] which suggested a link between brain circulation and metabolism, interest in this line of research virtually ceased during the first quarter of the twentieth century. Undoubtedly, this was due in part to a lack of tools sufficiently sophisticated to pursue this type of research. In addition, the research of Leonard Hill, Hunterian Professor of the Royal College of Surgeons in England, was very influential.[9] His eminence as a physiologist overshadowed the inadequacy of his own experiments, which led him to conclude that no relationship existed between brain function and brain circulation.

There was no serious challenge to Leonard Hill's views until a remarkable clinical study was reported by John Fulton in the 1928 issue of Brain.[10] At the time of the report Fulton was a resident in neurosurgery under Harvey Cushing at the Peter Bent Brigham Hospital in Boston. A patient presented to Cushing's service with gradually decreasing vision due to an arteriovenous malformation of the occipital cortex. Surgical removal of the malformation was attempted but unsuccessful, leaving the patient with a bony defect over primary visual cortex. Fulton elicited a history of a cranial bruit audible to the patient whenever he engaged in a visual task. Based on this history, Fulton pursued a detailed investigation of the behavior of the bruit which he could osculate and record over occipital cortex. Remarkably consistent changes in the character of the bruit could be appreciated depending upon the visual activities of the patient. Whereas opening the eyes produced only modest increases in the intensity of the bruit, reading produced striking increases. The changes in cortical blood flow related to the complexity of the visual task and the attention of the subject to that task anticipated findings and concepts that have only recently been addressed with modern functional imaging techniques.[11] Fulton left his neurosurgical residency and studies of the cerebral circulation never to return and pursued a career in neurophysiology initially under the tutelage of Sir Charles Sherrington and later, for many years, at Yale University.

At the close of World War II, Seymour Kety and colleagues opened the next chapter in studies of brain circulation and metabolism (for a review see ref. 12). Working with Lou Sokoloff and others, Kety developed the first quantitative methods for measuring *whole* brain blood flow and metabolism in humans. The introduction of an *in vivo* tissue autoradiographic measurement of regional blood flow in laboratory animals by Kety's group[13,14] provided the first glimpse of quantitative changes in blood flow in the brain related directly to brain function. Given the later importance of derivatives of this technique to functional brain imaging with both PET and fMRI, it is interesting to note the (dis)regard the developers had for this technique as a means of assessing brain functional organization. To quote from the comments of William Landau to the members of the American Neurological Association meeting in Atlantic City[13]:

> Of course we recognize that this is a very secondhand way of determining physiological activity; it is rather like trying to measure what a factory does by measuring the intake of water and the output of sewage. This is only a problem of plumbing and only secondary inferences can be made about function. We would not suggest that this is a substitute for electrical recording in terms of easy evaluation of what is going on.

With the introduction of the deoxyglucose technique for the regional measurement of glucose metabolism in laboratory animals[15] and its later adaptation for PET,[16] enthusiasm was much greater for the potential of such measurements to enhance our knowledge of brain function (for review see ref. 12).

Soon after Kety and colleagues introduced their quantitative methods for measuring whole brain blood flow and metabolism in humans, David Ingvar, Neils Lassen and their Scandinavian colleagues introduced methods applicable to man that permitted regional blood flow measurements to be made using scintillation detectors arrayed like a helmet over the head.[17] They demonstrated directly in normal human subjects that blood flow changed regionally during changes in brain functional activity (for review see ref. 12). The first study of functionally induced regional changes in blood flow using these techniques in normal humans was actually reported by Ingvar and Risberg at an early meeting on brain blood and metabolism[18] and was greeted with cautious enthusiasm and a clear sense of its potential importance for studies of human brain function by Seymour Kety.[19] However, despite many studies of functionally induced changes in regional cerebral blood that followed (for review see ref. 20), this approach was not embraced by the majority of neuroscientists studying humans or laboratory animals. It is interesting to note that this indifference was to disappear almost completely in the 1980s, a subject to which we will return shortly.

In 1973[21] Godfrey Hounsfield introduced X-ray computed tomography (CT), a technique based upon principles presented earlier by Alan Cormack.[22,23] Overnight the way in which we looked at the human brain changed. Immediately, researchers envisioned another type of tomography, PET, which created *in vivo* autoradiograms of brain function.[24,25] A new era of functional brain mapping began. The autoradiographic techniques for the measurement of blood flow[13] and glucose metabolism[15] in laboratory animals could now be performed safely in humans.[26,16] Additionally, quantitative techniques were developed[27,28] and, importantly, validated[28,29] for the measurement of oxygen consumption.

Soon it was realized that highly accurate measurements of brain function in humans could be performed with PET (for review see ref. 30). Although this could be accomplished with either measurements of blood flow or metabolism (for review see ref. 12), blood flow became the favored technique because it could be measured quickly (<1 min) using an easily produced radiopharmaceutical ($H_2^{15}O$) with a short half-life (123 s), which allowed many repeat measurements in the same subject.

The study of human cognition with PET was aided greatly by the involvement of cognitive psychologists in the 1980s whose experimental designs for dissecting human behaviors using information processing theory fit extremely well with the emerging functional brain imaging strategies (for review see ref. 30). It may well have been the combination of cognitive science and systems neuroscience with brain imaging that lifted this work from a state of indifference and obscurity in the neuroscience community in the 1970s (see above) to its current role of prominence in cognitive neuroscience.

Another technology—MRI—also emerged along with PET and CT. It was based upon yet another set of physical principles discovered independently by Block[31] and Purcell and colleagues[32] and expanded to imaging by Paul Lauterbur.[33] Initially MRI provided superb anatomical information, but important metabolic and physiological information was also inherent in the data. An opening for MRI in the area of functional brain imaging emerged when it was discovered that during changes in neuronal activity there are local changes in the amount of oxygen in the tissue.[34,35] By combining this observation with a much earlier observation by Pauling and Coryell[36] that changing the amount of oxygen carried by hemoglobin changes the degree to which hemoglobin disturbs a magnetic field, Ogawa and colleagues[37] were able to demonstrate that *in vivo* changes in blood oxygenation could be detected with MRI. The MRI signal (technically known as T2* or "tee-two-star") arising from this unique combination of brain physiology[34] and nuclear magnetic resonance physics[36,38] became known as the blood oxygen level dependent or BOLD signal.[37] There quickly followed several demonstrations of BOLD signal changes in normal humans during functional brain activation,[39–41] giving birth to the field of functional MRI or fMRI.

In the discussion to follow it is important to keep in mind that when a BOLD signal is detected blood flow to a region of brain has changed out of proportion to the change in oxygen consumpton.[42] When blood flow changes more than oxygen consumption, in either direction, there is a reciprocal change in the amount of deoxyhemoglobin present locally in the tissue changing the local magnetic field properties. Both increases and decreases occur in the BOLD signal in the normal human brain.

METABOLIC REQUIREMENTS OF COGNITION

While many had assumed that behaviorally induced *increases* in local blood flow would be reflected in local increases in the oxidative metabolism of glucose,[2] evidence from brain imaging studies with PET[34,35] and fMRI[42] have indicated otherwise. Fox and his colleagues[34,35] demonstrated that in normal, awake adult humans, stimulation of the visual or somatosensory cortices results in dramatic increases in blood flow but minimal increases in *oxygen consumption*. Increases in *glucose utilization* occur in parallel with blood flow,[35] an observation fully anticipated by the work of others (e.g., see refs. 43 and 44). However, changes in blood flow and glucose utilization were much in excess of the changes in oxygen consumption, an observation contrary to most popularly held notions of brain energy metabolism.[2] These results suggested that the additional metabolic requirements associated with increased neuronal activity might be supplied largely through glycolysis alone.

Another element of the relationship between brain circulation and brain function that was not appreciated prior to the advent of functional brain imaging was the fact that regional blood flow and the fMRI BOLD signal not only increase in areas of the brain appropriate to task performance but also decrease from a resting baseline in areas of the brain uninvolved in a particular task.[45] An appreciation of these decreases requires explanation.

Physiologists have long recognized that neurons in the cerebral cortex can both increase or decrease their activities from a resting, baseline firing pattern depending upon task conditions. Examples abound in the neurophysiological literature (e.g., see Fig. 2 in ref. 46). A parsimonious view of these decreases in neuronal activity is that they reflect the activity of inhibitory interneurons acting within local circuits of the cerebral cortex. Because inhibition is considered to be energy requiring,[47] it has not been viewed as possible to distinguish inhibitory from excitatory cellular activity on the basis of changes in either blood flow or metabolism. Thus, on this view a local increase in *inhibitory* activity would be as likely to increase blood flow and the fMRI BOLD signal as would a local increase in *excitatory* activity. How, then, might decreases in blood flow or the fMRI BOLD signal arise?

To understand the possible significance of decreases in blood flow in functional imaging studies it is important to distinguish two separate conditions in which they might arise. The less interesting and more usually referred to circumstance arises when two images are compared in which one contains a regional increase in blood flow due to some type of task activity (e.g., hand movement producing increases in contralateral motor cortex blood flow) and the control image that does not (i.e., in this example, no hand movement). In our example, subtracting the image associated with no hand movement from the image associated with hand movement reveals the expected increase in blood flow in motor cortex. Simply reversing the subtraction produces an image with a decrease in the same area. Although this example may seem trivial and obvious, such subtraction reversals are often presented in the analysis of very complex tasks and in such a manner as to be quite confusing even to those working the field.

The second circumstance in which decreases in blood flow and the fMRI BOLD signal appear is not due to the above type of data manipulations (i.e., an active task image subtracted from a passive state image). Rather, blood flow and the fMRI BOLD signal decrease from a resting baseline (i.e., the activity in a region of brain has not been first elevated by a task). The usual baseline conditions from which this occurs consist of lying quietly but fully awake in an MRI or PET scanner with eyes closed or passively viewing a television monitor. In the examples discussed by Shulman,[45] areas of the medial orbital frontal cortex and the region of the posterior cingulate cortex and precuneus consistently showed decreased blood flow when subjects actively processed a wide variety of visual stimuli as compared to a passive baseline condition. There was no indication that these areas of decrease were activated in the passive, baseline condition.

The metabolic accompaniments of functionally induced decreases in blood flow were not initially explored, and it was tacitly assumed by those who even bothered to think about it that such reductions would probably be accompanied by coupled reductions in oxygen consumption. Therefore, it came as a surprise that the fMRI BOLD signal, based on tissue oxygen availability, detected both increases and decreases during functional activation. Decreases have been widely appreciated by investigators using fMRI although, surprisingly, no formal publications on the subject have yet appeared.

Complimenting these observations from functional brain imaging on the relationship between oxygen consumption and blood flow during decreases are earlier quantitative metabolic studies of a phenomenon known as cerebellar diaschisis.[48,49] In this condition, there is a reduction in blood flow and metabolism in the hemisphere of the cerebellum contralateral to an injury to the cerebral cortex, usually a stroke. Of particular interest is that blood flow is reduced significantly more than oxygen consumption.[48,49] These changes in the cerebellum are thought to reflect a reduction in neuronal activity within the cerebellum due to reduced input from the cerebral cortex. One can reasonably hypothesize that similar, large-scale reductions in systems-level activity are occurring during the course of normal functional brain activity.[45] The recognition of such changes probably represents a unique contribution of functional brain imaging and should stimulate increased interest in the manner in which brain resources are allocated on a large systems level during task performance.

Taken together, the data we have at hand suggest that blood flow changes more than oxygen consumption in the face of increases as well as decreases in local neuronal activity (FIG. 1). Glucose utilization also changes more than oxygen consumption during increases in brain activity (we presently have no data on decreases

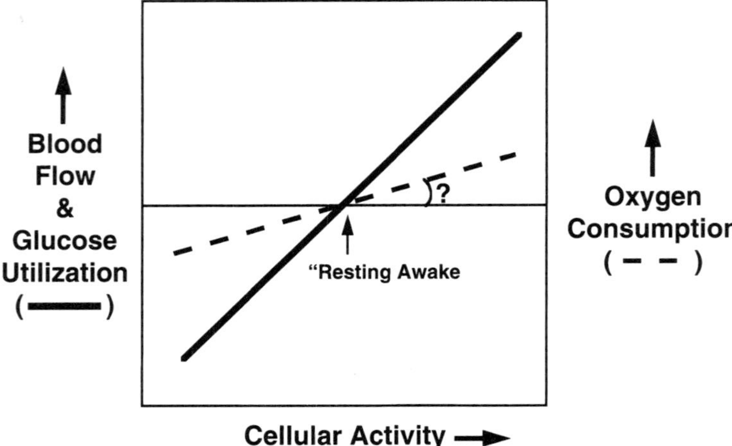

FIGURE 1. Relationship of blood flow, glucose utilization, and oxygen consumption to the cellular activity of the brain during changes in functional activity. This relationship is characterized by parallel changes in blood flow and glucose utilization in excess of any changes in oxygen consumption. The degree to which oxygen consumption actually changes at all remains to be determined. The literature supporting this summary is reviewed in the text.

in glucose utilization) and may equal the changes in blood flow in both magnitude and spatial extent. Although surprising to many, these results were not entirely unanticipated. Experimental studies of epilepsy in *well-oxygenated, passively venti-lated* experimental animals[b] [50] had indicated that blood flow increased in excess of the oxygen requirements of the tissue. During the increased neuronal activity of a seizure discharge increase in the brain, venous oxygen content was routinely observed.[50] Because of the increase in blood pressure associated with the seizure discharge, the fact that blood flow exceeded the oxygen requirements of the tissue was attributed to a loss of cerebral autoregulation.[50] A similar concern was expressed about equally prescient experiments involving brain blood flow changes during sciatic nerve stimulation in rodents.[52,53] However, experiments by Ray Cooper and colleagues largely circumvented that concern.[54,55] They demonstrated that oxygen availability measured locally in the cerebral cortex of awake patients undergoing surgery for the treatment of intractable epilepsy increased during changes in behavioral activity (e.g., looking at pictures, manual dexterity, reading). These changes in oxygen availability occurred in the absence of any change in blood pressure and were observed during normal brain function in humans. Surprisingly, these observations were largely ignored until the work of Fox and his colleagues called attention to the phenomenon in normal human subjects with PET.[34,35]

---

[b] Wilder Penfield is frequently given credit for the observation that venous oxygenation increases during a seizure discharge (i.e., so-called red veins on the cortex). Careful reading of his many descriptions of the cortical surface of the human brain during a seizure fail to disclose such a description. Rather, he describes quite clearly the *infrequent* appearance of arterial blood locally in pial veins *after* a focal cortical seizure.[51] ". . . the almost invariable objective alteration in the exposed hemisphere coincident with the onset of the fit is a cessation of pulsation in the brain" (ref. 51, p. 607).

Interpretation of these blood flow-metabolism relationships during changes in functional brain activity is presently controversial. Several schools of thought have emerged. One hypothesis which addresses the role of glycolysis in brain functional activation is most eloquently articulated by Pierre Magistretti and colleagues based on their work with cultured astrocytes (for review see refs. 56 and 57). In this theory increases in neuronal activity stimulated by the excitatory amino acid transmitter glutamate result in relatively large increases in glycolytic metabolism in astrocytes. The energy supplied through glycolysis in the astrocyte is used to metabolize glutamate to glutamine before being recycled to neurons (for review see refs. 56 and 57). Coupled with estimates that increased firing rates of neurons require little additional energy over and above that required for the normal maintenance of ionic gradients[58] leads to the hypothesis that the primary metabolic change associated with changes (at least increases) in neuronal activity are glycolytic and occur in astrocytes.

In somewhat greater detail, neuronal activation results in sodium ion influx and potassium efflux. This is accompanied by an influx of protons into neurons, initially alkalinizing the extracellular space, which results in alkalinization of the astrocyte.[59] Alkalinization of the astrocyte results in stimulation of glycolysis[60] with the breakdown of glycogen[44,61] and the production of both pyruvate and lactate in excess of astrocyte metabolic needs and despite normal tissue oxygenation. The lactate can then leave the astrocyte and be taken up by neurons to be oxidatively metabolized by neurons.[62] Because glucose metabolism exceeds oxygen consumption during increases in neuronal activity,[35] another fate for lactate must also be sought. This might possibly occur through enhanced removal from the brain by flowing blood, an hypothesis for which no evidence presently exists, or reincorporation into astrocytic glycogen.[63]

Additional support for this hypothesis comes from *in vivo* observations that increases in neuronal activity are associated with glycogenolysis in astrocytes,[61] a convenient source of readily available energy for such a process, located in a cell uniquely equipped enzymatically for the process.[57,64] Finally, measurements of tissue lactate with magnetic resonance spectroscopy (MRS) in humans[65–67] and with substrate-induced bioluminescence in laboratory animals[68] has shown localized increases in tissue lactate during physiologically induced increases in neuronal activity.

Not surprisingly, the above hypothesis has been challenged and alternatives offered to explain the observed discrepancy between changes in blood flow and glucose utilization, which appear to change in parallel, and oxygen consumption, which changes much less than blood flow or glucose utilization. One suggestion is that the observed discrepancy is transient (e.g., see ref. 67). Measuring brain glucose and lactate concentrations and blood oxygenation with MRI and MRS in normal human volunteers, Frahm and colleagues[67] observed a rise in visual cortex lactate concentration that peaked after 3 min of visual stimulation and returned to baseline after 6 min of continuous stimulation. During this same period of time, blood oxygen concentration was initially elevated but also returned to baseline by the end of the stimulation period. In a complementary study R. G. Shulman and colleagues[69] similarly suggested, on the basis of MRS studies of *anesthetized* rats during forepaw stimulation that "oxidative CMRglu supplies the majority of energy during *sustained* brain activation. However, in a very careful study of this question by Bandettini and associates in awake humans,[70] they concluded from their own data and a careful analysis of the literature that BOLD signal changes and blood flow remained elevated during prolonged periods of brain activation provided that there was no *habituation* to the presented stimulus. This conclusion is entirely consistent with the original observations of Fox and Raichle.[34]

Another popular hypothesis is based on optical imaging work of physiologically stimulated visual cortex by Grinvald and associates.[71] In their work they measure changes in reflected light from the surface of visual cortex in *anesthetized* cats. Using wavelengths of light sensitive to deoxyhemoglobin and oxyhemoglobin, they note an almost immediate *increase* in deoxyhemoglobin concentration followed, after a brief interval, by an *increase* in oxyhemoglobin which is greater in magnitude and extends over a much larger area of the cortex than do the changes in deoxyhemoglobin.[71] They interpret these results to mean that increases in neuronal activity are associated with highly localized increases in oxygen consumption which stimulate a vascular response, delayed by several seconds, that is large in relation to both the magnitude of the increase in oxygen consumption and the area of cerebral cortex that is actually active. In other words, by their theory increases in neuronal activity in the cerebral cortex are associated with a delayed (1–3 s) reactive hyperemia which delivers oxygen in excess of metabolic needs to the active area of cortex and its surroundings. This hypothesis has stimulated much interest in the use of high-field strength MRI systems to detect the initial but small increases in deoxyhemoglobin.[72] The hope would be that both spatial and temporal resolution of fMRI would be improved by focusing on this early and spatially confined event.

Support for the hypothesis of Grinvald and his associates[71] comes from theoretical work by Buxton and Frank.[73] In their modeling work they show that in an idealized capillary tissue cylinder in the brain, an increase in blood flow in excess of the increased oxygen metabolic demands of the tissue is needed in order to maintain proper oxygenation of the tissue. This results from the poor diffusivity and solubility of oxygen in brain tissue. In this theory, blood flow remains coupled to oxidative metabolism, but in a nonlinear fashion designed to overcome the diffusion and solubility limitations of oxygen in brain tissue in order to maintain adequate tissue oxygenation.

Although the hypothesis that reactive hyperemia is a normal consequence of increased neuronal activity merits careful consideration, several observations remained unexplained. First, it does not account for the increased glucose utilization which parallels the change in blood flow observed in normal humans[35] and laboratory animals.[68,74] Second, it does not agree with the observations of Woolsey and associates[74] who have done detailed studies of the vasculature and its response to changes in neuronal activity in the rodent whisker-barrel system. In these studies, using several techniques to characterize the functional and anatomic relationships between a whisker-barrel and its vasculature, Woolsey and associates[74] have demonstrated a remarkably tight spatial relationship between changes in neuronal activity within a single barrel and the response of the vascular supply to that barrel. There is little evidence in these studies for spatially diffuse reactive hyperemia surrounding the stimulated area of cortex. Third, the supporting hypothesis put forth by Buxton and Frank[73] does not provide an explanation for the observation that blood flow and oxygen utilization do not change in the face of increasing hypoxia until a PaO_2 of approximately 30 mmHg is reached (e.g., see ref. 75). Fourth, the initial rise in deoxyhemoglobin seen in the experiments of Malonek and Grinvald[71] is not accompanied by a fall in oxyhemoglobin as would be expected with a sudden rise in local oxygen consumption which preceded the onset of the vascular response (see Fig. 3A, ref. 71). In the absence of any evidence of capillary recruitment in brain[76,77] which could explain their findings, we should exercise caution in accepting the data of Malonek and Grinvald[71] until an explanation for this particular discrepancy is found and better concordance is achieved with other experiments. Clearly, more information is needed on the exact nature of the vascular events surrounding functional brain activation. Finally, we are left without an explanation for the observation that when blood flow decreases below a resting baseline, as it frequently does in functional brain imaging studies,[45] a negative BOLD signal arises because blood flow decreases more than oxygen consumption.

One final caveat should be mentioned. From the perspective of this review it would be easy to assume that because blood flow and glucose utilization appear to increase together and more than oxygen utilization during increases in neuronal activity, the increase in blood flow serves to deliver needed glucose. Recent data from Powers and colleagues[78] suggest otherwise. They noted no change in the magnitude of the normalized regional blood flow response to physiological stimulation of the human brain during stepped hypoglycemia. They concluded that the increase in blood flow associated with physiological brain activation was not regulated by a mechanism that matched local cerebral glucose supply to local cerebral glucose demand.[78]

So what are we to conclude at this point? Any theory designed to explain functional brain imaging signals must accommodate three observations. First, local increases and decreases in brain activity are reliably accompanied by changes in blood flow. Second, these blood flow changes exceed any accompanying change in the oxygen consumption. If this were not the case, fMRI based on BOLD signal changes could not exist. Third, although paired data on glucose metabolism and blood flow are limited, they suggest that blood flow changes are accompanied by changes in glucose metabolism of approximately equal magnitude and spatial extent. Additionally, evaluation of extant data and design of future experiments must carefully consider the effect of anesthesia on laboratory animals (a factor in many of the animal experiments discussed in this review). Finally, habituation to certain types of stimuli[70] may well complicate the interpretation of the resulting data as well as rapid, practice-induced *shifts in the neuronal circuitry* used for the performance of a task[79] if these phenomena are overlooked.

We do not presently know why blood flow changes so dramatically and reliably during changes in brain activity or how these vascular responses are so beautifully orchestrated. These questions have confronted us for more than a century and remain incompletely answered. At no time have answers been more important or intriguing than at the present time because of the immense interest focused on them by the use of functional brain imaging with PET and fMRI. We have at hand tools with the potential to provide unparalleled insights into some of the most important scientific, medical, and social questions facing mankind. Understanding those tools is clearly a high priority. Following the example of Fred Plum, we will obtain that understanding.

ACKNOWLEDGMENTS

I would like to acknowledge my deep sense of gratitude to Fred Plum who inspired me as a first year medical student at the University of Washington to pursue a career in neuroscience and has supported and encouraged me ever since. Mentorship of this type sets a high standard for those to follow. In addition, I would like to acknowledge many years of generous support from The National Institute of Neurological Disorders and Stroke, the National Heart, Lung and Blood Institute, The McDonnell Center for Studies of Higher Brain Function at Washington University, as well as The John D. and Katherine T. MacArthur Foundation and The Charles A. Dana Foundation. Finally, none of the personal work referred to in this review would have been possible without the collaboration and support of many valued colleagues and students with whom I have worked over the past 28 years.

REFERENCES

1. ROY, C. S. & C. S. SHERRINGTON. 1890. On the regulation of the blood supply of the brain. J. Physiol. (Lond.) **11:** 85–108.
2. SIESJO, B. K. 1978. Brain Energy Metabolism. John Wiley & Sons. New York.
3. JAMES, W. 1890 Principles of Psychology. : 97–99. Henry Holt & Co. New York.
4. MOSSO, A. 1881. Ueber den Kreislauf des Blutes im Menschlichen Gehirn. Verlag von Veit & Co. Leipzig.
5. BROCA, P. 1879. Sur la temperatures morbides locales. Bull. Acad. Med. (Paris) **2S:** 1331–1347.
6. BROCA, P. 1861. Remarques sur le siege de la faculte du langage articule; suivies d'une observation d'aphemie (perte de la parole). Bull. Soc. Anatom. (Paris) **6:** 330–357, 398–407.
7. MOSSO, A. 1894. La Temperatura del Cervello. Fratelli Treves, Editori. Milano.
8. BERGER, H. 1901. Zur Lehre von der Blutzirkulation in der Schadelhohle des Menschen. Verlag von Gustav Fischer. Jena, Germany.
9. HILL, L. 1896. The Physiology and Pathology of the Cerebral Circulation. An Experimental Research. J & A Churchill. London.
10. FULTON, J. F. 1928. Observations upon the vascularity of the human occipital lobe during visual activity. Brain **51:** 310–320.
11. SHULMAN, G. L., M. CORBETTA, R. L. BUCKNER, M. E. RAICHLE, J. A. FIEZ, F. M. MIEZIN & S. E. PETERSEN. 1997. Top-down modulation of early sensory cortex. Cereb. Cortex **7:** 193–206.
12. RAICHLE, M. E. 1987. Circulatory and metabolic correlates of brain function in normal humans. *In* Handbook of Physiology, The Nervous System. V. Higher Functions of the Brain. F. Plum, Ed.: 643–674. American Physiological Society. Bethesda, MD.
13. LANDAU, W. M., W. H. FREYGANG, JR., L. P. ROLAND, L. SOKOLOFF & S. KETY. 1955. The local circulation of the living brain: Values in the unanesthetized and anesthetized cat. Trans. Am. Neurol. Assoc. **80:** 125–129.
14. KETY, S. 1960. Measurement of local blood flow by the exchange of an inert diffusible substance. Methods Med. Res. **8:** 228–236.
15. SOKOLOFF, L., M. REIVICH, C. KENNEDY, M. H. DES ROSIERS, C. S. PATLAK, K. D. PETTIGREW, O. SAKURADA & M. SHINOHARA. 1977. The [^{14}C]deoxyglucose method for the measurement of local glucose utilization: Theory, procedure and normal values in the conscious and anesthetized albino rat. J. Neurochem. **28:** 897–916.
16. REIVICH, M., D. KUHL, A. WOLF, J. GREENBERG, M. PHELPS, T. IDO, V. CASELLA, J. FOWLER, E. HOFFMAN, A. ALAVI, P. SOM & L. SOKOLOFF. 1979. The [^{18}F]fluorodeoxyglucose method for the measurement of local glucose utilization in man. Circ. Res. **44:** 127–137.
17. LASSEN, N. A., K. HOEDT-RASMUSSEN, S. C. SORENSEN, E. SKINHOJ, B. CRONQUIST, E. BODFORSS & D. H. INGVAR. 1963. Regional cerebral blood flow in man determined by Krypton-85. Neurology **13:** 719–727.
18. INGVAR, D. H. & J. RISBERG. 1965. Influence of mental activity upon regional cerebral blood flow in man. Acta Neurol. Scand. Suppl. **14:** 183–186.
19. KETY, S. 1965. Closing comments. Acta Neurol. Scand. Suppl. **14:** 197.
20. LASSEN, N. A., D. H. INGVAR & E. SKINHOJ. 1978. Brain function and blood flow. Sci. Am. **239:** 62–71.
21. HOUNSFIELD, G. N. 1973. Computerized transverse axial scanning (tomography): Part I. Description of system. Br. J. Radiol. **46:** 1016–1022.
22. CORMACK, A. M. 1963. Representation of a function by its line integrals, with some radiological applications. J. Appl. Phys. **34:** 2722–2727.
23. CORMACK, A. M. 1973. Reconstruction of densities from their projections, with applications in radiological physics. Phys. Med. Biol. **18:** 195–207.
24. TER-POGOSSIAN, M. M., M. E. PHELPS, E. J. HOFFMAN & N. A. MULLANI. 1975. A positron-emission tomograph for nuclear imaging (PETT). Radiology **114:** 89–98.
25. HOFFMAN, E. J., M. E. PHELPS, N. A. MULLANI, C. S. HIGGINS & M. M. TER-POGOSSIAN.

1976. Design and performance characteristics of a whole-body positron tranaxial tomograph. J. Nucl. Med. **17:** 493–502.

26. RAICHLE, M. E., W. R. W. MARTIN, P. HERSCOVITCH, M. A. MINTUN & J. MARKHAM. 1983. Brain blood flow measured with intravenous $H_2^{15}O$. II. Implementation and validation. J. Nucl. Med. **24:** 790–798.

27. FRACKOWIAK, R. S. J., G. L. LENZI, T. JONES & J. D. HEATHER. 1980. Quantitative measurement of regional cerebral blood flow and oxygen metabolism in man using ^{15}O and positron emission tomography: Theory, procedure and normal values. J. Comp. Tomogr. **4:** 727–736.

28. MINTUN, M. A., M. E. RAICHLE, W. R. W. MARTIN & P. HERSCOVITCH. 1984. Brain oxygen utilization measured with O-15 radiotracers and positron emission tomography. J. Nucl. Med. **25:** 177–187.

29. ALTMAN, D. I., L. L. LICH & W. J. POWERS. 1991. Brief inhalation method to measure cerebral oxygen extraction fraction with PET: Accuracy determination under pathologic conditions. J. Nucl. Med. **32:** 1738–1741.

30. POSNER, M. I. & M. E. RAICHLE. 1994. Images of Mind. W. H. Freeman & Co. New York.

31. BLOCK, F. 1946. Nuclear induction. Phys. Rev. **70:** 460–474.

32. PURCELL, E. M., H. C. TORRY & C. V. POUND. 1946. Resonance absorption by nuclear magnetic moments in solid. Phys. Rev. **69:** 37.

33. LAUTERBUR, P. 1973. Image formation by induced local interactions: Examples employing nuclear magnetic resonance. Nature **242:** 190–191.

34. FOX, P. T. & M. E. RAICHLE. 1986. Focal physiological uncoupling of cerebral blood flow and oxidative metabolism during somatosensory stimulation in human subjects. Proc. Natl. Acad. Sci. USA **83:** 1140–1144.

35. FOX, P. T., M. E. RAICHLE, M. A. MINTUN & C. DENCE. 1988. Nonoxidative glucose consumption during focal physiologic neural activity. Science **241:** 462–464.

36. PAULING, L. & C. D. CORYELL. 1936. The magnetic properties and structure of hemoglobin, oxyhemoglobin and caronmonoxyhemoglobin. Proc. Natl. Acad. Sci. USA **22:** 210–216.

37. OGAWA, S., T. M. LEE, A. R. KAY & D. W. TANK. 1990. Brain magnetic resonance imaging with contrast dependent on blood oxygenation. Proc. Natl. Acad. Sci. USA **87:** 9868–9872.

38. THULBORN, K. R., J. C. WATERTON, P. M. MATTHEWS & G. K. RADDA. 1982. Oxygenation dependence of the transverse relaxation time of water protons in whole blood at high field. Biochim. Biophys. Acta **714:** 265–270.

39. OGAWA, S., D. TANK, R. MENON, J. M. ELLERMANN, S.-G. KIM, H. MERKLE & K. UGURBIL. 1992. Intrinsic signal changes accompanying sensory stimulation: Functional brain mapping with magnetic resonance imaging. Proc. Natl. Acad. Sci. USA **89:** 5951–5955.

40. KWONG, K., J. W. BELLIVEAU, D. A. CHESLER, I. E. GOLDBERG, R. M. WEISSKOFF, B. P. PONCELET, D. N. DENNEDY, B. E. HOPPEL, M. S. COHEN, R. TURNER, H-M. CHENG, T. J. BRADY & B. R. ROSEN. 1992. Dynamic magnetic resonance imaging of human brain activity during primary sensory stimulation. Proc. Natl. Acad. Sci. USA **89:** 5675–5679.

41. BANDETTINI, P. A., E. C. WONG, R. S. HINKS, R. S. TIKOFSKY & J. S. HYDE. 1992. Time course EPI of human brain function during task activation. Magn. Reson. Med. **25:** 390–397.

42. KIM, S. G. & K. UGURBIL. 1997. Comparison of blood oxygenation and cerebral blood flow effects in fMRI: Estimation of relative oxygen consumption change. Magn. Reson. Med. **38:** 59–65.

43. SOKOLOFF, L. 1981. Relationships among local functional activity, energy metabolism, and blood flow in the central nervous system. Fed. Proc. **40:** 2311–2316.

44. YAROWSKY, P., M. KADEKARO & L. SOKOLOFF. 1983. Frequency-dependent activation of glucose utilization in the superior cervical ganglion by electrical stimulation of cervical sympathetic trunk. Proc. Natl. Acad. Sci. USA **80:** 4179–4183.

45. SHULMAN, G. L., J. A. FIEZ, M. CORBETTA, R. L. BUCKNER, F. M. MIEZEN, M. E.

RAICHLE & S. E. PETERSEN. 1997. Common blood flow changes across visual tasks: II. Decreases in cerebral cortex. J. Cognit. Neurosci. In press.

46. GEORGOPOULOS, A. P., J. F. KALASKA, R. CAMINITI & J. T. MASSEY. 1982. On the relations between the direction of two-dimensional arm movements and cell discharge in primate motor cortex. J. Neurosci. **2:** 1527–1537.

47. ACKERMAN, R. F., D. M. FINCH, T. L. BABB & J. ENGEL, JR. 1984. Increased glucose metabolism during long-duration recurrent inhibition of hippocampal pyramidal cells. J. Neurosci. **4:** 251–264.

48. MARTIN, W. R. W. & M. E. RAICHLE. 1983. Cerebellar blood flow and metabolism in cerebral hemisphere infarction. Ann. Neurol. **14:** 168–176.

49. YAMAUCHI, H., H. FUKUYAMA & J. KIMURA. 1992. Hemodynamic and metabolic changes in crossed cerebellar hypoperfusion. Stroke **23:** 855–860.

50. PLUM, F., J. B. POSNER & B. TROY. 1968. Cerebral metabolic and circulatory responses to induced convulsions in animals. Arch. Neurol. **18:** 1–13.

51. PENFIELD, W. 1937. The circulation of the epileptic brain. Res. Publ. Assoc. Res. Nerv. Ment. Dis. **18:** 605–637.

52. HOWSE, D. C., F. PLUM, T. E. DUFFY & L. G. SALFORD. 1973. Cerebral energy metabolism and the regulation of cerebral blood flow. Trans. Am. Neurol. Assoc. **98:** 153–155.

53. SALFORD, L. G., T. E. DUFFY & F. PLUM. 1975. Association of blood flow and acid-base change in brain during afferent stimulation. *In* Cerebral Circulation and Metabolism. T. W. Langfitt, L. C. McHenry, M. Reivich & H. Wollman, Eds.: 380–382. Springer-Verlag. New York.

54. COOPER, R., H. J. CROW, W. G. WALTER & A. L. WINTER. 1966. Regional control of cerebral vascular reactivity and oxygen supply in man. Brain Res. **3:** 174–191.

55. COOPER, R., D. PAPAKOSTOPOULOS & H. J. CROW. 1975. Rapid changes of cortical oxygen associated with motor and cognitive function in man. *In* Blood Flow and Metabolism in the Brain. A. M. Harper, W. B. Jennett, J. D. Miller & J. O. Rowan, Eds.: 14.8–14.9. Churchill Livingstone. New York.

56. TSACOPOULOS, M. & P. J. MAGISTRETTI. 1996. Metabolic coupling between glia and neurons. J. Neurosci. **16:** 877–885.

57. BITTAR, P. G., Y. CHARNAY, L. PELLERIN, C. BOURAS & P. MAGISTRETTI. 1996. Selective distribution of lactate dehydrogenase isoenzymes in neurons and astrocytes of human brain. J. Cereb. Blood Flow Metab. **16:** 1079–1089.

58. CREUTZFELDT, O. D. 1975. Neurophysiological correlates of different functional states of the brain. *In* Brain Work. The Coupling of Function, Metabolism and Blood Flow in the Brain. D. H. Ingvar & N. A. Lassen, Eds.: 21–46. Munksgaard. Copenhagen.

59. CHESLER, M. & R. P. KRAIG. 1987. Intracellular pH of astrocytes increases rapidly with cortical stimulation. Am. J. Physiol. **253:** R666–R670.

60. HOCHACHKA, P. W. & T. P. MOMMSEN. 1983. Protons and anaerobiosis. Science **219:** 1391–1397.

61. SWANSON, R. A., M. M. MORTON, S. M. SAGAR & F. R. SHARP. 1992. Sensory stimulation induces local cerebral glycogenolysis: Demonstration by autoradiography. Neuroscience **51:** 451–461.

62. DRINGEN, R., H. WIESINGER & B. HAMPRECHT. 1993. Uptake of L-lactate by cultured rat brain neurons. Neurosci. Lett. **163:** 5–7.

63. DRINGEN, R., D. SCHMOLL, M. CESAR & B. HAMPRECHT. 1993. Incorporation of radioactivity from [^{14}C]lactate into the glycogen of cultured mouse astroglial cells. Evidence for gluconeogenesis in brain cells. Biol. Chem. Hoppe-Seyler **374:** 343–347.

64. HARLEY, C. A. & C. H. BIELAJEW. 1992. A comparison of glycogen phosphorylase *a* and cytochrome oxidase histochemical staining in rat brain. J. Comp. Neurol. **322:** 377–389.

65. PRICHARD, J. W., D. L. ROTHMAN, E. NOVOTNY, C. C. HANSTOCK & R. G. SHULMAN. 1991. Lactate rise detected by ^{1}H NMR in human visual cortex during physiologic stimulation. Proc. Natl. Acad. Sci. USA **88:** 5829–5831.

66. SAPPEY-MARINIER, D., G. CALABRESE, G. FEIN, J. W. HUGG, C. BIGGINS & M. W. WEINER. 1992. Effect of photic stimulation on human visual cortex lactate and phosphates using ^{1}H and ^{31}P magnetic resonance spectroscopy. J. Cereb. Blood Flow Metab. **12:** 584–592.

67. FRAHM, J., G. KRUGER, K.-D. MERBOLDT & A. KLEINSCHMIDT. 1996. Dynamic uncoupling

and recoupling of perfusion and oxidative metabolism during focal brain activation in man. Magn. Reson. Med. **35:** 143–148.

68. UEKI, M., F. LINN & K.-A. HOSSMANN. 1988. Functional activation of cerebral blood flow and metabolism before and after global ischemia of rat brain. J. Cereb. Blood Flow Metab. **8:** 486–494.

69. HYDER, F., J. R. CHASE, K. L. BEHAR, G. F. MASON, D. L. ROTHMAN & R. G. SHULMAN. 1996. Increased tricarboxylic acid cycle flux in rat brain during forepaw stimulation detected with 1H[^{13}C]NMR. Proc. Natl. Acad. Sci. USA **93:** 7612–7617.

70. BANDETTINI, P. A., K. K. KWONG, T. L. DAVIS, R. B. H. TOOTELL, E. C. WONG, P. T. FOX, J. W. BELLIVEAU, R. M. WEISSKOFF & B. R. ROSEN. 1997. Characterization of cerebral blood oxygenation and flow changes during prolonged brain activation. Hum. Brain Mapping **5:** 93–109.

71. MALONEK, D. & A. GRINVALD. 1996. Interactions between electrical activity and cortical microcirculation revealed by imaging spectroscopy: Implications for function brain mapping. Science **272:** 551–554.

72. MENON, R. S., S. OGAWA, X. HU, J. P. STRUPP, P. ANDERSON & K. UGURBIL. 1995. BOLD based function MRI at 4 Tesla includes a capillary bed contribution: Echo-planar imaging correlates with previous optical imaging using intrinsic signals. Magn. Reson. Med. **33:** 453–459.

73. BUXTON, R. B. & L. R. FRANK. 1997. A model for the coupling between cerebral blood flow and oxygen metabolism during neural stimulation. J. Cereb. Blood Flow Metab. **17:** 64–72.

74. WOOLSEY, T. A., C. M. ROVAINEN, S. B. COX, M. H. HENEGAR, G. E. LIANG, D. LIU, Y. E. MOSKALENKO, J. SUI & L. WEI. 1996. Neuronal units linked to microvascular modules in cerebral cortex: Response elements for imaging the brain. Cereb. Cortex **6:** 647–660.

75. SHIMOJYO, S., P. SCHEINBERG, K. KOGURE & O. M. REINMUTH. 1968. The effects of graded hypoxia upon transient cerebral blood flow and oxygen consumption. Neurology **18:** 127–133.

76. VILLRINGER, A., J. PLANCK, C. HOCK, L. SCHLEINKOFER & U. DIRNAGL. 1993. Near infrared spectroscopy (NIRS): A new tool to study hemodynamic changes during activation of brain function in human adults. Neurosci. Lett. **154:** 101–104.

77. VILLRINGER, A., A. THEM, U. LINDAUER & U. DIRNAGL. 1994. Capillary perfusion in the rat brain cortex. An in vivo confocal microscopy study. Circ. Res. **75:** 55–62.

78. POWERS, W. J., I. B. HIRSCH & P. E. CRYER. 1996. Effect of stepped hypoglycemia on regional cerebral blood flow response to physiological brain activation. Am. J. Physiol. **270** (Heart Circ. Physiol. **39**): H554–H559.

79. RAICHLE, M. E., J. A. FIEZ, T. O. VIDEEN, A. M. K. MACLEOD, J. V. PARDO, P. T. FOX & S. E. PETERSEN. 1994. Practiced-related changes in human brain functional anatomy during non-motor learning. Cereb. Cortex **4:** 8–26.

The Persistent Vegetative State:
A View across the Legal Divide

H. RICHARD BERESFORD[a]

Cornell Law School
Ithaca, New York
and
Department of Neurology
University of Rochester School of Medicine
Rochester, New York

Praise for Fred Plum can take many forms: for pedagogical dynamism, for depth and breadth of contributions to neurology and neuroscience, for sure-handed guidance of a department that has infused neurology with today's and tomorrow's leaders, and for a truly uncanny ability to fan a drive to excel in those he has touched. Mindful of his admonition to be substantive in what one says and does, my praise will embody a few reflections on the enduring legal and social impact of the "point of view" he and Bryan Jennett authored for the journal *Lancet* in 1972.[1]

THE *LANCET* PAPER

Recognizing the need for an acceptable term to describe patients who are "neither unconscious nor in coma in the usual sense of these terms," Jennett and Plum proposed the term "persistent vegetative state" (hereinafter PVS). It was of course not the choice of label that made their effort important—although it bears noting that, to this day and despite various attempts to come up with a better descriptor, the term enjoys general acceptance in both medical[2] and legal[3] forums. What Jennett and Plum accomplished is a particularly vivid reminder that some severely brain-injured persons may have "wakefulness without awareness." Such individuals may exhibit coordinated motor responses after noxious stimuli or even spontaneously, and may utter sounds, move their eyes, grimace, smile, or even swallow food or liquids placed in their mouths. Yet it is impossible to demonstrate that they respond in a discernibly conscious way to specific auditory, visual or other sensory inputs. In short, there is, despite an apparent wakefulness, the "absence of any evidence of a functioning mind which is either receiving or projecting information."[1]

The fact that subcortical and brain-stem structures remain functional allows prolonged survivals if caregivers attend to nutrition and hygiene. This potential for indefinite survival, observed Jennett and Plum, "presents a problem with humanitarian and socioeconomic implications which society as a whole will have to confront."[1] The problem is indeed profound and has generated—and will continue to generate—practical and conceptual dilemmas for physicians and the legal system.

[a] Address correspondence to H. Richard Beresford, Cornell Law School, Myron Taylor Hall, Ithaca, NY 24853-4901. E-mail: bersford@law.mail.cornell.edu

THE *QUINLAN* LITIGATION

The PVS became a center of legal controversy in 1976 when Fred Plum and others testified that Karen Quinlan was in a PVS and would remain that way. What the court failed to hear—or at least failed to grasp—was his additional testimony that her survival was not necessarily dependent on use of a mechanical ventilator. Whether this judicial misconception affected the ultimate decision by the New Jersey Supreme Court is speculative. However, both the trial court and the state supreme court assumed that removal of the ventilator would shortly lead to her death.

The judiciary in *Quinlan* conceived its role as determining the lawfulness of allowing Ms. Quinlan to die by reason of removal of her life support. To this end, it sought assurance from medical experts who testified that she was surely permanently unconscious, and heard testimony from her father, physicians, theologians and others about the moral basis for authorizing her father to request removal of the respirator. Having appraised this evidence, the New Jersey Supreme Court ultimately ruled that if her physicians agreed there was "clear and convincing" evidence she was permanently unconscious and a hospital ethics committee concurred in this prognosis, her father could, under the legal doctrine of substituted judgment, lawfully exercise her constitutional right of privacy to refuse the ventilator.[4] As many readers know, the ventilator was then discontinued and Ms. Quinlan survived nearly 10 years—as Fred Plum might have predicted. A recent report in The New England Journal of Medicine described the neuropathological findings in her brain.[5] Although cortical scarring was present (especially in parietal and occipital regions), the most extensive scarring was in the thalami. Basal forebrain, brain stem and hypothalamus were largely intact.

In rationalizing its decision, the New Jersey court opined that allowing Ms. Quinlan to live in a PVS was akin to asking her to "endure the unendurable."[4] It hypothesized that if she were granted a brief lucid interval to gauge her plight, she might readily conclude that continuing survival was something she would choose to forego. The court thus viewed PVS as a condition that at least some sapient persons would regard as equivalent to death. Consistent with this view, the court discounted the assertion of Ms.Quinlan's attending neurologist that his reluctance to remove the respirator stemmed from uncertainty over whether this was a medically appropriate action. The court—without supporting evidence—simply assumed that his reluctance reflected fear of adverse legal consequences. In other words, it must have seemed axiomatic to the court that an informed physician would not allow a commitment to protecting human life to engender treatments that would do no more than extend a life of perpetual unawareness.

Responding to concerns that it was authorizing euthanasia, the court offered two defenses. First, it declared that if Ms. Quinlan died after removal of the ventilator, the cause of death would be the brain disorder that caused her to be in a PVS, not the withdrawal of support for respiration. Second, even if there were a causal link between death and removal of treatment, the court viewed any "homicide" as justifiable because it would implement her constitutional right to decline medical treatment.

LITIGATION AFTER *QUINLAN*

Since the decision in *Quinlan*, many courts have approved requests to end life support for persons in PVS.[6-8] Although dissenting judges have occasionally vociferated about the devaluation of "life" that these decisions imply,[8] a consensus has developed that permanent unconsciousness is a cogent justification for ending life support. Legal controversies now tend to center on whether life support can lawfully be withdrawn from individuals whose preferences are unknown or unknowable, on whether severe neurological afflictions with preservation of rudimentary awareness should be approached in the same way as PVS, and on whether a legally meaningful distinction exists between removal of a mechanical life support and removal of fluids and nutrition. Of these, the first two draw the most attention and will be highlighted in the brief discussion that follows.

The Conroy Litigation

Several years after the *Quinlan* decision, the New Jersey Supreme Court was asked to rule on the request by the nephew of the severely brain-injured Claire Conroy to remove her feeding tube. Ms. Conroy was not in a PVS—her physicians had detected modest behavioral responses to sensory stimuli. She was, however, severely demented, incontinent, and bedbound in a nursing home and had no prospects for clinical improvement. Her wishes about use of the feeding tube were unknown, but her nephew believed that removal of the tube was consistent with her previously exhibited attitudes and values. After prolonged litigation, the court ruled—after her death—in *In re Conroy*[9] that the medical facts did not justify granting the nephew the authority he sought. However, the court did prescribe a procedure for use in nursing homes that would permit withdrawal of life support from severely impaired residents whose preferences are unknown.

Under the *Conroy* court's formula, life support could be stopped if there is "clear and convincing" evidence that the burdens of sustaining life exceed the benefits of continuing survival. In making this "objective" determination, the court indicated that physical pain is the operative burden and that proof of intractable pain is necessary before the burden of survival should be taken as outweighing the benefits of remaining alive. An individual would thus need enough awareness to experience demonstrably intractable pain before life support could be stopped under this "objective" prong of the *Conroy* formula, a requirement that obviously excludes individuals in a PVS.

The Cruzan Case

The primacy of autonomous choice in end-of-life decisions is exemplified in the U.S. Supreme Court's recent decision in *Cruzan v. Director*.[3] The core of the dispute between family and caregivers was not over whether Nancy Cruzan was in a PVS. The testifying neurological experts largely agreed on that point, and the Court exhibited no qualms about the idea that a competent individual might prefer death over life in a PVS. However, the Court upheld a Missouri statute that required "clear and convincing" proof that this was indeed Ms. Cruzan's choice. It would not concede that being in a PVS is in itself a lawful justification for ending life support. In other words, the Court was unwilling to presume that Nancy Cruzan—or anyone else for that matter—would actually choose to reject a feeding tube in such a circumstance. Although there are data on which the Court could have relied in adopting such a presumption, its refusal was consistent with prevailing law.[10] The Court's decision in *Cruzan* thus underscores the powerful impact of the autonomy principle in deliberations about whether to continue life support for individuals in PVS or with other severe neurological impairments.

The Supreme Court did not say that it is unlawful in all circumstances to end life support for individuals in a PVS if their wishes cannot be ascertained. But it did indicate that a state's interest in protecting the life of its citizens empowers the state, in a constitutional sense, to require convincing proof that ending life support is what the afflicted person would have chosen, whether by written advance directive or by unambiguous oral statements. In a separate opinion, moreover, Justice Scalia even suggested that a state legislature could, in the interests of upholding the preeminent value of life, bar removal of life support from those in a PVS—even if this constraint is contrary to their autonomously expressed wishes. These threads suggest that the Court will be inclined to defer to democratically enacted laws concerning decisions about removal of life support. If this interpretation is correct, state lawmakers should have considerable leeway in developing standards and rules for end-of-life decisions affecting individuals with severe neurological impairments. It thus seems appropriate to consider non-autonomy based justifications state lawmakers might use to guide their policy choices.

JUSTIFYING LIFE-ENDING DECISIONS

PVS as Death

As Plum and colleagues have shown with positron emission tomography, cerebral blood flow and metabolism can be profoundly impaired in the PVS.[11] Law professor David Smith has used this information to buttress an argument that PVS should be treated for legal purposes as equivalent to brain death.[12] He is not the first to propose that a permanent loss of consciousness be regarded as a death of the human person, and that ethical and legal rules should be modified to take this into account, but he is the first to rely substantially on advances in neuroscience to reorient societal attitudes about the relationship between consciousness and human life. Although his proposal has not attracted wide support, it challenges the many who readily accept the notion of brain death to explain why the two types of permanent unawareness, brain death and PVS, should have different legal connotations.

An obvious response is that, in the present state of the art of neurology, brain death is an absolute indicator of permanent unconsciousness, whereas a diagnosis of PVS carries with it a small but somewhat quantifiable chance that some awareness will return.[2,13] Another response might be that using consciousness as the measure of life risks indeterminacy because of the difficulties that inhere in arriving at an agreement on definition of the term,[14] even among physicians.[15] It is arguably easier to rely on a demonstrated presence or absence of brain-stem functions as the measure of human life. In this construct, the concept of mind plays no role in the definition of life; it is the brain stem that counts, no matter what the state of the neocortex.

PVS as Diminished Life

Even if the PVS is not the same as death, there is an emerging consensus that traditional constraints on decisions about life support apply less stringently to persons in a PVS than to persons with lesser impairments. For example, the New

York Do Not Rescucitate law includes permanent unconsciousness as one of four grounds for writing a DNR order,[16] and the federal child abuse law would allow ending life support for neonates who are "irreversibly comatose."[17] Also, the *Quinlan* court explicitly declared that the state's interest in protecting life wanes in proportion to the prognosis for regaining awareness.[4] In other words, not all lives are equal when it comes to applying protective legal and ethical rules. The slippery slope concerns here are obvious. Although these concerns should help to constrain temptations to expand the definition of diminished life, they also probably assure that the legal system will continue to be called on to resolve uncertainties about the rightness of withdrawing care from some individuals with severe neurological impairments.

PVS and the Beneficence Principle

A professional obligation of physicians is to provide treatments that help their patients and withhold treatments that burden or do not help. For PVS and other severe neurological impairments, the universe of demonstrably helpful treatments is small once adequate nutrition and hygiene have been provided. Yet is is also difficult to envision treatments that are burdensome to such individuals. They are, by definition, too neurologically compromised to experience quantifiable suffering. Thus, applying a traditional benefit/burden analysis to evaluate what care to provide or withhold is not a fruitful enterprise. If we take into account the suffering of caregivers or the strength of public attitudes about what ought or ought not to be done, then it might be possible to arrive at a calculus of benefits or burdens. However, this would have little to do with the interests of the afflicted individual unless, for example, he or she had once strongly expressed a wish not to be a financial or emotional burden on others. In this scenario, it might be defensible to hold that prolonging survival is indeed a burden that could be weighed against the contestable benefit of remaining alive.

PVS and Resource Allocation

The social costs of caring for individuals with severe neurological impairments are already substantial. Moreover, for the near term at least, developing treatments are more likely to extend life span than to achieve meaningful neurological improvement. The polity therefore faces increasingly hard choices about how many resources to allocate to persons who will never improve or achieve any capacity for social participation. One option is to do as Oregon has done: formally and explicitly establish categories of illnesses or individuals to whom few or no public resources are allocated.[18] This sort of rationing is contentious anywhere, but especially so in a society as wealthy as ours. Nevertheless, the current drive to constrain health care costs through greater reliance on market forces and reduced public expenditures will almost inevitably result in fewer resources being available to care for those with severe and permanent neurological impairments.

The legal system in the United States affords no constitutional or other formal entitlement to health care—although federal and state legislation do offer a variety of safety nets—and the public seems quite tolerant of the fact that millions of citizens lack health insurance or secure access to minimally adequate health services. In this cultural setting, it is not difficult to foresee a growing public willingess to skimp on care for the severely brain injured. A simple ethical justification for this attitude is that health resources are finite and must be expended where they do the most good. Individuals with severe neurological impairments arguably have a weak claim on these limited resources because they have so little to gain from treatment. Whatever claim they have would rest on the principle that all human lives have instrinsic value and that a moral society will expend a decent minimum of resources to sustain those lives. Yet, as we have seen, the judiciary and much of the public have accepted the proposition that society's obligation to the severely brain injured does not include use of all available life-extending resources. Against this backdrop, it may be worthwhile to look at the role of clinical neurologists in decisional processes that could eventuate in ending life support for the severely brain injured.

NEUROLOGISTS AND PVS

Formal Ethical Standards

The American Academy of Neurology holds that it is ethical to withdraw life support (including fluids and nutrition) from a patient in a PVS, provided the diagnosis is secure and there is evidence this accords with the patient's wishes.[19] The Academy's position rests on the considered belief that the PVS, as defined by Jennett and Plum, is diagnosable and that its salient feature is an irreversible loss of awareness. It further reflects an assumption that consciousness is what confers special value on human life.

In a sense, the Academy position on PVS is inconsistent with its later declaration that the taking of vital organs from anencephalic infants for purposes of transplantation is unethical because it violates the "dead donor" rule.[20] Individuals in a PVS and anencephalic infants are both permanently unconscious, and it is arguably illogical to suggest that actions which cause their deaths—removal of a feeding tube or removal of both kidneys—are ethical for one but not the other. Several counterarguments can be raised, however. The most straightforward is that the Uniform Anatomical Gift Act,[21] which regulates organ transplantation, requires that heart-beating donors be brain dead before their organs can be removed. Also, surgical removal of organs is a far more invasive, coarse, and immediate cause of death than removal of a feeding tube or respirator. Moreover, society has always treated newborns with a special solicitude and using them as organ sources, even for the most altruistic of purposes, may be too crass to contemplate.

Whatever the inconsistency between the two statements, they stress the need for careful and rigorous assessments of severely brain-injured individuals and concurrent sensitivity to legal and social overtones. In these respects, the statements recognize that both clinical expertise and enlightened citizenship should be brought to bear, a call that Jennett and Plum heralded in the *Lancet* paper. However, conflating applications of neurological expertise with ethical and social policy choices can be problematic.[22]

Without offering a definition of consciousness, the Academy's position statement on the PVS declares that permanent unconsciousness can be reliably identified. A recent comprehensive review of published studies[21] lends support to this view. It cites two types of evidence. One type constitutes the accumulated experience of neurological clinicians applying established criteria for the diagnosis of PVS, coupled with outcome data which reveal that individuals vegetative for longer than one year rarely regain awareness. The second type of evidence derives from *in vivo* neuroimaging and postmortem neuropathology. The imaging studies demonstrate profound cortical hypometabolism in PVS, and autopsy studies typically reveal extensive neocortical injury. It thus appears that neurologists can offer a tenable diagnosis of PVS by applying appropriately rigorous clinical standards, but it is less clear that they can offer expert guidance to those who must actually decide whether to withdraw life support.

Boundaries of Neurological Expertise

Assume for the moment that an accurate diagnosis of PVS can be made. Does it then follow that neurologists' opinions about what ought to be done should be given special weight by families or other decision makers? For example, can neurologists confidently assure decision makers that individuals whose eyes are open and who move and make sounds nevertheless cannot experience pain or pleasure? Can they accurately predict how long the individuals will survive? Can they communicate a sense of what it is to be "unconscious"? Can they inform decision makers as to what constitutes an appropriate allocation of resources for one in a PVS? If not, the neurologist's role appears narrow, albeit pivotal. It is narrow in the sense that the ethical issue of whether life support *ought* to be stopped must be resolved by others (for example, families, primary providers, courts). It is pivotal because the issue of whether to end life support is not ripe for discussion until there is no more than trivial uncertainty about diagnosis or prognosis.

If making a diagnosis of PVS is indeed the principal contribution neurologists can make in resolving the ethical and legal dilemma, the reliability of the diagnosis assumes overriding importance. The 1994 review,[2] noted above, concluded that recovery of consciousness in adults who have been vegetative for more than one year is "exceedingly rare." The few persons who did regain consciousness after that interval, including one who had been vegetative for 36 months, were totally dependent and had severe residual neurological impairments. A more recent report in the same journal described a patient who regained consciousness after 17 months in a vegetative state.[13] After reviewing available data describing recovery of awareness after one year in a vegetative state, the authors estimated that the probability of regaining some awareness was 14 percent. If this figure is accurate, the question then emerges as to how certain neurologists can be when they offer their opinions to families, primary providers, ethics committees or courts.

Available data clearly would support an opinion that an adult who has been vegetative for more than one year will *probably* not regain consciousness. These data may also amount to "clear and convincing" evidence, a more exacting legal standard. However, they do not appear to support an opinion that meets the most rigorous legal standard of "beyond a reasonable doubt." This standard requires something akin to moral certainty about the accuracy of an opinion. At minimum, a neurologist could still testify with moral certainty that a person in a PVS for more than one year will have severe neurological disabilities and will be incapable of independent living, whether or not consciousness returns.

Decision makers may or may not rely on neurological opinions that rest on less than moral certainty. They could, for example, accept opinions based on the sort of probabilities clinicians ordinarily apply in their clinical practices. These seldom add up to moral certainty, and may not even meet a "clear and convincing" test of legal probity. On the other hand, where reliance on an opinion may lead to a decision to cause or hasten the death of an individual, decision makers may insist that opinions rest on a moral certainty as to their accuracy. These considerations have clear significance for neurologists asked to venture opinions about individuals in PVS. They should try to determine what standard of certainty they are expected to meet, and should self-critically evaluate whether their opinions will satisfy that standard. Since the data available to support an opinion are somewhat "soft," the challenge may be daunting; however, trying to sidestep the challenge could deform an ethically sensitive decisional process that calls for the best that neurological clinicians have to offer.

CONCLUDING REMARKS

The debate over what justifies ending life support for individuals with severe neurological impairments will continue. Wider use of advance directives and a growing willingness of lawmakers to countenance autonomous life-ending choices will temper the debate. However, the public is likely to remain uneasy about slippery slopes and about threats to the sanctity of life it may perceive in efforts to calibrate legal and ethical protections by reference to the status of the neocortex. In this context, the contributions of Fred Plum stand out. By stressing the defining role of higher cortical functions for the human condition and by challenging clinicians, lawmakers and others to engage over the meaning of irretrievable loss of these functions, he has both framed and richly informed the debate.

REFERENCES

1. JENNETT, B. & F. PLUM. 1972. Persistent vegetative state after brain damage. Lancet **1:** 734–737.
2. MULTI-SOCIETY TASK FORCE. 1994. Medical aspects of the persistent vegetative state. N. Engl. J. Med. **330:** 1499–1508, 1572–1579.
3. Cruzan v. Director, 497 U.S. 261 (Supreme Ct. 1990).
4. *In re* Quinlan, 70 N.J. 10, 355 A. 2d 647 (N.J. Sup. Ct. 1976), *cert. den. sub nom* Garger v. N.J., 429 U.S. 922 (Supreme Ct. 1976).
5. KINNEY, H. C., J. KOREIN, A. PANIGRAPHY, *et al.* 1994. Neuropathological findings in the brain of Karen Ann Quinlan. N. Engl. J. Med. **330:** 1469–1475.
6. RHODEN, N. R. 1988. Litigating life and death. Harvard Law Rev. **102:** 375–446.
7. Council Report. 1990. Persistent vegetative state and the decision to withdraw or withhold life support. JAMA **263:** 426–430.
8. BERESFORD, H. R. 1989. Legal aspects of termination of treatment decisions. Neurol. Clin. **7(4):** 775–787.
9. *In re* Conroy, 486 A. 2d 1209 (N.J. Sup. Ct. 1985).
10. LINDGREN, J. 1993. Death by default. Law Contemp. Prob. **56:** 187–254.
11. LEVY, D. E., J. J. SIDTIS, D. A. ROTTENBERG, *et al.* 1987. Differences in cerebral blood flow and glucose utilization in vegetative versus locked-in patients. Ann. Neurol. **22:** 673–682.
12. SMITH, D. R. 1986. Legal recognition of neocortical death. Cornell Law Rev. **71:** 850–888.
13. CHILDS, N. L. & W. N. MERCER. 1996. Late improvement in consciousness after post-traumatic vegetative state. N. Engl. J. Med. **334:** 24–25.
14. SEARLE, J. R. 1995. The mystery of consciousness. New York Review 11/2/95: 60–66, 11/16/95: 54–62.
15. PAYNE, K., R. M. TAYLOR, C. STOCKING & G. A. SACHS. 1996. Physicians' attitudes about the care of patients in the persistent vegetative state: A national survey. Ann. Intern. Med. **125:** 104–110.
16. N.Y. Public Health Law, Article 29-B—Orders Not to Resuscitate, McKinney's Consol. Laws NY, 1989.
17. Child Abuse Prevention and Treatment Act, U.S. Code Annot., section 5102, as amended.

18. THOMAS, W. J. 1993. The Oregon Medicaid proposal: Ethical paralysis, tragic democracy, and the fate of a utilitarian health care program. Oregon Law Rev. **72:** 147–196.
19. EXECUTIVE BOARD of the AMERICAN ACADEMY of NEUROLOGY. 1989. Position of the American Academy of Neurology on certain aspects of the care and management of the persistent vegetative state. Neurology **39:** 125–126.
20. Resolution of Executive Board of the American Academy of Neurology 7/8/95, copy on file with author.
21. Uniform Anatomical Gift Act. 8 Uniform Laws Annot. 15 (1972).
22. BERESFORD, H. R. 1996. Ethics in neuroscience: Mind over matter? Poynter Lecture 1996. Indiana University Foundation. Bloomington, IN. p. 21.

Emerging Concepts in Sports Neurology

BARRY D. JORDAN[a]

Reed Neurological Research Center
UCLA School of Medicine
and
Biobehavioral Research Center
Charles R. Drew University of Medicine and Science
Los Angeles, California

Within the past decade, sports neurology has surfaced as a distinct and viable medical subspecialty. The importance of sports neurology as a discipline has resulted from the public health concerns and clinical syndromes highlighted within the context of this chapter. The emerging concepts of this new neurological subspecialty will be discussed.

SPORTS NEUROEPIDEMIOLOGY

Sports neuroepidemiology is the study of the distribution and dynamics of neurological injuries in sports and the factors that affect these characteristics. Although injury to the nervous system is a relatively uncommon consequence of athletic endeavor and sports participation, the majority of catastrophic injuries in sports are neurological. Overall estimates of the prevalence, incidence, and mortality associated with brain and spinal cord injury in sports are largely unavailable. Accordingly, sports neuroepidemiology will become an important discipline to document the public health burden of catastrophic neurological injuries in sports. If one considers all of the sports and recreational athletic activities engaged in by today's society (TABLE 1), speculation as to the potential magnitude of various neurological injuries is astonishing. In general, neurological injuries are expected in contact/collision sports such as football, boxing, ice hockey, martial arts, etc. However, catastrophic brain and spinal cord injury may be encountered in almost any sport, especially high-velocity vehicular sports and those associated with falls (e.g., hang gliding, mountain climbing, gymnastics, roller blading, skiing).

The magnitude of sports-related neurological injury can only be estimated from existing large population-based epidemiological studies of traumatic injury to the central nervous system (CNS). Worldwide estimates of the incidence of traumatic brain injury from all causes ranges from 152 to 430 cases per 100,000 population per year.[1] The percentage of brain injuries related to sports ranges anywhere from 3 to 25%.[1] Using these figures, the rates of sports-related brain injuries could theoretically range from 4.6 to 67.5 cases per 100,000 population per annum. This estimate may be conservative if one includes bicycling and motorcycling as sports. Worldwide incidence of spinal cord injury ranges from 150 to 500 cases per 100,000 population.[1] The percentage of spinal cord injuries related to recreation ranges from 3 to 19%.[1] Accordingly, the frequency of sports-related spinal cord injury

---

[a] Address correspondence to Barry D. Jordan, M.D., M.P.H., Charles R. Drew University of Medicine and Science, 1621 E. 120th Street, MP 19B, Los Angeles, CA 90059.

TABLE 1. Various Sports and Athletic Activities in Today's Society

Archery, autoracing, baseball, basketball, bowling, Bungee jumping, canoeing and kayaking, cycling, dance/ballet, diving, equestrian sports, football, golf, gymnastics, hang gliding, ice hockey, jogging, lacrosse, mountain climbing, parachuting/sky diving, roller blading/roller skating, rugby, skateboard, skiing and winter sports, swimming and water sports, shooting, tennis/racquet sports, weightlifting, wrestling

could range from 4.5 to 95 cases per 100,000 population. The estimated frequency of sports-related CNS injuries covers a wide range because of methodological differences in data collection among the various epidemiologial investigations.

There are inherent difficulties associated with delineating the frequency of catastrophic neurological injuries in sports. First, a well-established population-based sport injury surveillance and data collection system is lacking. Sport and recreational athletic activity is diffusely and vastly integrated into out society. These activities can be team versus individual, amateur versus professional, scholastic versus non-scholastic or organized versus unorganized. Accordingly, a centralized surveillance system that can accurately identify all sporting injuries is extremely problematic. One method of tracking injuries would have to be the local, state, and federal government. A second inherent problem in the documentation of neurologial injuries in sports is the calculation of incidence, prevalence, and mortality data. Without knowledge of the number of participants in each sport, only the absolute number of specific injuries can be determined. The absolute number of neurological injuries in sports may provide an indication of the public health burden, but cannot afford the opportunity to calculate injury rates and identify high-risk endeavors. A third difficulty in the assessment of neurological injuries in sports is making adequate comparisons between sports because athletic exposures vary according to the sport. For example, football exposure may be documented by quarters or games, boxing exposure may be determined by bouts or rounds, and cycling exposure may be determined by miles. Thus, all athletic exposures among sports are not equivalent. This factor has to be incorporated into any exposure and injury analysis among sports. Accordingly, sports neuroepidemiology will become a vital discipline in establishing the true public health burden and magnitude of neurological injury in sports and recreational athletic activity.

ACUTE TRAUMATIC BRAIN INJURY

The diagnosis, management, and prevention of acute traumatic brain injuries (ATBI) in sports have become an increasing concern. A wide variety of ATBI may be encountered in sports (TABLE 2); however, the overwhelming majority of

TABLE 2. Types of Acute Traumatic Brain Injury

Diffuse	Focal
Concussion	Intracerebral hematoma
Diffuse Axonal Injury	Subdural hematoma
	Epidural hematoma
	Cerebral contusion

TABLE 3. Glasgow Coma Scale

	Response	Score
	Verbal	1
	None	2
	Incomprehensible sounds	3
	Inappropriate words	4
	Confused	5
	Oriented	
	Eye Opening	1
	None	2
	To pain	3
	To speech	4
	Spontaneously	
	Motor	1
	None	2
	Abnormal extension	3
	Abnormal flexion	4
	Withdraws	5
	Localizes	6
	Obeys	

traumatic brain injuries (TBI) is the cerebral concussion. To date, a variety of grading scales have been used to classify ATBI in sports. The most universally accepted scale is the Glasgow Coma Scale (GCS).[2] Although this scale was not initially intended specifically for sports, it is very appropriate in evaluating the head-traumatized athlete. The most commonly utilized scales that have been devised specifically for sports-related head trauma is the Cantu scale[3] and the Colorado Medical Society (CMS) scale.[4] The current author has also devised a scale[5] that combines the elements from both the Cantu and CMS scales. More recently, the American Academy of Neurology (AAN) has published a revised CMS scale for the diagnosis and management of concussion in sports.[6]

Glasglow Coma Scale

The GCS assesses verbal response, motor response, and eye opening and provides a practical means of monitoring changes in the level of consciousness. The scores of the GCS range from 3 to 15 (TABLE 3) and can be classified into mild, moderate, and severe injury. Limitations of the GCS are that it does not take into account pupillary reaction and extraocular eye movements, or historical aspects of head trauma (e.g., headache, amnesia, etc.). It relies primarily on findings noted on neurological examination.

A score of 13 to 15 on the GCS signifies a mild head trauma. An athlete experiencing this type of trauma will at least be able to utter incomprehensible words, open eyes in response to pain, and will be able to withdraw to pain. An athlete who experiences a mild head trauma should have prompt serial examinations. Failure to rapidly recover to normal (i.e., score of 15) within a reasonable amount of time (e.g., 15 min) should necessitate further investigation. The athlete who has an initial score of 15 at the time of injury (without loss of consciousness or amnesia)

TABLE 4. Cantu Grading System for Concussion in Sports

Grade and Symptoms	Criteria for Return to Play
1 **Mild:** No loss of consciousness; posttraumatic amnesia less than 30 min	May return to play if asymptomatic for one week
2 **Moderate:** Loss of consciousness less than 5 min in duration or posttraumatic amnesia lasting longer than 30 min, but less than 24 h in duration	May return to play if asymptomatic for one week
3 **Severe:** Loss of consciousness for more than 5 min or posttraumatic amnesia for more than 24 h	Should not be allowed to play for at least one month. May then return to play if asymptomatic for one week

and is neurologically asymptomatic (for at least 20 min) may be allowed to return to competition that same day. No athlete should be allowed to return to competition if his or her score is less than 15.

Moderate head injury scores are in the range of 9 to 12. Any athlete that scores in this range should be removed from competition and undergo a neurological evaluation including neuroimaging (i.e., CT or MRI scan). This athlete should be considered as experiencing a significant injury and will probably require hospitalization for observation. An athlete who sustains a moderate head injury according to the GCS and does not have a focal brain lesion or skull fracture should have a rest period before being allowed to return to competition. The duration of this mandatory rest period is determined by the time required for the GCS score to normalize and the duration of associated neurological symptoms. An athlete who exhibits a moderate injury according to the GCS should be cautiously advised regarding participation is contact sports.

An athlete who scores in the range of 3 to 8 on the GCS is considered to have a severe head injury and a relatively poorer prognosis. Such an athlete should be emergently transported to a hospital for a prompt neurological and/or neurosurgical consultation. A reasonable percentage of those experiencing a severe head injury will probably exhibit some residual neurological deficits, which would be a contraindication to participation in contact/collision sports. An athlete who sustains a severe head trauma and recovers should be advised against continued participation in contact/collision sports.

Cantu Scale

The Cantu grading system (TABLE 4) for head trauma has been widely used in sports.[4] This scale grades concussion as either mild, moderate, or severe. The criteria for the various grades are determined by the level of consciousness and/or the duration of posttraumatic amnesia. Mild (grade 1) concussion on the Cantu scale is characterized by no loss of consciousness and posttraumatic amnesia lasting less than 30 min. The athlete may be dazed, stunned, and/or confused and may exhibit cognitive impairment. Since a mild concussion according to the Cantu scale is not associated with loss of consciousness, it may be difficult to recognize and may go undetected. An athlete with a mild concussion should be removed from competition. It is recommeded that an athlete with a mild concussion be asymptomatic for one week before returning to competition. A second grade 1 concussion necessitates a

TABLE 5. Colorado Medical Society Grading System for Concussion in Sports

Grade and Symptoms	Criteria for Return to Play
1 **Mild:** Confusion without amnesia; no loss of consciousness	May return to play if asymptomatic at rest and exertion after observation of at least 20 min
2 **Moderate:** Confusion with amnesia; no loss of consciousness	May return to play if asymptomatic for one week
3 **Severe:** Loss of consciousness	Should not be allowed to play for at least one month. May then return to play if asymptomatic for two weeks

two-week rest period and requires the athlete to be asymptomatic for one week. Three grade 1 concussions in one season should result in the termination of play during that season.

A moderate concussion on the Cantu scale is defined as unconsciousness lasting less than 5 min or posttraumatic amnesia lasting more than 30 min but less than 24 h. The advantage of the Cantu scale is that it does not lump all cases of unconsciousness together. An athlete who experiences a brief loss of consciousness and regains neurological function quickly may not require emergency transportation. The athlete with a grade 2 concussion should be removed from competition and undergo a neurological evaluation. An athlete who sustains a moderate concussion may be allowed to return to competition if he is asymptomatic for one week. Athletes who sustain two moderate concussions in one season should be held from competition for one month and be allowed to return when asymptomatic for one week.

A grade 3 (severe) concussion on the Cantu scale is characterized by loss of consciousness lasting more than 5 min or posttraumatic amnesia lasting 24 h or longer. The unconscious athlete should be emergently transported to the hospital on a spine board with the head and neck immobilized. Any athlete who sustains a severe concussion should undergo a detailed neurological evaluation. He should not return to competition earlier than one month after the injury. A second severe concussion in one season should terminate the season for that athlete.

Colorado Medical Society

The CMS[5] scale (TABLE 5) represents a simple grading system to classify head injury and comprises three grades: (1) mild, (2) moderate, and (3) severe. The criteria for each grade and recommendations for return to contact sports are described below.

Grade 1 (mild) head injury on the CMS scale is characterize by momentary confusion without amnesia or loss of consciousness. The athlete exhibiting a grade 1 concussion may be dazed or be labeled as having his "bell rung," "dinged," or "seeing stars." This type of concussion represents the most common type of head injury encountered in sports. The athlete is often able to continue his performance and the diagnosis may only be detected either by specific questioning or by the athlete behaving confused (e.g., missing assignments on plays or walking to the incorrect sidelines). The athlete may be allowed to return to play after at least 20 min of observation and is found to be asymptomatic (i.e., not experiencing posttraumatic/postconcussion syndrome characterized by headache, confusion, impaired memory, etc., at rest and during exertion). It is recommended than an athlete experiencing a second grade 1 concussion be removed from activity. Three grade 1 concussions in a season should terminate the season for the athlete. An advantage to this classification of head injury is that it enables an athlete to return to competition that same day if he experiences a mild (grade 1) concussion that is relatively short-lived and is asymptomatic for 20 min.

Grade 2 (moderate) head injury on the CMS scale is characterized by confusion with amnesia (anterograde and/or retrograde). The athlete exhibiting a grade 2 concussion should be considered as experiencing a significant head trauma and should not be allowed to return to competition that day. Unlike the Cantu scale, the CMS scale does not specify the duration of amnesia and essentially categorizes all amnesias together. Similar to the grade 1 head trauma, the athlete does not experience loss of consciousness. The athlete with a grade 2 concussion should have repeated evaluations by a health care provider or be carefully observed over the next 24 h by a reasponsible adult who is informed regarding symptoms of evolving neurological deterioration. If neurological symptoms worsen or persist for longer than one week, then a CT or MRI scan is recommended. An athlete with a grade 2 concussion may return to competition after one week of being asymptomatic. An athlete experiencing two grade 2 concussions should not be allowed to return to competition for at least one month, and possible termination of the season should be considered. Obviously, if an athlete has three grade 2 concussions during one season, he or she should not return to competition that season.

Grade 3 (severe) head trauma on the CMS scale is the most devastating type of concussion and is categorized by loss of consciousness. Grade 3 concussions include all cases of loss of consciousness together, regardless of duration. It is recommended that any athlete experiencing a loss of consciousness be transported to the hospital for further neurological evaluation, which can include a CT or MRI scan. Hospitalization is recommended for persistent neurological symptoms or if evidence of intracranial pathology is detected. An athlete that sustains a grade 3 concussion may return to competition after one month after having been asymptomatic for two weeks. A season is terminated when there are two grade 3 concussions or evidence of intracranial pathology (i.e., contusion or intracranial hemorrhage).

Combined Scale

A four-grade scale (TABLE 6) was proposed to combine the advantages of the Cantu and CMS scales. This scale classifies head trauma as (1) mild, (2) mild–moderate, (3) moderate–severe, and (4) severe.[5]

Grade 1 (mild) head trauma on the combined scale is similar to grade 1 (mild) head injury on the CMS scale. This is characterized by confusion without amnesia and no loss of consciousness. Similar to the CMS scale, an athlete may return to competition the same day if he recovers quickly and completely and provided that he is asymptomatic at rest and exertion for 20 min.

Grade 2 (mild–moderate) head injury on the combined scale is a combination of mild (grade 1) and moderate (grade 2) on the Cantu scale and a moderate (grade 2) on the CMS scale. The athlete exhibits confusion without loss of consciousness but also experiences amnesia that lasts less than 24 h. An athlete who suffers a grade 2 (mild–moderate) concussion should be removed from competition and should not return to competition unless he is asymptomatic for a week. The evalua-

TABLE 6. Combined Clinical Grading System for Head Trauma in Sports

Grade and Symptoms	Criteria for Return to Play
1 **Mild:** Confusion without amnesia; no loss of consciousness	May return to play if asymptomatic at rest and exertion after observation of at least 20 min
2 **Mild–Moderate:** Confusion with amnesia lasting less than 24 h; no loss of consciousness	May return to play if asymptomatic for one week
3 **Moderate–Severe:** Loss of consciousness with an altered level of consciousness not exceeding 2–3 min; posttraumatic amnesia lasting more than 24 h	Should not be allowed to play for at least one month. May then return to play if asymptomatic for one week
4 **Severe:** Loss of consciousness with an altered level of consciousness not exceeding 2–3 min	Should not be allowed to return to play for at least one month. May then return to play if asymptomatic for two weeks

tion of a grade 2 concussion should include a neurological examination and neuroimaging, if indicated.

An athlete with a grade 3 (moderate–severe) concussion on the combined scale exhibits loss of consciousness not exceeding 2–3 min or posttraumatic amnesia lasting longer than 24 h. If the athlete experiences loss of consciousness, it is usually brief and recovery is rapid—so rapid that the athlete may not require immediate transport to the hospital. Nonetheless, he should undergo a detailed neurological evaluation and observe a mandatory rest period. The athlete should not return to competition before one month and should be asymptomatic for at least one week. The neurological evaluation should include a neurological examination and neuroimaging (i.e., CT or MRI).

A grade 4 (severe) head trauma on the combined scale should be considered a medical emergency. The athlete experiences loss of consciousness without a rapid recovery (i.e., a few minutes). In the athlete who fails to response rapidly, a more severe catastrophic injury should be presumed until proven otherwise. This athlete should be transported to a hospital on a spine board, if indicated, and undergo a neurological and/or neurological consultation including immediate neuroimaging. An athlete who suffers from a severe acute brain injury should not be allowed to return to competition before one month and should be asymptomatic for two weeks. Depending upon the type and severity of the injury, future participation in contact sports may be contraindicated.

American Academy of Neurology Scale

More recently, the AAN has adopted a modification of the previously developed CMS scale (TABLE 7).[6] The AAN scale classifies concussion into mild (grade 1), moderate (grade 2), and severe (grade 3).

Mild (grade 1) concussion on the AAN scale is characterized by transient confusion and/or transient concussive symptoms without loss of consciousness. To be classified as a mild concussion these symptoms should resolve within 15 min. However, if symptoms persist longer than 15 min, then the athlete is classified as having a moderate (grade 2) concussion. The athlete experiencing a mild (grade 1) concus-

TABLE 7. American Academy of Neurology Grading Scale

Grade and Symptoms	Criteria for Return to Play
1 **Mild:** Transient confusion; no loss of consciousness, concussive symptoms or mental status abnormalities resolving within 15 min	May return to contest if asymptomatic
2 **Moderate:** Transient confusion; no loss of consciousness, concussive symptoms or mental status abnormalities resolving after 15 min	May return to competition after one full week without symptoms
3 **Severe:** Loss of consciousness	
(a) Brief (seconds)	May return to competition if asymptomatic for one week
(b) Prolonged (minutes)	May return to competition if asymptomatic for two weeks

sion can be allowed to return to competititon if he is asymptomatic at rest and with exertion. An athlete who experiences postconcussive symptoms lasting longer than 15 min (i.e., moderate—grade 2) should not be allowed to return to competition the same day. He should be removed from the competition and undergo a follow-up evaluation at the site of competition on the following day. An athlete with a moderate (grade 2) concussion may return to competition only after being asymptomatic for one full week.

Severe (grade 3) concussions are associated with LOC. Because all cases of LOC should not be lumped together, grade 3 concussions are further subdivided into (a) brief (seconds) and (b) prolonged (minutes). An athlete who experiences LOC without rapid recovery or who exhibits persistent or progressive neurological signs should be emergently transferred to the nearest hospital via ambulance. According to the AAN scale, an athlete experiencing a brief LOC (grade 3a) should be held from competition until asymptomatic for one week. The athlete who experiences prolonged LOC (grade 3b) should be asymptomatic for two weeks before being allowed to participate again in contact sports.

The advantage of the AAN scale is that it provides a time frame in which postconcussive symptoms should resolve in order to be considered mild versus moderate. The previous CMS scale[4] did not have a duration of time or cutoff period that distinguished a mild concussion from more severe ones. A potential limitation of the AAN scale is that it does not distinguish between confusion without amnesia and confusion with amnesia. Although this distinction may be more theoretical than practical, an athlete who is confused but does not exhibit amnesia (if physiologically possible) should not be considered in the same classification of severity as an athlete with amnesia. Amnesia implies that the athlete is unable to learn new information and represents a more severe injury than an athlete who is dazed. Another potential limitation of the AAN scale is that it does not really differentiate a moderate (grade 2) from a severe concussion with a brief LOC (grade 3a) in regard to return to play. True LOC is an infrequent consequence of athletic concussion and implies bilateral cerebral hemispheric or brain-stem dysfunction. Accordingly, an athlete who experiences LOC (no matter how brief) should not be classified in the same category as an athlete who has postconcussive symptoms lasting longer than 15 min. Another potential limitation of the AAN scale is that the suggested rest period for athletes experiencing LOC may be too short.

TABLE 8. Indications for Neurological Evaluation after Head Injury in Sports

- Loss of consciousness lasting longer than 2 to 3 min
- Persistent neurological symptoms lasting longer than 24 h
- Focal neurological symptoms lasting longer than 24 h
- Seizures (focal or generalized)
- Clinical evidence of a skull fracture (e.g., Battle's sign, raccoon eyes, or cranial nerve palsies)

General Principles of Management

Regardless of the rating scale used to assess the severity of head trauma, certain general principles of management pertain. It must be realized that the scales mentioned above are general guidelines for health care providers and should not supersede good clinical judgment.

One difficulty inherent in the assessment of ATBI in sports is the documentation of mild TBI not associated with LOC. The distinction between the classical "ding" and the more concerning concussion with amnesia may be difficult to discern. In the "ding" or acute confusional state without LOC, the athlete is dazed and confused. The athlete cannot be evaluated for possible amnesia until the confusion has resolved. Once the athlete's confusion has cleared, that athlete can be assessed to determine if he or she experienced any amnesia. The assessment of amnesia should inquire about memory of events after (anterograde) and before (retrograde) the traumatic brain insult. A concussion with retrograde and anterograde injury implies a more serious injury than anterograde amnesia alone. Any athlete who exhibits amnesia should not return to completion in a contact/collision sport that same day.

There are certain situations in the management of head injury in sports that should alert the team physician or trainer that further neurological evaluation is indicated (TABLE 8). First, any athlete who is rendered unconscious and does not respond within a few minutes should be immediately evaluated in the hospital and considered for overnight observation. If an athlete exhibits a focal neurological deficit after a head injury, he or she should be considered a medical emergency and expeditiously transported to the hospital. Focal neurological deficits include hemiparesis, hemisensory loss, aphasia, or unilateral hyperreflexia. The presence of a focal neurological deficit is suggestive of a focal brain lesion such as an intracranial hemorrhage. The persistence of neurological symptoms in the head-injured athlete who is not rendered unconscious deserves special comment. If an athlete is still experiencing neurological symptoms (e.g., headache, dizziness, or impaired memory) 24 h after head trauma, then this athlete should also undergo neurological evaluation.

The clinical suspicion of a skull fracture should be another major indication for the neurological evaluation of the head-injured athlete. A basilar skull fracture should be suspected if the athlete develops a Battle's sign (a postauricular hematoma), otorrhea (cerebrospinal fluid bleeding from the ear canal), rhinorrhea (cerebrospinal fluid leaking from the nose), raccoon eyes (periorbital ecchymosis sec-ondary to leakage of blood from the anterior fossa into periorbital tissues), hemotympanum (blood behind the eardrum) or injuries to certain cranial nerves (e.g., the facial nerve). A skull fracture may also be suspected if there is a palpable malalignment of the calvarium.

TABLE 9. Contraindications to Returning to Contact Sports after Head Trauma

- Residual neurological deficits
- Prolonged coma
- Intracranial hemorrhage
- Cerebral contusion
- Posttraumatic epilepsy
- Skull fracture (relative contraindication)

Contraindications to Returning to Contact Sports

Certain situations exist when an athlete should not be allowed to return to contact sports after head trauma (TABLE 9). Any athlete who exhibits residual neurological impairment (e.g., language dysfunction, hemiparesis, tremor or movement disorders) should not be allowed to return to contact sports. The rationale for this is based on the potential risk for exacerbating existing neurological impairment. Furthermore, any athlete who is experiencing persistent cognitive impairment or behavioral abnormalities should also be considered in this category. Any athlete who experiences posttraumatic epilepsy should also not be allowed to return to contact sports, especially boxing.

Prolonged unconsciousness (6 h or longer) in the absence of a focal brain lesion (i.e., contusion, intracranial hemorrhage) is suggestive of diffuse axonal injury (DAI). Any athlete who has exhibited clinical evidence of DAI should not be allowed to participate in contact sports. Radiological support of DAI may be new white matter changes noted on MRI. The clinical significance of nonspecific white matter changes in the athlete who has not experienced prolonged unconsciousness remains to be determined. Although participation in contact sports should be determined on an individual basis, an athlete with white matter changes on MRI is theoretically and potentially at risk.

Participation in contact sports after a skull fracture is controversial. Obviously, if a skull fracture is complicated by intracranial hemorrhage, a cerebral contusion, or DAI, the athlete should not be allowed to participate. Individuals that have experienced previous intracranial hemorrhages or cerebral contusions are presumably at risk of reinjury. The athlete who had uncomplicated skull fracture that has well healed after one year may be considered for participation in contact sports. However, this policy is highly debatable and should probably be determined on an individual basis with consideration given to protective headgear, risk of head trauma, and prior neurological history (e.g., prior episodes of head trauma, history of posttraumatic seizures).

SECOND IMPACT SYNDROME

The second impact syndrome (SIS) represents an infrequent, but potentially catastrophic, neurological outcome associated with head trauma.[7,8] This syndrome has been primarily described in football, hockey, and boxing. However, it could be anticipated in any contact/collision sport where head trauma is not infrequent. SIS can be considered as an exaggerated response to a second relatively minor head trauma when an athlete is symptomatic from an earlier head trauma. Typically an athlete is then allowed to return to competition while symptomatic from the previous concussion (e.g., headache, dizziness, memory impairment, decreased concentration, etc.). The athlete then sustains a second (typically, minor) head trauma that results in increased intracranial pressure which leads to brain herniation, brain stem compromise, coma respiratory failure, and/or death. The mechanism is felt to be secondary to loss in vasomotor autoregulation. The SIS can be prevented by not allowing an athlete to return to contact/collision sports while symptomatic from concussion.

CHRONIC TRAUMATIC BRAIN INJURY

Chronic traumatic brain injury (CTBI) in sports represents the long-term cumulative effect of multiple concussive and subconcussive blows to the head. This condition has been described, mostly among retired boxers, as the "punch-drunk" syndrome, dementia pugilistic, or chronic traumatic encephalopathy. However, a milder form has been described among soccer players who may "head" the soccer ball with a high frequency.[9] Theoretically, this clinical syndrome can also be anticipated in American football.

Approximately 20% of retired professional boxers exhibit CTBI.[10] They tend to be less skilled boxers, have poor defensive skills, and are notorious for their ability to take a punch.[11] However, more highly skilled scientific boxers can also develop this syndrome with long exposure in boxing. Documented risk factors for CTBI in boxing include later retirement (over 28 years of age), increased duration of career (more than 10 years), and a greater number of bouts (more than 150 fights).[10] Boxers afflicted with CTBI may experience personality changes or impaired intellectual function, ranging from slow mentation or forgetfulness to severe dementia, and motor disturbances may include cerebellar dysfunction, extrapyramidal disorder of the Parkinson type, slurred speech, and ataxia.[10–13] Pathologically, these boxers exhibit varying combinations of brain atrophy, cavum septum pellucidum, degeneration of the substantia nigra, and Purkinje cell reduction in the cerebellum.[14] Pathologically, CTBI associated with boxing also resembles Alzheimer's disease by the presence of neurofibrillary tangles and beta-amyloid protein deposition in diffuse plaques.[15] Milder or subclinical chronic brain injury may be encountered in active amateur and professional boxers. Clinically, these boxers may exhibit mild difficulties with memory, concentration, and attention identifiable by neuropsychological testing. Neuroimaging techniques such as CT or MRI may demonstrate brain atrophy or progressive changes indicative of the cumulative effect of head trauma.[16–18] Recent evidence suggests that possession of the apoliprotein E (APOE) e4 allele may be associated with increased severity of chronic neurological deficits in high-exposure boxers.[19]

Soccer players have been observed to exhibit abnormalities on CT, electroencephalography (EEG), and neuropsychological testing similar to those encountered among boxers.[9,20,21] On CT scanning approximately one-third of retired soccer players demonstrated brain atrophy.[20] Also of note, cavum septum pellucid were noted in 6% of retired soccer players. It also has been demonstrated that soccer players display a higher frequency of EEG disturbances than does the normal population,[21] and that 80% of soccer players experience mild to severe neuropsychological impairment involving attention, concentration, memory, and judgment.[9]

TRANSIENT QUADRIPARESIS

Transient quadriparesis is a well-described clinical entity that has been primarily encountered in American football; however, it may be anticipated in any contact or collision sport. Symptoms associated with neuropraxia of the cervical spinal cord may include sensory dysfunction characterized by burning pain, numbness, and/or tingling of the extremities associated with variable motor impairment ranging from mild weakness to complete paralysis.[22] Neurological symptoms are typically transient and complete recovery usually occurs within 10–15 min; cases of prolonged neurological dysfunction occurring over a period of 36–48 h have been reported.[22]

The pathogenic mechanism of transient quadriparesis is thought to be secondary to neuropraxia of the cervical spinal cord. Neuropraxia of the cord is more likely to occur in individuals with a decreased anteroposterior diameter of the spinal canal.[22] Predisposing conditions that are associated with a decreased anteroposterior spinal canal include developmental or congenital spinal stenosis, congenital fusion, cervical instability, or protrusion of an intervertebral disc.[22]

Any athlete experiencing a transient quadriparesis should undergo a detailed neurological evaluation to determine the extent and etiology of the injury in order to make recommendations for future play. This neurological evaluation should include a comprehensive neurological examination, plain radiographs of the cervical spine, and an MRI of the cervical spine.[23,24] CT/myelography and electrophysiological testing can also provide additional information if the aforementioned are inconclusive. Plain radiographs of the cervical spine should be obtained immediately in any athlete experiencing an episode of transient quadriparesis. These plain radiographs are to ensure that the player has not sustained a fracture of the cervical spine nor displays any evidence of cervical instability, both of which require emergency medical management. Cervical spine radiographs are also necesary to detect congenital anomalies of the cervical spine which may predispose athletes to transient quadriparesis.

MRI can provide a noninvasive means of evaluating injury to the spinal cord or roots. It can serve as a useful guide for the physician to determine whether additional diagnostic studies should be performed and assist in establishing whether conservative or aggressive management should be pursued. If MRI is unavailable, then CT scanning, with or without metrizimide myelography, may be done. CT has the ability to better define skeletal architecture of the cervical spine. Both MRI and CT are useful in documenting cervical spinal stenosis which may predispose an athlete to neuropraxia of the cord.

The determination of cervical spinal stenosis has previously been established by using the ratio method.[22] This measure represents the ratio of the sagittal diameter of the cervical canal divided by the sagittal diameter of the adjacent cervical body as seen in a lateral cervical spine radiograph. A normal ratio is 1.00 or greater and a ratio less than 0.80 is considered stenotic.[22] The significance of this theoretical ratio has been challenged because it may raise inappropriate caution in contact sports in the absence of spinal stenosis.[23,24] The MRI scan has the distinct advantage of establishing how stenotic a spinal canal is around the cervical spinal cord and does not depend on hypothetical ratios. Accordingly, it is suggested that the MRI should serve as a noninvasive, yet accurate, means of determining the existence of cervical spinal stenosis[23,24] which can potentially increase the risk of injury to the cervical spine. A grading scale for cervical spinal stenosis by MRI is shown in TABLE 10.

Electrophysiological testing can provide additional documentation of extent of neurological injury. Spinal somatosensory evoked potentials can determine if there is delayed conduction in the spinal cord. Electromyography/nerve conduction velocities (EMG/NCV) can also document whether the cervical roots are compromised.

The management of the athlete who experiences transient neurological symptoms attributable to the cervical spinal cord, cervical nerve roots, or brachial plexus

TABLE 10. Grading Scale for Cervical Spinal Stenosis by Magnetic
Resonance Imaging

Grade 1	Normal: No evidence of spinal stenosis. A full CSF reserve around the cervical spinal cord.
Grade 2	Borderline/Mild: Impingement of the thecal sac with some decrease reserve of the CSF reserve around the cervical spinal cord. No spinal cord compression.
Grade 3	Significant: Almost complete obliteration of the CSF reserve secondary to compression of the thecal sac with or without spinal cord compression.

CSF, cerebrospinal fluid.

requires careful consideration. It is essential that the team physician be able to distinguish the usually benign "stingers" or "burners" (stretch injuries to the brachial plexus or cervical nerve roots) from the more ominous transient neuropraxia of the cervical spinal cord. Characteristic clinical presentation of neuropraxia of the cervical spinal cord is transient paresthesia of all four extremities with or without transient quadriparesis. Typically these symptoms last approximately 10 to 15 min and resolve completely. Incomplete resolution of symptoms by 24 to 48 h suggests more serious injury to the cervical spine. Any athlete who experiences this transient neuropraxia of the cervical spinal cord should be removed from play and treated as a cervical spine fracture until plain radiographs fail to demonstrate a fracture or cervical instability. Once it has been established that the athlete has a stable cervical spine, without fracture, an MRI scan of the cervical spine should be obtained. This imaging technique will identify those athletes with structural lesions, such as disk herniation or osteophyte formation, which significantly encroach upon and narrow the cervical spinal canal, causing a developmental spinal stenosis.

Controversy exists as to whether athletes with a normal MRI or mild spinal stenosis with a normal neurological examination should be allowed to return to play after an episode of transient quadriparesis. Obviously the decision is difficult, and each case should be interpreted individually. However, individuals with significant spinal stenosis should not be allowed to play in contact or collision sports.

Although it is not clear whether transient quadriparesis predisposes to catastrophic cervical spine injury, it is probably justifiable to exercise caution and prohibit continued participation in football, especially for those athletes who have experienced multiple episodes. The spear tackler's spine represents a clinical subset of football players where participation in tackle sports and other collision activities is contraindicated.[25] These athletes display the following characteristics:

- Developmental cervical spinal stenosis
- Persistent straightening or reversal of the normal cervical lordotic nerve on lateral plain films
- Concomitant preexisting posttraumatic roentogenographic abnormalities of the cervical spine
- Documentation of having employed spear-tackling techniques

Participation in collision sports is precluded in this subset because the combination of the above-mentioned features predisposes the athlete to axial loading of the cervical spine. This axial loading could potentially result in permanent neurological sequelae such as quadriplegia.

CONCLUSION

Sports neurology has developed into an important medical subspecialty that is vital to protecting the health of the athlete. The future will require that neurologists become more familiar with sports medicine and that sports medicine physicians become adept at treating neurological conditions in the athlete.

REFERENCES

1. KRAUS, J. F. 1991. Epidemiologic features of injuries to the central nervous system. *In* Neuroepidemiology: A Tribute to Bruce Schoenberg. D. W. Anderson, Ed.: 333–357. CRC Press. Boca Raton, FL.
2. TEASDALE, G. & B. JENNETT. 1974. Assessment of coma and impaired consciousness: A practical scale. Lancet **1:** 81–84.
3. CANTU, R. C. 1986. Guidelines for return to contact sports after a cerebral concussion. Physician Sportsmed. **14(10):** 75–83.
4. KELLY, J. P., J. S. NICHOLS, C. M. FILLEY, *et al.* 1991. Concussion in sports: Guidelines for prevention of catastrophic outcome. JAMA **266:** 2867–2869.
5. JORDAN, B. D. 1994. Sports injuries. *In* Current Diagnosis in Neurology. E. Feldman, Ed.: 253–256. Mosby Year Book. St. Louis, MO.
6. QUALITY STANDARD SUBCOMMITTEES. 1997. Practice parameter: The management of concussion in sports (summary statement). Neurology **48:** 581–585.
7. SANDERS, R. L. & R. E. HARBOUGH. 1984. The second impact in catastrophic contact-sports head trauma. JAMA **252:** 538–539.
8. CANTU, R. C. & R. VOY. 1995. Second impact syndrome: A risk in any sport. Physician Sportsmed. **23(6):** 27–34.
9. TYSVAER, A. T. & E. A. LOCHEN. 1991. Soccer injuries to the brain: A neuropsychologic study of former soccer players. Am. J. Sports Med. **19:** 56–59.
10. ROBERTS, A. H. 1969. Brain Damage in Boxers. Pitman Medical Scientific Publishing Co. London.
11. CRITCHLEY, M. 1957. Medical aspects of boxing particularly from a neurological standpoint. Br. Med. J. **1:** 357–362.
12. JORDAN, B. D. 1993. Chronic neurologic injuries in boxing. *In* Medical Aspects of Boxing. B. D. Jordan, Ed.: 177–185. CRC Press. Boca Raton, FL.
13. MENDEZ, M. F. 1995. The neuropsychiatric aspects of boxing. Int. J. Psychiatry **25:** 249–262.
14. CORSELLIS, J. A. N., C. J. BRUTON & D. FREEMAN-BROWNE. 1973. The aftermath of boxing. Psychol. Med. **3:** 270–303.
15. ROBERTS, G. W., D. ALLSOP & C. BRUTON. 1990. The occult aftermath of boxing. J. Neurol. Neursurg. Psychiatry **53:** 373–378.
16. JORDAN, B. D., C. JOHRE, W. A. HAUSER, *et al.* 1992. CT of 338 active professional boxers. Radiology **185:** 509–512.
17. JORDAN, B. D. & R. D. ZIMMERMAN. 1990. Computed tomography and magnetic resonance imaging comparisons in boxers. JAMA **263:** 1670–1674.
18. JORDAN, B. D. 1992. Serial computed tomography in professional boxers. J. Neuroimag. **2:** 181–185.
19. JORDAN, B. D., N. R. RELKIN, L. D. RAVDIN, *et al.* 1997. Apolipoprotein (Ee4) associated with chronic traumatic brain injury in boxing. JAMA **278:** 136–140.
20. SORTLAND, O. & A. T. TYSVAER. 1989. Brain damage in former association football players: An evaluation by cerebral computed tomography. Neurovad. **31:** 44–48.
21. TYSVAER, A. T., O. V. STORLI & N. I. BACKEN. 1989. Soccer injuries to the brain: A neurologic and electroencephalographic study of former players. Acta Neurol. Scand. **80:** 151–156.
22. TORG, J. S., H. PAVLOV, S. E. GENUARIO, *et al.* 1986. Neuropraxia of the cervical spinal cord with transient quadriplegia. J. Bone Jt. Surg. Am. **68:** 1354–1370.

23. JORDAN, B. D., R. F. WARREN, P. TSAIRIS, *et al.* 1992. How to evaluate transient quadriparesis. Physician Sports Med. **20(2):** 83–90.
24. CANTU, R. C. 1997. Transient quadriparesis. *In* Sports Neurology, 2nd edit. B. D. Jordan, P. Tsairis & R. F. Warren, Eds. Lippincott–Raven. Philadelphia, PA. In press.
25. TORG, J. S., B. SENNETT & H. PAVLOV. 1993. Spear tackler's spine. An entity precluding participation in the tackle football and collision activities that expose the cervical spine to axial energy impacts. Am. J. Sports Med. **21:** 640–649.

Symptom Localization in Neuropsychiatry

A Functional Neuroimaging Approach

DAVID A. SILBERSWEIG[a] AND EMILY STERN[b]

Functional Neuroimaging Laboratory
The New York Hospital–Cornell Medical Center (Box 171)
525 East 68th Street
New York, New York 10021

INTRODUCTION

One hundred years ago, there was little distinction between neurology and psychiatry. Great physician-scientists such as Jackson, Charcot, Kraepelin, and Freud made seminal observations linking abnormalities of perception, cognition, emotion, and behavior to brain dysfunction. However, even as these pioneers had profound insights into the workings of the human mind, they knew that they lacked the neuroscientific tools to understand its neurobiologic substrate in a detailed fashion. Perhaps as a result, psychiatry and neurology drifted apart. Disorders were classified as psychiatric if they were "nonfocal" disturbances of mentation or behavior for which no clear brain lesion could be found.

The explosion of neuroscientific investigation over the past few decades, fueled by technological advances, has helped to dissolve this dichotomous conception of diseases as purely "neurologic" or "psychiatric." As a result, patients are better served, and there has been a renewed exploration of the interface between human brain and mental function, in both the normal and the diseased state.

One approach to the brain-mind interface is to link particular clinical or behavioral abnormalities to specific brain regions or systems through the use of specialized methodologies. This chapter describes the use of one of these methods, positron emission tomography (PET), to localize the systems-level brain dysfunction underlying psychiatric symptoms. Our work in this context owes much to Fred Plum, who in this century has greatly contributed to, and transmitted, the neurobehavioral tradition of careful clinical-neuropathological correlation. Dr. Plum's work, probing the neural substrates of consciousness through the careful observation and study of unconscious disease states, set a powerful example. He likewise called upon his trainees to pay careful attention to the phenomenology of clinical signs and symptoms—even those affecting the highest of human functions—and to gather relevant neurobiological data so as to localize them in the neuraxis. We therefore hope that our work constitutes a suitable expression of our gratitude, in the form that Dr. Plum would most appreciate.

[a,b] E-mail: dasilber@med.cornell.edu; estern@med.cornell.edu

RATIONALE FOR SYMPTOM-ORIENTED APPROACH

When attempting to identify the brain circuits underlying neuropsychiatric diseases, a symptom-oriented strategy can be particularly effective. Many psychiatric disorders are still descriptive,[1] representing heterogeneous combinations of symptoms; and particular symptoms, such as delusions, may occur in different psychiatric syndromes, such as schizophrenia or affective disorders. Moreover, psychopharmacologic agents, such as neuroleptics, successfully treat particular symptoms, such as delusions, whether in the setting of schizophrenia or affective disorders.[2] Although between-group functional neuroimaging studies of patients with psychiatric syndromes versus control subjects have been quite informative, within-group studies of symptoms can reduce the potential sources of confounding variance. The direct study of symptoms is also more likely to yield pathophysiologically meaningful information than the valuable but indirect approach of employing a neuropsychological task that is hypothesized to (but may not) relate to symptom formation.

Because individual symptom states are more likely to map onto brain states than are heterogeneous descriptive syndromes, we and our colleagues from London have developed and validated functional neuroimaging techniques that allow the detection of patterns of neuronal activity specific to the naturalistic occurrence of neuropsychiatric symptoms. We chose to study the "positive" symptoms of hallucinations in schizophrenia and tics in Tourette's syndrome because (1) clinically, they represent striking, disabling manifestations of classic neuropsychiatric disorders, the pathophysiologies of which are not understood; (2) neurobiologically, they represent afferent and efferent instances (respectively) of recurrent, transient, involuntary intrusions within the ongoing stream of neural processing; and (3) methodologically, their study constitutes a challenge, requiring the integration of knowledge from clinical neuropsychiatry, physiology, physics, and mathematics that makes functional neuroimaging research such an interdisciplinary and rewarding endeavor.

Here we will describe our work examining the systems-level functional neuroanatomy of neuropsychiatric symptom states (occurring at the exact time of imaging). In addition, we will discuss the work of our colleagues, identifying the basal (or "resting") pattern of neural activity correlating with trait measurements of neuropsychiatric symptoms (taken within days or weeks of imaging) in schizophrenia and major depression.

METHODS

Functional neuroimaging provides an *in vivo* approach to examine pathologic symptoms in neuropsychiatric disease. This direct measure of brain function complements and extends other neuroscientific investigative methods. Studies of neurotransmitter metabolites in the blood and spinal fluid, for example, are helpful but indirect. Studies of the brain at autopsy are of interest but are often confounded by changes due to preterminal medical events and by tissue processing. Structural imaging methods are useful for measuring volumes of particular structures as well as morphology, but do not supply direct information about brain function. Finally, no adequate animal models exist for most neuropsychiatric diseases, which affect the highest forms of human mentation and behavior.

Positron emission tomography (PET), single photon emission computed tomography (SPECT), functional magnetic resonance imaging (fMRI), magnetoencephalography (MEG), and electroencephalography (EEG) all provide *in vivo* measures of brain function, each with its own strengths and weaknesses. Although techniques such as fMRI are extremely promising and rapidly developing,[3,4] to date, some of the most sophisticated experiments dealing with neuropsychiatric disease have been performed with PET. PET can be used to examine brain metabolism (with [^{18}F]fluorodeoxyglucose; [^{18}F]FDG), blood flow (with ^{15}O), and neurochemistry (with specific radioactively labeled ligands). The studies described below have been performed with $H_2{}^{15}O$ PET, a technique which uses radioactively labeled water to measure blood flow as an index of neuronal activity.[5]

$H_2{}^{15}O$ PET can be used to measure the basal "resting state," which may itself reflect underlying trait-like aspects of psychopathology. In addition, because of its short half-life (2.07 min), it can be used to examine the brain in repeated "activated" conditions that are either experimentally imposed or that occur due to particular symptom states that are present at the time of the scan. In the former, study design is crucial to developing a mental task that isolates the specific cognitive process of interest.[6] Often, another experimental condition, which acts as a sensory-motor control state, is used to control for the afferent and efferent components of the activation condition. In the latter, a more naturalistic approach aims to image the symptom of interest as it occurs.[7]

Appropriate image processing and analyses are critical to extract statistical information from functional imaging data. For PET, the images are realigned to correct for slight head movement between scans. Often the images are smoothed with a spatial filter and transformed into the standardized, stereotactic coordinate space of Talairach and Tournoux[8] to increase signal-to-noise and accommodate the normal variability in gyral anatomy across subjects. Alternatively, MRI scans of each individual can be coregistered with the PET data for additional, detailed neuroanatomic reference, or the images can be interpreted in the context of a composite probabilistic atlas of neuroanatomy.[9] Normalization for differences in global blood flow across conditions and subjects is performed, and categorical (*t* test), correlational (regression), principal component (PCA), or other statistical analyses are then performed.[10]

PET can be used to image the neural correlates of symptom traits as well as symptom states. To examine symptom traits, one approach has been to measure the symptoms of interest using clinical tools, such as symptom rating scales, in many different patients. Resting scans are then used to find brain areas in which rCBF correlates positively or negatively with the symptom measures across subjects. Two examples of this, which examine the symptoms of schizophrenia and major depression, are described below. The study of symptom states requires either eliciting the symptom of interest using an activation task or using methods that can capture an image of the brain as the symptom occurs. Two examples of the latter approach, examining hallucinations in schizophrenia and tics in Tourette's syndrome, are also described.

TRAIT STUDIES

Many basal measurements of brain activity in schizophrenic patients have been performed with SPECT and [^{18}F]FDG PET. The majority have demonstrated a relative decrease in frontal activity compared to normal control subjects; however, some have not shown hypofrontality and a few have even demonstrated hyperfrontality.[11-13] Until relatively recently, such studies were characterized by between-group subtraction designs and region-of-interest analyses. With an increase in sophistication in study design, image acquisition, and image analysis, it has been possible to more fully explore brain function and dysfunction in schizophrenia, including the identification of brain areas implicated in specific symptoms.

In an elegant study by Liddle and colleagues,[14] the neural correlates of clinical traits were identified in a group of 30 chronic schizophrenic patients. Their symptoms were assessed within two weeks of scanning using section 2 of the Comprehensive Assessment of Symptoms and History (CASH).[15] Syndrome scores (reflecting the presence of related or co-occurring symptoms) were then obtained by a factor analysis of the symptom scores. The items used for this analysis included measures of both positive and negative symptoms such as delusions, hallucinations, positive formal thought disorder, poverty of speech, poverty of content of speech, decreased spontaneous movement, inappropriate affect, and a score for affective flattening (which incorporated scores for lack of facial expression, affective nonresponsivity, paucity of expressive gestures, and decreased vocal inflection, by taking their mean). Resting regional cerebral blood flow (rCBF) was measured with a steady state ^{15}O-inhalation technique. For each syndrome, a statistical parametric map (SPM,[10] a map of statistical significance) of the correlation between syndrome score and rCBF at each pixel was generated. This was done for both positive and negative correlations.

The analysis of symptom scores revealed three factors accounting for 75.9% of the variance in symptom scores. The three factors identified were psychomotor poverty, disorganization, and reality distortion. Each of the three syndromes was correlated with a specific distributed pattern of rCBF.

The syndrome of psychomotor poverty was negatively correlated with rCBF in the prefrontal cortex (especially on the left, extending from dorsolateral prefrontal cortex to medial prefrontal cortex and into contiguous anterior cingulate cortex) and the left parietal association cortex. Significant positive correlations were present in the head of the caudate bilaterally.

Disorganization was positively correlated with rCBF in the anterior cingulate and contiguous medial prefrontal cortices (especially on the right), the left superior temporal sulcus, and the dorsomedial nucleus of the thalamus. Negative correlations between disorganization and rCBF were present in the right ventral prefrontal cortex/insular cortex, in Broca's area, and bilaterally in the posterior portion of the angular gyrus.

Reality distortion was positively correlated with rCBF in the left temporal and frontal regions, especially the left parahippocampal region, but also including the left superior temporal pole and the left lateral prefrontal cortex. Positive correlations were also present in the left ventral striatum. Negative correlations were present in the right posterior cingulate, posterior superior temporal region and adjacent supramarginal gyrus, and the head of caudate.

In a related study, Friston *et al.* used directed and nondirected (canonical) correlational analyses to examine the relationship between overall psychopathology in schizophrenia and rCBF.[16] The highest positive correlations were found in the left temporal region (especially the parahippocampal region), the left midbrain, the thalamus, and the left striatum. Less significant, negative correlations were present in the right insula/frontal operculum, and in bilateral superior parietal association cortex.

In a study by Bench *et al.* similar methods were used to examine the neural correlates of symptoms in major depression.[17] A factor analysis was performed on patients' psychiatric and cognitive symptom ratings. Scores from the resulting three-factor solution were then correlated with rCBF. The first factor had high loadings for anxiety and corresponded to a combination of psychic and somatic anxiety, insomnia, and psychomotor agitation. The score for this factor correlated positively with rCBF in the right posterior cingulate cortex and the inferior parietal lobule bilaterally. The second factor corresponded to psychomotor retardation and depressed mood and showed negative correlations with rCBF in the left inferior and dorsolateral prefrontal cortex, the left superior temporal gyrus, and the left inferior parietal lobule (including supramarginal and angular gyri). Less significant positive correlations were present in left ventral striatum and precuneus as well as right inferior temporo-occipital cortex. The third factor had high loadings for cognitive performance and psychomotor agitation (which were inversely related). Cognitive impairment was correlated with decreased rCBF in the left medial prefrontal cortex, the right anterior thalamus, the right superior temporal gyrus, the right postcentral gyrus, and the posterior cingulate cortices bilaterally.

These trait study findings increase our understanding of the brain circuits in which basal dysfunction may predispose to neuropsychiatric symptom formation. The state studies, in contrast, provide information about the brain circuits in which dysfunction underlies symptom expression. After a descripton of the state studies, the trait and state findings will be integrated, and the implications for neuropsychiatric symptom localization will be discussed.

STATE STUDIES

An approach that we have taken to the localization of neuropsychiatric symptoms has been to perform functional neuroimaging experiments which specifically isolate the symptom of interest by imaging it as it occurs in a naturalistic fashion. A number of neuropsychiatric symptoms are involuntary, transient, randomly occurring, and idiosyncratic. Because of these characteristics, defining the brain areas which are active specifically during these events has been difficult. We have developed and validated PET techniques to image such symptom states.[18,19] These methods were then applied to the study of hallucinations in schizophrenia and tics in Tourette's syndrome.

Hallucinations are perceptions in the absence of external stimuli. They are present in up to 74% of patients with schizophrenia.[20] Auditory-verbal hallucinations are most common; however, visual and other sensory modality hallucinations can be present. They usually comprise voices talking to or about the patient in a derogatory fashion. Unlike the hallucinations of traditional neurologic disorders, they are often experienced as real and of emotional relevance.[21] These factors make this symptom extremely debilitating.

Earlier functional imaging studies have suggested a number of frontal, temporal, and striatal brain areas that may be involved in the predisposition to hallucinate.[22-27] They did not, however, have the temporal discrimination necessary to isolate the brain state associated with the transient, randomly occurring hallucinating state. Using the specifically designed methods of PET image acquisition and analysis noted above, we studied five schizophrenic patients with classic auditory-verbal hallucinations despite medication, and one drug-naive patient with both visual and auditory-linguistic hallucinations.[28] The patients were asked to report the occurrence of each hallucination during the scanning protocol, and the exact timing of the hallucinations was noted relative to radiotracer delivery to the brain. An analysis[19] was then performed to locate the brain regions in which activity was highly correlated with the occurrence of hallucinations.

In the individual subject with visual and auditory-verbal hallucinations, prominent activity was detected in bilateral (left > right) visual and auditory-linguistic association cortices, and in left posterior cingulate, right parahippocampal/mesotemporal and temporal pole (para)limbic regions, as well as in right striatum. The regions of activation common to the group of five patients with auditory-verbal hallucinations were deep (para)limbic and subcortical structures, including the bilateral hippocampus and parahippocampal gyrus, right anterior cingulate gyrus, bilateral thalamus, and right ventral striatum. There were no prominent frontal activations in these group analyses.

The same methodology was employed to identify the brain circuits associated with tics in Tourette's syndrome. Tourette's syndrome is a striking neuropsychiatric disorder characterized by multiple motor and vocal tics, which may be simple or complex in nature. Although basal ganglia dysfunction has been implicated due to the occurrence of tics in conditions such as carbon monoxide poisoning and encephalitis lethargica, the neural correlates of tics had not previously been defined. Six right-handed male patients with Tourette's syndrome and frequent tics were studied.[29] Tics were monitored with video cameras as well as a throat microphone and tape recorder. Information about the exact timing of the tics relative to radiotracer delivery to the brain was used to identify brain regions in which activity was highly correlated with the occurrence of tics.

Increased brain activity highly correlated with involuntary tic behavior was detected in executive motor cortices (supplementary motor, premotor, anterior cingulate, and dorsolateral prefrontal), primary motor cortices, language cortices (including Broca's area), other paralimbic cortices (posterior cingulate, and insula), and subcortical regions (lentiform nucleus and midbrain tegmentum). Activations in auditory and post-rolandic heteromodal association cortices were also detected.

DISCUSSION

The results presented above, obtained through the careful use of functional neuroimaging techniques, have implications for a "neurologic" model of neuropsychiatric symptomatology.

The symptom trait studies of Liddle and Bench demonstrate the ability to utilize within-group variance in symptom profiles to identify patterns of resting brain activity that correlate with a predisposition to individual symptoms or symptom factors. Comparing the results across these two studies reveals another important finding: that the similar symptoms of psychomotor poverty in schizophrenia and psychomotor retardation in depression have similar profiles of dorsolateral prefrontal hypoactivity, despite the marked difference in DSM (Diagnostic and Statistical Manual of Mental Disorders) diagnosis.[30]

Our symptom state studies suggest that dysfunction in specific neural circuits is associated with the occurrence of major positive neuropsychiatric symptoms. These circuits are distributed and have neocortical, paralimbic, limbic, and subcortical components. They also show somatotopic and/or modality specificity that is consistent with the clinical phenomenology of the symptom. The perceptual symptom of hallucinations, for example, is correlated with activity in afferent post-rolandic cortices, whereas the behavioral symptom of tics is correlated with activity predominantly in efferent pre-rolandic cortices. Furthermore, auditory-verbal and visual hallucinations in the individual patient analysis were associated with activity in auditory-linguistic and visual association cortices, respectively. Similarly, vocal and motor tics in the patients with Tourette's syndrome were associated with activity in Broca's area and motor cortices.

Perhaps most interesting and relevant from the vantage point of pathogenesis, however, is not the neocortical activity, but the activity detected in the (para)limbic and subcortical regions. Here, the findings from our state studies and Liddle's trait studies of positive symptoms converge. These deeper, phylogenetically older regions are highly interconnected and have convergent and divergent connections from and to widespread areas of cortex.[31] They thereby constitute a foundation for mnemonic, attentional, emotional, and intentional processing, and are necessary for the organism to label and evaluate the relevance of sensory data and to select an appropriate action.[32] It is therefore not unreasonable that dysfunction in these regions or the interactions (or functional connectivity[33]) among them can contribute to the inappropriate labeling of percepts in hallucinations and the inappropriate initiation of actions in tics. Elsewhere we have discussed the details of possible functional contributions of specific activated brain regions (such as the hippocampus, ventral striatum, and thalamus) to symptom formation, and the implications of these findings for an understanding of pathophysiology of disorders such as schizophrenia.[34] In this paper we will continue to focus upon the implications of the findings for a contemporary conceptualization of neuropsychiatric disorders.

The neuroanatomic symptom specificity demonstrated in the above studies, within and across descriptive psychiatric syndromes, suggests not only a more biologically based approach to differential diagnosis and therapeutics, but also a more neurologic model of pathophysiology, in which psychiatric symptoms can be localized. The model is supported by the convergence of clinical lesion, structural imaging, electrophysiologic, and functional imaging studies that suggest similar localizations for particular psychiatric symptoms, whether due to "idiopathic" psychiatric disorders or to known neurologic conditions. Depression, for example, has been associated with left frontal strokes in structural MRI studies,[35] and with left frontal hypoactivity on PET studies of patients with primary major depression (as noted above) or with depression secondary to movement disorders.[36] Furthermore, specific psychomotor and cognitive subsyndromes within the depressive spectrum have been associated with dorsolateral and medial prefrontal regions respectively, as noted above.[17] Another example of conceptual convergence is the implication of left mesotemporal dysfunction in the pathogenesis of psychosis, by functional neuroimaging studies of schizophrenia such as those described above, and by the clinical and electrophysiological characterization of patients with partial complex seizure disorders.[37] This "neurologic" mapping of psychiatric symptomatology is also consistent with the traditional lesion literature and the rapidly expanding functional imaging literature indicating that even subtle cognitive and behavioral operations can be mapped,[38,39] and that many of these operations involve parallel distributed, cortical-subcortical brain circuits.[40-42]

The neurologic model would therefore suggest that neuropsychiatric disorders of diverse etiology could cause a similar symptom by affecting a particular final common neuroanatomic pathway, much the same way as a stroke, tumor or abscess could all cause a contralateral hemiparesis if they involved the telencephalic motor system. Furthermore, the particular expression of the symptom could indicate the specific node in the distributed system/circuit that is affected (or the specific nodes that are disconnected), much as pyramidal and extrapyramidal movement disorders, or cortical and subcortical (including striatal vs. thalamic) aphasias can now be discriminated.[43]

Hallucinations, for example, may be visual or auditory, formed or unformed, lateralized or nonlateralized, linguistic or musical. Each of these clinical characteristics has neurologic localizing value in the context of hallucinations secondary to complex partial epilepsy foci, peduncular hallucinosis, stroke, etc.[44] The results of our state studies and Liddle's trait studies of schizophrenic hallucinations suggest that the higher-order phenomenology of schizophrenic hallucinations, such as stereotypical auditory-linguistic content and emotional/motivational relevance, may be localizable as well. This is the case even in the absence of gross structural pathology, although more subtle morphometric abnormalities have recently been described.[45] Regional cytoarchitectonic and neurochemical abnormalities associated with schizophrenia in the regions detected with functional neuroimaging provide plausible basic mechanisms (including abnormal GABA-glutamate-dopamine (D4) connectivity and interactions in interneuron populations) that could underlie symptom formation.[46–48]

The findings from our Tourette's syndrome-tic study provide another example of the localization of a neuropsychiatric symptom to a distributed neural system. In this case, two of the executive motor cortico-striato-pallido-thalamo-cortical circuits described by Alexander and colleagues,[49] the motor/putamen and anterior cingulate/ventral striatal circuits, are implicated. Activity in executive motor structures, usually associated with volitional behavior,[50] can explain the urge or will to move that is often associated with tics in Tourette's syndrome. Within these circuits, the direct and indirect pathways provide a balance of excitation and inhibition that may be disrupted.[51] The particular, somatotopically specific cortical regions that are entrained by this disruption may determine the phenomenology of the unvoluntary behavior. Dopaminergic projections from the midbrain tegmentum, a region activated in the study, are involved in the modulation of these circuits.[49] This may help to explain why dopaminergic excess exacerbates tics, whereas dopaminergic blockade attenuates them.[52]

In this context, it is notable that in functional neuroimaging studies of obsessive-compulsive disorder (OCD, which has symptomatology that often occurs with tics and Tourette's syndrome), the adjacent, parallel orbitofrontal/head of caudate circuit (more associated with cognitive-emotional integration) is implicated.[53] By combining the tic and OCD results, one can begin to localize symptom subtypes within the spectrum of repetitive, unvoluntary behaviors in a manner consistent with the known connectivity and increasingly understood functions of prefrontal subsystems.

The information obtained with these imaging techniques can therefore clarify the systems-level pathophysiology of neuropsychiatric disorders by identifying the brain regions and systems in which dysfunction is necessary or sufficient to cause specific symptoms. More basic cellular and molecular neuroscientific techniques can then be used in a complementary fashion to clarify the etiology of that localized dysfunction in patients with specific clinical syndromes. This convergent approach can provide a foundation for the development of more targeted, biologically based diagnostic and therapeutic strategies.

The localizationist approach that we are advocating here is also illustrated or supported by functional neuroimaging studies of phobic anxiety symptoms,[54] theories of attention deficit-hyperactivity disorder,[55] and some recent textbooks of neuropsychiatry.[44] We would like to think that it is consistent with Dr. Plum's exhortations to make psychiatric thinking more neurologic and to use scientific data to do so. Indeed, it is not dissimilar to the approach taken by Drs. Plum and Posner in The Diagnosis of Stupor and Coma,[56] in which they clarified those neural systems in which dysfunction was necessary and sufficient to cause impairments in consciousness, the varieties of signs and symptoms that followed disruption of specific parts of those systems, and the various etiologies or disorders that could produce those characteristic neuropathologic and clinical presentations. We hope to have shown how functional neuroimaging techniques are beginning to allow the extension of such neurologic localization approaches to psychiatric disorders which, not long ago, were thought to be "psychological" in nature due to their striking symptomatology and the apparent lack of associated gross brain lesions.

REFERENCES

1. DSM-IV. 1994. Diagnostic and Statistical Manual of Mental Disorders. American Psychiatric Association. 4th edit. Washington, D.C.
2. KAPLAN, H. I. & B. J. SADOCK. 1993. Pocket Handbook of Psychiatric Drug Treatment. Williams & Wilkins. Baltimore, MD.
3. OGAWA, S., D. W. TANK, R. MENON, *et al.* 1992. Intrinsic signal changes accompanying sensory stimulation: Functional brain mapping with magnetic resonance imaging. Proc. Natl. Acad. Sci. USA **89(13):** 5951–5955.
4. BANDETTINI, P. A., A. JESMANOWICZ, E. C. WONG & J. S. HYDE. 1993. Processing strategies for time-course data sets in functional MRI of the human brain. Magn. Reson. Med. **30(2):** 161–173.
5. RAICHLE, M. E., W. R. MARTIN, P. HERSCOVITCH, M. A. MINTUN & J. MARKHAM. 1983. Brain blood flow measured with intravenous H2(15)O. II. Implementation and validation. J. Nucl. Med. **24(9):** 790–798.
6. POSNER, M. I., S. E. PETERSEN, P. T. FOX & M. E. RAICHLE. 1988. Localization of cognitive operations in the human brain. Science **240:** 1627–1631.
7. JONES, T., D. A. SILBERSWEIG, E. STERN, *et al.* 1996. The development of in vivo tracer methods to obtain new information about human disease: A study of the hallucinating brain. Eur. J. Nucl. Med. **23(3):** 332–335.
8. TALAIRACH, J. & P. TOURNOUX. 1988. Co-Planar Stereotaxic Atlas of the Human Brain. Thieme Medical Publishers. Stuttgart.
9. PAUS, T., N. OTAKY, Z. CARAMANOS, *et al.* 1996. In vivo morphometry of the intrasulcal gray matter in the human cingulate, paracingulate, and superior-rostral sulci: Hemispheric asymmetries, gender differences and probability maps. J. Comp. Neurol. **376(4):** 664–673.
10. FRISTON, K. J., A. P. HOLMES, K. J. WORSLEY, J.-P. POLINE, C. D. FRITH & R. S. J. FRACKOWIAK. 1995. Statistical parametric maps in functional imaging: A general linear approach. Hum. Brain Mapping **2(4):** 189–210.
11. FRISTON, K. J. 1992. The dorsolateral prefrontal cortex, schizophrenia and PET. J. Neural Transm. Suppl. **37:** 79–93.
12. DE LISI, L. E., M. S. BUCHSBAUM, H. H. HOLCOMB, *et al.* 1985. Clinical correlates of decreased anteroposterior metabolic gradients in positron emission tomography (PET) of schizophrenic patients. Am. J. Psychiatry **142(1):** 78–81.
13. SZECHTMAN, H., C. NAHMIAS, E. S. GARNETT, *et al.* 1988. Effect of neuroleptics on altered cerebral glucose metabolism in schizophrenia. Arch. Gen. Psychiatry **45(6):** 523–532.
14. LIDDLE, P. F., K. J. FRISTON, C. D. FRITH, S. R. HIRSCH, T. JONES & R. S. FRACKOWIAK. 1992. Patterns of cerebral blood flow in schizophrenia. Br. J. Psychiatry **160:** 179–186.
15. ANDREASEN, N. C. 1987. Comprehensive assessment of symptoms and history. University College of Iowa College of Medicine. Iowa.
16. FRISTON, K. J., P. F. LIDDLE, C. D. FRITH, S. R. HIRSCH & R. S. FRACKOWIAK. 1992. The left medial temporal region and schizophrenia. A PET study. Brain **115(Pt. 2):** 367–382.
17. BENCH, C. J., K. J. FRISTON, R. G. BROWN, R. S. FRACKOWIAK & R. J. DOLAN. 1993. Regional cerebral blood flow in depression measured by positron emission tomography: The relationship with clinical dimensions. Psychol. Med. **23(3):** 579–590.
18. SILBERSWEIG, D. A., E. STERN, C. D. FRITH, *et al.* 1993. Detection of thirty-second cognitive activations in single subjects with positron emission tomography: A new low-dose H2(15)O regional cerebral blood flow three-dimensional imaging technique. J. Cereb. Blood Flow Metab. **13(4):** 617–629.
19. SILBERSWEIG, D. A., E. STERN, L. SCHNORR, *et al.* 1994. Imaging transient, randomly occurring neuropsychological events in single subjects with positron emission to-

mography: An event-related count rate correlational analysis. J. Cereb. Blood Flow Metab. **14(5):** 771–782.

20. WING, J. K., J. E. COOPER & N. SARTORIUS. 1974. Measurement and Classification of Psychiatric Symptoms. Cambridge University Press. Cambridge, UK.

21. SCHNEIDER, K. 1959. Clinical Psychopathology. Grune & Stratton. New York.

22. CLEGHORN, J. M., E. S. GARNETT, C. NAHMIAS, *et al.* 1990. Regional brain metabolism during auditory hallucinations in chronic schizophrenia. Br. J. Psychiatry **157:** 562–570.

23. CLEGHORN, J. M., S. FRANCO, B. SZECHTMAN, *et al.* 1992. Toward a brain map of auditory hallucinations. Am. J. Psychiatry **149(8):** 1062–1069.

24. VOLKOW, N. D., A. P. WOLF, P. VAN GELDER, *et al.* 1987. Phenomenological correlates of metabolic activity in 18 patients with chronic schizophrenia. Am. J. Psychiatry **144(2):** 151–158.

25. DE LISI, L. E., M. S. BUCHSBAUM, H. H. HOLCOMB, *et al.* 1989. Increased temporal lobe glucose use in chronic schizophrenic patients. Biol. Psychiatry **25(7):** 835–851.

26. SUZUKI, M., S. YUASA, Y. MINABE, M. MURATA & M. KURACHI. 1993. Left superior temporal blood flow increases in schizophrenic and schizophreniform patients with auditory hallucination: A longitudinal case study using 123I-IMP SPECT. Eur. Arch. Psychiatry Clin. Neurosci. **242(5):** 257–261.

27. MCGUIRE, P. K., G. M. SHAH & R. M. MURRAY. 1993. Increased blood flow in Broca's area during auditory hallucinations in schizophrenia. Lancet **342:** 703–706.

28. SILBERSWEIG, D. A., E. STERN, C. FRITH, *et al.* 1995. A functional neuroanatomy of hallucinations in schizophrenia. Nature **378:** 176–179.

29. STERN, E., D. A. SILBERSWEIG, K.-Y. CHEE, C. D. FRITH, R. S. J. FRACKOWIAK & R. J. DOLAN. 1996. A functional neuroanatomy of involuntary action in Tourette's syndrome. Neuroimage **3(3):** S600.

30. DOLAN, R. J., C. J. BENCH, P. F. LIDDLE, *et al.* 1993. Dorsolateral prefrontal cortex dysfunction in the major psychoses; symptom or disease specificity? J. Neurol. Neurosurg. Psychiatry **56(12):** 1290–1294.

31. PANDYA, D. N. & E. H. YETERIAN. 1985. Architecture and Connections of Cortical Association Areas. *In* Cerebral Cortex, vol. 4. A. Peters & E. G. Jones, Eds. Plenum. New York.

32. MESULAM, M.-M. 1985. Principles of Behavioral Neurology (F. Plum, Ed., Contemporary Neurology). F. A. Davis Company. Philadelphia, PA.

33. FRISTON, K. J. & C. D. FRITH. 1995. Schizophrenia: A disconnection syndrome? Clin. Neurosci. **3(2):** 89–97.

34. SILBERSWEIG, D. & E. STERN. 1996. Functional neuroimaging of hallucinations in schizophrenia: Toward an integration of bottom-up and top-down approaches. Mol. Psychiatry **1:** 367–375.

35. STARKSTEIN, S. E., R. G. ROBINSON & T. R. PRICE. 1987. Comparison of cortical and subcortical lesions in the production of poststroke mood disorders. Brain **110(Pt. 4):** 1045–1059.

36. MAYBERG, H. S. 1994. Frontal lobe dysfunction in secondary depression. J. Neuropsychiatry Clin. Neurosci. **6(4):** 428–442.

37. TRIMBLE, M. R. 1991. The Psychoses of Epilepsy. Raven Press. New York.

38. DAMASIO, A. R. & D. TRANEL. 1992. Knowledge systems. Curr. Opin. Neurobiol. **2(2):** 186–190.

39. POSNER, M. I. & S. DEHAENE. 1994. Attentional networks. Trends Neurosci. **17(2):** 75–79.

40. MESULAM, M.-M. 1990. Large-scale neurocognitive networks and distributed processing for attention, language, and memory. Ann. Neurol. **28(5):** 597–613.

41. ALEXANDER, G. E., M. D. CRUTCHER & M. R. DE LONG. 1990. Basal ganglia-thalamocortical circuits: Parallel substrates for motor, oculomotor, "prefrontal" and "limbic" functions. Prog. Brain Res. **85:** 119–146.

42. GOLDMAN-RAKIC, P. S. 1988. Changing concepts of cortical connectivity: Parallel distributed cortical networks. *In* Neurobiology of Neocortex. P. Rakic & W. Singer, Eds.: 177–202. John Wiley & Sons. New York.

43. DAMASIO, A. R., H. DAMASIO, M. RIZZO, N. VARNEY & F. GERSH. 1982. Aphasia with

nonhemorrhagic lesions in the basal ganglia and internal capsule. Arch. Neurol. **39(1):** 15–24.

44. CUMMINGS, J. L. 1985. Clinical Neuropsychiatry. Grune & Stratton, Inc. Orlando, FL.

45. BARTA. P. E., G. D. PEARLSON, R. E. POWERS, S. S. RICHARDS & L. E. TUNE. 1990. Auditory hallucinations and smaller superior temporal gyral volume in schizophrenia. Am. J. Psychiatry **147(11):** 1457–1462.

46. BENES, F. M., S. L. VINCENT, G. ALSTERBERG, E. D. BIRD & J. P. SAN GIOVANNI. 1992. Increased GABAA receptor binding in superficial layers of cingulate cortex in schizophrenics. J. Neurosci. **12(3):** 924–929.

47. OLNEY, J. W. & N. B. FARBER. 1995. Glutamate receptor dysfunction and schizophrenia. Arch. Gen. Psychiatry **52(12):** 998–1007.

48. MRZLJAK, L., C. BERGSON, M. PAPPY, R. HUFF, R. LEVENSON & P. S. GOLDMAN-RAKIC. 1996. Localization of dopamine D4 receptors in GABAergic neurons of the primate brain. Nature **381:** 245–248.

49. ALEXANDER, G. E., M. R. DE LONG & P. L. STRICK. 1986. Parallel organization of functionally segregated circuits linking basal ganglia and cortex. Annu. Rev. Neurosci. **9:** 357–381.

50. DEIBER, M. P., R. E. PASSINGHAM, J. G. COLEBATCH, K. J. FRISTON, P. D. NIXON & R. S. FRACKOWIAK. 1991. Cortical areas and the selection of movement: A study with positron emission tomography. Exp. Brain Res. **84(2):** 393–402.

51. PARENT, A. & L. N. HAZRATI. 1995. Functional anatomy of the basal ganglia. II. The place of subthalamic nucleus and external pallidum in basal ganglia circuitry. Brain Res. Rev. **20(1):** 128–154.

52. ROBERTSON, M. M. 1989. The Gilles de la Tourette syndrome: The current status. Br. J. Psychiatry **154:** 147–169.

53. BAXTER, L. R., JR., J. M. SCHWARTZ, J. C. MAZZIOTTA, *et al.* 1988. Cerebral glucose metabolic rates in nondepressed patients with obsessive-compulsive disorder. Am. J. Psychiatry **145(12):** 1560–1563.

54. RAUCH, S. L., C. R. SAVAGE, N. M. ALPERT, *et al.* 1995. A positron emission tomographic study of simple phobic symptom provocation. Arch. Gen. Psychiatry **52(1):** 20–28.

55. VOELLER, K. K. 1991. What can neurological models of attention, intention, and arousal tell us about attention-deficit hyperactivity disorder? J. Neuropsychiatry Clin. Neurosci. **3(2):** 209–216.

56. PLUM, F. & J. B. POSNER. 1982. The Diagnosis of Stupor and Coma. 3rd edit. F. A. Davis Co. Philadelphia, PA.

Index of Contributors